FIFTH EDITION

The MD Anderson Surgical Oncology Handbook

Editors

Barry W. Feig, MD
C. Denise Ching, MD

MD Anderson Cancer Center
Department of Surgical Oncology
Houston, Texas

Wolters Kluwer | Lippincott Williams & Wilkins
Health

Philadelphia · Baltimore · New York · London
Buenos Aires · Hong Kong · Sydney · Tokyo

Acquisitions Editor: Brian Brown
Product Manager: Brendan Huffman
Production Manager: Alicia Jackson
Senior Manufacturing Manager: Benjamin Rivera
Marketing Manager: Lisa Lawrence
Design Coordinator: Doug Smock
Production Service: Aptara, Inc.

Library of Congress Cataloging-in-Publication Data
   The MD Anderson surgical oncology handbook / MD Anderson Cancer Center, Department of Surgical Oncology ; editors, Barry W. Feig, C. Denise Ching. — 5th ed.
      p. ; cm.
   Surgical oncology handbook
   Includes bibliographical references and index.
      ISBN 978-1-60831-284-9 (pbk.)
   I. Feig, Barry W., 1959– II. Ching, C. Denise (Christine Denise)   III. University of Texas MD Anderson Cancer Center. Dept. of Surgical Oncology.   IV. Title: Surgical oncology handbook.
   [DNLM: 1. Neoplasms—surgery—Handbooks. QZ 39]
   LC classification not assigned
   616.99′4059—dc23

                                                                          2011033093

Care has been taken to confirm the accuracy of the information presented and to describe generally accepted practices. However, the authors, editors, and publisher are not responsible for errors or omissions or for any consequences from application of the information in this book and make no warranty, expressed or implied, with respect to the currency, completeness, or accuracy of the contents of the publication. Application of the information in a particular situation remains the professional responsibility of the practitioner.

   The authors, editors, and publisher have exerted every effort to ensure that drug selection and dosage set forth in this text are in accordance with current recommendations and practice at the time of publication. However, in view of ongoing research, changes in government regulations, and the constant flow of information relating to drug therapy and drug reactions, the reader is urged to check the package insert for each drug for any change in indications and dosage and for added warnings and precautions. This is particularly important when the recommended agent is a new or infrequently employed drug.

   Some drugs and medical devices presented in the publication have Food and Drug Administration (FDA) clearance for limited use in restricted research settings. It is the responsibility of the health care providers to ascertain the FDA status of each drug or device planned for use in their clinical practice.

   To purchase additional copies of this book, call our customer service department at (800) 638-3030 or fax orders to (301) 223-2320. International customers should call (301) 223-2300.

   Visit Lippincott Williams & Wilkins on the Internet: at LWW.com. Lippincott Williams & Wilkins customer service representatives are available from 8:30 am to 6 pm, EST.

To our dear friends and families, for their support,
enthusiasm, and patience through our many years
of training and continued long hours spent
in the care of patients with cancer.

CONTRIBUTORS

John D. Abad, MD
Assistant Professor
Department of Surgery
Indiana University School of
    Medicine
Surgical Oncologist
Cancer Care Partners
South Bend, Indiana

Eddie K. Abdalla, MD, FACS
Assistant Professor
Department of Surgical Oncology
The University of Texas MD
    Anderson Cancer Center
Houston, Texas

Keith D. Amos, MD
Assistant Professor
Department of Surgery
Division of Surgical Oncology
University of North Carolina
Chapel Hill, North Carolina

**Robert Hans Ingemar Andtbacka,
MD, CM, FRCSC**
Assistant Professor of Surgery
Department of Surgery
University of Utah
Assistant Professor
Huntsman Cancer Institute
Salt Lake City, UT

Brian Badgwell, MD, MS
Assistant Professor of Surgery
Division of Surgical Oncology
Winthrop P. Rockefeller Cancer
    Institute
The University of Arkansas for
    Medical Sciences
Little Rock, Arkansas

Donald P. Baumann, MD, FACS
Associate Professor
Department of Plastic Surgery
Division of Surgery
The University of Texas MD
    Anderson Cancer Center
Houston, Texas

**Shanda H. Blackmon, MD, MPH,
FACS**
Section Head
Thoracic Surgery
The Methodist Hospital Assistant
    Professor
Weill Cornell Medical College
Clinical Specialist
MD Anderson

Debashish Bose, MD, PhD
Assistant Professor of Surgery
Department of Surgical Oncology
MD Anderson Cancer Center
    Orlando
Orlando, Florida

Tawnya L. Bowles, MD
Clinical Assistant Professor
Department of Surgery
University of Utah and
    Intermountain Medical Center
Salt Lake City, Utah

Abigail S. Caudle, MD
Assistant Professor
Department of Surgical Oncology
The University of Texas MD
    Anderson Cancer Center
Houston, Texas

George J. Chang, MD, MS, FACS, FASCRS
Associate Professor of Surgical
    Oncology
Associate Medical Director
Colorectal Center
U.T. MD Anderson Cancer Center
Houston, Texas

C. Denise Ching, MD
Surgical Oncologist
Department of Breast Health and
    Surgical Oncology
Palo Alto Medical Foundation
Palo Alto, California

Eugene A. Choi, MD
Surgical Oncologist
University of Chicago Medical
    Center
Chicago, IL

Carlo M. Contreras, MD
Department of Surgery
University of South Alabama
USA Mitchell Cancer Institute
Alabama

Janice N. Cormier, MD, MPH
Associate Professor
Department of Surgical Oncology
The University of Texas MD
    Anderson Cancer Center
Houston, Texas

Christopher H. Crane, MD
Professor
Program Director and Section Chief
Gastrointestinal Section
U.T. MD Anderson Cancer Center
Houston, Texas

Melissa A. Crosby, MD, FACS
Assistant Professor
Department of Plastic Surgery
Division of Surgery
The University of Texas MD
    Anderson Cancer Center
Houston, Texas

Keith A. Delman
Assistant Professor
Department of Surgery
Emory University
Atlanta, Georgia

Barry W. Feig, MD
Professor of Surgery
Department of Surgical Oncology
U.T MD Anderson Cancer Center
Houston, Texas

Jason B. Fleming, MD
Associate Professor
Department of Surgical Oncology
Division of Surgery
The University of Texas MD
    Anderson Cancer Center
Houston, Texas

Jason B. Fleming, MD, FACS
Associate Professor
Chief Pancreas Surgery
Director Surgical Oncology
   Fellowship
Deputy Chairman
Department of Surgical Oncology
The University of Texas MD
   Anderson Cancer Center
Houston, Texas

Jeffrey E. Gershenwald, MD, FACS
Professor of Surgery and Cancer
   Biology
Departments of Surgical Oncology
   and Cancer Biology
The University of Texas MD
   Anderson Cancer Center
Houston, Texas

Elizabeth G. Grubbs, MD, FACS
Assistant Professor of Surgery
Department of Surgical Oncology
The University of Texas MD
   Anderson Cancer Center
Houston, Texas

Mouhammed A. Habra, MD
Assistant Professor
Department of Endocrine Neoplasia
   and Hormonal Disorders
The University of Texas MD
   Anderson Cancer Center
Houston, Texas

Liz Y. Han, MD, MPH
Attending Gynecologic Oncologist
Department of Obstetrics and
   Gynecology
Kaiser Permanente
Oakland, California

Matthew M. Hanasono, MD
Assistant Professor
Department of Plastic Surgery
The University of Texas MD
   Anderson Cancer Center
Houston, Texas

Kelly L. Herne, MD
Volunteer faculty
Department of Dermatology
The University of Texas Houston
   Medical School
Houston, Texas

Wayne L. Hofstetter, MD
Associate Professor of Surgery
Director of Esophageal Surgery
Department of Thoracic and
   Cardiovascular Surgery
The University of Texas MD
   Anderson Cancer Center
Houston, Texas

F. Christopher Holsinger, MD, FACS
Associate Professor
Department of Head and Neck
   Surgery
Director
Program in Minimally Invasive
   Head and Neck Surgery
The University of Texas MD
   Anderson Cancer Center
Houston, Texas

Cary Hsu, MD
Surgical Oncology Fellow
The University of Texas MD
   Anderson Cancer Center
Houston, Texas

Kelly K. Hunt, MD, FACS
Hamill Foundation Distinguished
    Professor of Surgery in Honor of
    Dr. Richard G. Martin
Sr. Professor of Surgical Oncology
Chief
Surgical Breast Oncology
The University of Texas MD
    Anderson Cancer Center
Houston, Texas

Rosa F. Hwang, MD
Associate Professor
Department of Surgical Oncology
The University of Texas MD
    Anderson Cancer Center
Houston, Texas

Sharon Renae Hymes, MD
Associate Professor
Department of Dermatology
The University of Texas MD
    Anderson Cancer Center
Houston, Texas

Jose A. Karam, MD
Assistant Professor
Faculty Physician/Surgeon
Department of Urology
U.T. MD Anderson Cancer Center
Houston, Texas

Matthew H. Katz, MD
Assistant Professor
Department of Surgical Oncology
Division of Surgery
The University of Texas MD
    Anderson Cancer Center
Houston, Texas

Catherine M. Kelly,
Department of Medical Oncology
Mater Misericordiae University
    Hospital
Institute for Cancer Research
Dublin, Ireland

David S. Kwon,
Division of Surgery
Department of Surgical Oncology
Henry Ford Health System
Detroit, Michigan

Christine S. Landry, MD
Surgical Oncologist
Department of Surgical Oncology
Banner MD Anderson Cancer
    Center
Gilbert, Arizona

Jeffrey E. Lee, MD
Professor and Chair
Irving and Nadine Mansfield and
    Robert David Levitt Cancer
    Research
Chair
Department of Surgical Oncology
Division of Surgery
U.T. MD Anderson Cancer Center,
    Houston, Texas

Joshua M.V. Mammen, MD, PhD, MBA
Assistant Professor of Surgery
Adjunct Professor of Molecular &
    Integrative Physiology
Associate Program Director
Surgery Residency
University of Kansas
Kansas City, Kansas

Paul F. Mansfield, MD
Professor of Surgery
Division of Surgery
Department of Surgical Oncology
Vice President
Acute Care Services
The University of Texas MD
    Anderson Cancer Center
Houston, Texas

Priscilla F. McAuliffe, MD, PhD
Assistant Professor of Surgery
Department of Surgery
University of Pittsburgh
Surgeon
Magee Women's Hospital of UPMC
Pittsburgh, Pennsylvania

Ian E. McCutcheon, MD, FRCS(C)
Professor of Neurosurgery
Director
Neuroendocrine Program
Department of Neurosurgery
The University of Texas MD
    Anderson Cancer Center
Houston, Texas

Melinda M. Mortenson, MD
Surgical Oncology
Department of Surgery
Sacramento Medical Center
Sacramento, CA

Kenneth A. Newkirk, MD
Assistant Professor
Department of Otolaryngology–
    Head and Neck Surgery
Georgetown University Medical
    Center

**Andrea Landgraf Oholendt, PharmD,
BCOP**
Clinical Pharmacy Specialist
Division of Pharmacy
The University of Texas MD
    Anderson Cancer Center
Houston, Texas

Nancy D. Perrier, MD, FACS
Professor of Surgery
Chief
Section of Surgical Endocrinology
Department of Surgical Oncology
The University of Texas MD
    Anderson Cancer Center
Houston, Texas

Geoffrey L. Robb, MD
Chairman
Department of Plastic Surgery
Professor
Department of Plastic Surgery
University of Texas MD Anderson
    Cancer Center
Houston, Texas

Emily K. Robinson, MD, FACS
Associate Professor of Surgery
Surgeon
Department of Surgery
The University of Texas Medical
    School at Houston
Houston, Texas

Jorge A. Romaguera
Professor
Department of Lymphoma and
    Myeloma
The University of Texas MD
    Anderson Cancer Center
Houston, Texas

Maria Citarella Russell, MD
Surgical Oncology Fellow
MD Anderson Cancer Center
Houston, Texas

Justin M. Sacks, MD
Assistant Professor
Department of Plastic and
    Reconstructive Surgery
The Johns Hopkins University
    School of Medicine
Baltimore, Maryland

Eric J. Silberfein, MD
Assistant Professor of Surgery
Michael E. DeBakey Department of
    Surgery
Division of Surgical Oncology
Baylor College of Medicine
Ben Taub General Hospital
Houston, Texas

Brian M. Slomovitz, MD, MPH
Attending Gynecologic Oncologist
Department of Obstetrics and
    Gynecology
Women's Cancer Center of
    Morristown Memorial Hospital
Morristown, New Jersey

Pamela T. Soliman, MD, MPH
Assistant Professor
Department of Gynecologic
    Oncology
The University of Texas MD
    Anderson Cancer Center
Houston, Texas

Ryan M. Thomas, MD
Fellow
Department of Surgical Oncology
The University of Texas MD
    Anderson Cancer Center
Houston, Texas

Mark J. Truty, MD, MSc
Surgical Oncology Fellow
The University of Texas MD
    Anderson Cancer Center
Houston, Texas

Vanja Vaccaro, MD
Research Fellow
Department of Medical Oncology
Regina Elena National Cancer
    Institute
Rome, Italy

Ara A. Vaporciyan, MD, FACS
Professor of Surgery and Deputy
    Chair
Director of Clinical Education &
    Training
Department of Thoracic and
    Cardiovascular Surgery
The University of Texas MD
    Anderson Cancer Center
Houston, Texas

Gauri R. Varadhachary, MD
Associate Professor
GI Medical Oncology
U.T. MD Anderson Cancer Center
Houston, Texas

Jula Veerapong, MD
Assistant Professor of Surgery
Department of Surgery
Saint Louis University
Saint Louis, Missouri

Mark T. Villa, MD
Assistant Professor
Department of Plastic Surgery
Division of Surgery
The University of Texas MD
    Anderson Cancer Center
Houston, Texas

Judith K. Wolf, MD
Chief
Department of Surgery
Banner MD Anderson Cancer
    Center
Gilbert, Arizona

Christopher G. Wood, MD
Professor
Faculty Physician/Surgeon
Department of Urology
U.T. MD Anderson Cancer Center
Houston, Texas

Yi-Qian Nancy You, MD, MHSc
Assistant Professor
Department of Surgical Oncology
Division of Surgery
The University of Texas MD
    Anderson Cancer Center
Houston, Texas

Welcome to the fifth edition of *The MD Anderson Surgical Oncology Handbook*! Since the publication of the first edition, the field of surgical oncology, the surgical care of patients with cancer, has grown from an avocation practiced by a few committed surgeons, usually trained in general surgery, to a defined and vigorous specialty with its own subspecialties, including those of breast, colorectal, melanoma, sarcoma, and hepatobiliary surgery.

Since the first edition of *The Handbook*, there have been major advances that have transformed the field. These have included advances in surgical techniques that have minimized patient morbidity and at the same time allowed refinement in surgical indications. Such advances have included the introduction of sentinel lymph node biopsy, especially for patients with melanoma and breast cancer; and advances in minimally invasive surgery, initially in the staging and palliative treatment of patients with gastrointestinal malignancies but now established as a standard of care for selected patients with various early-stage tumors, including colon cancer and adrenal tumors. Advances have also included technical innovations, including in liver, pancreatic, peritoneal, soft tissue, and reconstructive surgery that have allowed surgical care to be extended to patients not previously considered surgical candidates, including patients with bilobar liver tumors, those with involvement of major abdominal vasculature, and carcinomatosis. Advances in imaging, including the introduction of PET/CT as well as high-resolution CT and MRI, have allowed for more accurate preoperative staging, facilitating surgical treatment planning and permitting a more selective approach to surgical care of patients with various cancers. Major progress in our understanding of the molecular biology and the natural history of many solid tumors, through investigations often led by surgical oncologists, have resulted in a much deeper and more profound understanding of the mechanisms responsible for cancer incidence and progression. These advances have led not just to more accurate staging of patients with these cancers but to more accurate selection of patients for surgical treatment, and in some cases more effective and less toxic systemic therapies. Finally, integration of cancer-specific diagnostic treatment and outcomes data with information on patient quality of life, socioeconomic factors, and on costs and side effects of therapy, through the disciplines of health services, outcomes, and disparities research, are of increasing importance in obtaining the best possible result in individual patients while at the same time minimizing toxicity, waste, and overall cost.

The current edition of *The Handbook* provides an overview of current care of patients with cancer diagnoses commonly evaluated and treated by surgical oncologists and in doing so continues to align such care with the underlying philosophy of the Department of Surgical Oncology at MD Anderson: multidisciplinary, cooperative care is the ideal way to manage patients with cancer. Such care begins with an understanding of the underlying tumor biology and natural history of the disease and includes technical excellence in the delivery of indicated surgical treatment. It also demands integration of essential information from the available literature on currently preferred treatment modalities and emphasizes appropriate inclusion of adjunctive specialty care, including medical oncology, radiation oncology, interventional radiology, palliative care, pain management, physical therapy, nutritional support, social services, and nursing.

I am confident that you will find the current edition of *The Handbook* useful, whether you are a medical student on a surgical rotation, a surgical resident, a surgical oncology fellow, or an interested specialist in a related discipline. Especially for those of you early in your training, I hope that your exposure to the exciting and deeply rewarding field of surgical oncology through your surgical rotations and this handbook will interest some of you in pursuing the surgical care of patients with cancer as a career. I am delighted to be able to introduce the current edition of *The Handbook* to you and honored to have been a small part of it since the first edition. The dynamic nature of the field of surgical oncology will demand that we continue to revise and update its contents; it is exciting to know that some of you reading this will contribute to future editions!

Jeffrey E. Lee, MD
Chair, Department of Surgical Oncology
MD Anderson Cancer Center
Houston, Texas

PREFACE

The concept for the *MD Anderson Surgical Oncology Handbook* was originally conceived 16 years ago with the original objective being an attempt to document the philosophies and practices of the Department of Surgical Oncology at the MD Anderson Cancer Center. Since that time, through four editions, the book has become a practical guide for residents, fellows, and attending staff, to the established surgical oncology principles for treating cancer as it involves each organ system in the body. The purpose of the book is to outline management approaches based on our experience with surgical oncology problems at MD Anderson.

Consistent with the original concept, this book is written by current and former surgical oncology fellows at MD Anderson. Although the target audience for the first edition was surgical house staff and surgical oncology trainees, we found that there was a significantly wider appeal for the book across multiple disciplines and at various levels of training and experience. The handbook continues to maintain this appeal, despite various subsequent publications of similar intent, within other specialties. The authors represent various disciplines within oncology and training programs, and they have spent at least 2 years at the MD Anderson Cancer Center studying only surgical oncology. The diversity of authors allows us to present the current opinions and practices of the MD Anderson Department of Surgical Oncology, along with other opinions and treatment options practiced in a wider range of surgical training programs. By maintaining the emphasis of the book from the perspective of the surgical oncology fellows, we hope to prevent the book from becoming overly dogmatic in our medical opinions and practices.

This handbook is not meant to encompass all aspects of oncology in minute detail. Rather, it is an attempt to address commonly encountered as well as controversial issues in surgical oncology. While other authors present their opinions and approaches as firmly established, we have tried to point out controversies and show alternative approaches to these problems besides our own.

We particularly thank the patients seen and treated at MD Anderson for their warmth and appreciation of our care, as well as for their patience and understanding of the learning process. We are all aware that there is still a significant amount of learning that we all must entail in order to achieve our mission of eradicating cancer.

B.W.F.
C.D.C.

CONTENTS

Noninvasive Breast Cancer

Priscilla F. McAuliffe, Robert H. I. Andtbacka,
Emily K. Robinson, and Kelly K. Hunt

Noninvasive breast cancer comprises two separate entities: ductal carcinoma in situ (DCIS) and lobular carcinoma in situ (LCIS). DCIS is defined as a proliferation of epithelial cells confined to the mammary ducts, whereas LCIS is defined as a proliferation of epithelial cells confined to the lobules. Neither DCIS nor LCIS has demonstrable evidence of invasion through the basement membrane. Because they are noninvasive, DCIS and LCIS do not pose a risk of metastasis.

DUCTAL CARCINOMA IN SITU

Epidemiology

Before the introduction of screening mammography, most cases of DCIS remained undetected until a palpable mass formed. However, widespread use of screening mammography has resulted in a 10-fold increase in the reported incidence of DCIS since the mid-1980s. In the United States, the incidence is now 25 to 35 per 100,000 woman-years. The reported prevalence of DCIS has increased as the quality and sensitivity of mammography have improved, and DCIS currently accounts for 25% of all new screen-detected breast neoplasms in the United States, with 1.7 cases of DCIS detected per 1,000 screening mammograms. The incidence of detection of DCIS is higher in autopsy studies than in the general population, suggesting that not all DCIS lesions become clinically significant.

The median age reported for patients with DCIS ranges from 47 to 63 years, similar to that reported for patients with invasive carcinoma. However, the peak incidence of DCIS, 96.7 per 100,000 women, occurs at ages 65 to 69 years, which is younger than that for invasive breast cancer, in which the peak occurs at ages 75 to 79 years, with 453.1 per 100,000 women. The frequency of a family history of breast cancer among first-degree relatives of patients with DCIS (i.e., 10% to 35%) is the same as that reported for women with invasive breast malignancies. Other risk factors for DCIS are the same as those for invasive breast cancer, including older age, proliferative breast disease, increased breast density, nulliparity, and older age at the time of first full-term pregnancy.

Pathology

DCIS is a proliferation of malignant cells that have not breached the ductal basement membrane. They arise from ductal epithelium in the region of the terminal ductal–lobular unit. DCIS has traditionally been considered one stage in the continuum of histologic progression from atypical ductal hyperplasia to invasive carcinoma. DCIS comprises a heterogeneous group of lesions with variable histologic architecture, molecular and cellular characteristics, and clinical behavior. Malignant cells proliferate until the ductal lumen is obliterated, and there may be associated breakdown of the myoepithelial cell layer of the basement membrane surrounding the ductal lumen. Also, DCIS has been linked with changes in the surrounding stroma resulting in fibroblast proliferation, lymphocyte infiltration, and angiogenesis. Although the process is poorly understood, most invasive ductal carcinomas are believed to arise from DCIS.

Classification of DCIS

DCIS is generally classified as one of five subtypes—comedo, solid, cribriform, micropapillary, and papillary—based on the differences in the architectural pattern of the cancer cells and nuclear features. Cribriform, comedo, and micropapillary are the most common subtypes, although two or more patterns coexist in up to 50% of cases.

The classification of noninvasive breast cancer stratifies lesions based on their likelihood of recurrence and incorporates prognostic factors. Lagios et al. (1989) identified high nuclear grade and comedo necrosis as factors predictive of local recurrence. At 8 years, patients whose tumors had a high nuclear grade and comedo necrosis had a 20% local recurrence rate after breast conservation surgery and irradiation, compared with 5% for those patients whose tumors did not have necrosis and were a lower nuclear grade. Subsequently, Silverstein et al. (1995) developed the Van Nuys classification in which three risk groups were distinguished on the basis of the presence or absence of high nuclear grade and comedo-type necrosis: (a) non–high-grade DCIS without comedo-type necrosis, (b) non–high-grade DCIS with comedo-type necrosis, and (c) high-grade DCIS with or without comedo-type necrosis. Silverstein et al. found 31 cases of local recurrence among 238 patients who underwent breast-conserving surgery; the local recurrence rate was 3.8% in group 1, 11.1% in group 2, and 26.5% in group 3. The 8-year actuarial disease-free survival rate was 93% for group 1, 84% for group 2, and 61% for group 3. Other classification systems have been proposed; however, no single classification system has been universally accepted.

Multifocality

Multifocal DCIS is generally defined as DCIS present in two or more foci separated by 5 mm in the same breast quadrant. Most investigators believe that multifocal disease in fact represents intraductal spread from a single focus of DCIS. By careful serial subsectioning, Holland et al. (1990) demonstrated that multifocal lesions that appeared to be separate using traditional pathologic techniques actually originated from the same focus in 81 of 82 mastectomy specimens.

Multicentricity

Multicentric DCIS is defined as DCIS presenting as separate, discontinuous foci of disease involving more than one quadrant. The reported incidence of multicentricity may depend on the extent of the pathological review and therefore varies from 18% to 60%. Because mammary lobules are not constrained by the artificially imposed quadrant segregations, cursory pathological examination may incorrectly interpret contiguous intraductal spread as multicentricity. Approximately 96% of all local recurrences after treatment of DCIS occur in the same quadrant as the index lesion, implicating residual untreated disease rather than multicentricity, and raising questions about the importance of multicentricity.

Microinvasion

The American Joint Committee on Cancer (AJCC) staging system (Hayes, 2010) defines microinvasion as invasion of breast cancer cells through the basement membrane at one or more foci, none of which exceeds a dimension of 1 mm. A breast cancer with microinvasion is classified as a "T1mic" tumor, whereas DCIS is classified as "T0." Microinvasion upstages the cancer from stage 0 to stage 1 in the AJCC staging system. By definition, DCIS does not have the ability to metastasize to axillary lymph nodes or distant sites, whereas DCIS with microinvasion does. Axillary metastasis has been reported in 0% to 20% of patients with DCIS with microinvasion.

The incidence of microinvasion in DCIS varies according to the size and extent of the index lesion. Lagios et al. (1989) reported a 2% incidence of microinvasion in patients with DCIS measuring less than 25 mm in diameter, compared with a 29% incidence of microinvasion in lesions larger than 26 mm. The incidence of microinvasion is also higher in patients with high-grade or comedo-type DCIS with necrosis and in patients with DCIS who present with a palpable mass or nipple discharge.

Patients with DCIS with microinvasion have a worse prognosis compared with those who have DCIS alone. Mirza et al. (2000) reported the long-term results of breast-conserving therapy in patients with DCIS, DCIS with microinvasion, and T1 invasive breast cancers. The 20-year disease-specific survival rates in patients with DCIS were better than those among patients with DCIS with microinvasion or with T1 invasive tumors. Patients with microinvasion and those with T1 tumors had similar survival rates. In a retrospective study of 1,248 serially sectioned DCIS tumors, de Mascarel et al. (2002) reported a 10.1% incidence of axillary metastases in cases of DCIS with microinvasion. Patients with DCIS had a better 10-year distant metastasis-free survival rate than patients with DCIS with microinvasion (98% and 91%, respectively). The overall survival rate was also better in patients with DCIS (96.5% vs. 88.4%). However, the metastasis-free and overall survival rates were worse in patients with invasive ductal carcinoma than those with DCIS with microinvasion. These results suggest that DCIS with microinvasion should be characterized as a small invasive tumor with a good outcome and that the therapeutic approach for these patients should be similar to that for patients with invasive cancer. However, further study is needed to investigate the biology of microinvasion.

Diagnosis
Clinical Presentation
Before the implementation of routine screening mammography, most patients with DCIS presented with a palpable mass, nipple thickening or discharge, or Paget's disease of the nipple. Occasionally, DCIS was an incidental finding in an otherwise benign breast biopsy specimen. In patients with palpable lesions, up to 25% demonstrated foci of invasive disease. Now that screening mammography is more prevalent, most cases of DCIS are diagnosed when the tumor is still clinically occult. Patients with abnormalities detected by mammography should always undergo imaging of the contralateral breast because 0.5% to 3.0% of patients have synchronous occult abnormalities or cancers in the contralateral breast. Mammographic images should be compared with previous images, if available, to establish interval changes.

Mammographic Features
On a mammogram, DCIS can present as microcalcifications, a soft-tissue density, or both. Microcalcifications are the most common mammographic manifestation of DCIS (80% to 90%). DCIS accounts for 80% of all breast carcinomas presenting with calcifications. Any interval change from a previous mammogram is associated with malignancy in 15% to 20% of cases and most often indicates in situ disease. Holland et al. (1990) described two different classes of microcalcifications: (a) linear branching-type microcalcifications, which are more often associated with high–nuclear-grade, comedo-type lesions; and (b) fine, granular calcifications, which are primarily associated with micropapillary or cribriform lesions of lower nuclear grade that do not show necrosis. Although the morphology of microcalcifications suggests the architectural type of DCIS, it is not always reliable. Holland et al. also demonstrated that the mammographic findings significantly underestimated the pathological extent of disease, particularly in cases of micropapillary DCIS. Lesions were more than 2 cm larger by histologic examination than by mammographic estimation in 44% of micropapillary lesions, compared with

only 12% of cases of the pure comedo subtype. However, when magnification views were used in the mammographic examination, the extent of disease was underestimated in only 14% of cases of micropapillary tumors. Hence, magnification views increase the image resolution and are better able to detect the microcalcification shape, number, and extent when compared with mammography alone and should be used routinely in the evaluation of suspicious mammographic findings.

Magnetic Resonance Imaging

Mammography remains the standard for radiographic evaluation of DCIS. The cost and accessibility of magnetic resonance imaging (MRI) make it less feasible as an effective screening method. However, there is evidence that patients at high risk for breast cancer or those with very dense breasts may benefit from screening with MRI. Contrast-enhanced MRI is more sensitive than mammography in the detection of both DCIS and invasive cancer. However, because DCIS can mimic fibrocystic change and other benign findings on MRI, it can also lead to unnecessary biopsies. MRI is increasingly being utilized after initial diagnosis in the preoperative evaluation to identify multicentric and contralateral lesions, because presence of either of these may change the surgical treatment strategy. Hollingsworth et al. (2008) reported that MRI detected multicentric disease, defined as a separate focus of cancer more than 5 cm away from the index lesion or discontinuous growth to another breast quadrant, in 4.3% of 149 patients who presented with DCIS. Lehman et al. (2007) reported the utility of MRI in detecting contralateral breast cancer in a group of 969 patients with unilateral breast cancer, 196 of whom had DCIS. Of the patients with DCIS, MRI prompted biopsy in 18 patients. Contralateral breast cancer was detected in 5 patients (28% of those biopsied and 2.6% of those with DCIS). The sensitivity of detecting contralateral breast cancer was 71%; the specificity was 90%. There is ongoing research interest in using MRI to predict the presence of invasive disease among patients initially diagnosed with DCIS on core needle biopsy.

Diagnostic Biopsy

Stereotactic core-needle or vacuum-assisted biopsy is the preferred method for diagnosing DCIS. Calcifications that appear faint on mammogram or that are deep in the breast and close to the chest wall may be difficult to target with stereotactic biopsy. In addition, use of stereotactic biopsy in patients above the weight limit of the stereotactic system (about 135 kg) and in patients with small breasts, may be impossible. Patients who cannot remain prone or who cannot cooperate for the duration of the procedure are also not good candidates for stereotactic biopsy. Bleeding disorders and the concomitant use of anticoagulants are relative contraindications. Biopsy specimens should be radiographed to document the sampling of suspicious microcalcifications. Care should be taken to mark the biopsy site with a metallic clip in the event that all microcalcifications are removed with the biopsy procedure.

Because stereotactic core-needle and vacuum-assisted biopsy specimens represent only a sample of an abnormality observed on mammography, the results are subject to sampling error. Invasive carcinoma is found on excisional biopsy in 20% of patients in whom DCIS was diagnosed by a stereotactic core-needle biopsy. If the core-needle biopsy results are discordant with the findings of imaging studies, a needle-localized excisional biopsy should be performed to establish the diagnosis. After diagnosis using stereotactic core-needle biopsy, approximately 30% of patients with atypical ductal hyperplasia and up to 20% of patients with radial scar are found to have a coexistent carcinoma near the site of the biopsy when complete excision is performed. Therefore, when the final pathological studies from core-needle biopsy procedures indicate either of these diagnoses, consideration should be made for further excisional biopsy.

Patients who are not candidates for stereotactic biopsy or who have stereotactic biopsy results that are inconclusive or discordant with the mammographic findings should undergo excisional biopsy. This technique is performed with the assistance of preoperative needle localization of the mammographic abnormality or of the previously placed metallic clip marking the biopsy site. Specimen radiography is essential to confirm the removal of microcalcifications of interest. The excisional biopsy should be performed with the aim of obtaining a margin-negative resection that can serve as a definitive surgery.

Treatment

The diagnosis of DCIS is followed by surgical treatment with a mastectomy or breast-conserving surgery (also referred to as segmental mastectomy, lumpectomy, or wide local excision). Most patients who undergo breast-conserving surgery receive postoperative radiation therapy to improve local control. Postoperative endocrine therapy with tamoxifen should also be considered for those patients whose tumors are estrogen receptor positive.

Mastectomy Versus Breast-conserving Therapy

Traditionally, DCIS was treated with mastectomy. The rationale for performing total mastectomy in patients with DCIS was based on the high incidence of multifocality and multicentricity, as well as on the risk of occult invasion associated with the disease. Thus, mastectomy remains the standard with which other proposed therapeutic modalities are compared. However, in patients with DCIS, there are no prospective trials comparing outcomes after mastectomy with those after breast-conserving surgery. A retrospective review by Balch et al. (1993) documented a local relapse rate of 3.1% and a mortality rate of 2.3% after mastectomy for DCIS. The cancer-related mortality rate following mastectomy for DCIS was 1.7% in a series reported by Fowble (1989) and ranged from 0% to 8% in a review by Vezeridis and Bland (1994).

In one of the largest studies comparing breast-conserving therapy with mastectomy, Silverstein et al. (1992) examined 227 cases of DCIS without microinvasion. In this nonrandomized study, patients with tumors smaller than 4 cm with microscopically clear margins underwent breast-conserving surgery and radiation therapy, whereas patients with tumors larger than 4 cm or with positive margins underwent mastectomy. The rate of disease-free survival at 7 years was 98% in the mastectomy group compared with 84% in the breast-conserving surgery group ($P = 0.038$), with no difference in overall survival rates. In a meta-analysis, Boyages et al. (1999) reported a recurrence rate of 22.5%, 8.9%, and 1.4% following breast-conserving surgery alone, breast-conserving surgery with radiation therapy, and mastectomy, respectively. In patients who underwent breast-conserving surgery alone, approximately 50% of the recurrences were invasive cancers. Although recurrence rates are higher in patients who undergo breast-conserving surgery than in patients who undergo mastectomy, no survival advantage has been shown for patients treated with mastectomy.

Technique of Breast-conserving Surgery

The goal of breast-conserving surgery is to remove all suspicious calcifications and obtain negative surgical margins. Because DCIS is usually nonpalpable, breast-conserving surgery is most often performed with mammographic needle localization. Intraoperative orientation of the specimen with two or more marking sutures is critical for margin analysis. In addition, specimen radiography is essential to confirm the removal of all microcalcifications. In patients with extensive calcifications, bracketing of the calcifications with two or more wires may assist in the excision of all suspicious calcifications.

After whole-specimen radiography, the specimen should be inked and then serially sectioned for pathological examination to evaluate the margin status and extent of disease. Chagpar et al. (2003) demonstrated that intraoperative margin assessment with the use of sectioned-specimen radiography enabled re-excisions to be performed at the same surgery if the microcalcifications extended to the cut edge of the specimen, minimizing the need for second procedures for margin control. After the intraoperative margins are deemed adequate, the boundary of the resection cavity is marked with radiopaque clips to aid in the planning of postoperative radiation therapy and in mammographic follow-up.

The goal of breast-conserving surgery is to obtain tumor-free margins. A detailed pathologic study of DCIS, reported by Holland et al. (1990), demonstrated that up to 44% of lesions extended more than 2 cm further on histologic examination than that estimated by mammography. However, in most women, a 1 to 2 cm margin around the lesion is not feasible since the cosmetic result would be poor. Therefore, what constitutes an adequate margin for DCIS remains controversial. Most surgeons advocate re-excision for positive surgical margins, and many surgeons advocate re-excision for close margins, using varying thresholds of less than 1, 2, or 5 mm. Neuschatz et al. (2002) reported that residual tumor was found on re-excision in 41% of patients with DCIS with 0- to 1-mm margins, 31% of patients with 1- to 2-mm margins, and 0% of patients with greater than 2-mm margins. Lesion size was another predictor of residual DCIS.

Radiation Therapy

Most patients with DCIS who undergo breast-conserving surgery receive postoperative radiation therapy. Three prospective randomized studies have evaluated the role of radiation therapy following breast-conserving surgery for DCIS. In the National Surgical Adjuvant Breast and Bowel Project (NSABP) B-17 trial, 818 women with localized DCIS were randomized to breast-conserving surgery or breast-conserving surgery plus radiation therapy after margin-negative resections. At a follow-up time of 12 years, radiation therapy was associated with a reduction in the cumulative incidence of noninvasive ipsilateral breast tumors from 14.6% to 8% and with a reduction in the incidence of invasive ipsilateral breast tumors from 16.8% to 7.7%. There was no difference in the 12-year overall survival rate in the two groups, with 86% of women alive in the breast-conserving surgery group and 87% alive in the breast-conserving surgery plus radiation therapy group. However, 58% of all deaths occurred before any breast cancer event, and the death of 12 patients (3.0%) in the breast-conserving surgery group and 15 patients (3.6%) in the breast-conserving surgery plus radiation therapy group was attributed to invasive breast cancer.

The overall benefit of radiation therapy for patients with DCIS was also observed in the European Organization for Research and Treatment of Cancer 10853 trial (Julien et al., 2000). In this trial, 1,010 women with DCIS were randomized to breast-conserving surgery or breast-conserving surgery plus radiation therapy. At a median follow-up time of 4.25 years, radiation therapy was associated with a reduction in the incidence of noninvasive ipsilateral breast tumors from 8.8% to 5.8% and with a reduction in the incidence of invasive ipsilateral breast tumors from 8.0% to 4.8%. The lower recurrence rates in this trial when compared with those in the NSABP B-17 were attributed to the shorter follow-up time.

A third trial, which was conducted by the United Kingdom Coordinating Committee on Cancer Research, also confirmed the benefits of radiation therapy for local control (Houghton et al., 2003). After a median follow-up time of 4.4 years, there was a reduction in the incidence of noninvasive ipsilateral breast tumors from 7% to 3% and a reduction in the incidence of invasive ipsilateral tumors from 6% to 3%. Taken together, these three prospective randomized trials demonstrate that the addition of radiation therapy following breast-conserving therapy for DCIS results in an approximately 50% relative reduction in breast cancer recurrence.

Whole-breast radiation has been the standard for patients undergoing breast-conserving surgery and is generally tolerated well. The most common morbidity is radiation-induced skin changes including discoloration, fibrosis, and telangiectasias. Rare, severe side effects include damage to the heart and lungs, and a radiation-induced secondary malignancy, angiosarcoma.

Partial Breast Irradiation
In patients not receiving radiation therapy, local recurrences in the breast tend to occur in the immediate vicinity of the surgical resection cavity. Hence, the impact of whole-breast irradiation in reducing local recurrence may be limited to the immediate area surrounding the original tumor bed. On the basis of this knowledge, some have suggested that equivalent local control can be achieved by using partial breast irradiation focusing the treatment on the tissue surrounding the surgical resection cavity. Accelerated partial breast irradiation is a technique where high-dose radiation is delivered over a shorter period of time to a limited region of the breast surrounding the primary tumor site. The treatment is completed over 4 to 5 days, whereas conventional whole-breast external beam radiation therapy typically requires 5 to 6 weeks. Several methods of partial breast irradiation have been described, including brachytherapy via multiple catheters placed in the breast parenchyma, localized conformal external beam radiation therapy, brachytherapy via bead or seed implants, single-dose intraoperative radiation therapy, and brachytherapy via a balloon catheter inserted into the cavity after breast-conserving surgery. Jeruss (2010) recently reported an update on the American Society of Breast Surgeons Accelerated Partial Breast Irradiation Registry Trial. Of 194 patients with DCIS enrolled, 63 had at least 5 years of follow-up. Of these, 92% had favorable cosmetic results. The 5-year actuarial locoregional recurrence rate of 3.39% favorably compares with that of 7.5% reported using whole-breast radiation in the NSABP B-17 trial. The NSABP B-39/RTOG 0413 trial, which opened in 2005, will provide additional information about the potential role for accelerated partial breast irradiation in patients with DCIS and those with invasive breast cancer as well. Patients with no more than 3-cm DCIS or invasive stage I or II breast cancer who undergo margin-negative breast-conserving surgery are being randomized to standard adjuvant whole-breast external beam radiation therapy or accelerated partial breast irradiation. Patients will receive chemotherapy and endocrine therapy at the discretion of their treating physician. The primary endpoint is local tumor control, and the secondary endpoints are disease-free and overall survival, cosmetic results, and treatment toxicity.

Omitting Radiation Therapy
An estimated 20% of women undergoing breast-conserving surgery who would benefit from radiation therapy do not receive it as part of their treatment. The rates of radiation therapy use have been shown to vary, depending on the region of the country that the patient lives in and the age of the patient. Also, many patients choose mastectomy over breast-conserving surgery for DCIS because they are not able to complete 6 weeks of daily radiation therapy because of social or health considerations. Other patients who are candidates for breast-conserving surgery choose to undergo a mastectomy because of concerns about postirradiation complications. Breast-conserving surgery alone (i.e., without radiation therapy) may be sufficient in a select subgroup of patients with DCIS. Initial data that supported the use of breast-conserving surgery alone in the treatment of DCIS came from a study by Lagios et al. (1989) in which 79 patients with mammographically detected DCIS underwent margin-negative excision alone. After a follow-up time of 124 months, the local recurrence rate was 16% overall—33% for the subgroup of patients with

high-grade lesions and comedo necrosis versus only 2% for the patients with low- or intermediate-grade lesions.

Silverstein et al. (1996) developed the Van Nuys Prognostic Index (VNPI) by combining three statistically significant predictors of local recurrence: tumor size, margin width, and pathological classification. This index was recently modified to include patient age as a statistically significant predictor of local recurrence and is now referred to as the University of Southern California (USC)/VNPI (Silverstein, 2003). Numerical values ranging from 1 (best prognosis) to 3 (worst prognosis) are assigned for each of the four predictors. A size score of 1, 2, and 3 is given to small tumors (≤15 mm), intermediate tumors (16 to 40 mm), and large tumors (≥41 mm), respectively. Margin width is assigned a score of 1 if 10 mm or greater, 2 if 1 to 9 mm, and 3 if less than 1 mm. The pathological classification is 1 for non–high-grade DCIS without necrosis, 2 for non–high-grade DCIS with necrosis, and 3 for high-grade DCIS with or without necrosis. Patient age is assigned a score of 1 for greater than 60 years, 2 for 40 to 60 years, and 3 for less than 40 years. The sum of these results is the USC/VNPI score, with 4 being the lowest possible score and 12 the highest possible score. In a retrospective study of 706 patients with DCIS treated with or without radiation therapy after breast-conserving surgery, those patients with a USC/VNPI score of 4, 5, or 6, did not appear to benefit from the addition of radiation therapy for local recurrence-free survival compared with excision alone. In contrast, for patients with a USC/VNPI score of 7, 8, or 9, the absolute 12-year local recurrence-free survival rate was 12% higher among those who underwent radiation therapy and excision compared with those who underwent excision alone (73% vs. 61%). Although patients with a USC/VNPI score of 10, 11, or 12 showed the greatest benefit with the addition of radiation therapy, local recurrence rates still exceeded 40% at 8 years regardless of irradiation. On the basis of the USC/VNPI score, Silverstein (2003) proposed the following treatment schema for DCIS: wide local excision alone for patients with a USC/VNPI score of 4 to 6, excision plus radiation therapy for patients with a USC/VNPI score of 7 to 9, and mastectomy for patients with a USC/VNPI score of 10 to 12. The USC/VNPI score may be a useful adjunct in therapeutic decision making; however, multiple attempts at independently validating the utility of this risk stratification scheme have not been consistent.

While margin width is an independent prognostic factor for recurrence using the USC/VNPI score, it is unlikely that margin width alone can identify the patients with DCIS treated with breast conservation for whom radiation therapy can be safely omitted. In a retrospective analysis of 469 patients with DCIS who underwent breast conservation with margins that were at least 10 mm, Silverstein et al. (1999) did not detect a lower recurrence rate when postoperative radiation therapy was employed. In contrast, even on reanalysis of the NSABP B-17 data, all patient cohorts benefited from radiation therapy, regardless of the clinical or mammographic tumor characteristics. Furthermore, Wong et al. (2003) reported the early termination of a prospective single-arm trial conducted at the Dana-Farber/Harvard Cancer Center in which radiation therapy was omitted in patients with grade 1 to 2 DCIS that was no more than 25 mm and excised with 10 mm or greater margins. At a median follow-up of 3.3 years, the number of local recurrences observed was 2.5% per patient-year, corresponding to a 5-year rate of 12.5%.

More recently, Rudloff et al. (2010) proposed a multivariable nomogram to estimate risk for local recurrence in women with DCIS treated with breast-conserving surgery. The nomogram incorporates commonly available factors which have previously been shown to affect risk of ipsilateral breast tumor recurrence. These include age at diagnosis, family history, type of patient presentation (radiologic or clinical), nuclear grade, necrosis, margins, number of excisions, and receipt of radiation and/or adjuvant endocrine therapy. The nomogram calculates an actual, individualized estimate of absolute risk of ipsilateral breast tumor recurrence at 5 or 10 years, which can be weighed against the use of available adjuvant treatment options.

There are two large prospective studies designed to investigate the role of observation versus radiation therapy after breast-conserving therapy in patients with DCIS. In the Eastern Cooperative Oncology Group E-5194 trial, patients with low- or intermediate-grade DCIS smaller than 25 mm, or high-grade DCIS smaller than 10 mm, with excisional margins of at least 3 mm, underwent breast-conserving surgery without radiation therapy. Hughes (2009) reported the much lower 5-year rate of ipsilateral breast events in the 565 patients in the low/intermediate grade group of 6.1%, whereas the incidence for the 105 patients in the high-grade group was 15.3%. Long-term follow-up of this cohort is ongoing. Similarly, the Radiation Therapy Oncology Group (RTOG) 9804 trial randomized patients with low- or intermediate-grade DCIS less than 25 mm, excised with margins of at least 3 mm to postoperative radiation therapy or observation with the option of tamoxifen use in each group. This trial was closed early due to poor accrual.

Endocrine Therapy

Two prospective randomized trials have evaluated the effect of tamoxifen on outcome in patients with DCIS treated with breast-conserving therapy. In the NSABP B-24 trial, 1,804 women with DCIS were randomly assigned to breast-conserving surgery and radiation therapy followed by either tamoxifen at 20 mg/day or a placebo for 5 years. Sixteen percent of the women in this study had positive resection margins. At 7 years of follow-up, women who received tamoxifen had fewer breast cancer events than did the placebo group (10.0% vs. 16.9%). Among those who received tamoxifen, the rate of ipsilateral invasive breast cancer was 2.6% at 7 years compared with 5.3% in the control group. Tamoxifen also decreased the 7-year cumulative incidence of contralateral breast neoplasms (invasive and noninvasive) to 2.3% compared with 4.9% in the control group. The benefit of tamoxifen therapy also extended to patients with positive margins or margins of unknown status. There was no difference in the 7-year overall survival rate, which was 95% in both the tamoxifen and the placebo groups. Most deaths occurred before recurrence developed and were not necessarily related to breast cancer. A subgroup analysis, based on estrogen receptor status, indicated that women with estrogen receptor-positive DCIS who received tamoxifen had a 59% reduction in their relative risk of breast cancer events when compared with those who received the placebo. Among patients with estrogen receptor-negative DCIS, there was no added benefit from tamoxifen.

In a second prospective randomized trial (United Kingdom Coordinating Committee on Cancer Research), patients who underwent breast-conserving surgery were randomized to no adjuvant treatment, adjuvant radiation therapy or tamoxifen, or adjuvant radiation therapy plus tamoxifen. Patients with positive margins were excluded from this trial, and only 10% of the women were younger than 50 years old, compared with 33% in the NSABP B-24 trial. After a median follow-up time of 4.4 years, Houghton et al. (2003) reported that radiation therapy had the greatest impact on reducing ipsilateral breast cancer events, whereas tamoxifen added to radiation therapy did not result in a significant additional benefit. The relatively short follow-up time and complex design of this trial makes interpretation of the results in direct comparison to the NSABP B-24 trial difficult.

The decision of whether to use adjuvant tamoxifen for patients with DCIS should be made on an individual basis. The use of tamoxifen has been associated with vasomotor symptoms, deep vein thrombosis, pulmonary embolism, and increased cataract formation. The risk of endometrial cancer is increased two to seven times among patients who receive the drug. Tamoxifen is also associated with increased rates of stroke and benign ovarian cysts. Therefore, the effects of tamoxifen to reduce ipsilateral breast tumors and to prevent contralateral breast disease should be weighed against the risk of tamoxifen use in each patient. In addition, tamoxifen should be reserved for patients with estrogen receptor-positive tumors.

Aromatase inhibitors have been shown to be beneficial in the adjuvant treatment of invasive breast cancer in postmenopausal women with estrogen receptor-positive disease. These agents have fewer cardiovascular side effects than tamoxifen and may be beneficial in the adjuvant treatment of patients with DCIS following breast-conserving surgery. Two randomized prospective clinical trials opened in 2003—NSABP B-35 and the International Breast Cancer Intervention Study (IBIS-II)—compared the adjuvant use of tamoxifen versus anastrozole following breast-conserving surgery in patients with a diagnosis of DCIS. Results from these trials have not been reported but will help to define the role of aromatase inhibitors in the adjuvant treatment of DCIS.

Axillary Node Staging

Because DCIS is a noninvasive disease, lymph node involvement is not expected. Thus, the role for axillary lymph node dissection is limited, and node dissection should not be performed on a routine basis. In cases where patients have large tumors (>4 cm) or extensive microcalcifications, a focus of invasion can be missed because of limited pathological sampling (as discussed earlier, a 20% rate of concomitant invasive cancers has been reported on final pathology in patients who were diagnosed with DCIS on stereotactic biopsy). Such patients are at higher risk for lymph node metastasis. Hence, patients who undergo mastectomy for large, high-grade DCIS should be considered for intraoperative lymphatic mapping and sentinel lymph node dissection because it is not possible to perform lymphatic mapping after a mastectomy if invasive cancer is found in the mastectomy specimen. Patients with large, high-grade, or palpable DCIS who are undergoing breast-conserving surgery are also potential candidates for intraoperative lymphatic mapping and sentinel lymph node dissection (discussed in Chapter 2). In a study by Cox et al. (1998), the combination of hematoxylin–eosin staining and immunohistochemistry revealed that 6% of patients with newly diagnosed DCIS had metastatic disease in the sentinel nodes. Klauber-DeMore et al. (2000) found that sentinel lymph nodes were positive for cancer among 12% of patients with DCIS considered to be at high risk for invasion and among 10% of patients who had DCIS with microinvasion. This risk must be weighed against the risk of lymphedema associated with sentinel node dissection in each patient.

Predictors of Local Relapse

Several features of DCIS are associated with a less favorable clinical course. Traditional pathological variables, such as large tumor size (>3 cm), high nuclear grade, comedo-type necrosis, and positive margins, are associated with a greater risk of local recurrence, as previously discussed. Involved margins of resection constitute the most important independent prognostic variable for predicting local relapse. As described previously, the USC/VNPI combines four significant predictors of local recurrence: tumor size, margin width, pathological classification, and younger patient age (<50 years). A strong family history of breast cancer is associated with an increased risk of local recurrence; however, these factors are not considered contraindications for breast-conserving therapy. Molecular markers, such as overexpression of HER-2/*neu*, nm23, heat shock protein, and metallothionein; low expression of p21, Waf1, and Bcl2; and DNA aneuploidy have been reported to be associated with high-grade comedo lesions, but their importance as independent prognostic variables in DCIS have not been clarified.

Treatment and Outcome of Local Recurrence

The overall survival rate in patients with DCIS is excellent. In the NSABP B-17 trial, only 27 deaths (3.3%) attributed to breast cancer occurred after a median follow-up time of 12 years. In the NSABP B-24 trial, 0.8% of the patients died as a consequence of their breast cancer after 7 years of follow-up. In both trials, and in other studies, approximately 50% of all local recurrences were invasive cancers. The management of local recurrence depends on the therapy the patient received for the primary cancer. In cases of local recurrence in patients who underwent breast-conserving surgery without radiation therapy, re-excision with negative margins and postoperative radiation therapy is recommended. For patients who have recurrent breast cancer after receiving breast-conserving surgery and radiation therapy, mastectomy is usually the preferred treatment. If the recurrent tumor is invasive, staging of the axillary nodes is performed with lymphatic mapping and sentinel lymph node dissection.

The prognosis after treatment of local recurrence depends on whether the recurrence is invasive or noninvasive. Silverstein et al. (1998) found that among patients with invasive recurrences, the 8-year disease-specific mortality rate was 14.4%, and the distant disease probability was 27.1%. In a follow-up study, Romero et al. (2004) reported a 10-year disease-specific mortality rate of 15% in patients with invasive recurrence. Although most patients with recurrent disease after DCIS do survive, an invasive recurrence is a serious event. Patients with DCIS should undergo long-term follow-up for both recurrent disease and development of new ipsilateral or contralateral primary tumors.

Surveillance

Following breast-conserving surgery, a mammogram should be obtained prior to radiation therapy to rule out residual microcalcifications. In addition, a mammogram should be obtained 4 to 6 months after the completion of radiation therapy to establish a new baseline. Follow-up of patients after breast-conserving surgery with or without radiation therapy should include annual or biannual physical examination and annual mammography for the first 5 years, with an annual physical examination and mammogram thereafter. The National Comprehensive Cancer Network treatment guidelines recommend a physical examination every 6 months for 5 years and annually thereafter. Whether this improves the detection of recurrence and outcome is not known. Both patients who undergo breast-conserving therapy and those who undergo mastectomy should be monitored for the development of new primary cancers in the contralateral breast. The risk of development of a new primary cancer in the contralateral breast after treatment of DCIS is two to five times greater than the risk of development of a first primary breast cancer and is approximately the same as the risk of development of a new contralateral primary cancer after invasive cancer.

Current Management of DCIS at the University of Texas M. D. Anderson Cancer Center

An algorithm for the current treatment of DCIS at the M. D. Anderson Cancer Center is outlined in Figure 1.1. Patients diagnosed with a mammographic abnormality undergo bilateral diagnostic mammography, and the mammograms are compared with previous images, if available. Magnification views are routinely used to delineate the abnormality in the index breast. Ultrasound is also frequently used to assess tumor size, multicentricity, and nodal status. Diagnostic biopsy is performed by using a vacuum-assisted stereotactic core-needle biopsy technique. When DCIS is diagnosed, the pathological evaluation details the tumor type and grade, any evidence of microinvasion, and the status of both the estrogen and the progesterone receptors. MRI is not routinely employed in the preoperative evaluation of

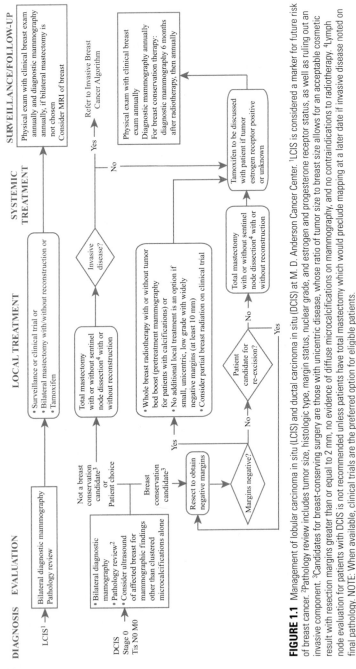

FIGURE 1.1 Management of lobular carcinoma in situ (LCIS) and ductal carcinoma in situ (DCIS) at M. D. Anderson Cancer Center. [1]LCIS is considered a marker for future risk of breast cancer. [2]Pathology review includes tumor size, histologic type, margin status, nuclear grade, and estrogen and progesterone receptor status, as well as ruling out an invasive component. [3]Candidates for breast-conserving surgery are those with unicentric disease, whose ratio of tumor size to breast size allows for an acceptable cosmetic result with resection margins greater than or equal to 2 mm, no evidence of diffuse microcalcifications on mammography, and no contraindications to radiotherapy. [4]Lymph node evaluation for patients with DCIS is not recommended unless patients have total mastectomy which would preclude mapping at a later date if invasive disease noted on final pathology. NOTE: When available, clinical trials are the preferred option for eligible patients.

patients with DCIS. The decision to use MRI is based on the density of the breasts and the findings on mammographic imaging.

The choice of surgical therapy for an individual patient is based on several factors, including tumor size and grade, margin width, mammographic appearance, and patient preference. The benefits and risks of breast-conserving surgery and mastectomy should be discussed in detail with each patient. Most patients with DCIS are candidates for breast-conserving therapy, and this is the preferred method of local treatment since it offers similar overall survival outcomes compared with mastectomy. Mastectomy is indicated in patients with diffuse, malignant-appearing calcifications in the breast and/or persistent positive margins after attempts at surgical excision, and those with a contraindication to postoperative radiation therapy. Although tumor size is not an absolute indication for mastectomy, mastectomy is often preferred for patients with large (>4 cm in diameter), high-grade DCIS. There are few data available on the efficacy of breast-conserving surgery for DCIS with index lesions greater than 4 cm in diameter. Mastectomy may also be a better choice when a patient's anxiety over the possibility of recurrence outweighs the impact a mastectomy would have on her quality of life. Immediate breast reconstruction should be considered for all patients who require or elect mastectomy. Intraoperative margin assessment with sectioned-specimen radiography is used in patients undergoing breast-conserving surgery and for patients with extensive calcifications undergoing skin-sparing mastectomy. Re-excision is usually recommended for patients who have margins less than 2 mm on final pathological examination after breast-conserving surgery.

Patients who undergo mastectomy for DCIS routinely undergo intraoperative lymphatic mapping and sentinel lymph node dissection. In patients who undergo breast-conserving surgery, sentinel lymph node dissection is performed on an individual basis and primarily reserved for cases where the DCIS is palpable, high grade or exhibits comedo-type necrosis.

Adjuvant radiation therapy is recommended to reduce the risk of local recurrence in patients who undergo breast-conserving surgery. Breast-conserving surgery alone (without radiation therapy) is considered for selected patients with small (<1 cm in diameter), low-grade lesions that have been excised with margins of at least 5 to 10 mm and who can be observed diligently for recurrence. Partial breast irradiation is offered for selected patients. Tamoxifen is offered for 5 years to women with estrogen receptor-positive DCIS who do not have a history of venous thromboembolism or stroke.

Following surgical resection, patients undergo annual physical and clinical breast examinations. Patients who receive breast-conserving surgery and radiation therapy undergo a diagnostic mammogram after surgery to ensure removal of all suspicious calcifications, 6 months after the completion of radiation therapy and annual bilateral mammograms thereafter. If a mastectomy is performed, the patient is followed with an annual diagnostic mammography of the contralateral breast.

All patients with DCIS are considered for clinical trials, which are the preferred treatment options for eligible patients.

LOBULAR CARCINOMA IN SITU

LCIS was first described in 1941. During the era that followed, the treatment of LCIS was the same as that of invasive carcinoma—radical mastectomy. Haagensen et al. (1978) is credited with altering the treatment philosophy for LCIS. In a review of 211 cases, a 17% incidence of subsequent invasive carcinoma was found among women with LCIS treated by observation alone (without surgery). The risk of developing a subsequent carcinoma was equal for both breasts, and only six patients died of breast cancer. Haagensen concluded that close observation for LCIS allowed for early detection of subsequent malignancy, with associated high cure rates. Haagensen's rationale for observation of LCIS was based on his view that patients with LCIS were at increased risk for invasive breast cancer but that LCIS itself did not progress into a malignancy. However, more recent work has indicated that certain types of LCIS may be indolent precursors of infiltrating lobular cancer and that surgical resection should be considered in selected subtypes of LCIS.

Epidemiology

The incidence of LCIS is difficult to estimate because the diagnosis is most often made as an incidental finding. LCIS is often not detectable by palpation, gross pathological examination, or mammography. On evaluation of mammographic abnormalities, LCIS is found in 0.5% to 1.3% of breast core-needle biopsy specimens and 0.5% to 3.9% of excisional breast biopsy specimens. Traditionally, LCIS was more commonly reported in premenopausal women than in postmenopausal women. In Haagensen's series, 90% of the patients were premenopausal. However, in a review of the Surveillance, Epidemiology, and End Results program database, Li et al. (2002) reported that from 1978 to 1998, the incidence of LCIS increased in all age groups, but it increased the most in women 50 to 79 years old. The increase in incidence in women 40 to 49 years old continued up until 1989 but then stabilized, whereas the incidence in women 50 years of age or older increased throughout the study period. Between 1996 and 1998, the incidence of LCIS was the highest in women 50 to 59 years old (11.47/100,000 person-years) followed by women 60 to 69 years old (8.14/100,000 person-years). The reason for this increase in LCIS seen in women 50 years of age or older is multifactorial. Increased use of screening mammography led to an increased number of biopsies performed, increasing the identification rate of LCIS. Furthermore, as estrogen is hypothesized to play a role in the pathogenesis of LCIS, hormone replacement therapy in postmenopausal women may also account for the increased incidence of LCIS in this age group.

The theory that LCIS represents a marker of increased risk of invasive breast carcinoma is supported by the fact that the mean age at diagnosis is 10 to 15 years younger than that for invasive cancer. However, in women 50 years of age or older, as the incidence of LCIS has increased, the incidence of infiltrating lobular carcinoma has increased concurrently in this age group, whereas women younger than 50 years old have not experienced an increase in invasive lobular carcinoma. Recently, some have suggested that LCIS is morphologically and biologically more heterogeneous than previously reported. Although classic LCIS may not be associated with invasive lobular carcinoma, cases of larger, more pleomorphic LCIS lesions may represent clonal proliferation of cells that may progress to invasive lobular carcinoma. Molecular analysis of LCIS and invasive lobular carcinoma has revealed decreased expression or loss of the cell surface adhesion molecule E-cadherin in both tumor types. This contrasts with ductal carcinoma, in which E-cadherin expression is usually maintained. LCIS and invasive ductal carcinoma have also been shown to exhibit similar loss of heterozygosity. In addition, in an analysis of 180 patients with LCIS treated with breast-conserving therapy, Fisher et al. (2004) reported that eight of nine patients (89%) with invasive ipsilateral breast carcinoma recurrence had a recurrence of the lobular type. These data further strengthen the theory that LCIS is not only a marker for increased risk of invasive breast cancer, but also a direct precursor of invasive lobular carcinoma.

Pathology

LCIS is characterized by intraepithelial proliferation of the terminal ductal–lobular unit. The cells are slightly larger and paler than those that line the normal acini, but the lobular architecture remains intact. The cells have a homogeneous morphology and do not display prominent chromatin. The cytoplasm-to-nucleus ratio is normal, with infrequent mitoses and no necrosis. The proliferating cells do not penetrate the basement membrane. Recently, a pleomorphic variant of LCIS with larger nuclei, central necrosis, and calcifications was described. This variant may be more prone to progressing to invasive lobular carcinoma.

The diagnosis of LCIS involves the differentiation of LCIS from other forms of benign disease and from invasive lesions. In the absence of complete replacement of the lobular unit, "atypical lobular hyperplasia" is the designated pathological term. Papillomatosis in the terminal ducts may resemble LCIS but lacks the characteristic involvement of the acini. DCIS may extend retrograde into the acini, but it has a more characteristic anaplastic cell morphology and generally expresses E-cadherin. LCIS is contained within the basement membrane and is thus distinguished from invasive lobular carcinoma.

Numerous studies have documented that LCIS is multifocal and multicentric. If diligently sought, foci can be found elsewhere in the breast in almost all cases. In addition, LCIS is identified in the contralateral breast in 50% to 90% of cases. Thus, the presence of LCIS reflects a phenotypic manifestation of a generalized abnormality present throughout both breasts. As a result, the treatment of LCIS should be directed not only at the index lesion, but also at both breasts.

Diagnosis
Clinical Presentation

Because LCIS is usually not detectable by physical examination or mammography, it is most commonly diagnosed as an incidental finding in a breast biopsy specimen. Therefore, the clinical presentation of patients with LCIS is similar to that of patients requiring breast biopsy for fibroadenoma, benign ductal disease, DCIS, or invasive breast cancer. Patients diagnosed with LCIS should undergo bilateral diagnostic mammography to exclude other abnormalities in the breast. Ultrasound is also useful in evaluating suspicious findings.

Treatment
Surgery

The optimal clinical management of patients diagnosed with LCIS identified on core-needle biopsy remains controversial. In the past, many surgeons opted to observe such patients because a diagnosis of LCIS was considered a marker for increased risk of breast cancer rather than a precursor of invasive cancer. However, recent studies by Arpino et al. (2004) and others have reported a 0% to 10% risk of synchronous invasive breast cancer and a 0% to 50% risk of synchronous DCIS in patients diagnosed with LCIS by core-needle biopsy specimens. Hence, patients with LCIS with high-risk features, such as pleomorphic LCIS, diagnosed by core-needle biopsy specimens are now recommended to undergo surgical excision to rule out synchronous invasive cancer and DCIS.

In contrast with DCIS, there is a lack of prospective randomized trials evaluating adjuvant treatment following surgical excision of LCIS. Most of the patients diagnosed with LCIS since the mid-1970s have undergone clinical observation alone based on the recommendations of Haagensen. In a study of patients who underwent observation alone after margin-negative surgical excision of LCIS, Fisher et al. (2004) reported an overall 14.4% ipsilateral and 7.8% contralateral breast cancer event rate after 12 years. Nearly 85% of ipsilateral breast tumors were detected by mammography, and the risk of ipsilateral tumors was approximately 1.6% per year. More than 96% of all ipsilateral tumors occurred in the same quadrant as the original LCIS. Nine of 26 (34.6% [5.0% of the total]) patients with ipsilateral tumors had an invasive breast cancer, an incidence that was similar to that in patients with contralateral breast tumors (5.6% of the total). However, the contralateral breast tumors occurred later. Only 2 of the 180 patients in the study died from breast cancer, resulting in a breast cancer-specific mortality rate of 1.1% at 12 years of follow-up time. The free excision margins were believed to have contributed to the low rate of invasive ipsilateral breast tumors. In another study of 100 patients with LCIS, Ottesen et al. (2000) reported a 13% invasive ipsilateral breast cancer event rate and a 16% overall rate of breast cancers. In this study, margin status was not evaluated, and the invasive ipsilateral breast tumor event rate was more than double that observed by Fisher. Hence, complete excision of LCIS with negative margins may result in decreased occurrence of invasive breast cancer. On the other hand, Ciocca et al. (2008) reported a retrospective analysis of 2,894 patients who underwent breast-conserving surgery for DCIS or stage I or II breast cancer between 1980 and 2007, 10% of whom had LCIS within the lumpectomy specimen, 90% of whom did not. In the group with LCIS in the lumpectomy specimen, approximately one-third had LCIS at the margin. The crude local recurrence rate of the patients with LCIS within the specimen (4.5%) was not statistically different from that in the group with no LCIS (3.8%). Furthermore, there was also no statistical difference in actuarial 5- and 10-year local recurrence rates if LCIS was present at the margin (6% and 6%), if LCIS was present, but not at the margin (1% and 15%), or if no LCIS was present (2% and 6%). Because the presence of LCIS did not impact recurrence, Ciocca did not recommend re-excision if LCIS was identified at or close to margin surfaces and concluded that LCIS was likely not a precursor to the development of invasive lesions. At the present time, there are insufficient data to recommend re-excision to achieve negative margins for LCIS. Further study of the various LCIS subtypes is needed to determine whether patients with some subtypes would indeed benefit from re-excision.

Contralateral mirror-image breast biopsy, a procedure advocated for patients with LCIS in the past, has fallen out of favor because a mirror-image biopsy negative for LCIS does not eliminate the need for close observation of the remaining breast tissue in the contralateral breast. A viable therapeutic option for LCIS is bilateral prophylactic mastectomy. This approach is usually reserved for patients who have additional risk factors for breast cancer or who experience extreme anxiety regarding the observation and/or chemoprevention options. Because LCIS poses no risk of regional metastasis, axillary node dissection is not required. Immediate breast reconstruction should be offered for patients who undergo prophylactic mastectomy for LCIS.

Endocrine Therapy and Chemoprevention

Another treatment option for patients with a diagnosis of LCIS is chemoprevention with tamoxifen. In the NSABP P-1 breast cancer prevention trial, Fisher et al. (1998) observed a 56% decrease in the incidence of invasive breast cancers in a subset of women with LCIS who received tamoxifen as compared with women with LCIS who underwent observation alone. The annual hazard rate of invasive cancer was 5.69 per 1,000 women who received tamoxifen compared with 12.99 per 1,000 women who did not. In the NSABP P-2 trial, postmenopausal women with LCIS were eligible to be randomized between tamoxifen and raloxifene. Vogel et al. (2006) reported that the two agents offered an equivalent risk reduction for invasive breast cancer (incidence 4.30 per 1,000, vs. 4.41 per 1,000, for tamoxifen and raloxifene, respectively). Patients receiving raloxifene had a lower risk of thromboembolic events and cataracts. There was no statistical difference in risk of other cancers, fractures, ischemic heart disease, and stroke for the two drugs. A 2010 update, at 81 months of median follow-up, revealed that raloxifene was 78% as effective as tamoxifen at preventing invasive disease, but had far fewer toxicities, with statistically significantly fewer endometrial cancers. Vogel et al. concluded that depending on an individual's personal risk factors, both raloxifene and tamoxifen are valuable for breast cancer risk reduction. Raloxifene may be particularly beneficial to a postmenopausal woman with an intact uterus who also faces a risk of osteoporosis; tamoxifen would be an appropriate choice for high-risk postmenopausal women.

Radiation Therapy
Adjuvant radiation therapy has not been evaluated specifically for the treatment of LCIS, and data are currently insufficient to recommend this treatment on a routine basis. If synchronous DCIS or invasive breast cancer is found in an excised LCIS specimen, the patient will benefit from radiation therapy and should receive treatment according to the guidelines for DCIS or invasive breast cancer.

Surveillance
Following breast-conserving therapy for LCIS, patients should undergo annual or biannual physical examinations with bilateral breast examinations. They should also undergo annual bilateral diagnostic mammography. Use of screening ultrasound in patients with LCIS is being evaluated. Also, patients who undergo a bilateral mastectomy with or without reconstruction should undergo an annual physical examination, and any suspicious lesions should be evaluated with ultrasound and biopsy analysis.

Current Treatment of LCIS at M. D. Anderson Cancer Center
The algorithm for treatment of patients with LCIS at M. D. Anderson Cancer Center is outlined in Figure 1.1. If not performed prior to obtaining the biopsy specimen, patients found to have LCIS are evaluated with bilateral diagnostic mammography. The new mammograms are compared with previous images, if available. Suspicious lesions are further evaluated with ultrasound, and additional core-needle biopsy specimens are obtained when appropriate.

Patients found to have a suspicious abnormality on mammography or ultrasound undergo breast-conserving therapy with excision of the abnormality under needle localization. If they are found to have synchronous DCIS or invasive breast cancer, subsequent treatment is administered according to the guidelines for these tumors. Re-excision to attain negative margins is not routinely performed in patients found to have isolated classical LCIS in an excised specimen. If necessary, re-excision is performed to achieve negative margins in patients with a diagnosis of pleomorphic LCIS. Bilateral prophylactic mastectomy is reserved for patients with additional risk factors for breast cancer and patients who experience extreme anxiety regarding the observation and/or chemoprevention options.

Patients who undergo breast-conserving therapy for LCIS do not routinely receive radiation therapy but are offered tamoxifen or raloxifene if they are suitable candidates for risk reduction with antiestrogen therapy.

After breast-conserving surgery, patients undergo annual physical examinations and bilateral diagnostic mammography. Following a bilateral prophylactic mastectomy with or without reconstruction, patients are evaluated with the use of annual physical examinations, and any suspicious lesions are investigated by using ultrasound and biopsy when appropriate.

All patients with LCIS are considered for clinical trials, which are the preferred treatment options for eligible patients.

Recommended Readings

Arpino G, Allred DC, Mohsin SK, et al. Lobular neoplasia on core-needle biopsy—clinical significance. *Cancer.* 2004;101(2): 242–250.

Balch CM, Singletary SE, Bland KI. Clinical decision-making in early breast cancer. *Ann Surg.* 1993;217(3):207–225.

Boyages J, Delaney G, Taylor R. Predictors of local recurrence after treatment of ductal carcinoma in situ: a meta-analysis. *Cancer.* 1999;85(3):616–628.

Brinton LA, Sherman ME, Carreon JD, et al. Recent trends in breast cancer among younger women in the United States. *J Natl Cancer Inst.* 2008;100(22):1643–1648.

Chagpar A, Yen T, Sahin A, et al. Intraoperative margin assessment reduces reexcision rates in patients with ductal carcinoma in situ treated with breast-conserving surgery. *Am J Surg.* 2003;186(4): 371–377.

Ciocca RM, Li T, Freedman GM, et al. Presence of lobular carcinoma in situ does not increase local recurrence in patients treated with breast-conserving therapy. *Ann Surg Oncol.* 2008;15(8):2263–2271.

Cox CE, Pendas S, Cox JM, et al. Guidelines for sentinel node biopsy and lymphatic mapping of patients with breast cancer. *Ann Surg.* 1998;227(5):645–651; discussion 651–653.

de Mascarel I, MacGrogan G, Mathoulin-Pelissier S, et al. Breast ductal carcinoma in situ with microinvasion: a definition supported by a long-term study of 1248 serially sectioned ductal carcinomas. *Cancer.* 2002;94(8):2134–2142.

El-Tamer M, Chun J, Gill M, et al. Incidence and clinical significance of lymph node metastasis detected by cytokeratin immunohistochemical staining in ductal carcinoma in situ. *Ann Surg Oncol.* 2005;12(3):254–259.

Fisher B, Costantino J, Redmond C, et al. Lumpectomy compared with lumpectomy and radiation therapy for the treatment of intraductal breast cancer. *N Engl J Med.* 1993;328(22):1581–1586.

Fisher B, Costantino JP, Wickerham DL, et al. Tamoxifen for prevention of breast cancer: report of the National Surgical Adjuvant Breast and Bowel Project P-1 Study. *J Natl Cancer Inst.* 1998;90(18):1371–1388.

Fisher B, Dignam J, Wolmark N, et al. Tamoxifen in treatment of intraductal breast cancer: National Surgical Adjuvant Breast and Bowel Project B-24 randomised controlled trial. *Lancet.* 1999;353(9169):1993–2000.

Fisher B, Land S, Mamounas E, et al. Prevention of invasive breast cancer in women with ductal carcinoma in situ: an update of the National Surgical Adjuvant Breast and Bowel Project experience. *Semin Oncol.* 2001;28(4):400–418.

Fisher ER, Costantino J, Fisher B, et al. Pathologic findings from the National Surgical Adjuvant Breast Project (NSABP) Protocol B-17. Intraductal carcinoma (ductal carcinoma in situ). The National Surgical Adjuvant Breast and Bowel Project Collaborating Investigators. *Cancer.* 1995; 75(6):1310–1319.

Fisher ER, Land SR, Fisher B, et al. Pathologic findings from the National Surgical Adjuvant Breast and Bowel Project: twelve-year observations concerning lobular carcinoma in situ. *Cancer.* 2004;100(2): 238–244.

Fowble B. Intraductal noninvasive breast cancer: a comparison of three local treatments. *Oncology (Williston Park).* 1989;3(6):51–58; discussion 63–64, 66, 69.

Gill JK, Maskarinec G, Pagano I, et al. The association of mammographic density with ductal carcinoma in situ of the breast: the Multiethnic Cohort. *Breast Cancer Res.* 2006;8(3):R30.

Haagensen CD, Lane N, Lattes R, et al. Lobular neoplasia (so-called lobular carcinoma in situ) of the breast. *Cancer.* 1978;42(2):737–769.

Holland R, Hendriks JH, Vebeek AL, et al. Extent, distribution, and mammographic/histological correlations of breast ductal carcinoma in situ. *Lancet.* 1990;335(8688):519–522.

Hollingsworth AB, Stough RG, O'Dell CA, et al. Breast magnetic resonance imaging for preoperative locoregional staging. *Am J Surg.* 2008;196(3):389–397.

Houghton J, George WD, Cuzick J, et al. Radiotherapy and tamoxifen in women with completely excised ductal carcinoma in situ of the breast in the UK, Australia, and New Zealand: randomised controlled trial. *Lancet.* 2003;362 (9378):95–102.

Hughes LL, Wang M, Page DL, et al. Local excision alone without irradiation for ductal carcinoma in situ of the breast: a trial of the Eastern Cooperative Oncology Group. *J Clin Oncol.* 2009;27(32):5319–5324.

Jeruss JS, Kuerer HM, Beitsch PD, et al. Update on DCIS outcomes from the American Society of Breast Surgeons accelerated partial breast irradiation registry trial. *Ann Surg Oncol.* 2011;18(1):65–71.

Julien JP, Bijker N, Fentiman IS, et al. Radiotherapy in breast-conserving treatment for ductal carcinoma in situ: first results of the EORTC randomised phase III trial 10853. EORTC Breast Cancer Cooperative Group and EORTC Radiotherapy Group. *Lancet.* 2000;355(9203):528–533.

Klauber-DeMore N, Tan LK, Liberman L, et al. Sentinel lymph node biopsy: is it indicated in patients with high-risk ductal carcinoma-in-situ and ductal carcinoma-in-situ with microinvasion? *Ann Surg Oncol.* 2000;7(9):636–642.

Lagios MD, Margolin FR, Westdahl PR, et al. Mammographically detected duct carcinoma in situ. Frequency of local recurrence following tylectomy and prognostic effect of nuclear grade on local recurrence. *Cancer.* 1989;63(4):618–624.

Land SR, Wickerham DL, Costantino JP, et al. Patient-reported symptoms and quality of life during treatment with tamoxifen or raloxifene for breast cancer prevention: the NSABP Study of Tamoxifen and Raloxifene (STAR) P-2 trial. *JAMA.* 2006;295(23):2742–2751.

Lehman CD, Gatsonis C, Kuhl CK, et al. MRI evaluation of the contralateral breast in women with recently diagnosed breast cancer. *N Engl J Med.* 2007;356(13):1295–1303.

Li CI, Anderson BO, Daling JR, et al. Changing incidence of lobular carcinoma in situ of the breast. *Breast Cancer Res Treat.* 2002;75(3):259–268.

Mirza NQ, Vlastos G, Meric F, et al. Ductal carcinoma-in-situ: long-term results of breast-conserving therapy. *Ann Surg Oncol.* 2000;7(9):656–664.

Neuschatz AC, DiPetrillo T, Steinhoff M, et al. The value of breast lumpectomy margin assessment as a predictor of residual tumor burden in ductal carcinoma in situ of the breast. *Cancer.* 2002;94(7):1917–1924.

Nielsen M, Thomsen JL, Primdahl S, et al. Breast cancer and atypia among young and middle-aged women: a study of 110 medicolegal autopsies. *Br J Cancer.* 1987;56(6):814–819.

Ottesen GL, Graversen HP, Blichert-Toft M, et al. Carcinoma in situ of the female breast. 10 year follow-up results of a prospective nationwide study. *Breast Cancer Res Treat.* 2000;62(3):197–210.

Page DL, Dupont WD, Rogers LW, et al. Continued local recurrence of carcinoma 15–25 years after a diagnosis of low grade ductal carcinoma in situ of the breast treated only by biopsy. *Cancer.* 1995;76(7):1197–1200.

Romero L, Klein L, Ye W, et al. Outcome after invasive recurrence in patients with ductal carcinoma in situ of the breast. *Am J Surg.* 2004;188(4):371–376.

Rudloff U, Jacks LM, Goldberg JI, et al. Nomogram for predicting the risk of local recurrence after breast-conserving surgery for ductal carcinoma in situ. *J Clin Oncol.* 2010;28(23):3762–3769.

Silverstein MJ. The University of Southern California/Van Nuys prognostic index for ductal carcinoma in situ of the breast. *Am J Surg.* 2003;186(4):337–343.

Silverstein MJ, Cohlan BF, Gierson ED, et al. Duct carcinoma in situ: 227 cases without microinvasion. *Eur J Cancer.* 1992;28(2–3):630–634.

Silverstein MJ, Lagios MD, Craig PH, et al. A prognostic index for ductal carcinoma in situ of the breast. *Cancer.* 1996;77(11):2267–2274.

Silverstein MJ, Lagios MD, Groshen S, et al. The influence of margin width on local control of ductal carcinoma in situ of the breast. *N Engl J Med.* 1999;340(19):1455–1461.

Silverstein MJ, Lagios MD, Martino S, et al. Outcome after invasive local recurrence in patients with ductal carcinoma in situ of the breast. *J Clin Oncol.* 1998;16(4):1367–1373.

Silverstein MJ, Poller DN, Waisman JR, et al. Prognostic classification of breast ductal carcinoma-in-situ. *Lancet.* 1995;345(8958):1154–1157.

Vezeridis MP, Bland KI. Management of ductal carcinoma in situ. *Surg Oncol.* 1994; 3(6):309–325.

Vigeland E, Klaasen H, Klingen TA, et al. Full-field digital mammography compared to screen film mammography in the prevalent round of a population-based screening programme: the Vestfold County Study. *Eur Radiol.* 2008;18(1):183–191.

Vogel VG, Costantino JP, Wickerham DL, et al. Effects of tamoxifen vs raloxifene on the risk of developing invasive breast cancer and other disease outcomes: the NSABP Study of Tamoxifen and Raloxifene (STAR) P-2 trial. *JAMA.* 2006;295(23):2727–2741.

Vogel VG, Costantino JP, Wickerham DL, et al. Update of the National Surgical Adjuvant Breast and Bowel Project Study of Tamoxifen And Raloxifene (STAR) P-2 Trial: preventing breast cancer. *Cancer Prev Res (Phila Pa).* 2010;3(6):696–706.

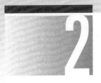

Invasive Breast Cancer

David S. Kwon, Catherine M. Kelly,
and C. Denise Ching

EPIDEMIOLOGY

Breast cancer is the most common cancer diagnosed and the second most common cause of cancer-related mortalities among women in the United States. In 2010, approximately 209,060 new cases were diagnosed, and nearly 40,230 (Cancer Facts and Figures 2010, American Cancer Society) breast cancer–related deaths occurred. For an American woman, the lifetime risk of being diagnosed with breast cancer is 1 in 8% or 12%, and the lifetime risk of dying from breast cancer is approximately 2.4%.

In the late 1980s, rates of regional disease at diagnosis decreased among women older than 40 years. This decrease likely reflects the increased use of mammography in the early 1980s that continues through the present day. In contrast, the increase in survival rates in this same time period, particularly for women with regional disease, likely reflects continued improvements in systemic adjuvant therapy. Therefore, both screening mammography and improved therapy have likely contributed to the decline in breast cancer mortality rates in the United States.

RISK FACTORS

Multiple factors are associated with an increased risk of developing breast cancer, including genetic predisposition, a history of proliferative breast disease or prior radiation, a personal or family history of breast cancer, and hormone exposure. A simplified version of previously summarized risk factors for breast cancer is provided in Table 2.1.

Personal Factors

Gender, age, and a personal or family history of breast cancer are all significant personal factors associated with an increased risk for breast cancer. The most important risk factor for the development of breast cancer is gender. The female-to-male ratio for breast cancer is 100:1. Therefore, this section focuses on risk factors among women.

Age is also an important risk factor. According to the National Cancer Institute's Surveillance, Epidemiology, and End Results Program, the incidence of breast cancer increases rapidly during the fourth decade of life. After menopause, the incidence continues to increase but at a much slower rate, peaking in the fifth and sixth decades of life and slowly leveling off during the sixth and seventh decades. Approximately 1 out of 8 invasive breast cancers will be found in women younger than 45 years; approximately 2/3 invasive breast cancers are found in women older than 55 years.

A family history of breast cancer has been recognized to increase a woman's risk of breast cancer. The overall risk depends on the number of relatives with cancer, their ages at diagnosis, and whether the disease was unilateral or bilateral. The highest risk is associated with a young first-degree relative with bilateral breast cancer. For example, the cumulative breast cancer risk for a 30-year-old woman

TABLE 2.1	Risk Factors for Breast Cancer and Associated Relative Risks	
Risk Factor	**Category at Risk**	**Relative Risk**
Germline mutations	*BRCA1* and younger than 40 years old	200
	BRCA1 and 60–69 years old	15
Proliferative breast disease	Lobular carcinoma in situ	16.4
	Ductal carcinoma in situ	17.3
Personal history of breast cancer	Invasive breast cancer	6.8
Ionizing radiation exposure	Hodgkin disease	5.2
Family history	First-degree relative with pre-menopausal breast cancer	3.3
	First-degree relative with post-menopausal breast cancer	1.8
Age at first childbirth	Older than 30 years	1.7–1.9
Hormone replacement therapy with estrogen and progesterone	Current user for at least 5 years	1.3
Early menarche	Younger than 12 years	1.3
Late menopause	Older than 55 years	1.2–1.5

Singletary SE. Rating the risk factors for breast cancer. *Ann Surg* 2003;237:474.

whose sister had bilateral breast cancer before age 50 is 55% by age 70. This risk decreases to 8% for a 30-year-old woman whose sister developed unilateral breast cancer after age 50. Overall, the risk of developing breast cancer is increased approximately 1.5- to 3-fold if a woman has a first degree relative (mother or sister) with breast cancer.

A personal history of breast cancer is a significant risk factor for the development of cancer in the contralateral breast. The incidence of contralateral breast cancer is 0.5% to 1.0% per year of follow-up.

Genetic Predisposition

While genetic mutations can be associated with a risk for breast cancer as high as 60% to 80%, only 5% to 10% of all breast cancers among Caucasian women are believed to result from an inherited gene mutation. Autosomal dominant conditions associated with an increased risk for breast cancer include Li-Fraumeni syndrome, *BRCA1* and *BRCA2* mutations, Muir-Torre syndrome, Cowden disease, and Peutz-Jeghers syndrome (Table 2.2). Although autosomal dominant, these conditions do not always exhibit 100% penetrance. Another inherited condition that may be associated with breast cancer is the autosomal recessive disorder ataxia-telangiectasia. *PTEN* and *TP53* are other genetic mutations associated with breast cancer risk, accounting for less than 1% of cases.

Mutations in the breast cancer susceptibility genes *BRCA1*, located on the long arm of chromosome 17q, and *BRCA2*, found on chromosome 13, are associated with an increased risk of breast cancer and ovarian cancers. The estimated lifetime risk of breast cancer development in mutation carriers ranges from 37% to 87% by age 70 for breast cancer, and the risk of ovarian cancer from 16% to 63% and 10% to 27%, respectively, for carriers of *BRCA1* and *BRCA2*.

TABLE 2.2   Autosomal Dominant Conditions Associated with Possible Development of Breast Cancer

Syndrome	Defect	Associated Condition or Increased Risk for ...
BRCA1	Mutation of chromosome 17q	Malignancies of the breast, ovaries, and possibly prostate and colon
BRCA2	Mutation of chromosome 13q	Malignancies of the breast (including male), ovaries, prostate, larynx, and pancreas
Li-Fraumeni	Mutation in the p53 gene on chromosome 17p	Malignancies of the breast, brain, and adrenal glands; soft-tissue sarcomas
Muir-Torre	Mutation in DNA mismatch repair genes (hMLH1 and hMSH2) on chromosome 2p	Malignancies of the breast and gastrointestinal (GI) and genitourinary tracts; sebaceous tumors (i.e., hyperplasia, adenoma, epithelioma, carcinoma), keratoacanthoma
Cowden disease	Mutation in the PTEN gene on chromosome 10q	Malignancies of the breast, colon, uterus, thyroid, lung, and bladder; hamartomatous polyps in GI tract
Peutz-Jeghers	Mutation in the STK11 gene on chromosome 19p	Malignancies of the breast and pancreas; mucocutaneous melanin deposition, hamartomas of the GI tract

Proliferative Breast Disease

Nonproliferative breast diseases such as adenosis, fibroadenomas, apocrine changes, duct ectasia, and mild hyperplasia carry no increased risk of breast cancer whereas proliferative breast diseases are associated with breast cancer to various degrees (RR is 1.5 to 2.0). Moderate or florid hyperplasias without atypia, papillomas, and sclerosing adenosis carry a slightly increased risk of breast cancer (1.5 to 2 times that of the general population). Atypical ductal or lobular hyperplasia is associated with a moderately increased risk of developing breast cancer (4 to 5 times). Lobular carcinoma in situ is associated with a high risk of breast cancer (8 to 10 times). These risks apply equally to both breasts, even if the proliferative breast disease was unilateral.

Prior Radiation Exposure

Therapeutic radiation exposure to treat disease can be a significant cause of radiation-induced carcinogenesis; the highest associated risk is seen with higher doses of radiation given at the time of treatment and radiation treatment given at a young age, that is, the increased risk of breast cancer if the exposure was before age 30 (relative risk is 5.2). This has been observed in women receiving mantle irradiation for treatment of Hodgkin disease.

Endocrine Factors

Endogenous Hormone Exposure

Endogenous endocrine factors have also been implicated as risk factors in breast cancer. Early age at menarche and the establishment of regular ovulatory cycles may have an effect on risk. Women who start regular ovulatory cycles before age 13 have a fourfold greater risk for breast cancer than those whose menarche occurred after age 13 and who had a 5-year delay to the development of regular cycles. Although age at menarche is important, age at onset of regular menses may have a larger effect on risk.

Nulliparity and advanced age at first childbirth increase the risk of developing breast cancer. Compared to a woman with a first live birth at age younger than 20, the relative risk for a nulliparous woman is 1.67, and for a woman giving birth older than age 30 is 2.23. Women who have their first child between ages 30 and 34 have the same risk as nulliparous women; women older than 35 years have a greater risk than nulliparous women.

The risk of breast cancer for women who experience menopause after age 55 is twice that of women who experience menopause before age 44. The cumulative duration of menstruation may also be important. Women who menstruate for more than 30 years are at greater risk than those who menstruate for less than 30 years. These observations indicate that the hormonal milieu at different times in a woman's life may affect her risk of breast cancer, and the total duration of exposure to endogenous estrogen is an important factor in breast cancer risk.

Exogenous Hormone Exposure

Exogenous hormone replacement therapy is known to increase a woman's risk of breast cancer (relative risk after 5 years of treatment is 1.3). The Women's Health Initiative, a large-scale prospective study, was abruptly halted in 2002 because interim analysis of the data indicated that the risks of continuing hormonal replacement therapy outweighed the benefits. Data demonstrated a 26% increase in the risk of breast cancer over a 5-year period. In addition, the study confirmed the increased risk of stroke as well as an unexpected increased risk in coronary artery disease. However, the benefits associated with hormone replacement therapy include increased bone density and fewer postmenopausal symptoms. Therefore, treating physicians should thoroughly discuss the risks and benefits of this therapy with their patients.

A number of models exist that assess the risk of developing breast cancer. The Breast Cancer Risk Assessment Tool, a publicly available resource, was developed by scientists at the National Cancer Institute and the National Surgical Adjuvant Breast and Bowel Project (NSABP). It is based on a statistical model known as the GAIL model. The model uses a woman's own personal medical history (number of previous breast biopsies and the presence of atypia in those biopsies), her own reproductive history (age at the start of menstruation and age at the first live birth), and the history of breast cancer among her first-degree relatives (mother, sisters, daughters) to estimate her risk of developing invasive breast cancer over a 5-year period and over a lifetime.

PATHOLOGY

Invasive carcinomas of the breast tend to be histologically heterogeneous tumors. The vast majority of these tumors are adenocarcinomas that arise from the terminal ducts. There are five common histologic variants of mammary adenocarcinoma:

1. *Infiltrating ductal carcinoma* accounts for 75% of all breast cancers. This lesion is characterized by the absence of special histologic features. It is hard on palpation and gritty when transected. It is associated with various degrees of fibrotic response. Often there is associated ductal carcinoma in situ (DCIS) within the specimen. Infiltrating ductal carcinomas commonly metastasize to axillary lymph nodes. The prognosis for patients with these tumors is poorer than that for patients with some of the other histologic subtypes (i.e., mucinous, colloid, tubular, and medullary). Distant metastases are found most often in the bones, lungs, liver, and brain.

2. *Infiltrating lobular carcinoma* is seen in 5% to 10% of breast cancer cases. Clinically, this lesion often has an area of ill-defined thickening within the

breast. Microscopically, small cells in a single- or Indian-file pattern are characteristically seen. Infiltrating lobular cancers tend to grow around ducts and lobules. Multicentricity and bilaterality are observed more frequently in infiltrating lobular carcinoma than in infiltrating ductal carcinoma. The prognosis for lobular carcinoma is similar to that for infiltrating ductal carcinoma. In addition to metastasizing to axillary lymph nodes, lobular carcinoma is known to metastasize to unusual sites (e.g., meninges and serosal surfaces) more often than other forms of breast cancer.

3. *Tubular carcinoma* accounts for only 2% of breast carcinomas. The diagnosis of tubular carcinoma is made only when more than 75% of the tumor demonstrates tubule formation. Axillary nodal metastases are uncommon with this type of tumor. The prognosis for patients with tubular carcinoma is considerably better than that for patients with other types of breast cancer.

4. *Medullary carcinoma* accounts for 5% to 7% of breast cancers. Histologically, the lesion is characterized by poorly differentiated nuclei, a syncytial growth pattern, a well-circumscribed border, intense infiltration with small lymphocytes and plasma cells, and little or no DCIS. The prognosis for patients with pure medullary carcinoma is favorable; however, mixed variants with invasive ductal components will have prognoses similar to invasive ductal carcinoma.

5. *Mucinous or colloid carcinoma* constitutes approximately 3% of breast cancers. It is characterized by an abundant accumulation of extracellular mucin surrounding clusters of tumor cells. Colloid carcinoma is slow growing and tends to be bulky. If a breast carcinoma is predominantly mucinous, the prognosis is favorable.

6. *Rare histologic types* of breast malignancy include papillary, apocrine, secretory, squamous cell and spindle cell carcinomas, and metaplastic carcinoma. Infiltrating ductal carcinomas occasionally have small areas containing one or more of these special histologic types. Tumors with these mixed histologic appearances behave similarly to pure infiltrating ductal carcinomas.

DIAGNOSIS

History and Physical Examination

The diagnosis of breast cancer has undergone a dramatic evolution over the past 25 years. Previously, 50% to 75% of all breast cancers were detected by self-examination. With the widespread availability of mammographic screening, there has been a greater shift toward the diagnosis of nonpalpable lesions. With this trend, evaluation of a woman for breast cancer relies on a careful history, radiologic screening, and physical examination.

The history is directed at assessing cancer risk and establishing the presence or absence of symptoms indicative of breast disease. It should include age at menarche, menopausal status, previous pregnancies, and use of oral contraceptives or postmenopausal replacement estrogens. A personal history of breast cancer and the age at diagnosis, as well as a personal history of other cancers treated with radiation (e.g., Hodgkin disease) is important. In addition, the family history of breast cancer or ovarian cancer in first-degree relatives (i.e., mother or sister) should be established. Any significant prior breast history should be elucidated including previous breast biopsies, especially if done for atypical disease, breast augmentation/reduction, breast problems, and any imaging history. After the risk for breast cancer has been determined, the patient should be assessed for specific symptoms. Breast pain and nipple discharge are often, but not always, associated with benign processes such as fibrocystic disease and intraductal papilloma. Malaise, bony pain, and weight loss are rare but may indicate metastatic disease.

Physical examination by the health care provider should take into consideration the comfort and emotional well-being of the patient. Examination is initiated by careful visual inspection with the patient sitting upright. Nipple changes, gross asymmetry, and obvious masses are all noted. The skin must be inspected for subtle changes; these can range from slight dimpling to the more dramatic *peau d'orange*, an erythematous and thickened appearance associated with locally advanced or inflammatory breast cancer. In large or ptotic breasts, the breasts should be lifted to facilitate inspection of the inferior portion of the breast and the inframammary fold. After careful inspection and with the patient remaining in the sitting position, the cervical, occipital, and periclavicular nodal basins are examined for potential disease. Both axillae are then carefully palpated. If palpable, nodes should be characterized as to their number, size, and mobility. Examination of the axilla always includes palpation of the axillary tail of the breast; assessment of this area is often overlooked once the patient is placed in a supine position. Palpation of the breast parenchyma itself is accomplished with the patient supine and the ipsilateral arm placed over the head. The subareolar tissues and each quadrant of both breasts are systematically palpated. Masses are noted with respect to their size, shape, location, consistency, and mobility.

Critical analysis of physical examinations has shown that the examinations are often inadequate for differentiating benign and malignant breast masses. Various series have identified a 20% to 40% error rate, even among experienced examiners. Because of the high rate of inaccuracy, any persistent breast mass requires additional evaluation. Furthermore, for the differentiation of a locally advanced or inflammatory breast carcinoma, a multidisciplinary team consisting of a medical oncologist, surgeon, and radiation oncologist should be consulted to obtain consensus as to the patient's diagnosis and the most appropriate treatment regimen.

Diagnostic Imaging

The choice of initial diagnostic evaluation after the detection of a breast mass should be individualized for each patient according to age, perceived cancer risk, and characteristics of the lesion. For most patients, mammographic evaluation is the essential initial step. Mammography serves two purposes to assess the risk of malignancy for the palpable lesion and to screen both breasts for other nonpalpable lesions. Bilateral synchronous cancers occur in approximately 3% of all cases; at least half of these lesions are nonpalpable.

The American College of Radiology developed the breast imaging reporting and data system (BI-RADS), which categorizes mammographic findings as follows: I, negative (no findings); II, benign appearance; III, probably benign appearance (<2% chance of malignancy); IV, findings suspicious for breast cancer (further divided into IVa, mildly suspicious, and IVb, moderately suspicious); and V, findings highly suspicious for breast cancer (>90% chance of breast cancer). On the basis of these findings, recommendations are made for either short- or long-term surveillance versus further immediate work up. For lesions interpreted as "probably benign" (BI-RADS 3) such as well-defined, solitary masses, careful counseling, and short-term follow-up with repeat radiographic studies in 6 months may be undertaken in patients at low risk for breast cancer. Conversely, if a mammogram identifies a stellate or spiculated mass typical of malignancy, immediate work up may be required.

Mammographic signs of malignancy can be divided into two main categories: microcalcifications and density changes. Microcalcifications can be clustered or scattered. Density changes include discrete masses, architectural distortions, and asymmetries. The most predictive mammographic findings of malignancy are spiculated masses with associated architectural distortion, clustered microcalcifications in a linear or branching array, and microcalcifications associated with a mass. Additional suspicious findings on mammogram include nipple changes, and axillary adenopathy. The presence or absence of these mammographic findings can predict malignancy with an accuracy of 70% to 80%. Mammography is least accurate in younger patients with dense breasts; for this reason, it is rarely used in patients younger than the age of 35 years for screening.

Once screening mammography demonstrates a suspicious lesion, further evaluation is necessary for diagnosis. Breast ultrasound is now an important adjunct to mammograms, and helps with clinical decision making. In young women with dense breast tissue, where a mammogram can misidentify suspicious lesions, ultrasound is often used to further study suspicious areas or palpable lesions. For all ages, it is regularly included in the initial evaluation and work up of mammographically indeterminate lesions, solid and cystic lesions, as well as the evaluation of axillary lymph nodes. Ultrasound is routinely used at the M. D. Anderson Cancer Center (MDACC) to evaluate the axillary nodal basin and any suspicious infraclavicular, supraclavicular, or internal mammary adenopathy. Suspicious nodes are sampled by ultrasound-guided fine-needle aspiration (FNA).

Breast MRI has been gaining in popularity for the diagnosis and surgical planning of breast cancer. While its utility is somewhat controversial, in certain circumstances, breast MRI has been found to be a useful adjunct for evaluating inconclusive findings on conventional imaging. Clinical indications for breast MRI include patients who have a moderate to high-risk for developing breast cancer (Table 2.3). High-risk patients who should undergo breast MRI include women with a history of mantle radiation; documented BRCA1 or BRCA2 gene mutation; first-degree relative with a BRCA1 or BRCA2 mutation that have not yet themselves been tested; or a documented risk of greater than 20% to 25% lifetime risk of developing breast cancer. Studies evaluating high-risk patients with an overall cumulative lifetime risk of developing breast cancer of approximately 30% show that MRI is able to detect cancer in approximately 1% to 3% of patients. MRI is also recommended for women with invasive lobular cancer, which may not be optimally assessed with mammograms.

TABLE 2.3	Indications for Breast MRI

High-Risk Patients
1. Documented BRCA1 or BRCA2 gene mutation
2. First degree relative with BRCA1 or BRCA2 gene mutation who have not had genetic testing performed
3. History of mantle radiation
4. History of breast cancer syndromes, such as Li-Fraumeni, Cowden, or Bannayan-Riley-Ruvalcaba

Moderate-Risk Patients (must be determined on an individual basis with treating clinician)

1. Lifetime risk of breast cancer of 15%–20% (defined by the BRCAPRO or other models (Gail model, Claus model) dependent on family history)
2. Personal history of breast cancer, ductal carcinoma in situ (DCIS), lobular carcinoma in situ (LCIS), atypical ductal hyperplasia (ADH), or atypical lobular hyperplasia (ALH)
3. Dense breasts or unevenly dense breasts when viewed by mammograms

TISSUE ACQUISITION

Evaluation of Palpable Breast Mass

After mammographic evaluation, palpable masses suspected to be malignant should undergo FNA biopsy or, preferably, core-needle biopsy. Some clinicians advocate needle biopsy at the time of initial evaluation (i.e., before mammography). For most patients being treated at MDACC, biopsy is deferred until after mammographic examination is completed because a postbiopsy hematoma can occasionally obscure subsequent radiographic evaluation. See Figure 2.1 for the MDACC algorithm for palpable breast masses.

For young patients with dense breasts for whom mammography is not ideal, needle biopsy with or without the aid of ultrasonography is the primary mode of evaluation. However, if the lesion can be visualized under ultrasound, an ultrasound-guided needle biopsy allowing visual confirmation is preferred.

FNA with a 22-gauge needle allows for accurate differentiation between cystic and solid masses and provides material for cytologic examination but does not establish an invasive component if a breast cancer diagnosis is made. Cystic lesions cannot be differentiated from solid lesions by mammography but are very well characterized by ultrasonography. Benign simple cysts typically are round, oval, and smooth edged on ultrasound; they yield non-bloody fluid and become nonpalpable after aspiration. Complex cysts have septations, are multiloculated, and can have internal debris; they can be associated with bloody or benign serous appearing fluid on aspiration. Bloody aspirate should be submitted for cytologic analysis. The incidence of malignancy among breast cysts is approximately 1% and is limited almost exclusively to complex cysts that yield bloody or serous fluid on aspiration, or have a residual mass after aspiration. For simple cysts, aspiration is often curative; only one in five breast cysts will recur, and most of these are obliterated with a

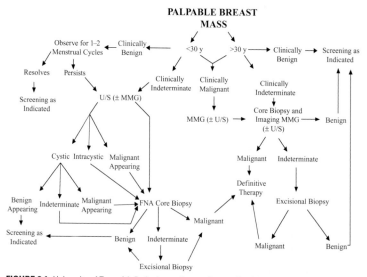

FIGURE 2.1 University of Texas M. D. Anderson Cancer Center algorithm for the workup of a palpable breast mass.

second drainage. If a cyst persists in spite of multiple aspiration attempts, excision is usually recommended.

For solid lesions, both fine needle and core needle biopsies are used for biopsy. Core needle biopsy is preferred for evaluation of suspected malignant lesions as it allows for better preservation of histologic architecture on pathologic review. For FNA, several passes through the lesion with the syringe under constant negative pressure will typically yield ample material for cytologic evaluation. The material is evacuated onto a microscopic slide and immediately fixed in 95% ethanol. Multiple studies have demonstrated that FNA is simple, safe, and accurate in evaluating benign and malignant breast masses. However, for lesions interpreted as malignant, cytologic evaluation is unable to differentiate between in situ and invasive carcinoma. Although physical examination, mammography, and needle biopsy all carry a risk of error when used alone, the combination of these three modalities is extremely accurate in predicting whether a palpable lesion is benign or malignant. For lesions with equivocal or contradictory results, open biopsy is the definitive test.

Evaluation of Nonpalpable Lesions

With the rise of mammographic screening programs, the diagnosis of nonpalpable breast cancer has risen rapidly in the United States. The MDACC approach to nonpalpable breast masses is outlined in Figure 2.2. For any suspicious lesion, diagnostic biopsy is warranted. Ultrasound-guided biopsy is not useful for evaluating microcalcifications because they are generally not visible sonographically. Mammography-guided stereotactic breast biopsy is a useful technique for obtaining tissue for diagnosis from nonpalpable lesions and microcalcifications.

Tissue sampling can be obtained with stereotactic-guided imaging to obtain multiple core-needle biopsies via a vacuum-assisted cutting device placed through a small 1/4-in incision removing or sampling the lesion in question and often some surrounding tissue.

SURGICAL BREAST BIOPSY CONSIDERATIONS

Excisional Biopsy

When core-needle biopsy or FNA is impossible or inappropriate, excisional breast biopsy with or without needle localization may be performed and serves as both diagnostic and local treatment purposes. The entire suspicious mass and a surrounding 1-cm rim of normal tissue should be excised. An excisional biopsy such as this will fulfill the requirements for lumpectomy and avoid subsequent re-excision. Needle biopsy is preferred over excisional biopsy if at all possible.

For either palpable or nonpalpable suspicious lesions, planning an optimal open biopsy mandates careful consideration of at least three issues. First, the biopsy site may require future re-excision for breast conservation treatment. Second, the incision of the biopsy procedure must be able to be incorporated into a future mastectomy incision if this form of treatment is chosen. Third, the biopsy must be constructed in a cosmetically optimal manner without compromising oncologic principles. All breast biopsies should be performed with the assumption that the target lesion is malignant.

Biopsies are typically performed in an outpatient setting. Curvilinear incisions are often used to take advantage of decreased lines of tension along Langer's lines. Radial scars are generally avoided except in the extreme medial (lower) aspect of the breast, where mastectomy incisions become radially oriented or in the extreme lateral position at the 2 or 3 o'clock position, where less skin will need to be sacrificed for a skin-sparing mastectomy (SSM).

NONPALPABLE BREAST ABNORMALITY

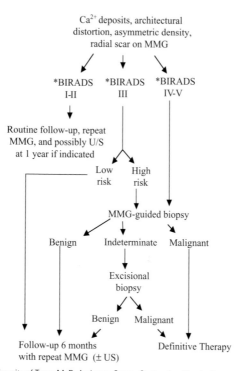

FIGURE 2.2 University of Texas M. D. Anderson Cancer Center algorithm for the workup of a nonpalpable breast mass. BIRADS, breast imaging reporting and data system.

Circumareolar incisions have an obvious cosmetic advantage but may lead to sacrifice of areolar tissue if re-excision is required. Although a small amount of peripheral tunneling is acceptable to maintain an incision within a potential mastectomy scar, extreme tunneling to the periphery of the breast from a central periareolar incision must be avoided. Situating the incision well away from the abnormality for cosmetic reasons not only makes it virtually impossible to identify the tumor bed if re-excision is required, but also results in the removal of an inordinate amount of breast tissue. Therefore, the incision should generally be placed directly over the malignant lesion to avoid excessive tissue removal that may compromise cosmetic outcome or to prevent being unable to locate the tumor bed if re-excision is required. Patients who undergo breast-conserving surgery should have a separate axillary incision that is not contiguous with the breast incision. Separating these incisions provides a better cosmetic outcome (the axillary drain will cause the biopsy cavity to become distorted if they are not separated).

Needle-Localized Excisional Biopsy

For nonpalpable lesions, preoperative needle localization with a self-retaining hook wire is required. This procedure requires careful communication between the radiologist and the surgeon. For most lesions, the localizing needle is placed under mammographic or ultrasound guidance into the breast via the shortest direct path to the lesion. The self-retaining wire is placed through the needle, and then the needle may or may not be removed at the discretion of the surgeon. Postlocalization mammograms of the wire are reviewed to confirm that the wire is within the targeted area. Excisional biopsy is then performed by excising breast tissue around the wire tip. For superficial lesions, an ellipse of skin at the point of wire insertion may be removed en bloc with the underlying breast tissue. Postexcision specimen radiographs are essential to confirm the localized target was removed. Often, the entry site of the wire is not directly over the targeted lesion, and this trajectory should be accounted for when the incision is placed on the breast.

Once the biopsy specimen has been excised, it must be handled carefully. The surgeon should note the orientation of the excised breast tissue and then hand deliver the specimen to the pathology department. For marking borders on a lumpectomy specimen, three sides must be marked to allow correct localization by pathology (i.e., the surgeon should place a short stitch on the superior margin, a long stitch on the lateral border and a single stitch on the anterior margin). In pathology, and at times in the OR, the lateral, medial, superior, inferior, superficial, and deep margins should be inked in a color-coded manner. Material is then further examined by pathology and should be additionally processed for receptor analysis and flow cytometry.

Closure of the biopsy incision requires meticulous hemostasis. Drains are not used in the breast. The skin is closed with a subcuticular suture, and Dermabond or a light dressing is placed.

STAGING

After a breast cancer has been diagnosed, the patient is clinically staged using the American Joint Committee on Cancer (AJCC) guidelines. The AJCC TNM breast cancer staging system was updated in 2010 and published in the seventh edition of the *AJCC Cancer Staging Manual*. The TNM classifications and stage groupings are summarized in Tables 2.4 and 2.5. In the seventh edition, there have been adjustments to the T, N, and M categories reflecting new clinical outcome data since the publication of the previous edition.

In the sixth edition, there were problems implementing isolated tumor cells (ITCs) and micrometastases into appropriate staging; breast cancer cases with exclusively nodal micrometastases (pN1mi) were grouped as having the same prognostic significance as macrometastases. More stringent classification of ITCs and single cells has been made in the seventh edition. Analysis of the SEER database revealed that when nodal tumor deposits less than 2.0 mm are the only finding in lymph nodes and the primary tumor is less than 2 cm, the incremental decrease in survival at 5 and 10 years was only 1% compared to patients with no nodal metastases detected. The most significant change in the seventh edition involves the reclassification of T0 and T1 tumors with nodal micrometastases. Stage IA refers to all invasive tumors less than 2 cm with no spread outside the breast. Stage IB refers to invasive breast cancers less than 2 cm with micrometastatic disease found in the lymph nodes (nodal disease greater than 0.2 mm but less than 2 mm).

A second change in the seventh edition involves the pM staging of breast cancer. The seventh edition now separates out incidentally detected breast cancer less than 0.2 mm found in nonregional nodal tissue with no clinical or radiological evidence of metastasis. This disease should be now designated M0(i+) and not M1.

Current AJCC TNM Classification and Stage Grouping for Breast Carcinoma

Classification and Stage Grouping	Definition
Primary Tumor (T)	
TX	Primary tumor cannot be assessed
T0	No evidence of primary tumor
Tis	Carcinoma in situ
Tis (DCIS)	Ductal carcinoma in situ
Tis (LCIS)	Lobular carcinoma in situ
Tis (Paget)	Paget disease of the nipple with no tumor
T1	Tumor 2 cm or less in greatest dimension
T1mic	Microinvasion 0.1 cm or less in greatest dimension
T1a	Tumor more than 0.1 cm but not more than 0.5 cm in greatest dimension
T1b	Tumor more than 0.5 cm but not more than 1 cm in greatest dimension
T1c	Tumor more than 1 cm but not more than 2 cm in greatest dimension
T2	Tumor more than 2 cm but not more than 5 cm in greatest dimension
T3	Tumor more than 5 cm in greatest dimension
T4	Tumor of any size with direct extension to (a) chest wall or (b) skin, only as described as follows
T4a	Extension to chest wall, not including pectoralis muscle
T4b	Edema (including *peau d'orange*) or ulceration of the skin of the breast, or satellite skin nodules confined to the same breast
T4c	Both T4a and T4b
T4d	Inflammatory carcinoma
Regional Lymph Nodes (N)	
NX	Regional lymph nodes cannot be assessed (e.g., previously removed)
N0	No regional lymph node metastasis
N1	Metastasis in movable ipsilateral axillary lymph node(s) (levels I and II)
N2	Metastases in ipsilateral axillary lymph nodes fixed or matted, or in clinically apparent ipsilateral internal mammary nodes in the *absence* of clinically evident axillary lymph node metastasis
N2a	Metastasis in ipsilateral axillary lymph nodes fixed to one another (matted) or to other structures
N2b	Metastasis only in clinically apparent ipsilateral internal mammary nodes and in the *absence* of clinically evident axillary lymph node metastasis

(*continued*)

TABLE 2.4 Current AJCC TNM Classification and Stage Grouping for Breast Carcinoma (*continued*)

Classification and Stage Grouping	Definition
N3	Metastasis in ipsilateral infraclavicular lymph node(s), or in clinically apparent ipsilateral internal mammary lymph node(s) and in the *presence* of clinically evident axillary lymph node metastasis; or metastasis in ipsilateral supraclavicular lymph node(s) with or without axillary or internal mammary lymph node involvement
N3a	Metastasis in ipsilateral infraclavicular lymph node(s) and axillary lymph node(s)
N3b	Metastasis in ipsilateral internal mammary lymph node(s) and axillary lymph node(s)
N3c	Metastasis in ipsilateral supraclavicular lymph node(s)
Regional Lymph Nodes (pN)	
pNX	Regional lymph nodes cannot be assessed (e.g., previously removed, not removed for pathological study)
pN0	No regional lymph node metastasis histologically, no additional examination for isolated tumor cells
pN0(i−)	No regional lymph node metastasis histologically, negative IHC
pN0(i+)	No regional lymph node metastasis histologically, positive IHC, no IHC cluster greater than 0.2 mm
pN0(mol−)	No regional lymph node metastasis histologically, negative molecular findings (RT-PCR)
pN0(mol+)	No regional lymph node metastasis histologically, positive molecular findings (RT-PCR)
pN1mi	Micrometastasis (greater than 0.2 mm, none greater than 2.0 mm)
pN1	Metastasis in 1–3 axillary lymph nodes, and/or in internal mammary nodes with microscopic disease detected by sentinel lymph node dissection but not clinically apparent
pN1a	Metastasis in 1–3 axillary lymph nodes
pN1b	Metastasis in internal mammary nodes with microscopic disease detected by sentinel lymph node dissection but not clinically apparent
pN1c	Metastasis in 1–3 axillary lymph nodes and in internal mammary lymph nodes with microscopic disease detected by sentinel lymph node dissection but not clinically apparent
pN2	Metastasis in 4–9 axillary lymph nodes, or in clinically apparent internal mammary lymph nodes in the *absence* of axillary lymph node metastasis
pN2a	Metastasis in 4–9 axillary lymph nodes (at least one tumor deposit greater than 2.0 mm)
pN2b	Metastasis in clinically apparent internal mammary lymph nodes in the *absence* of axillary lymph node metastasis

(*continued*)

TABLE 2.4	Current AJCC TNM Classification and Stage Grouping for Breast Carcinoma (*continued*)

Classification and Stage Grouping	Definition
pN3	Metastasis in 10 or more axillary lymph nodes, or in infraclavicular lymph nodes, or in clinically apparent ipsilateral internal mammary lymph nodes in the *presence* of 1 or more positive axillary lymph nodes; or in more than 3 axillary lymph nodes with clinically negative microscopic metastasis in internal mammary lymph nodes; or in ipsilateral supraclavicular lymph nodes
pN3a	Metastasis in 10 or more axillary lymph nodes (at least one tumor deposit greater than 2.0 mm), or metastasis to the infraclavicular lymph nodes
pN3b	Metastasis in clinically apparent ipsilateral internal mammary lymph nodes in the *presence* of 1 or more positive axillary lymph nodes; or in more than 3 axillary lymph nodes and in internal mammary lymph nodes with microscopic disease detected by sentinel lymph node dissection but not clinically apparent
pN3c	Metastasis in ipsilateral supraclavicular lymph nodes
Distant Metastasis (M)	
MX	Distant metastasis cannot be assessed
M0	No distant metastasis
M1	Distant metastasis

Note: Paget disease associated with a tumor is classified according to the size of the tumor.
DCIS, ductal carcinoma in situ; LCIS, lobular carcinoma in situ; IHC, immunohistochemistry; RT-PCR, reverse transcriptase-polymerase chain reaction.
Adapted from American Joint Committee on Cancer (AJCC). *AJCC Cancer Staging Manual.* 7th ed. 2010.

Early-Stage Breast Cancer (T1, T2, N0, N1, N1mi)

Approximately 75% of patients with breast cancer present with tumors less than 5 cm in diameter and no evidence of fixed or matted nodes. Workup for patients with clinical stage I or stage II breast cancer is usually limited to a complete history and physical examination, a chest radiograph, and evaluation of serum liver chemistries. In the absence of increased serum liver chemistries or palpable hepatomegaly, liver imaging is not used routinely in the preoperative evaluation of patients with early-stage disease. The routine use of bone scans in asymptomatic patients with apparent early-stage breast cancer carries is not generally indicated; studies have demonstrated only a 2% incidence of positive scan results in this setting.

Surgery for patients with early-stage breast cancer reflects treatment options addressing both disease in the breast as well as evaluating and treating for disease in the local regional lymph nodes. It includes options for breast conservation therapy including segmental mastectomy and radiation therapy or total mastectomy with or without reconstruction. During the same surgery, the regional nodes are evaluated in the form of sentinel lymph node (SLN) dissection with the possibility of axillary node dissection if SLNs are found to harbor malignancy. See the MDACC approach to early-stage breast cancer in Figure 2.3.

■T■A■B■L■E■ 2.5	Anatomic Stage/Prognostic Groups		
Stage 0	Tis	N0	M0
Stage IA	T1[a]	N0	M0
Stage IB	T0	N1mi	M0
	T1[a]	N1mi	M0
Stage IIA	T0	N1[b]	M0
	T1[a]	N1[b]	M0
	T2	N0	M0
Stage IIB	T2	N1	M0
	T3	N0	M0
Stage IIIA	T0	N2	M0
	T1[a]	N2	M0
	T2	N2	M0
	T3	N1	M0
	T3	N2	M0
Stage IIIB	T4	N0	M0
	T4	N1	M0
	T4	N2	M0
Stage IIIC	Any T	N3	M0
Stage IV	Any T	Any N	M1

[a]T1 includes T1mi.
[b]T0 and T1 tumors with nodal micrometastases only are excluded from Stage IIA and are classified in Stage IB; M0 includes M0(i+).

Locally Advanced Breast Cancers (TxN2, T3Nx, T4Nx)

Locally advanced breast cancer encompasses tumors with a broad range of biological behaviors. This category includes tumors that are large and/or have extensive regional lymph node involvement without evidence of distant metastatic disease at initial presentation. Approximately 10% to 20% of all patients with breast cancer have stage III disease, which includes T0, T1 or T2 with N2 disease; T3 tumors with N1 or N2 disease, T4 tumors with any N classification; or any T classification with N3 regional lymph node involvement. Approximately 25% to 30% of stage III breast cancers are inoperable at the time of diagnosis.

Many locally advanced breast cancers are discovered by a patient or her spouse. The remaining is discovered during routine physical examination. On occasion, a discrete mass may not be present; rather, there is a diffuse infiltration of the breast tissue. These patients present with a breast, that is, asymmetric, immobile, and different in consistency from the contralateral breast. Seventy-five percent of patients with stage III disease will have clinically palpable axillary or supraclavicular lymph nodes at the time of diagnosis. This clinical finding is confirmed on pathological examination in 66% to 90% of patients. Of the patients with positive nodes, 50% will have more than four nodes involved. When appropriate staging is performed, 20% of patients with stage III disease are found to have distant metastases at presentation. Distant metastases are also the most frequent form of treatment failure and usually appear within 2 years of the initial diagnosis.

Workup in this patient population includes similar studies and laboratory work as in early-stage breast cancer as well as bone scan and computer tomography scan of the chest, abdomen, and pelvis +/− PET to rule out metastatic disease, typically to the lung, liver, and bone (Figs. 2.3 and 2.4). Up to 25% of asymptomatic

Note: Consider Clinical Trials as treatment options for eligible patients.

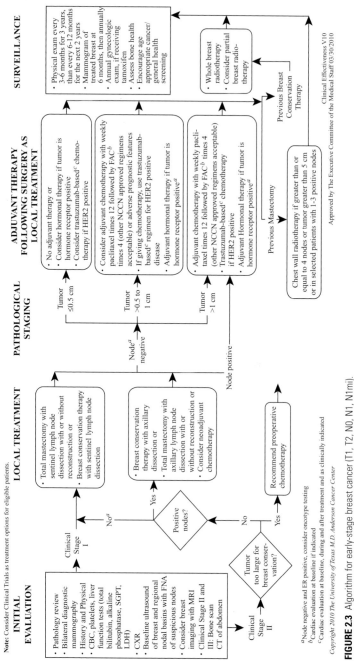

FIGURE 2.3 Algorithm for early-stage breast cancer (T1, T2, N0, N1, N1mi).

INITIAL EVALUATION

- Pathology review
- Bilateral diagnostic mammography
- History and Physical
- CBC, platelets, liver function tests (total bilirubin, alkaline phosphatase, SGPT, LDH)
- CXR
- Baseline ultrasound of breast and regional nodal basins with FNA of suspicious nodes
- Consider breast imaging with MRI
- Clinical Stage II and III: Bone scan CT of abdomen

Clinical Stage I

Clinical Stage II

LOCAL TREATMENT

Tumor too large for breast conservation?

No → Positive nodes?

Yes → Recommend preoperative chemotherapy

Positive nodes?
No[a] →
- Total mastectomy with sentinel lymph node dissection with or without reconstruction or
- Breast conservation therapy with sentinel lymph node dissection

Yes →
- Breast conservation therapy with axillary lymph node dissection or
- Total mastectomy with axillary lymph node dissection with or without reconstruction or
- Consider neoadjuvant chemotherapy

PATHOLOGICAL STAGING

Node[a] negative

Node positive

Tumor ≤0.5 cm

Tumor >0.5 to 1 cm

Tumor >1 cm

ADJUVANT THERAPY FOLLOWING SURGERY AS LOCAL TREATMENT

- No adjuvant therapy or
- Consider hormonal therapy if tumor is hormone receptor positive
- Consider trastuzumab-based[c] chemotherapy if HER2 positive

- Consider adjuvant chemotherapy with weekly paclitaxel times 12 followed by FAC[b] times 4 (other NCCN approved regimens acceptable) or adverse prognostic features
- If giving chemotherapy, use trastuzumab-based[c] regimen for HER2 positive disease
- Adjuvant hormonal therapy if tumor is hormone receptor positive[a]

- Adjuvant chemotherapy with weekly paclitaxel times 12 followed by FAC[b] times 4 (other NCCN approved regimens acceptable)
- Trastuzumab-based[c] chemotherapy if HER2 positive
- Adjuvant Hormonal therapy if tumor is hormone receptor positive[a]

Previous Mastectomy

Chest wall radiotherapy if greater than or equal to 4 nodes or tumor greater than 5 cm or in selected patients with 1-3 positive nodes

Previous Breast Conservation Therapy

- Whole breast radiotherapy
- Consider partial breast radiotherapy

SURVEILLANCE

- Physical exam every 3-6 months for 3 years, then every 6-12 months for the next 2 years, then annually
- Mammogram of treated breast at 6 months, then annually
- Annual gynecologic exam, if receiving tamoxifen
- Assess bone health
- Encourage age appropriate cancer/general health screening

[a] Node negative and ER positive, consider oncotype testing
[b] Cardiac evaluation at baseline if indicated
[c] Cardiac evaluation at baseline, during and after treatment and as clinically indicated

Copyright 2010 The University of Texas M.D. Anderson Cancer Center

Clinical Effectiveness V10
03/30/2010

Approved by The Executive Committee of the Medical Staff

Note: Consider Clinical Trials as treatment options for eligible patients.

EVALUATION FOR METASTASIS

TREATMENT METASTASIS

Note: All patients with bone metastases should also be treated with bisphosphonate, if life expectancy is longer than 12 weeks and creatinine clearance is 30 or greater.

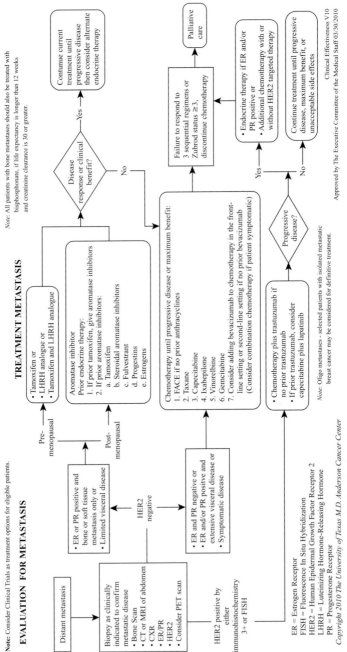

ER = Estrogen Receptor
FISH = Fluorescence In Situ Hybridization
HER2 = Human Epidermal Growth Factor Receptor 2
LHRH = Luteinizing Hormone-Releasing Hormone
PR = Progesterone Receptor
Copyright 2010 The University of Texas M.D. Anderson Cancer Center

Clinical Effectiveness V10
Approved by The Executive Committee of the Medical Staff 03/30/2010

FIGURE 2.4 Evaluation for metastasis in locally advanced breast cancer.

patients with apparent stage III cancer have positive bone scan results; thus, routine scanning in this population appears worthwhile.

Patients with locally advanced breast cancer are typically treated with an anthracycline-based regimen and a taxane before surgery or sandwiched around surgery. If postoperative chemotherapy is planned, it should precede radiation therapy to avoid interrupting the treatment of systemic disease because distant metastases are the most frequent form of treatment failure. Adjuvant hormonal therapy is routinely offered to all patients with receptor-positive tumors.

Several cancer treatment centers have reported experiences with combined modality therapy for locally advanced disease. Although the protocols differ among institutions with respect to the specific chemotherapy regimens and the type of local treatment, the studies have used induction neoadjuvant chemotherapy followed by local treatment (i.e., surgery, radiation therapy, or both) and subsequent adjuvant chemotherapy. Many patients with locally advanced breast cancer are now being treated with this chemotherapy sandwich approach. See Figure 2.5 for the MDACC approach to locally invasive breast cancer.

Inflammatory Breast Cancer

Inflammatory breast cancer is a rare, aggressive form of locally advanced breast cancer. It represents 1% to 6% of all breast cancers and presents as erythema, warmth, and edema of the breast. Rapid onset of symptoms (within 3 months) is necessary to make the diagnosis of inflammatory carcinoma. The time course distinguishes it from locally advanced breast cancer with secondary lymphatic invasion, which usually progresses slowly over more than 3 months. Pain is also present in half of patients with inflammatory breast cancer. Initial diagnosis of these physical findings as sequelae of an infectious process often delays diagnosis and treatment. The characteristic pathologic finding is dermal lymphatic invasion by carcinoma therefore biopsy for diagnosis should include a segment of involved skin. Ultimately, the diagnosis of inflammatory breast carcinoma is based on the clinical evaluation, which includes the time frame for which the signs and symptoms appear and the absence of dermal lymphatic invasion pathologically does not exclude the diagnosis.

Inflammatory carcinoma, similar to other forms of locally advanced breast cancer, is a systemic disease. In a study of inflammatory carcinoma, local therapy as the only treatment modality resulted in poor outcomes; the median survival was less than 2 years, and the 5-year overall survival (OS) rate was 5%. The use of multimodality therapy in these patients has improved local control and OS rate over local therapy alone. Standard treatment is anthracycline- and then taxane-based chemotherapy, sandwiched around surgery. With the addition of chemotherapy to the treatment regimen, the 5-year OS rate is 40%, although this number has not improved since the 1970s. Patients with Her-2/Neu overexpression are candidates for trastuzumab and lapatinib. Radiation is administered after completion of all surgery and systemic therapy. Patients with disease progression during chemotherapy proceed to preoperative radiation therapy or, if the cancer is operable, surgery. If the patient is to undergo surgery, modified radical mastectomy, which improves local disease control, may remove potential chemoresistant foci, and may provide additional clinical information to guide future treatment.

MULTIDISCIPLINARY EVALUATION

Once the diagnosis of breast cancer has been made, the optimization of treatment decisions is best coordinated in a multidisciplinary fashion. The collaborative efforts of surgical oncologists with medical oncology, radiation oncology, geneticists, and plastic and reconstructive surgeons are used to address the

INITIAL EVALUATION

- Pathology review
- Bilateral diagnostic mammography
- History and Physical
- Bone scan
- CT or MRI of abdomen
- Baseline breast and nodal nodal ultrasound with FNA of suspicious nodes
- CXR
- CBC, platelets, liver function tests (total bilirubin, alkaline phosphatase, SGPT, LDH)

CLINICAL STAGE

Stage II[a] or Stage III[a] (including inflammatory breast cancer)

→ HER2 positive?

NEOADJUVANT THERAPY (See Appendix A)

Yes →
- Paclitaxel and Trastuzumab followed by FEC (75 mg/m²) and Trastuzumab[c]
- HER2 positive chemotherapy options from NCCN

No →
- Weekly Paclitaxel times 12, followed by FAC[b] times 4
- HER2 negative chemotherapy options from NCCN

→
- Assess tumor size within 6-8 weeks and completion of systemic treatment with physical exam, and additional imaging with mammogram and/or ultrasound
- Mammogram of involved breast
- If candidate for breast conservation therapy, place radio-opaque markers for tumors ≤ 2 cm unless tumor marked by calcification prior to systemic therapy

→ Breast conservation therapy candidate?

Yes →

LOCAL TREATMENT

- If clinically node negative at diagnosis, proceed with sentinel node biopsy followed by axillary node dissection if the sentinel node is positive.
- If clinically node positive, proceed with axillary node dissection

No →

Total mastectomy with nodal treatment as determined by initial status:
- clinically node negative at diagnosis, proceed with sentinel node biopsy followed by axillary node dissection if sentinel node is positive, or
- clinically node positive, proceed with axillary node dissection
- Consider reconstruction

PATHOLOGICAL FINDINGS

From local treatment →

Stage II disease, except T3N0, with 0-3 involved lymph node(s) →
- Whole breast radiotherapy for breast conservation therapy with or without regional lymphatics
- Discuss chest wall radiotherapy with or without regional lymphatics for patients with total mastectomy and 1-3 positive lymph nodes

Stage III disease or T3N0 or 4 or more involved lymph nodes; residual tumor >5 cm →
- Post mastectomy radiotherapy to chest wall and regional lymphatics
- Whole breast radiotherapy with regional lymphatics for breast conservation therapy

→ Endocrine therapy for ER+ and/or PR+ sequential after chemotherapy and local therapy →

SURVEILLANCE

Physical exam every 3-6 months for 3 years, then every 6-12 months for the next 2 years.
Annual gynecologic exam
Annual assessment of bone density if on Aromatase Inhibitors.
Encourage age appropriate cancer and general health guidelines

[a] If tumor meets criteria for breast conservation therapy, then consider page 1 for local treatment first.
[b] Cardiac evaluation at baseline if indicated
[c] Cardiac evaluation at baseline, during and after treatment and as clinically indicated

FIGURE 2.5 Algorithm for locally advanced breast cancer.

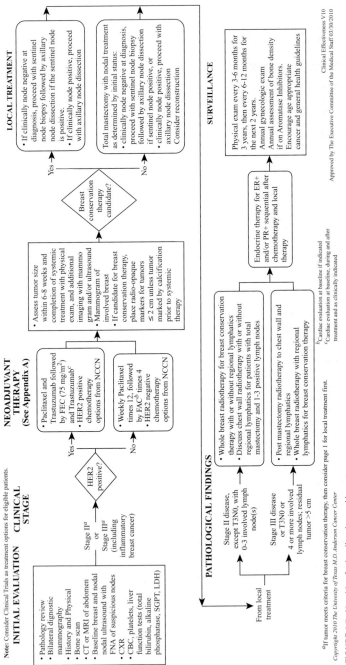

extent of breast resection, adjuvant and endocrine therapies, radiation options, and reconstructive choices.

SURGICAL TREATMENT

Many of the current recommendations regarding therapy for invasive breast cancer have been influenced by the results of randomized, prospective clinical trials performed by the NSABP. A summary of selected trials is presented in Table 2.6.

Breast Conservation Therapy versus Total Mastectomy

Many patients with breast cancer can be effectively treated with breast-conserving therapy (BCT), which entails completely removing the tumor with a concentric margin of surrounding tissue free of tumor, in combination with radiation therapy. Six prospective randomized trials comparing breast conservation strategies with radical or modified radical mastectomy have failed to demonstrate any survival benefit to the more aggressive approach. Among these trials, the two most widely known were conducted by Harris et al. at the National Cancer Institute in Milan, Italy, and by Fisher et al. in conjunction with the NSABP in the United States. The Milan trial was limited to patients with stage I breast cancer (tumor less than 2 cm and negative axillary lymph nodes) and compared radical mastectomy with a breast conservation strategy involving quadrantectomy, axillary lymph node dissection (ALND), and radiation therapy.

NSABP B-06 examined women with primary tumors up to 4 cm in diameter and N0 or N1 nodal status. Patients were randomly assigned to modified radical mastectomy, lumpectomy with ALND, or lumpectomy and ALND plus radiation therapy. Histologically, negative margins were required in the breast conservation groups. Disease-free and OS rates did not differ significantly among the three groups, but the local recurrence rate was markedly reduced at 10 years by radiation therapy (12% with radiation therapy vs. 53% without radiation therapy). These results upheld breast conservation surgery as an appropriate treatment for patients with stage I or stage II breast cancer and made it clear that radiation therapy is required as an integral part of any breast conservation strategy.

No significant differences in local control, disease-free survival (DFS), or OS rate have been noted, even in the most recent follow-up of these studies almost 20 years after their inception, indicating that survival for most breast cancer patients is not dependent on the choice of mastectomy versus BCT.

The standard for BCT at MDACC for local control of the breast is excision of the tumor with negative margins followed by radiation therapy. A radiation oncologist sees the patients after completion of surgery or adjuvant chemotherapy to determine radiation dosimetry and simulation, and radiation therapy is begun 3 to 4 weeks after surgery. A dose of 50 Gy is given to the whole breast, and then 10 Gy is given to the operative site as a boost using tangential ports and computerized dosimetry. The use of partial breast radiation therapy for BCT instead of whole breast irradiation with a boost to the tumor site has shown promising results.

Although BCT and mastectomy result in equivalent survival rates for patients with stage I or stage II disease, the decision for BCT must be made individually. Of utmost importance in the success of BCT is the patient's motivation and commitment to preserve the breast and prevent advanced recurrences. Daily outpatient radiation treatments over 5 to 6 weeks are required for total breast irradiation. More important is long-term follow-up of the preserved breast to detect breast cancer recurrences. Other factors that must be considered in making the choice between mastectomy and breast conservation surgery, are outlined in Table 2.7.

For extremely small breasts, the cosmetic result may be unacceptable following local excision, especially for patients with sizeable tumors. For large or pendulous

T A B L E 2.6	Summary of Selected NSABP Therapeutic Trials for Invasive Breast Cancer

Trial	Treatment	Outcome
NSABP B-04	Total mastectomy vs. total mastectomy with XRT vs. radical mastectomy	No significant difference in disease-free or overall survival rates
NSABP B-06	Total mastectomy vs. lumpectomy vs. lumpectomy with XRT	No significant difference in disease-free or overall survival rates; addition of XRT to lumpectomy reduced local recurrence rate from 39% to 10%
NSABP B-13	Surgery alone vs. surgery plus adjuvant chemotherapy in node-negative patients with estrogen receptor-negative tumors	Improved disease-free survival rate for adjuvant chemotherapy group
NSABP B-14	Surgery alone vs. surgery plus adjuvant tamoxifen in node-negative patients with estrogen receptor-positive tumors	Improved disease-free survival rate for adjuvant tamoxifen group
NSABP B-18	Neoadjuvant chemotherapy with doxorubicin, cyclophosphamide, or both for 4 cycles vs. the same regimen given postoperatively	No significant difference in overall survival or disease-free survival rates (53%–70% at 9 years in the postoperative group and 69% and 55% in the preoperative group)
NSABP B-21	Lumpectomy plus tamoxifen vs. lumpectomy plus tamoxifen plus XRT vs. lumpectomy plus XRT for node-negative tumors <1 cm	Combination of XRT and tamoxifen was more effective than either alone in reducing ipsilateral breast tumor recurrence
NSABP B-27	Neoadjuvant chemotherapy comparing AC × 4 cycles than surgery vs. AC × 4 cycles, docetaxel × 4 cycles than surgery vs. surgery between 4 cycles of AC and 4 cycles of docetaxel	Groups I and III were combined and compared with group II; clinical and pathological complete response rates increased significantly among patients who received preoperative AC and docetaxel
NSABP B-32	SLN biopsy followed by axillary dissection vs. SLN biopsy alone for clinically node-negative patients	SLN identification rate was similar in both groups, accuracy was high for both, negative predictive value was high for both

NSABP, National Surgical Adjuvant Breast and Bowel Project; XRT, radiation therapy; AC, doxorubicin (Adriamycin), cyclophosphamide; SLN, sentinel lymph node.

TABLE 2.7 Absolute and Relative Contraindications to Breast-Conserving Therapy

Absolute Contraindications

Prior radiotherapy to the breast or chest wall

Radiotherapy use during pregnancy

Diffuse suspicious or malignant-appearing microcalcifications

Multicentric disease

Positive pathological margin after multiple attempts to obtain negative margins

Relative Contraindications

Multifocal disease requiring two or more separate surgical incisions

Active connective tissue disease involving the skin (especially scleroderma and lupus)

Tumor size >5 cm (controversial)

Focally positive margins after multiple attempts to obtain negative margins

Adapted from National Comprehensive Cancer Network Guidelines, 2011.

breasts, lack of uniformity in radiation dosing may result in unattractive fibrosis and retraction. Patients may benefit from mastectomy plus reconstruction and perhaps surgical augmentation or reduction of the contralateral breast. Patients with larger tumors might also be best served by mastectomy because of the poor cosmetic outcome that results when a large area of the breast is removed. Very little data exist in a prospective randomized setting for the feasibility of BCT in patients with large tumors. Khanna et al. investigated the outcomes for 68 patients who underwent BCT without the use of neoadjuvant chemotherapy for 4- to 12-cm tumors. The mean tumor diameter was 5 cm, and the median follow-up was 48 months. The actuarial locoregional recurrence rate was 8.5%, and no recurrence occurred in patients who had negative surgical margins. No significant difference in DFS rates was noted for patients who underwent BCT and those who underwent mastectomy. Ninety-four percent of the patients who underwent BCT reported a favorable cosmetic outcome. Alternatively, a more attractive approach to treating T3 tumors, or for patients with unfavorable breast–tumor ratios, may be neoadjuvant chemotherapy, which may shrink the tumor to the point where breast conservation is feasible or cosmetically optimal.

Although there is no difference in OS for patients who undergo mastectomy or BCT for early-stage breast cancer, difference in recurrence rates between the two surgical treatment options exist. Attempts have been made to identify patients with a high rate of local recurrence after BCT on the basis of the histology of the primary tumor. The risk of local recurrence has been shown to be higher for women younger than 35 years and for women whose tumors are greater than 2 cm in diameter, regardless of lymph node status. For patients with positive lymph nodes, nuclear grade is also significantly correlated with recurrence. The local recurrence rates for BCT (as documented in the Milan study, NSABP B-06, and the Danish Breast Cancer Cooperative Group study) range from 2.6% to 18%, which is slightly higher than the range quoted for mastectomy (2.3% to 13%). In the Milan study, the 20-year crude incidence rate for recurrence was significantly higher for BCT than for mastectomy (8.8% vs. 2.3%; $P < 0.001$). However, there was no significant difference in OS rates between BCT and mastectomy in any of these studies. The ultimate goal of BCT for patients with early-stage breast cancer is to provide an optimal cosmetic result without compromising local control. Clearly, a multidisciplinary effort coupled with careful patient selection is critical for the successful outcomes of BCT.

Despite evidence documenting equivalent survival rates in BCT and mastectomy in early-stage breast cancer, patients have been gravitating toward total mastectomy. While many patients are candidates for BCT, it appears they desire total mastectomy based on preference, or in part out of concern for recurrence or being exposed to radiation therapy. The clinical indications for mastectomy include multicentric disease, large tumor to breast size ratio, pre-existing morbidities or conditions that preclude radiation therapy (i.e., prior history of radiation, pregnancy, etc.), and inflammatory breast cancer.

General trends in mastectomy have evolved toward the removal of decreasing amounts of tissue with equivalent local recurrence rates. Initially favoring the radical Halsted mastectomy which called for the removal of all breast tissue, the majority of skin overlying the breast tissue, all of the underlying muscles (pectoralis major and minor) and axillary nodal tissue, breast surgery then evolved to prefer the modified radical mastectomy which requires removal of the breast tissue, the majority of skin over the breast tissue, and axillary nodal contents, but leaves the underlying pectoralis muscle behind. Then with the advent of the sentinel node biopsy technique, simple mastectomies were performed removing just the breast tissue with the majority of the overlying skin, but leaving the majority of the axillary nodal contents and pectoralis muscle in place. In 1991, popularization of the SSM has transformed the way mastectomies are performed. SSM consists of a total mastectomy with resection of the nipple–areola complex, while allowing access to the axilla for possible dissection. It also preserves a significant amount of the native skin envelope and the inframammary fold, enhancing the aesthetic results of immediate breast reconstruction. Several retrospective reviews have documented the oncologic safety of this procedure, and in early stage breast cancer, the added benefit of immediate reconstruction provides the patient with psychological peace of mind. More recently at MDACC, local, regional, and systemic recurrence rates between patients undergoing SSM and conventional mastectomy did not differ significantly, and when adjusted for clinical staging and age, DFS rates were also not significantly different.

Currently there is rising interest in nipple sparing mastectomies (NSM) which allow for preservation of the nipple and areolar complex. NSMs were initially attempted over 45 years ago; however, they were subsequently abandoned secondary to complications and concerns regarding oncologic validity. More recently there has been an increase in reported experiences with NSM, showing the increasing renewed interest in NSMs. One study discussed the results of 192 procedures performed on 126 patients being evaluated. These 192 procedures included 54 women having unilateral mastectomies, and 69 undergoing bilateral mastectomies. In this study, 44 patients had invasive cancer, 20 had DCIS, and 4 had phyllodes tumors. In all patients, nipple tissue was cancer free on pathologic review. Median follow-up of 24.6 months resulted in 2 local recurrences, with none being at the nipple. These findings led to the conclusion what the risk of local relapse was very low, and that nipple sparing procedures could be considered in selected patients. However, it was recognized that additional prospective clinical trials would need to be performed before this procedure was truly validated. Current discussions revolve around careful patient selection. In most cases, NSM were performed in women who had tumors less than 3 cm in size, which were greater than 1 to 2 cm from the nipple. Importance in the technique of coring out the nipple papule so that only a 3-mm layer of tissue remains in the nipple is also emphasized. There are few reported long-term outcomes on the oncologic safety and the risk of cancer developing in the remaining tissue after surgery, and all reported experiences to this date remain relatively small. As such, there is no current consensus on the safety or absolute indications for this procedure.

Prophylactic Total Mastectomy

The efficacy of bilateral or contralateral prophylactic mastectomy (CPM) has been documented in reducing the incidence of breast cancer. In certain patient populations like those who have BRCA1 or BRCA2 mutation, prophylactic mastectomy may reduce the risk for developing breast cancer by 66% to 100%. In a larger multi-center study examining 483 women with BRCA1 or BRCA2 mutations, prophylactic mastectomy was associated with a 90% relative risk reduction in breast cancer risk, and the absolute risk reduction was found to be 46.8%.

There has recently been an increase in rates of CPMs performed in those patients with an index breast cancer who are not BRCA carriers. SEER database evaluations comparing rates of contralateral prophylactic mastectomies performed in the late 1990s versus the early 2000s for both invasive breast cancer and DCIS showed 150% and 148% increases respectively [IDC, 1998 (1.8%) to 2003 (4.5%); DCIS, 1998 (2.1%) to 2005 (5.2%)]. For most patients without a significant family history of BRCA mutation, the estimated risk of contralateral malignancy is estimated to be approximately 0.7% to 1% per year. In this setting, CPM has been shown to reduce the risk of contralateral breast cancer by 90%. However, there is little data to suggest whether this decreases breast cancer mortality and derives any survival benefit. Recently, Bedrosian et al. performed a population-based study examining survival outcomes of breast cancer patients undergoing CPM. Using data from the SEER registry, a causal relationship between survival and CPM could not be proven. A subset of women younger than 50 years with early-stage ER-negative tumors was found to have improved survival with CPM. However, the SEER database did not account for BRCA1 or BRCA2 mutations, high-risk family history, or data regarding chemotherapy, and could not be evaluated in this model.

Ultimately, the choice to undergo prophylactic mastectomy is a personal decision. It is, however, imperative that the practitioner counsel patients regarding factors associated with developing contralateral breast cancer, the role of endocrine therapy in reducing the risk of contralateral breast cancer, and psychosocial factors affecting patients' desires to undergo surgical prophylaxis.

AXILLARY STAGING

Axillary staging is performed in all patients with invasive breast cancer—axillary lymph node status is the single most prognostic factor in patients with invasive breast cancer. Identifying patients with metastases in the axillary lymph nodes is imperative for prognosis, regional treatment, and local control.

ALND was once considered the gold standard for evaluating the draining nodal basin for lymph node metastases. With earlier detection of breast cancer due to screening mammography, the probability of nodal involvement has decreased, and the routine use of ALND to determine axillary metastases has made it hard to justify this procedure in certain patient populations.

SLN Dissection

Lymphatic mapping with SLN dissection has become a well-established alternative to ALND. The SLN is defined as the first lymph node or group of nodes that receive lymphatic drainage from a primary breast cancer and, therefore, the node(s) most likely to contain metastatic tumor cells. SLN dissection has been proven to provide a reliable image of the tumor status of the remaining axillary lymph nodes. An added benefit of SLN dissection is that it limits the extent of axillary surgery and reduces the morbidity associated with the surgery, including pain and sensory deficits, decreased range of motion, seromas, and lymphedema.

In the hands of an experienced team consisting of a surgeon, nuclear medicine physician, pathologist, and operating room nurses and technicians, the finding of a tumor-free SLN almost invariably indicates that the patient has node-negative breast cancer and need not undergo further axillary dissection. Most studies report successful SLN detection in 94% to 98% of patients, an accuracy rate of 97% to 100%, and a false-negative rate of 0% to 15%. SLN biopsy should not be undertaken until the team has consistently documented a high rate of SLN identification and low rate of false-negative SLNs.

At MDACC, SLN dissection is performed utilizing intraoperative lymphatic mapping with or without vital blue dye (Lymphazurin). Preoperative lymphoscintigraphy, although not mandatory, can be used to identify the SLN and document patterns of lymphatic drainage. It should especially be considered in patients who may have issues with impaired lymphatic drainage to the axilla, such as that caused by prior breast and/or axillary surgery or radiation. Transcutaneous localization of increased radioactivity is performed with a handheld gamma counter, and visible blue dye may also be used intraoperatively to locate the SLN. Once the sentinel node(s) are removed, the axilla is examined to confirm a drop in radioactivity. A residual high level of radioactivity indicates that additional sentinel nodes remain in the nodal basin.

The incidence of finding a positive SLN increases as the primary tumor grows. A substantial proportion of patients with apparent early-stage breast cancer present with axillary nodal metastases. In one study, 17% of patients with clinically staged T1N0 disease had histologically positive nodes; this figure rose to 27% for patients with clinically T2N0 staged disease. Other studies have found that 10% of patients with tumors smaller than 0.5 cm have positive axillary lymph nodes. Tumors 0.5 to 1.0 cm are associated with positive axillary lymph nodes in 13% to 22% of patients, and 1.1- to 2.0-cm tumors are associated with lymph node metastases in up to 30% of patients.

SLN dissection may be unsuccessful in patients with certain clinical presentations (a) medial hemisphere location of the primary tumor where preoperative lymphoscintigraphy does not identify an axillary SLN, (b) previous axillary surgery because the lymphatic drainage from the primary may be distorted, and (c) in the obese and elderly, as they may have delayed or impaired drainage to the axilla.

In recent years, advances in the histopathologic evaluation of the sentinel node has increased the identification of a subset of patient with micrometastatic disease or small clusters of ITCs. The long-term clinical impact of ITC has yet to be determined; studies have resulted in opposing conclusions, and the prognostic and therapeutic implications remain unclear. Its impact on therapy is still unknown but has been reflected in the seventh edition of the AJCC.

De Boer et al. examined the disease-free and OS in the presence of ITCs or micrometastases with favorable primary-tumor characteristics that underwent a sentinel-node biopsy. They found that micrometastases or ITCs in the regional lymph nodes were associated with an absolute reduction in the 5-year rate of DFS of nearly 10 percentage points; among patients who received systemic adjuvant therapy, the 5-year rate of DFS was significantly improved, with an absolute benefit of nearly 10 percentage points. A better understanding of the natural history of the disease would help determine whether subsequent axillary dissection, axillary radiation therapy, or adjuvant chemotherapy is needed in patients with micrometastasis in the SLN.

Axillary Node Dissection

Traditionally, for patients who have biopsy-proven metastasis or who have a tumor-involved SLN, ALND has remained the gold standard. If axillary metastasis is confirmed, patients undergo standard ALND, consisting of en bloc removal of levels I and II nodal tissue, and if level III nodes are grossly or pathologically involved, removal of these nodes as well. However, removal of clinically negative level III lymph nodes is of little benefit with respect to staging because only 1% to 3% of stage I or stage II patients show level III involvement in the absence of level I or level II disease. Level III dissections carry a substantially higher risk of subsequent lymphedema, especially if radiation therapy is also used. The level I or level II ALND should preserve the long thoracic and thoracodorsal nerves and avoid stripping of the axillary vein. A closed-suction drain is placed and removed after the drainage has sufficiently decreased.

ALND achieves regional control, but its effect on survival remains controversial. Recently released data from the ACOSOG Z0011 study served to examine patients with clinically node-negative early-stage breast cancer (T1 or T2) who had three or fewer sentinel nodes with metastases as detected by hematoxylin and eosin staining. Patients were randomized to no further treatment versus axillary dissection. At a median follow-up of 6.3 years, local recurrence was reported in 3.6% of the ALND group versus 1.8% of the SLND-only group. After ALND alone, ipsilateral axillary recurrence was identified in 0.5% of patients versus 0.9% in the SLND-only arm. There was no significant difference in OS (ALND 91.9% vs. 92.5% in SLN-only; $P = 0.24$) or DFS (ALND 82.2% vs. 83.8% in SLN-only; $P = 0.13$) at 5 years. Although this study closed due to poor accrual, the results of this study suggest that in clinically node-negative patients, who will receive whole breast radiotherapy and systemic adjuvant therapy, ALND does not necessarily improve survival and SLN dissection alone with completed adjuvant therapy may offer excellent regional control in selected patients. Since the publication of these practice-changing results, at MDACC we now discuss with women that are clinically node-negative T1 or T2 breast cancer and planning to undergo breast-conservation therapy with whole breast irradiation, that if they subsequently are found to have two or fewer positive SLNs, completion of ALND appears to show no impact on OS or local–regional recurrence, and thus is not mandatory. Conversely, patients that plan to undergo mastectomy or breast-conserving surgery with accelerated partial-breast irradiation, or that will receive whole-breast irradiation in the prone position where the low axilla is not treated, and those patients who received neoadjuvant chemotherapy (patients cohorts excluded from ACOSOG Z0011), should still undergo completion of ALND when a positive SLN is identified.

BREAST RECONSTRUCTION

For patients who do not undergo breast conservation, breast reconstruction should be considered a standard option of cancer therapy. Reconstruction may involve autologous tissue, synthetic implants, or both. Chapter 24 expands on the technical details and potential options for breast reconstruction.

Although satisfactory results can be obtained with either immediate or delayed reconstruction, there has been increased interest in delayed reconstruction, especially since more patients are undergoing postmastectomy radiation therapy (PMRT). Acute and chronic complications and poor aesthetic outcomes have been identified in patients who undergo immediate reconstruction with placement of a permanent breast implant followed by postmastectomy radiation. In addition, some surgeons believe that immediate reconstruction may interfere with the delivery of radiation.

There has been recent data to suggest that delayed–immediate reconstruction allows patients who do not require postmastectomy radiation to receive the benefits of SSM similar to immediate reconstruction. This procedure entails a staged SSM with insertion of a saline-filled tissue expander that serves as an adjustable scaffolding to preserve a three-dimensional contour of the breast skin envelope. On the basis of the pathology, if the patient requires postmastectomy radiation, the tissue expander is deflated to allow radiation therapy, followed by delayed reconstruction approximately 3 months later. If no postmastectomy radiation is required, then the patient can undergo definitive reconstruction within 1 to 2 weeks.

MEDICAL TREATMENT

Chemotherapy

For node-positive and node-negative breast cancer patients, decisions regarding adjuvant chemotherapy must be individualized. The use of systemic therapy is effective in reducing the risk of recurrence and death from breast cancer. Age, tumor size, breast tumor characteristics, and lymph node status are all important factors that affect whether one should receive chemotherapy, either in a neoadjuvant or adjuvant setting. In the past decade, as our knowledge of the complexity of breast cancer grows, it is clear that breast cancer is no longer a single disease entity, but rather a group of molecularly distinct subtypes each with different prognoses, natural histories, and chemotherapeutic sensitivities, all of which factor into decisions regarding adjuvant chemotherapy.

Rationale for Adjuvant Chemotherapy

Adjuvant chemotherapy is directed at treating occult micrometastatic disease thereby reducing the risk of recurrence. Chemotherapy works most effectively when the tumor volume is small and still in the linear growth phase. This rationale led to some of the first adjuvant clinical trials of polychemotherapy versus observation in lymph node-positive breast cancer that showed improved disease-free (DFS) and OS. Subsequently, in 1988, based on the early results of several randomized trials evaluating systemic therapy in lymph node-negative breast cancer, the US National Cancer Institute (NCI) issued a "clinical alert" that resulted in the recommendation by the 2000 National Institutes of Health (NIH) Consensus Conference that chemotherapy should be considered in all women with tumors greater than 1 cm or positive lymph nodes.

The Early Breast Cancer Trialists' Collaborative Group (EBCTCG) meta-analyses (Oxford Overview, Overview Analyses) have provided extensive evidence illustrating the efficacy of adjuvant chemotherapy in early breast cancer. The most recent publication in 2005 was based on data from 60 randomized trials initiated before 1995 comparing polychemotherapy to no treatment. At 15 years there was a significant reduction in the absolute risk of recurrence and breast cancer mortality for polychemotherapy compared to none. The absolute benefits at 10 or 15 years were three times greater for younger compared to older women. The proportional reductions in recurrence and breast cancer mortality were similar in node-negative and node-positive patients. However, the absolute benefit was greater in node-positive patients. The Overview Analyses also indicate that the greatest effect of adjuvant chemotherapy occurs in the initial few years after therapy; however, the effects last for long periods of time, exceeding 15 to 20 years.

Further subgroup analysis showed that adjuvant chemotherapy was effective in both ER-negative and ER-positive breast cancer. However, the Overview Analyses and data from several Cancer and Leukemia Group B (CALGB) trials in patients with node-positive breast cancer indicate greater chemotherapy benefit in ER-negative compared to ER-positive disease. The first report from the 2005 to 2006 Overview Analyses specifically considered the benefit of chemotherapy in ER-negative tumors. In this analysis women with ER-negative breast cancer randomized to polychemotherapy versus none. Significant reductions were observed in the absolute risk of recurrence and cancer-specific mortality of 12.3% and 9.2%, and

8.6% and 6.1% for patients less than 50 years and between 50 to 69 years, respectively. These data are based on clinical trials conducted with older regimens and it is expected the proportional reductions observed for recurrence and mortality would be greater with contemporary chemotherapy.

Decisions regarding adjuvant chemotherapy are based on prognosis, that is, risk of breast cancer recurrence, and on the likelihood of benefiting from treatment. A risk of distant recurrence of greater than or equal to 10% is often used as the threshold at which systemic adjuvant chemotherapy is recommended. Tumor size and nodal status are important independent prognostic factors for survival for early stage breast cancer. Other important prognostic factors include histological grade (based on morphological features of the tumor), ER, PR (progesterone receptor), HER2 (human epidermal growth factor receptor 2), and the presence of lymphovascular invasion.

A number of consensus and evidence-based guidelines produced by the National Comprehensive Cancer Network (NCCN), the National Institutes of Health (NIH) Consensus Development criteria and the St. Gallen expert opinion criteria provide recommendations on the use of adjuvant chemotherapy in early breast cancer based on clinical data and tumor characteristics.

Adjuvant! Online (www.adjuvantonline.com) is a widely used freely available web-based tool. It considers multiple clinical and pathological factors and produces estimates for recurrence and mortality. In addition, this program incorporates the effect of co-morbid conditions in the determination of prognosis and benefit from various therapeutic interventions. Adjuvant! Online has been independently validated by Canadian investigators and the concordance with actual recurrence and mortality rates was within 1% of predictions based on this model.

Recently, a number of prognostic tests have been developed using gene expression profiling. The most widely used commercially available test in the United States is Oncotype DX (Genomic Health Inc, Redwood City, CA). This reverse-transcriptase-polymerase-chain-reaction (RT-PCR) assay is intended for use in HR-positive node-negative breast cancer patients who will receive 5 years of tamoxifen. It measures the gene expression of 16 cancer-related genes (including ER, PR, HER2, and Ki67) in paraffin-embedded tumor tissue and using a regression model calculates a recurrence score (RS) that is an estimate of the risk of developing a distant metastases at 10 years. Two suggested cut-off points categorize patients into low (RS < 18), intermediate (RS ≥ 18 < 31) and high (RS ≥ 31) risk groups corresponding to 6.8%, 14.3%, and 30.5% risk of distant recurrence at 10 years after 5 years of tamoxifen therapy, respectively. These risk estimates represent the range of distant recurrence rates for HR-positive, node-negative breast cancers treated with 5 years of tamoxifen. The TAILORx (Trial Assigning Individualized Options for Treatment) trial randomized patients with HR-positive, node-negative breast cancer and an intermediate RS to chemotherapy and endocrine therapy versus endocrine therapy only. The results of TAILORx, which is now closed to accrual, are eagerly awaited.

The FDA-approved 70-gene signature (MammaPrint, Agendia) was developed at The Netherlands Cancer Institute from a retrospective series of 78 patients younger than 55 years who received no adjuvant systemic therapy and had less than 5 cm, node-negative breast cancer. This assay stratifies patients into good and poor risk groups according to the risk of developing a distant metastasis. The prospective multicenter randomized MINDACT (microarray in node-negative disease may avoid chemotherapy) trial will test the clinical utility of MammaPrint in selecting patients with node-negative, HR-positive, or negative breast cancer for adjuvant chemotherapy.

There are multiple tools for estimating risk of treatment failure, with or without the use of adjuvant systemic therapies, and some may also predict the magnitude of benefit from endocrine or chemotherapy. All require determination of their clinical utility in prospective trials; while all of them seem to predict outcome, it is uncertain whether there is a "best" predictor.

Determining Adjuvant Chemotherapy Regimens

Adjuvant chemotherapy regimens contain non-cross-resistant agents with differing targets and mechanisms of action. There are many regimens considered "standard" and most were evaluated in clinical trials prior to the last decade when breast cancer when was considered a single disease entity (Table 2.8). Selecting the optimum

TABLE 2.8 Standard Chemotherapy Regimens Used in the Adjuvant Treatment of Breast Cancer

Regimen	Selected Standard Chemotherapy Regimens
Dose-dense AC-T	Doxorubicin 60 mg/m^2, cyclophosphamide 600 mg/m^2 IV, Day 1, every 14 days for 4 cycles; followed by paclitaxel 175 mg/m^2 IV, Day 1, every 14 days for 4 cycles
	Granulocyte colony stimulating factor (GCSF), Days 3–10 or pegfilgrastim, Day 2, cycles 1–8
TAC	Docetaxel 75 mg/m^2 IV, doxorubicin 50 mg/m^2, cyclophosphamide 500 mg/m^2 IV, Day 1, every 21 days for 6 cycles. GCSF, Days 3–10 or pegfilgrastim, Day 2, cycles 1–8
T + (FAC)	Paclitaxel 80 mg/m^2 IV weekly for 12 weeks; followed by fluorouracil 500 mg/m^2, doxorubicin 50 mg/m^2, cyclophosphamide 500 mg/m^2 IV, Day 1, every 21 days for 4 cycles
FEC + Docetaxel	Fluorouracil 500 mg/m^2, epirubicin 100 mg/m^2, cyclophosphamide 500 mg/m^2 IV, Day 1, every 21 days for 3 cycles; followed by docetaxel 100 mg/m^2, Day 1, every 21 days for 3 cycles
CEF (Canadian)	Cyclophosphamide 75 mg/m^2 PO, Days 1–14, epirubicin 60 mg/m^2 IV, Days 1 and 8, fluorouracil 500 mg/m^2 IV, Days 1 and 8, every 28 days for 6 cycles with co-trimoxazole support
CAF	Cyclophosphamide 100 mg/m^2, Day 1, doxorubicin 30 mg/m^2 IV, Days 1 and 8, fluorouracil 500 mg/m^2 IV, Days 1 and 8, every 28 days for 6 cycles
AC-T	Doxorubicin 60 mg/m^2 IV, Day 1, cyclophosphamide 600 mg/m^2 IV, Day 1; followed by paclitaxel 80 mg/m^2 IV, weekly for 12 weeks
TC	Docetaxel 75 mg/m^2 IV, Day 1, cyclophosphamide 600 mg/m^2 IV, Day 1, every 21 days for 4 cycles
AC	Doxorubicin 60 mg/m^2, cyclophosphamide 600 mg/m^2 IV, Day 1, every 21 days for 4 cycles
Oral (classic) CMF	Cyclophosphamide 100 mg/m^2 PO, Days 1–14, methotrexate 40 mg/m^2, Days 1–8, fluorouracil 600 mg/m^2, Days 1–8, every 28 days for 6 cycles
IV CMF	Cyclophosphamide 100 mg/m^2, methotrexate 40 mg/m^2, Day 1 and fluorouracil 600 mg/m^2 IV, Day 1, every 21 days for 9–12 cycles

Selected standard chemotherapeutic regimens listed in descending order of efficacy according to comparative randomized trials.

chemotherapy regimen takes into consideration the tumor biology (ER, PR, and HER2 status) and patient factors such as the presence of a co-morbidities (e.g., congestive heart failure, and peripheral neuropathy). The side effects and toxicities of modern adjuvant chemotherapy are largely transient and reversible; chronic, fortunately irreversible side effects such as cardiomyopathy, acute myelogenous leukemia, and myelodysplastic syndrome are rare.

Anthracyclines in the Adjuvant Treatment of Early Breast Cancer

Classic CMF (cyclophosphamide, methotrexate, fluorouracil) was one of the first adjuvant polychemotherapy regimens to significantly improve DFS and OS compared to observation in patients with node-positive breast cancer, and remains a widely used regimen. The anthracyclines (doxorubicin and epirubicin) have been extensively studied in the adjuvant setting beginning in the 1980s mostly in comparison to CMF. The EBCTCG meta-analyses of randomized trials showed that anthracycline-containing regimens were superior to first generation non-anthracycline-containing regimens such as CMF. Anthracycline-based regimens given for approximately 6 months were shown to reduce the annual breast cancer death rates by approximately 38% for women younger than 50 years at diagnosis and by approximately 20% for women aged between 50 and 69 years at diagnosis. The optimum doses of doxorubicin and epirubicin are considered to be 60 mg/m² and 100 mg/m², respectively. Anthracycline-induced cardiac toxicity has been well described. The incidence of congestive heart failure with cumulative doxorubicin doses of 240 to 360 mg/m² is between 1.6% and 2.1%. Data from adjuvant breast cancer trials indicate that the risk of congestive cardiac failure is low for women treated with an anthracycline.

Anthracyclines in HER2-Positive Breast Cancer

Over the past 15 years many studies have indicated that the incremental benefit from anthracycline-based therapy is largely confined to HER2-positive breast cancer. A recent meta-analysis reported significant benefit for anthracycline-based regimens in HER2-positive breast cancer in terms of DFS compared to HER2-negative disease. Co-amplification of topoisomerase-II-alpha (TOP2A) and HER2 has been proposed as the mechanism underlying anthracycline sensitivity in HER2-positive breast cancer. Topoisomerase-II-alpha is one of a number of targets for anthracyclines and lies in close proximity to HER2 on chromosome 17. Amplification or deletion of TOP2A appears to occur predominately in the HER2-positive breast cancer.

Preliminary data from the BCIRG 006 trial which randomized HER2-positive patients to a trastuzumab-containing regimen that contained an anthracycline versus a regimen that did not, reported similar efficacy for both, but fewer cardiac events and secondary leukemias in the non-anthracycline-containing arm. These data have prompted considerable debate regarding the role of anthracyclines in management of early breast cancer. However, due to the presence of conflicting data and the known existence of unpublished negative studies, HER2 and TOP2A are not considered ready for use in selecting patients for anthracycline therapy. Anthracycline-based regimens continue to be the standard of care.

Taxanes in the Adjuvant Treatment of Early Breast Cancer

Activity in the metastatic setting led to clinical trials designed to determine whether the addition of a taxane (paclitaxel or docetaxel) to anthracycline-containing regimens could improve outcome in the adjuvant treatment of breast cancer. These studies have examined sequential and concurrent taxane administration and taxanes as a substitute for an anthracycline. Several meta-analyses have shown small but statistically significant improvements in DFS and OS (~5% and ~3%

absolute benefit respectively) favoring the inclusion of a taxane compared to standard anthracycline-containing regimens. Improvements in outcome appear independent of the type of taxane, schedule of administration, hormone receptor, and nodal status.

Preliminary data from the EBCTCG overview analysis which included randomization to a taxane compared to non-taxane-containing regimen found an improvement in recurrence-free survival (HR, 0.83; $2P < 0.00001$) with the addition of a taxane to adjuvant chemotherapy. As with anthracyclines, there is considerable interest in identifying a subgroup particularly sensitive to these agents. Several retrospective studies have observed greater benefit from taxane administration in patients with HER2-positive breast cancer, however, others have not. At this time, HER2 status is not used to decide whether a taxane is included or omitted from the adjuvant chemotherapy regimen.

Taxane Scheduling

The ECOG 1199 study provided evidence that the scheduling of taxane treatment is important. In this study almost 5,000 patients with node-positive breast cancer were randomized in a 2 by 2 factorial design to four different taxane regimens. Improvements in OS were observed for weekly paclitaxel and three weekly docetaxel in comparison to paclitaxel given every 3 weeks. Toxicities in the weekly docetaxel arm, in particular hematological, led to administration of fewer cycles of treatment.

Tumor Biology and Choice of Adjuvant Chemotherapy

Important differences in the clinical behavior of estrogen receptor (ER)-positive and negative breast cancers have long been recognized. Gene expression profiling studies have identified at least four distinct molecular subtypes of breast cancer: basal-like, HER2-enriched, luminal A, and luminal B. In addition to differing biological and clinical behaviors they also have unique chemosensitivities. Gene expression profiling is not routinely performed so immunohistochemical surrogates are commonly used to determine subtype. In general, the basal-like and HER2-positive subtypes are predominately ER-negative, while the luminal subtypes are ER-positive. In the clinic, the triple negative phenotype is used to identify basal-like cancers; however, this misclassifies up to 30% of basal-like cancers.

Chemotherapy for ER-Positive Breast Cancer

Hormone-receptor-positive breast cancer comprises about 75% of all invasive breast cancers. Chemotherapy in addition to endocrine therapy is associated with an improvement in disease-free and OS compared to endocrine therapy alone. However, the overall benefit from chemotherapy is modest. Substantial molecular differences exist between good and poor risk ER-positive tumors and this has facilitated the development several gene expression-based prognostic predictors, Oncotype DX and MammaPrint, as aforementioned. Luminal A cancers (Oncotype Dx "low RS," MammaPrint "good risk") are characterized by high expression of ER and ER-related genes, and have low expression of proliferative markers such as Ki67 and are typically low grade. These patients have a good prognosis and high likelihood of benefit from endocrine therapy. In contrast, "luminal B" ("Oncotype DX high RS," "MammaPrint poor risk") cancers are characterized by lower expression of ER and ER-related genes, high expression of proliferation markers; these are typically high grade and have a poorer prognosis. Standard chemotherapeutic regimens and endocrine therapy should be considered for these patients.

Chemotherapy and Trastuzumab for HER2-Positive Breast Cancer

Between 20% and 25% of breast cancers are HER2-positive. Overexpression of HER2 is poor a prognostic marker. It is also predictive for response to trastuzumab

(Herceptin; Genentech, South San Francisco, CA) a humanized monoclonal antibody that targets the extracellular domain of the HER2 receptor. In the preoperative setting, pathological complete response rates of up to 65% have been reported with trastuzumab in combination with chemotherapy. The administration of chemotherapy in combination with 1 year of trastuzumab is associated with a 50% reduction in the risk of recurrence and about a 30% reduction in the risk of death. On the basis of several large randomized controlled trials 1 year of adjuvant trastuzumab has become a standard of care in for HER2-positive breast cancers.

The largest of these studies was HERA (Herceptin Adjuvant) an international study that randomized 5,102 women with HER2-positive breast cancer disease to observation versus 1 or 2 years of trastuzumab after completion of at least four cycles of chemotherapy. In this study, over half of the women accrued had node-positive disease and only 26% of patients in this study received both an anthracycline and a taxane. At a median follow-up of 23.5 months, 1 year of adjuvant trastuzumab was associated with a reduced risk of breast cancer recurrence (HR, 0.64; 95% CI, 0.54 to 0.76; $P < 0.0001$) and risk of death (HR, 0.66; 95% CI, 0.47 to 0.91; $P = 0.0115$) compared to observation alone.

The North Central Cancer Treatment Group trial (N9831) and NSABP B-31 examined the efficacy of adding trastuzumab to AC followed by paclitaxel. At a median follow-up of 2.9 years, AC followed by concurrent paclitaxel and trastuzumab resulted in a significant reduction in the risk of breast cancer recurrence (HR, 0.48; 95% CI, 0.41 to 0.57; $P < 0.0001$) and death (HR, 0.65; 95% CI, 0.51 to 0.84; $P = 0.0007$) compared with AC followed by paclitaxel alone.

The Finland Herceptin (FinHer) multicenter, open-label, study has attempted to identify the optimal duration of trastuzumab therapy. This study was designed to examine three weekly docetaxel compared to weekly vinorelbine followed by FEC in node-positive or high-risk node-negative patients. Patients with HER2-positive disease ($n = 232$) were randomized to receive 9 weeks of weekly trastuzumab administered with docetaxel or vinorelbine versus chemotherapy alone. At a median follow-up of 3 years there was a reduction in recurrence (HR, 0.42; 95% CI, 0.21 to 0.83; $P = 0.01$) and a trend toward improved survival (HR, 0.41; 95% CI, 0.16 to 1.08; $P = 0.07$) in the group receiving trastuzumab compared to those who did not. At the present time, 1 year of treatment is the standard of care; however, a shorter course as observed in the FinHER study may be adequate. There are currently four prospective studies addressing this question by randomizing women with HER2-positive breast cancer to 1 year versus 6 months (PHARE and PERSEPHONE) or 1 year versus 2 months (SOLD and SHORTER).

Considerable advances have been made in the treatment of HER2-positive breast cancer. Ongoing studies evaluating the role of lapatinib, a small tyrosine kinase inhibitor molecule targeting HER2 and EGFR, in the adjuvant/neoadjuvant setting (ALTTO, Neo-ALTTO, NSABP B-41, CALGB 40601, and TEACH) will provide further insight into the efficacy, resistance, and sensitivity of HER2-targeted agents.

Chemotherapy for Triple Negative Breast Cancer

The triple negative cancers are highly proliferative and carry a worse prognosis than other breast cancer subtypes. This subtype is uniquely sensitive to standard chemotherapy. Currently, DNA-damaging agents are being tested in this subgroup in order to exploit the strong association between these tumors and the presence of BRCA1 mutations. Homologous recombination, a high fidelity DNA repair pathway, relies on functioning BRCA1. When this pathway is dysfunctional the poly (ADP-ribose) polymerase (PARP) DNA repair mechanisms take over. PARP has been identified as an important drug target in order to bring about so called "synthetic lethality" of BRCA mutated tumors. PARP-inhibitors have been investigated in phase II studies for triple negative and

BRCA1/2-deficient cancers and results to date are promising. Epothilones, antiangiogenic agents, EGFR inhibitors, mTOR, PI3 kinase inhibitors, and agents that induce DNA double-strand breaks such as platinum agents are to be tested in clinical trials.

NEOADJUVANT CHEMOTHERAPY

Adjuvant chemotherapy is equally effective up to 12 weeks after definitive surgery but may be compromised by delays of more than 12 weeks after definitive surgery. Administering chemotherapy before primary surgery (neoadjuvant) with the same chemotherapy regimen has been shown to exhibit the same therapeutic effects. The use of neoadjuvant chemotherapy has its origins in the management of inoperable locally advanced breast cancer. Preoperative chemotherapy was initially introduced to downstage patients and enable successful local treatment. Subsequently, it was studied in patients with operable disease. Several phase II studies and eight randomized controlled trials have observed no difference in DFS or OS between adjuvant and neoadjuvant therapy. There are, however, increased rates of breast conserving therapy with the latter approach.

There are numerous factors to consider before using neoadjuvant chemotherapy to treat breast cancer:

1. Will administering neoadjuvant chemotherapy convert an otherwise large tumor requiring mastectomy into one manageable by BCT? If not, then neoadjuvant chemotherapy may not be desirable because a mastectomy will need to be performed either way, and much of the information (e.g., tumor size and lymph node involvement with metastases) useful in determining whether there is a role for further treatment with radiation may be lost.
2. The tumor in the breast must be carefully localized with a clip or permanent marker before chemotherapy to ensure proper localization of the tumor during surgery in the event that the chemotherapy produces a complete clinical response.
3. How much tissue should be removed during surgery after chemotherapy is completed? The answer is debatable, but generally all gross disease plus any other suspicious areas with a rim of normal-appearing tissue should be removed.
4. How should the nodal basin after neoadjuvant chemotherapy be managed? If there are either clinically suspicious nodes or nodes that appear to harbor disease based on imaging, ultrasound-guided FNA of the nodes in question or SLN dissection may be performed before the start of chemotherapy to confirm metastases. If the result of the biopsy is positive, then a formal ALND should be performed during definitive surgery. A negative ultrasound-guided FNA or SLN dissection result produces more of a dilemma. In this situation, whether to perform SLN dissection or ALND after chemotherapy is unclear and is currently being investigated by the American College of Surgeons Oncology Group. At MDACC, oncologists routinely perform SLN dissection after neoadjuvant chemotherapy during definitive surgery if the patients were clinically node negative by physical and ultrasound examinations prior to initiating chemotherapy.

Delivering chemotherapy in the preoperative setting allows the effects of treatment on the tumor burden to be directly observed. It can provide important prognostic information: firstly, the patients who achieve a pathologic complete response (pCR) have improved overall outcomes. Secondly, therapy can be altered based on tumor response and exposure to ineffective agents can be minimized. The effect of different chemotherapy regimens on tumor response can best be measured in the neoadjuvant setting because this may correlate to prognosis and to continued improvement of breast-conserving surgery rates. The results from NSABP B-27 clearly demonstrated that four cycles of AC preoperatively or four cycles of AC followed by surgery with four cycles of docetaxel postoperatively was not as efficacious in obtaining a clinical or pathological complete response as both four cycles of AC followed by four cycles of docetaxel in the neoadjuvant setting. The addition of docetaxel to AC increased the clinical complete response rate by 50% and nearly doubled the pathological complete response rate compared with AC alone. Finally, the use of neoadjuvant chemotherapy provides researchers with opportunities to improve chemotherapy use and patient outcomes based on tumor response. Newer techniques such as microarray gene profiling are being used to develop a method of classifying gene profiles associated with particular tumors that may correlate with pathological complete response. These data may eventually identify which patients will benefit from a particular regimen or which patients can be spared systemic therapy.

The disadvantages of using neoadjuvant chemotherapy include the possible delay of curative surgery, psychosocial factors, suboptimal clinical and radiologic assessment of the primary tumor, and the potential loss of prognostic information. Several other issues to be considered with this approach is addressing the timing of the SLN dissection (before or after preoperative chemotherapy) and whether a patient should receive postmastectomy irradiation if found to have three or less lymph nodes involved with metastases at the time of surgery.

ENDOCRINE THERAPY

Endocrine therapy has been associated with significant reductions in the risk of local recurrence, distant metastasis, and contralateral breast cancer. Tamoxifen, which was originally recommended for the treatment of postmenopausal women with ER-positive breast cancer, is now indicated for a much broader range of patients. Tamoxifen therapy is considered standard of care for premenopausal women with tumors expressing ER or PR hormone receptors, regardless of age or nodal status. Tamoxifen therapy is generally well tolerated; treatment-limiting adverse effects develop in less than 5% of patients. In addition to its antitumor properties, tamoxifen increases bone density and reduces serum cholesterol levels. However, tamoxifen also increases the incidence of endometrial cancer and thromboembolic events. Standard treatment with tamoxifen is 5 years. A meta-analysis of five randomized clinical trials showed that patients who were treated with tamoxifen for 3 to 5 years had a greater reduction in recurrence than did patients treated for 1 to 2 years (22% ± 8% vs. 7% ± 11). Data from NSABP B-14 indicated that 10 years of tamoxifen use offer no survival advantage over 5 years. Most recently, in the EBCTCG analysis, in women with ER-positive tumors were randomized to receive 5 years of adjuvant tamoxifen, there was a 41% proportional risk reduction of recurrence, and there was a 34% proportional risk reduction of mortality compared with those who did not receive tamoxifen. Currently, 5 years of adjuvant tamoxifen is considered standard therapy for premenopausal women.

Current ASCO recommendations for postmenopausal women include an aromatase inhibitor as a component of adjuvant endocrine therapy. The aromatase inhibitors anastrozole, letrozole, and exemestane work by inhibiting the aromatase enzyme that catalyzes the conversion of adrenal corticosteroids to estrogens and therefore decreases the conversion of precursor hormones to estrogen in adipose tissue. In the ATAC (Arimidex, Tamoxifen Alone or in Combination) trial, the efficacy and side effect profiles of anastrozole and tamoxifen were compared in postmenopausal women. For postmenopausal patients with early-stage breast cancer, anastrozole resulted in a higher DFS rate (86.9% vs. 84.5%) than tamoxifen, longer time to recurrence, and lower incidence of contralateral breast cancer. The results also demonstrated that the incidence of endometrial cancer, vaginal bleeding and discharge, cerebrovascular events, venous thromboembolic events, and hot flashes occurred significantly less frequently with anastrozole, whereas musculoskeletal disorders and fractures occurred less frequently with tamoxifen. As a result of the ATAC trial, anastrozole is now the preferred hormone therapy for postmenopausal patients with receptor-positive breast cancer.

For patients who have already been taking tamoxifen, studies have shown that switching to an aromatase inhibitor is safe. There have been demonstrable improvements in DFS rate after switching to aromatase inhibitors. It is unclear when an aromatase inhibitor should be initiated in postmenopausal women; ongoing trials (BIG 1 to 98) examining the timing and sequence of tamoxifen and aromatase inhibitors are currently being investigated. At a median follow-up of 76 months, there appears to be no significant differences in DFS, time to distant recurrence, or OS for sequential treatment versus letrozole monotherapy.

Ovarian suppression or ablation is another effective alternative adjuvant endocrine treatment in certain instances. However, there is currently no data to support the routine use of ovarian ablation over tamoxifen in premenopausal patients.

RADIATION TREATMENT

The role of radiation therapy in breast cancer has been well established. It is a useful adjunct in BCT, as adjuvant therapy after mastectomy, in the management of locoregional recurrence, and as palliative treatment in metastatic disease. In early-stage breast cancer, BCT with radiation therapy to the whole breast has been associated with equivalent long-term survival results versus mastectomy alone; recurrence rates are improved in all subsets of patients with the addition of radiation. Radiation therapy to the nodal basin helps achieve long-term regional control of microscopic disease.

When it comes to tumor recurrence with BCT, majority of relapses occur at or near the original tumor bed, rarely extending beyond 1 to 2 cm of the prior cavity. This has led to the rationale that accelerated partial breast irradiation (APBI) would deliver a homogenous dose of radiation within a confined space. Advantages of partial breast irradiation include shorter treatment (5 days vs. 6 weeks); less scatter radiation to the lungs, heart, and coronary vessels; and less skin burning and desquamation. Numerous studies are in progress to evaluate the dosimetry, side effect profiles, and efficacy of partial breast irradiation. While it is hoped that APBI may prove to have similar long-term effectiveness to whole breast irradiation for patients with early breast cancer, it will take time to optimize the appropriate patient population for whom this is suited. In addition, the delivery methods for partial breast irradiation currently under investigation and continue to evolve.

It is well known that PMRT reduces the risk of locoregional failure. Traditionally, the greatest benefit of PMRT is seen in those patients who are at highest risk for locoregional failure, defined as greater than 15%, due to greater than 4 positive lymph nodes, tumor size greater than or equal to 5 cm, T4 disease, or positive margins. Other factors associated with locoregional failure include age, histologic grade of tumors, lymphovascular invasion, and extracapsular spread of the lymph nodes. More recently, there has been considerable debate whether patients with 1 to 3 positive axillary lymph nodes would benefit from PMRT. There seems to be more data suggesting better outcomes with this subset population who undergo PMRT. But it has been unclear whether it is the effect of PMRT itself, or the improved delivery and efficacy of systemic therapy or better surgical technique that contribute to these results. Little data exists on present-day locoregional recurrence rates after mastectomy without PMRT. Sharma et al. examined early stage breast cancers with 1 to 3 positive axillary lymph nodes; one significant finding was that the 10-year risk of locoregional recurrence was not significantly different between patients without lymph node metastases and patients with one positive lymph node. They concluded that in this era of improved systemic therapy, any potential absolute locoregional recurrence (LRR) reduction and survival advantage that may be gained from the use of PMRT must be balanced against possible morbidities associated with radiation.

FOLLOW-UP AFTER PRIMARY TREATMENT OF INVASIVE BREAST CANCER

After primary therapy for invasive breast cancer, patients must be made aware of the long-term risk for recurrent or metastatic disease. Although most studies report that recurrences occur within 5 years after primary therapy, recurrences can occur more than 20 years after primary therapy.

The published American Society of Clinical Oncology guidelines for follow-up recommend scheduled visits every 3 to 6 months for Years 1 through 3, every 6 to 12 months for Years 4 through 5, and every 12 months thereafter. Monthly self-examination of the breasts is also recommended. Mammography is done 6 months after the completion of BCT to allow surgery- and radiation-induced changes to stabilize, and then yearly. For patients who have undergone mastectomy, a contralateral mammogram is obtained yearly. Routine bone scans, skeletal surveys, and computed tomographic scans of the abdomen and brain yield an extremely low rate of occult metastases in otherwise asymptomatic patients and is not cost-effective for patients with early-stage breast cancer (Table 2.9).

TREATMENT OF ADVANCED DISEASE

Locally Recurrent Breast Cancer

The time course, clinical significance, and prognosis of locally recurrent breast cancer vary dramatically between patients undergoing BCT and those undergoing mastectomy. Local recurrence rates of 5% to 10% at 8 to 10 years have been reported for patients with conserved breasts. Local recurrence typically occurs over a protracted time and is associated with systemic metastases in less than 10% of patients. Local recurrence following lumpectomy is curable in most cases; 50% to 63% of patients with local recurrence will remain disease-free 5 years after salvage mastectomy.

In contrast, local chest wall recurrence following mastectomy typically occurs within the first 2 to 3 years after surgery, and may even occur more than 10 years later. It is associated with distant metastases in as many as two-thirds of patients and results in eventual death for many. One-third of patients with chest wall recurrence will have concurrent distant metastatic disease, and within 1 year, half will have distant disease. The median survival in this setting is 2 to 3 years. However, initial node-negative status, time to chest wall recurrence more than 24 months, and treatment with radiation therapy for the recurrence were found to be independent predictors of improved disease-free and OS. Patients with these three favorable features had 10-year actuarial survival rate of 75.4%.

Any patient with a local recurrence, especially chest wall recurrences after mastectomy, should undergo complete restaging after detection of the recurrence (Fig. 2.6). For patients with a purely local recurrence, surgical excision plus radiation therapy provides better local control than does either modality alone. In patients with ER-positive recurrence, hormonal therapy may be considered as it has been shown to reduce second local failures at 5 years, although OS was not significantly changed.

Metastatic Breast Cancer

Metastatic breast cancer generally cannot be cured, and treatment is mainly palliative in order to control symptoms and prolong survival and quality of life. The

TABLE 2.9   Chemotherapy Recommendations for Patients with Locally Invasive Breast Carcinoma

Regimen	Drugs	Doses	Schedule	Frequency	Cycles
Adjuvant Pac-FAC (total 24 weeks)	Paclitaxel followed by	80 mg/m² IV over 1 hour	Weekly	Every 7 days	12 weeks
	5-Fluorouracil	500 mg/m² IV	Days 1 and 8[a]	Every 21 days	4
	Doxorubicin	50 mg/m² IV, continuous infusion	Day 1 (48–96 hours)	Every 21 days	4
	Cyclophosphamide	500 mg/m² IV	Day 1	Every 21 days	4
Trastuzumab-based adjuvant AC-PH-H[b]	Doxorubicin	60 mg/m² IV	Day 1	Every 21 days	4
	Cyclophosphamide followed by	600 mg/m² IV	Day 1	Every 21 days	4
	Paclitaxel with	80 mg/m² IV over 1 hour	Weekly	Every 7 days	12 weeks
	Trastuzumab followed by	4 mg/kg IV followed by 2 mg/kg IV	Weekly	Every 7 days	12 weeks
	Trastuzumab	2 mg/kg IV or 6 mg/kg IV	Weekly or Day 1	Every 7 days or every 21 days	Complete 1 year
Trastuzumab neoadjuvant PH-FEC(75)H	Paclitaxel	80 mg/m² IV over 1 hour	Weekly	Every 7 days	12 weeks
	Trastuzumab followed by	4 mg/kg IV followed by 2 mg/kg IV	Weekly	Every 7 days	12 weeks
	Fluorouracil	500 mg/m² IV	Day 1	Every 21 days	4
	Epirubicin	75 mg/m² IV	Day 1	Every 21 days	4
	Cyclophosphamide	500 mg/m² IV	Day 1	Every 21 days	4
	Trastuzumab	2 mg/kg IV	Weekly	Every 7 days	12 weeks

[a]If doxorubicin is given as a continuous infusion, the 5-fluorouracil is given on Day 1 and at the end of the infusion. For example, if doxorubicin is given over 72 hours, then the 5-fluorouracil is given on Days 1 and 4.
[b]Cardiac monitoring at baseline, 3, 6, and 9 months.
Copyright 2010 The University of Texas M.D. Anderson Cancer Center.

EVALUATION FOR RECURRENCE

TREATMENT FOR RECURRENCE

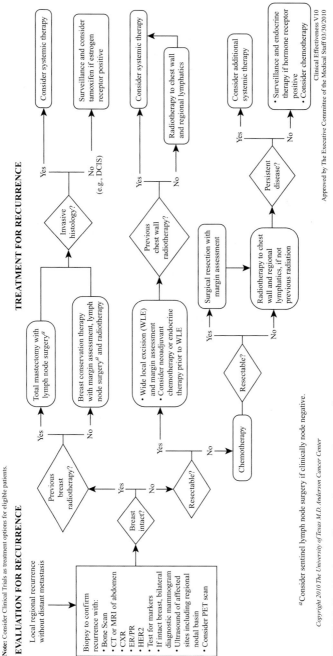

[a]Consider sentinel lymph node surgery if clinically node negative.

Copyright 2010 The University of Texas M.D. Anderson Cancer Center

Clinical Effectiveness V10
Approved by The Executive Committee of the Medical Staff 03/30/2010

FIGURE 2.6 Algorithm for surveillance and treatment of recurrent disease.

median survival after detection of distant metastases is 2 years, but some patients live for many years especially with the improvement in multimodality treatments. Chemotherapy rarely prolongs survival and is directed at improving tumor-related symptoms and slowing the spread of the tumor. The most common site of distant metastatic spread is the osseous skeleton; other common sites are the lungs, pleura, brain, liver, soft tissues, and lymph nodes. Certain subtypes of breast cancer present different patterns of metastases. For example, patients with rapidly growing, hormone receptor-negative, and poorly differentiated tumors are likely to have metastases to visceral organs (e.g., liver, lungs, and brain), whereas patients with slowly growing, hormone receptor-positive, and well-differentiated tumors are likely to develop metastases to bone and soft tissues and are less likely to exhibit early life-threatening manifestations.

For patients with metastases, the decision to treat with systemic chemotherapy or hormonal therapy rests on several issues: the site and extent of the disease, hormone receptor status, disease-free interval, age, and menopausal status. Patients with slow-growing tumors, limited disease, and non–life-threatening metastatic disease and hormone receptor-positive or known hormone-responsive tumors are generally offered hormonal therapy as the first therapeutic modality. Because all hormonal manipulations used today have a better therapeutic ratio than do cytotoxic therapies, the practical result of sequential hormonal therapies is that patients can be actively treated with few systemic side effects. When hormonal therapy is no longer effective, these patients proceed to chemotherapy. For patients with more extensive (i.e., symptomatic) or life-threatening disease and for all patients with hormone receptor-negative breast cancer, combination chemotherapy is the first treatment of choice. Anthracyclines (e.g., doxorubicin) and taxanes (e.g., paclitaxel and docetaxel) are currently the most effective antitumor agents against metastatic breast cancer.

The choice of initial chemotherapy depends on the patient's age, performance status, prior neoadjuvant and adjuvant chemotherapy, and disease-free interval. Anthracyclines or taxanes are options, as are capecitabine, vinorelbine, and gemcitabine. Because metastatic breast cancer is incurable with standard therapies, enrollment in clinical trials is always encouraged. Targeted agents against epidermal growth factor receptor, vascular endothelial growth factor, and other tumor-related proteins are actively under investigation. Trastuzumab-based chemotherapy is the standard of care for those with *HER-2/neu*-amplified tumors; however, for all other patients, combination chemotherapy has not been shown to prolong survival over sequential single agents, and it is associated with more intense side effects. Thus, outside of a clinical trial, patients with metastatic breast cancer are typically treated with sequential single agents.

In selected patients with controlled intact primary tumor and solitary metastases or multiple lesions at a single organ site, long disease-free period, and good performance status, consideration of metastasectomy may be considered, not as a standard of care, but in hopes of lengthening DFS times.

SPECIAL CONSIDERATIONS

Breast Cancer and Pregnancy

The definition of pregnancy-associated breast cancer is described as any breast carcinoma diagnosed during pregnancy, lactation, or during the first postpartum year. There is a low incidence of pregnancy-associated breast cancer, accounting for 2.8% of all breast malignancies, but breast cancer is one of the most common pregnancy-associated malignancies. Historically, the incidence is estimated at 1 in 3,000 pregnancies. These breast cancers are often identified in women at an earlier age, present as more advanced stage, and are often ER-negative, suggesting these tumors have other biologically distinct characteristics.

The diagnosis of pregnancy-associated breast cancer is typically more difficult because there is a low level of suspicion based on a comparatively young patient age, the relative frequency of nodular changes in the breast associated with pregnancy, and the increase in breast density during pregnancy that renders mammographic imaging less accurate. For these and other reasons, diagnosis of breast cancer in this population is frequently delayed. This delay may explain the advanced disease at presentation as well as relatively poor prognosis for women in which breast cancer is detected during pregnancy.

During gestation and lactation, breast examination reveals dense breast tissue that makes diagnosing breast cancer difficult. Palpation does not necessarily identify malignant from benign disease. The difficulties of the physical examination and hormonal changes associated with pregnancy account for a 2.5-fold increased risk for diagnosis at an advanced stage. Traditionally, mammography in young nonpregnant and nonlactating women reveals dense breast parenchyma that makes interpretation difficult, and based on such knowledge, the efficacy of mammography in pregnancy has been questioned. Both the safety and efficacy of mammography during pregnancy have been supported, with sensitivity rates from 78% to 90% in detecting suspicious features of malignancy. When the fetus is shielded adequately, the estimated fetal dose of radiation from a standard two-view mammogram is less than 0.004 Gy, and this is below the threshold exposure of 100 mGy that is associated with a 1% risk of fetal malformation and central nervous system problems published by the International Commission of Radiological Protection. Breast ultrasound is highly sensitive and specific in diagnosing during pregnancy and lactation, and is considered a standard method for the evaluation of a palpable breast mass. In addition, all persistent and suspicious breast masses should undergo evaluation by FNA, core-needle biopsy, or excisional biopsy. Excisional biopsy under local anesthesia is safe at any time during pregnancy.

Once a diagnosis of malignancy is established, treatment decisions are influenced by the specific trimester of pregnancy. See Figure 2.7 for the MDACC approach to pregnancy and breast cancer. The goal should be curative treatment of the breast cancer and preservation of pregnancy without injury to the fetus. The approach to each patient must be individualized, taking into account gestational age at presentation, stage of disease, and patient preference. Termination of pregnancy in the hope of minimizing hormonal stimulation of the tumor does not alter maternal survival and is not recommended. Genetic counseling is also recommended for all women with breast cancer during pregnancy.

Surgical treatment of gestational breast cancer is generally identical to that of nongestational breast cancer. There is no evidence that extra-abdominal surgical procedures are associated with premature labor or that the typically used anesthetic agents are teratogenic. Modified radical mastectomy or breast-conserving surgery with ALND as primary therapy can be undertaken at any point during pregnancy without undue risk to the mother or fetus. The safety of surgical intervention during pregnancy is well supported, but patients may defer until the 12th gestational week to avoid the risk of spontaneous abortion, which is highest in the first trimester. For cancer detected during the third trimester, delaying primary treatment for up to 4 weeks to allow for delivery before surgery is acceptable. If modified radical mastectomy is undertaken during pregnancy, breast reconstruction should not be performed simultaneously; reconstruction options, especially rectus or other myocutaneous flaps, are limited during pregnancy and the postpartum appearance of the contralateral breast is unknown until after pregnancy.

For women desiring breast conservation, treatment is complicated by the fact that radiation therapy is contraindicated during pregnancy during all trimesters. For cancers detected during the third trimester, lumpectomy and axillary dissection can be performed safely using general anesthesia, and radiation therapy can

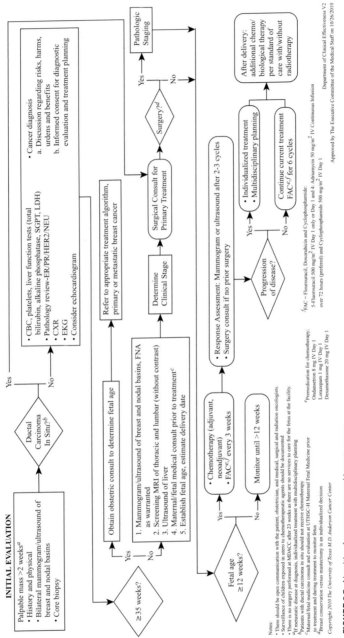

FIGURE 2.7 Algorithm for pregnancy and breast cancer.

be delayed until after delivery. Longer delays may be detrimental to maternal outcome, although the time limit within which radiation therapy must be carried out to minimize the risk of local recurrence is unknown.

The role of SLN dissection has not been proven to contribute significantly to improved prognosis. Controversy exists regarding the risk of fetal irradiation with radiocolloid administration. Several retrospective studies suggest fetal radiation absorption is negligible and that SLN biopsy may serve more of a role during pregnancy. However, it has not been evaluated systematically in pregnancy, and the complete efficacy, benefits, and risks of SLN biopsy in pregnancy remain unknown.

The decision to administer neoadjuvant or adjuvant chemotherapy is difficult, as fears of congenital malformations are a serious concern for the pregnant female. Most studies have demonstrated a safety profile and no increased risk of fetal malformation associated with chemotherapy administered during the second and third trimesters. In contrast, chemotherapy administration during the first trimester is associated with an increased incidence of spontaneous abortion, teratogenesis, or fetal malformations, especially in the setting of methotrexate.

The role of endocrine therapy is contraindicated secondary to teratogenicity and possible fetal malformation. There have been reports up to 20% fetal abnormalities, including craniofacial malformations and ambiguous genitalia, leading to the recommendation that endocrine therapy be delayed until pregnancy is over.

Published studies have found patients with pregnancy-associated breast cancer have similar survivals from those with nonpregnancy-associated breast cancer. These findings emphasize that definitive treatment and local control of breast cancer during pregnancy is not only feasible but also effective. Safe and effective treatment is available for many of these women with pregnancy-associated breast cancer.

CYSTOSARCOMA PHYLLODES

Cystosarcoma phyllodes represent an uncommon fibroepithelial breast neoplasm and accounts for only 0.5% to 1% of breast carcinomas. These tumors can occur in women of all ages, including adolescents and the elderly, but most arise in women between 35 and 55 years of age. Cystosarcoma phyllodes are typically quite large and have a mean diameter of 4 to 5 cm. Because phyllodes tumors and fibroadenomas are mammographically indistinguishable, the decision to perform excisional biopsy is usually based on large tumor size, a history of rapid growth, and patient age. Predicting the behavior of these tumors on the basis of histopathological features such as histotype (benign vs. indeterminate vs. malignant), margin status, stromal overgrowth, and size has been difficult partly because of their rarity. Common sites of metastases from malignant cystosarcoma phyllodes are lung, bone, and mediastinum.

Appropriate treatment for phyllodes tumors is complete surgical excision. Breast conservation surgery with appropriate margins is the preferred primary therapy. The incidence of local recurrence ranges from 5% to 15% for benign tumors and 20% to 30% for malignant tumors. Local recurrences are typically salvageable with total mastectomy and do not affect the OS rate. For all phyllodes tumors, the low incidence of axillary nodal metastases (less than 1%) obviates lymphadenectomy. The reported rates of distant metastasis for patients with malignant tumors range from 25% to 40%. The presence of stromal overgrowth may be the strongest predictor of distant metastasis and ultimate outcome. To date, no role for radiation therapy, chemotherapy, or hormonal therapy has been established for this disease.

Recommended Readings

Adjuvant therapy for breast cancer. *NIH Consens Statement.* 2000;17(4):1–35.

Anonymous, American Joint Committee on Cancer (AJCC). *AJCC Cancer Staging Manual.* 7th ed. New York, NY: Springer, Inc.; 2010.

Bedrosian I, Hu CY, Chang GJ. Population-based study of contralateral prophylactic mastectomy and survival outcomes of breast cancer patients. *J Natl Cancer Inst.* 2010;102(6):401–409.

Bedrosian I. The concept of prophylactic mastectomy. In: Henry M, Kuerer M, eds. *Kuerer's Breast Surgical Oncology.* New York, NY: McGraw-Hill Medical; 2010.

Bonadonna G, Brusamolino E, Valagussa P, et al. Combination chemotherapy as an adjuvant treatment in operable breast cancer. *N Engl J Med.* 1976;294(8):405–410.

Borner M, Bacchi M, Goldhirsch A, et al., for Swiss Group for Clinical Cancer Research. First isolated locoregional recurrence following mastectomy for breast cancer: results of a phase III multicenter study comparing systemic treatment with observation after excision and radiation. *J Clin Oncol.* 1994;12(10):2071–2077.

Bria E, Nistico C, Cuppone F, et al. Benefit of taxanes as adjuvant chemotherapy for early breast cancer: pooled analysis of 15,500 patients. *Cancer.* 2006;106(11):2337–2344.

Buzdar AU, Valero V, Ibrahim NK, et al. Neoadjuvant therapy with paclitaxel followed by 5-fluorouracil, epirubicin, and cyclophosphamide chemotherapy and concurrent trastuzumab in human epidermal growth factor receptor 2-positive operable breast cancer: an update of the initial randomized study population and data of additional patients treated with the same regimen. *Clin Cancer Res.* 2007; 13(1): 228–233.

Buzdar AU, Ibrahim NK, Francis D, et al. Significantly higher pathologic complete remission rate after neoadjuvant therapy with trastuzumab, paclitaxel, and epirubicin chemotherapy: results of a randomized trial in human epidermal growth factor receptor 2-positive operable breast cancer. *J Clin Oncol.* 2005;23(16):3676–3685.

Cancer Facts and Figures 2010, American Cancer Society [Available from: http://www.cancer.org/Research/CancerFactsFigures/CancerFactsFigures/cancer-facts-and-figures-2010]. See also SEER cancer registry database. 2010 [cited; Available from: www.seer.cancer.gov].

Carey LA, Dees EC, Sawyer L, et al. The triple negative paradox: primary tumor chemosensitivity of breast cancer subtypes. *Clin Cancer Res.* 2007;13(8):2329–2334.

Caudle AS, Hunt KK. The neoadjuvant approach in breast cancer treatment: it is not just about chemotherapy anymore. *Curr Opin Obstet Gynecol.* 2011;23(1):31–36.

Chagpar AB. Management of local recurrence after mastectomy. In: Henry M, Kuerer M, eds. *Kuerer's Breast Surgical Oncology.* New York, NY: McGraw-Hill Medical; 2010.

Cuzick J, Seslak I, Baum M, et al., on behalf of the ATAC/LATTE investigators. Effect of anastrozole and tamoxifen as adjuvant treatment for early-stage breast cancer: 10-year analysis of the ATAC trial. *Lancet Oncol.* 11(12):1135–1141.

de Boer M, van Dijck JAAM, Bult P, Borm GF, Tjan-Heijnen VCG. Breast cancer prognosis and occult lymph node metastases, isolated tumor cells, and micrometastases. *J Natl Cancer Inst.* 102(6): 410–425.

de Boer M, van Deurzen CH, van Dijck JA, et al. Micrometastases or isolated tumor cells and the outcome of breast cancer. *N Engl J Med.* 2009;361(7):653–663.

De Laurentiis M, Cancello G, D'Agostino D, et al. Taxane-based combinations as adjuvant chemotherapy of early breast cancer: a meta-analysis of randomized trials. *J Clin Oncol.* 2008;26(1):44–53.

Dent R, Trudeau M, Pritchard KI, et al. Triple-negative breast cancer: clinical features and patterns of recurrence. *Clin Cancer Res.* 2007;13(15 Pt 1):4429–4434.

Dhesy-Thind B, Pritchard KI, Messersmith H, O'Malley F, Elavathil L, Trudeau M. HER2/neu in systemic therapy for women with breast cancer: a systematic review. *Breast Cancer Res Treat.* 2008; 109(2):209–229.

Dressler LG, Berry DA, Broadwater G, et al. Comparison of HER2 status by fluorescence in situ hybridization and immunohistochemistry to predict benefit from dose escalation of adjuvant doxorubicin-based therapy in node-positive breast cancer patients. *J Clin Oncol.* 2005;23(19): 4287–4297.

Early Breast Cancer Trialists' Collaborative Group (EBCTCG). Effects of chemotherapy and hormonal therapy for early breast cancer on recurrence and 15-year survival: an overview of the randomised trials. *Lancet.* 2005;365(9472):1687–1717.

Early Breast Cancer Trialists' Collaborative Group. Polychemotherapy for early breast cancer: an overview of the randomised trials. *Lancet.* 1998;352(9132):930–942.

Esteva FJ, Hortobagyi GN. Topoisomerase II{alpha} amplification and anthracycline-based chemotherapy: the jury is still out. *J Clin Oncol.* 2009;27(21):3416–3417.

Fisher B, Bryant J, Wolmark N, et al. Effect of preoperative chemotherapy on the outcome of women with operable breast cancer. *J Clin Oncol.* 1998;16(8):2672–2685.

Fisher B, Jeong J-H, Dignam J, et al. Findings from recent National Surgical Adjuvant Breast and Bowel Project adjuvant studies in stage I breast cancer. *J Natl Cancer Inst Monogr.* 2001;(30):62–66.

Fisher B, Anderson S, Redmond CK, Wolmark N, Wickerham DL, Cronin WM. Reanalysis and results after 12 years of follow-up in a randomized clinical trial comparing total mastectomy with lumpectomy with or without irradiation in the treatment of breast cancer. *N Engl J Med.* 1995;333(22):1456–1461.

Fisher B, Anderson S, Tan-Chiu E, et al. Tamoxifen and chemotherapy for axillary node-negative, estrogen receptor-negative breast cancer: findings from National Surgical Adjuvant Breast and Bowel Project B-23. *J Clin Oncol.* 2001;19(4):931–942.

Fisher B, Jeong J-H, Bryant J, et al. Treatment of lymph-node-negative, oestrogen-receptor-positive breast cancer: long-term findings from National Surgical Adjuvant Breast and Bowel Project randomised clinical trials. *Lancet.* 2004;364(9437):858–868.

Fisher B, Brown AM, Dimitrov NV, et al. Two months of doxorubicin-cyclophosphamide with and without interval reduction therapy compared with 6 months of cyclophosphamide, methotrexate, and fluorouracil in positive-node breast cancer patients with tamoxifen-nonresponsive tumors: results from the National Surgical Adjuvant Breast and Bowel Project B-15. *J Clin Oncol.* 1990;8(9):1483–1496.

Fong PC, Boss DS, Yap TA, et al. Inhibition of poly(ADP-ribose) polymerase in tumors from BRCA mutation carriers. *N Engl J Med.* 2009;361(2):123–134.

Foulkes WD, Stefansson IM, Chappuis PO, et al. Germline BRCA1 mutations and a basal epithelial phenotype in breast cancer. *J Natl Cancer Inst.* 2003;95(19):1482–1485.

Gerber B, Krause A, Dieterich M, Kundt G, Reimer T. The oncological safety of skin sparing mastectomy with conservation of the nipple-areola complex and autologous reconstruction: an extended follow-up study. *Ann Surg.* 2009;249(3):461–468.

Giuliano AE, McCall L, Beitsch P, et al. Locoregional recurrence after sentinel lymph node dissection with or without axillary dissection in patients with sentinel lymph node metastases: the American College of Surgeons Oncology Group Z0011 randomized trial. *Ann Surg.* 2010;252(3):426–432; discussion 432–433.

Goldhirsch A, Ingle JN, Gelber RD, Coates AS, Thürlimann B, Senn H-J, and Panel members. Thresholds for therapies: highlights of the St Gallen International Expert Consensus on the primary therapy of early breast cancer 2009. *Ann Oncol.* 2009; 20(8):1319–1329.

Gonzalez-Angulo AM, Hennessy BT, Broglio K, et al. Trends for inflammatory breast cancer: is survival improving? *Oncologist.* 2007;12(8):904–912.

Green MC, Esteva FJ, Hortobagyi GN. Neoadjuvant Chemotherapy. *Breast Dis.* 2009; 21:23–31.

Hahn KM, Johnson PH, Gordon N, et al. Treatment of pregnant breast cancer patients and outcomes of children exposed to chemotherapy in utero. *Cancer.* 2006;107(6):1219–1226.

Harris JR, Lippman ME, Veronesi U, et al. Breast cancer. *N Engl J Med.* 1992;327(5):319–328.

Hayes DF, Thor AD, Dressler LG, et al. HER2 and response to paclitaxel in node-positive breast cancer. *N Engl J Med.* 2007;357(15):1496–1506.

Healey EA, Cook EF, Orav EJ, Schnitt SJ, Connolly JL, Harris JR. et al. Contralateral breast cancer: clinical characteristics and impact on prognosis. *J Clin Oncol.* 1993;11(8):1545–1552.

Hess KR, Pusztai L, Buzdar AU, Hortobagyi GN. Estrogen receptors and distinct patterns of breast cancer relapse. *Breast Cancer Res Treat.* 2003;78(1):105–118.

Hsueh EC, Hansen N, Giuliano AE. Intraoperative lymphatic mapping and sentinel lymph node dissection in breast cancer. *CA Cancer J Clin.* 2000;50(5):279–291.

Hsueh EC, Turner RR, Giuliano AE. Lymphoscintigraphy and lymphatic mapping for identification of sentinel lymph nodes. *World J Surg.* 2001;25(6):794–797.

Joensuu H, Bono P, Kataja V, et al. Fluorouracil, epirubicin, and cyclophosphamide with either docetaxel or vinorelbine, with or without trastuzumab, as adjuvant treatments of breast cancer: final results of the FinHer Trial. *J Clin Oncol.* 2009; 27(34): 5685–5692.

Joerger M, Thurlimann B. Update of the BIG 1–98 Trial: where do we stand? *Breast.* 2009;18(suppl 3):S78–S82.

Kang T, Yi M, Hunt KK, et al. Does blue dye contribute to success of sentinel node mapping for breast cancer? *Ann Surg Oncol.* 2010;17(suppl 3):280–285.

Khanna MM, Mark RJ, Silverstein MJ, et al. Breast conservation management of breast tumors 4 cm or larger. *Arch Surg.* 1992;127(9):1038–1041; discussion 1041–1043.

Kronowitz SJ. Delayed-immediate breast reconstruction: technical and timing considerations. *Plast Reconstr Surg.* 2010;125(2):463–474.

Kuerer HM, Hunt KK, Newman LA, Ross MI, Ames FC, Singletary SE. Neoadjuvant chemotherapy in women with invasive breast carcinoma: conceptual basis and fundamental surgical issues. *J Am Coll Surg.* 2000;190(3):350–363.

Kuhl CK. High-risk screening: multi-modality surveillance of women at high risk for breast cancer (proven or suspected carriers of a breast cancer susceptibility gene). *J Exp Clin Cancer Res.* 2002;21(suppl 3):103–106.

Kuhl CK. MR imaging for surveillance of women at high familial risk for breast cancer. *Magn Reson Imaging Clin N Am.* 2006;14(3):391–402, vii.

Kuhl CK, Schmutzler RK, Leutner CC, et al. Breast MR imaging screening in 192 women proved or suspected to be carriers of a breast cancer susceptibility gene: preliminary results. *Radiology.* 2000;215(1):267–279.

Kuhl CK, Schrading S, Leutner CC, et al. Mammography, breast ultrasound, and magnetic resonance imaging for surveillance of women at high familial risk for breast cancer. *J Clin Oncol.* 2005;23(33):8469–8476.

Kuhl CK, Schrading S, Weigel S, et al. The "EVA" Trial: evaluation of the efficacy of diagnostic methods (mammography, ultrasound, MRI) in the secondary and tertiary prevention of familial breast cancer. Preliminary results after the first half of the study period]. *Rofo.* 2005;177(6):818–827.

Kuhl CK, Kuhn W, Schild H. Management of women at high risk for breast cancer: new imaging beyond mammography. *Breast.* 2005;14(6):480–486.

Leach MO, Boggis CR, Dixon AK, et al. Screening with magnetic resonance imaging and mammography of a UK population at high familial risk of breast cancer: a prospective multicentre cohort study (MARIBS). *Lancet.* 2005;365 (9473):1769–1778.

Litton JK, Theriault RL. Breast cancer and pregnancy: current concepts in diagnosis and treatment. *Oncologist.* 2010;15(12):1238–1247.

Mansour EG, Gray R, Shatila AH, et al. Survival advantage of adjuvant chemotherapy in high-risk node-negative breast cancer: ten-year analysis—an intergroup study. *J Clin Oncol.* 1998;16(11):3486–3492.

Martin M, Rodríguez-Lescure Á, Ruiz A, et al. Randomized phase 3 trial of fluorouracil, epirubicin, and cyclophosphamide alone or followed by paclitaxel for early breast cancer. *J Natl Cancer Inst.* 2008;100(11):805–814.

McCredie JA, Inch WR, Alderson M. Consecutive primary carcinomas of the breast. *Cancer.* 1975;35(5):1472–1477.

Meijers-Heijboer H, van Geel B, van Putten WL, et al. Breast cancer after prophylactic bilateral mastectomy in women with a BRCA1 or BRCA2 mutation. *N Engl J Med.* 2001;345(3):159–164.

Middleton LP, Amin M, Gwyn K, Theriault R, Sahin A. Breast carcinoma in pregnant women: assessment of clinicopathologic and immunohistochemical features. *Cancer.* 2003;98(5): 1055–1060.

Mieog JS, van der Hage JA, van de Velde CJ. Neoadjuvant chemotherapy for operable breast cancer. *Br J Surg.* 2007;94(10):1189–1200.

National Comprehensive Cancer Network. *NCCN Clinical Practice Guidelines in Oncology®; Breast Cancer.* 2010 [cited January 19; Available from: http://www.nccn.org/professionals/physician_gls/PDF/breast.pdf.]

Nelson JC, Beitsch PD, Vicini FA, et al. Four-year clinical update from the American Society of Breast Surgeons MammoSite brachytherapy trial. *Am J Surg.* 2009; 198(1):83–91.

Norton L. A Gompertzian model of human breast cancer growth. *Cancer Res.* 1988; 48(24 Pt 1):7067–7071.

Olivotto IA, Bajdik CD, Ravdin PM, et al. Population-based validation of the prognostic model ADJUVANT! for early breast cancer. *J Clin Oncol.* 2005;23(12):2716–2725.

Pawlik TM, Kuerer HM. Accelerated partial breast irradiation as an alternative to whole breast irradiation in breast-conserving therapy for early-stage breast cancer. *Womens Health (Lond Engl).* 2005;1(1):59–71.

Perou CM, Sørlie T, Eisen MB, et al. Molecular portraits of human breast tumours. *Nature.* 2000;406(6797):747–752.

Piccart-Gebhart MJ, Procter M, Leyland-Jones B, et al. Trastuzumab after adjuvant chemotherapy in HER2-positive breast cancer. *N Engl J Med.* 2005;353(16): 1659–1672.

Pritchard KI, Shepherd LE, O'Malley FP, et al.; National Cancer Institute of Canada Clinical Trials Group. HER2 and responsiveness of breast cancer to adjuvant chemotherapy. *N Engl J Med.* 2006;354(20): 2103–2111.

Pritchard KI. Are HER2 and TOP2A useful as prognostic or predictive biomarkers for anthracycline-based adjuvant chemotherapy for breast cancer? *J Clin Oncol.* 2009;27(24):3875–3876.

Ravdin PM, Siminoff LA, Davis GJ, et al. Computer program to assist in making decisions about adjuvant therapy for women with early breast cancer. *J Clin Oncol.* 2001;19(4):980–991.

Rebbeck TR, Friebel T, Lynch HT, et al. Bilateral prophylactic mastectomy reduces breast cancer risk in BRCA1 and BRCA2 mutation carriers: the PROSE Study Group. *J Clin Oncol.* 2004;22(6):1055–1062.

Reintgen D, Giuliano R, Cox CE. Sentinel node biopsy in breast cancer: an overview. *Breast J.* 2000;6(5):299–305.

Romond EH, Perez EA, Bryant J, et al. Trastuzumab plus adjuvant chemotherapy for operable HER2-positive breast cancer. *N Engl J Med.* 2005;353(16):1673–1684.

Rouzier R, Perou CM, Symmans WF, et al. Breast cancer molecular subtypes respond differently to preoperative chemotherapy. *Clin Cancer Res.* 2005;11(16): 5678–5685.

Sacchini V, Pinotti JA, Barros AC, et al. Nipple-sparing mastectomy for breast cancer and risk reduction: oncologic or technical problem? *J Am Coll Surg.* 2006;203(5):704–714.

Salhab M, Al Sarakbi W, Joseph A, Sheards S, Trabers J, Mokbel K. Skin-sparing mastectomy and immediate breast reconstruction: patient satisfaction and clinical outcome. *Int J Clin Oncol.* 2006;11(1):51–54.

Schechter NR, Strom EA, Perkins GH, et al. Immediate breast reconstruction can impact postmastectomy irradiation. *Am J Clin Oncol.* 2005;28(5):485–494.

Sharma R, Bedrosian I, Lucci A, et al. Present-day locoregional control in patients with t1 or t2 breast cancer with 0 and 1 to 3 positive lymph nodes after mastectomy without radiotherapy. *Ann Surg Oncol.* 2010;17(11):2899–2908.

Singletary SE. Rating the risk factors for breast cancer. *Ann Surg.* 2003;237(4): 474–482.

Slamon, DJ, Press MF. Alterations in the TOP2A and HER2 genes: association with adjuvant anthracycline sensitivity in human breast cancers. *J Natl Cancer Inst.* 2009;101(9):615–618.

Slavin SA, Love SM, Goldwyn RM. Recurrent breast cancer following immediate reconstruction with myocutaneous flaps. *Plast Reconstr Surg.* 1994;93(6):1191–1204; discussion 1205–1207.

Solorzano CC, Ross MI, Delpassand E, et al. Utility of breast sentinel lymph node biopsy using day-before-surgery injection of high-dose 99mTc-labeled sulfur colloid. *Ann Surg Oncol.* 2001;8(10):821–827.

Sparano JA, Wang M, Martino S, et al. Weekly paclitaxel in the adjuvant treatment of breast cancer. *N Engl J Med.* 2008;358(16): 1663–1671.

Toth BA, Lappert P. Modified skin incisions for mastectomy: the need for plastic surgical input in preoperative planning. *Plast Reconstr Surg.* 1991;87(6): 1048–1053.

Wellisch DK, Schain WS, Noone RB, Little JW 3rd. The psychological contribution of nipple addition in breast reconstruction. *Plast Reconstr Surg.* 1987;80(5):699–704.

Wijayanayagam A, Kumar AS, Foster RD, Esserman LJ. Optimizing the total skin-sparing mastectomy. *Arch Surg.* 2008; 143(1):38–45; discussion 45.

Yi M, Kronowitz SJ, Meric-Bernstam F, et al. Local, regional, and systemic recurrence rates in patients undergoing skin-sparing mastectomy compared with conventional mastectomy. *Cancer.* 2011;117 (5):916–924.

Zambetti M, Moliterni A, Materazzo C, et al. Long-term cardiac sequelae in operable breast cancer patients given adjuvant chemotherapy with or without doxorubicin and breast irradiation. *J Clin Oncol.* 2001;19(1):37–43.

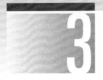

Melanoma

Joshua M.V. Mammen, C. Denise Ching, and
Jeffrey E. Gershenwald

EPIDEMIOLOGY

The incidence of invasive cutaneous melanoma in the United States has been rising by an average of 2.6% per year. An estimated 68,130 cases of invasive melanoma
were diagnosed in the United States in 2010. For Americans, the current estimated
lifetime risk of developing melanoma is 1 in 53; an estimated 8,700 people will have
died of melanoma in 2010. The incidence of melanoma has been increasing faster
than that of any other cancer, possibly secondary to sun exposure patterns and
changes in the ozone layer. The major environmental risk factor, exposure to ultraviolet B (UV-B) radiation, is reflected in geographic and ethnic patterns of melanoma rates. There have been changes in the distribution and stage of melanoma
at diagnosis, with an increasing percentage of thinner lesions. At present, many
melanomas diagnosed are less than 1 mm thick.

RISK FACTORS

Identifying risk factors and estimating an individual's risk of developing melanoma
can be clinically useful in determining primary prevention strategies and in direct-
ing the level of screening. Patients identified as being at high risk for melanoma
should be recruited to prevention trials.

Multiple factors can place a patient at risk for developing melanoma. Some
factors are modifiable while others are inherent to the individual.

1. *Skin type:* Caucasians have at least ten times the melanoma incidence of
   African Americans and seven times the melanoma incidence of American Hispanics. In addition, white patients with red or blond hair, light
   skin, or blue eyes are at increased risk for melanoma.
2. *Age:* The incidence of melanoma increases with age. The incidence of
   melanoma is 1.7-fold higher for women than men before 39 years of age.
   At greater than age 70, the incidence of melanoma is 2.2-fold higher for
   men than women.
3. *Gender:* In general, the incidence of melanoma is higher in men than in
   women. Specifically, a man's risk of melanoma development over his lifetime is 1.5 times higher than a woman's risk.
4. *Tanning bed use:* Tanning bed use more than ten times per year is associated with a doubling in the risk of melanoma for patients aged 30 years
   or older. Young patients who use tanning booths more than ten times
   annually have more than seven times the melanoma risk compared with
   individuals who do not use tanning booths. The risk for melanoma
   increases with the numbers of years, hours, and sessions. Since 2009, the
   World Health Organization lists tanning beds as a carcinogen.
5. *Previous melanoma:* A patient's risk of developing a second melanoma is
   3% to 7%; this risk is more than 900 times that of the general population.
6. *Sunlight exposure:* Sun exposure has been associated with an increased
   risk of melanoma. Unlike squamous cell cancer and basal cell cancer, a
   clear relationship has not been demonstrated with melanoma and

cumulative sun exposure. Rather, a more direct correlation appears to be present between the number of severe and painful sunburn episodes and the risk of melanoma; patients who have a history of greater than ten severe sunburns are more than twice as likely to develop a melanoma compared with patients who have no history of sunburns. It is important to note that even sunburns after the age of 20 may be associated with an increased risk of melanoma. The effect of sunlight has been attributed to exposure to UV-B radiation, which, according to hypothetical mechanisms of melanoma induction, may account for approximately two-thirds of melanomas. A potential role for UV-A radiation, however, has not been completely excluded.

7. *Benign nevi:* Although a benign nevus is most likely not a precursor of melanoma, the presence of large numbers of nevi has been consistently associated with an increased risk of melanoma. Persons with ≥50 nevi, all of which are >2 mm in diameter, have 5 to 17 times the melanoma risk of persons with fewer nevi. Also, individuals who tend to develop freckles have an increased risk of melanoma.

8. *Family history:* A family history of melanoma increases an individual's risk of melanoma by 3 to 8 times. Persons who have two or more family members with melanoma are at a particularly high risk for developing melanoma.

9. *Genetic predisposition:* Specific genetic alterations have been implicated in the pathogenesis of melanoma. A tumor suppressor gene located on chromosome 9p21 is probably involved in familial and sporadic cutaneous melanoma. Deletions or rearrangements of chromosomes 10 and 8p are also well documented in cutaneous melanoma. Also associated with an increase in melanoma incidence is the gain in copy number of chromosomes 2, 6p, 7, 8, 17, 19, and 20. A total of 8% to 12% of melanomas occur in individuals with a predisposition. These melanomas tend to present at an earlier age and individuals tend to have multiple primary lesions.

10. *Atypical mole and melanoma syndrome:* Previously known as dysplastic nevus syndrome, atypical mole and melanoma syndrome is characterized by the presence of multiple, large (>5 mm) atypical dysplastic nevi generally in areas covered by clothing that represent a distinct clinico-pathological type of melanocytic lesion. Melanomas can originate from either normal skin or from a dysplastic nevus. Since the actual frequency of an atypical mole progressing to melanoma is small, resection of the dysplastic nevi is not indicated.

CLINICAL PRESENTATION

Clinical features of melanoma include variegated color, irregular raised surface, irregular perimeter, and surface ulceration. A biopsy should be performed on any pigmented lesion that undergoes a change in size, configuration, or color. The so-called *ABCDE*s of early diagnosis are an easy mnemonic device to help physicians and laypersons remember the early signs of malignant melanoma. *A* denotes lesion asymmetry, *B* border irregularity, *C* color variegation, *D* diameter greater than 6 mm, and *E* a lesion that is elevating, evolving or enlarging.

When a patient presents with a lesion suggestive of melanoma, in addition to biopsy, a thorough physical examination must be performed, with particular emphasis on the skin (including the scalp, webspaces of digits, and intertriginous areas), all nodal basins, and subcutaneous tissues (see also "Staging" section later).

DIAGNOSIS

The choice of biopsy technique varies according to the anatomical site as well as the size and shape of the lesion. Particular attention, however, must be kept on the impact of the biopsy on options for definitive surgical treatment. Either an excisional biopsy or an incisional biopsy using a scalpel or punch is acceptable. Entire removal of the lesion is preferred to allow for accurate evaluation of the thickest part of the lesion. Punch biopsies can be performed for most lesions. Generally, they can be performed when lesions are located on areas where maximum preservation of surrounding skin is important, or can be completely excised with a punch. Punch biopsies should be performed at the most raised or darkest area of the lesion to sample the most aggressive area of the potential melanoma. Full-thickness biopsy into the subcutaneous tissue must be performed to permit proper staging of the lesion (see the T classification section later in this chapter). An excisional biopsy allows the pathologist to most accurately determine the thickness of the lesion since the entire lesion is available for evaluation. Excisional biopsies should be performed when the lesion is too large for a punch but still can be removed without excessive surgical intervention. For excisional biopsies, a narrow margin of normal-appearing skin (1 to 3 mm) is taken with the specimen. An elliptical incision is used to facilitate closure. The biopsy incision should be oriented to facilitate later wide local excision (e.g., longitudinally on extremities) and minimize the need for a skin graft to provide wound closure.

Shave biopsy is discouraged if a diagnosis of melanoma is being considered since the deep margin is often positive, making assessment of thickness limited. If a shave biopsy is performed, a deep shave is preferable. In general, we submit all pigmented lesions for permanent-section examination and perform definitive surgery at a later time.

Fine-needle aspiration biopsy may be used to document nodal and extranodal melanoma metastases but should not be used to diagnose primary melanomas.

PATHOLOGY

An experienced dermatopathologist should ideally review potential melanoma specimens due to the potential challenges associated with an accurate diagnosis. Although the pathologic analysis primarily consists of microscopic examination of hematoxylin-eosin–stained tumor, several melanocytic cell markers may also be useful in confirming the diagnosis of melanoma. Two antibodies that have been widely used in immunohistochemical evaluations are S-100 and HMB-45. S-100 is expressed not only by more than 90% of melanomas, but also by several other tumors and some normal tissues, including dendritic cells. In contrast, the monoclonal antibody HMB-45 is relatively specific (yet not as sensitive) for proliferative melanocytic cells and melanoma. It is therefore an excellent confirmatory stain for neoplastic cells when the diagnosis of melanoma is being considered. Anti-MART-1 staining has also been shown to be very useful in the diagnosis of melanoma. The major histomorphologic components that should be listed in a pathology report include Breslow thickness, Clark level, ulceration, margin status, and mitotic rate.

The major histomorphologic types of melanoma are as follows. While melanoma has been traditionally described in the following categories, prognosis is not dependent on the following descriptions, but rather upon TNM staging:

1. *Superficial spreading melanomas* constitute the majority of melanomas (approximately 70%) and generally arise in a pre-existing nevus.
2. *Nodular melanomas* are the second most common type (15% to 30%). Nodular melanomas progress to invasiveness more quickly than other types; however, when depth of the melanoma is controlled for, nodular melanomas are associated with the same prognosis as other lesions.

3. *Lentigo maligna melanomas* constitute a small percentage of melanomas (4% to 10%). These lesions occur in sun-exposed areas. Lentigo maligna melanomas are typically located on the faces of older white women. Many years can elapse before a lentigo maligna melanoma becomes invasive. In general, lentigo maligna melanomas are large (>3 cm at diagnosis), flat lesions and are uncommon in individuals younger than 50 years.

4. *Acral lentiginous melanomas* occur on the palms (palmar), soles (plantar), or beneath the nail beds (subungual), although not all palmar, plantar, and subungual melanomas are acral lentiginous melanomas. These melanomas account for only 2% to 8% of melanomas in white patients but for a substantially higher proportion of melanomas (35% to 60%) in darker-skinned patients. They are often large, with an average diameter of approximately 3 cm.

5. *Amelanotic melanomas* are melanomas that occur without pigmentation changes. These lesions are uncommon and are more difficult to diagnose because of their lack of pigmentation. Factors such as change in size, asymmetry, and irregular borders suggest malignancy and should prompt a biopsy.

Morphogenetic Correlates and Mutations in Melanoma

In addition to the classical descriptions of melanomas, recent molecular-based analyses have provided new insights into the pathogenesis of this disease. It follows that with knowledge of the specific molecular events within a tumor, scientists may translate this understanding into targeted therapies against such specific anomalies. Recent studies demonstrate that most melanomas have one or more mutations in essential kinase signaling pathways. Among the earliest kinase pathways found to be important in melanoma is the RAS-RAF-MEK-ERK kinase-signaling pathway. Studies have consistently found that more than 40% of cutaneous melanomas (particularly in superficial spreading melanoma) have mutations in a particular member of the RAF family known as BRAF. While more than 50 BRAF mutations have been identified, approximately 85% consist of a point mutation at V600E. Such a mutation leads to an approximately 400-fold increase in the activity of the BRAF protein. Interestingly, 80% of benign nevi also harbor BRAF mutations, suggesting that genetic alterations alone cannot fully explain the aggressive biology of melanoma. Nonetheless, BRAF has generated tremendous interest as a potential therapeutic target for melanoma (See Targeted Therapy section later). In the same kinase pathway, RAS has been found to be mutated in several malignancies; approximately 15% to 26% of melanomas are found to have an NRAS mutation. Similar to the BRAF mutation, NRAS mutation also leads to activation of the MAP kinase pathway. Interestingly, BRAF and NRAS mutations are rarely identified simultaneously in the same melanoma tumor.

The PI3 kinase-AKT pathway is the most common kinase pathway mutated in cancer. PTEN inhibits the activation of AKT; therefore, the loss of PTEN results in the constitutive activation of the AKT pathway. This mutation is seen in 10% to 30% of melanomas. Often, PTEN loss is found concurrently with NRAS mutations. Recently, mutations in AKT have also been identified in melanoma.

While MAP kinase signaling pathway mutations have been found commonly in cutaneous melanomas arising in sun-exposed areas, they are rather infrequent in mucosal and acral lentiginous melanomas. A missense mutation in the c-KIT gene has been found in more than 20% of mucosal melanomas and more than 10% of acral lentiginous melanomas. Despite these significant developments in detecting molecular anomalies, approximately 30% of patients with melanoma have no detectable abnormality in these genes; going forward, to improve outcomes in these patients, it will be essential to further unravel the molecular underpinnings of these tumors as well. Although not the focus of this chapter, more than 45% of uveal melanomas appear to have a mutation of another gene, the α-subunit of G-protein coupled receptors (*GNAQ*); a similar additional cohort harbor mutation of *GNA11*.

STAGING

The melanoma staging system has been revised numerous times as understanding of the disease has evolved. In 2009, the American Joint Committee on Cancer (AJCC) published a revised staging system for cutaneous melanoma in the seventh edition of the *AJCC Cancer Staging Manual*. The revisions reflect the results of an extensive survival analysis of prognostic factors conducted using data from more than 50,000 melanoma patients. Features of the revised system include mitotic rate becoming a key factor defining T1b lesions and immunohistochemistry being formally included in lymph node staging (Tables 3.1 and 3.2).

TABLE 3.1 2009 American Joint Committee on Cancer TNM Classification for Cutaneous Melanoma

T Classification	Thickness	Ulceration Status
T1	≤1.0 mm	a: Without ulceration and mitosis <1/mm^2 b: With ulceration or mitosis ≥1/mm^2
T2	1.01–2.0 mm	a: Without ulceration b: With ulceration
T3	2.01–4.0 mm	a: Without ulceration b: With ulceration
T4	>4.0 mm	a: Without ulceration b: With ulceration

N Classification	No. of Metastatic Nodes	Nodal Metastatic Mass
N1	1 node	a: Micrometastasis[a] b: Macrometastasis[b]
N2	2–3 nodes	a: Micrometastasis b: Macrometastasis c: In-transit met(s)/satellite(s) without metastatic nodes
N3	4 or more metastatic nodes, or matted nodes, or in-transit met(s)/satellite(s) with metastatic node(s)	

M Classification	Site	Serum Lactate Dehydrogenase Level
M1a	Distant skin, subcutaneous, or nodal metastases	Normal
M1b	Lung metastases	Normal
M1c	All other visceral metastases Any distant metastasis	Normal Elevated

[a]Micrometastases are diagnosed after sentinel lymph node biopsy.
[b]Macrometastases are defined as clinically detectable nodal metastases confirmed pathologically.
Adapted from Balch CM, Gershenwald JE, Soong SJ, et al. Final version of 2009 AJCC melanoma staging and classification. *J Clin Oncol.* 2009;27(36):6199–6206.

TABLE 3.2	2009 American Joint Committee on Cancer Stage Groupings for Cutaneous Melanoma					
	Clinical Staging[a]			**Pathological Staging**[b]		
	T	**N**	**M**	**T**	**N**	**M**
0	Tis	N0	M0	Tis	N0	M0
IA	T1a	N0	M0	T1a	N0	M0
IB	T1b	N0	M0	T1b	N0	M0
	T2a	N0	M0	T2a	N0	M0
IIA	T2b	N0	M0	T2b	N0	M0
	T3a	N0	M0	T3a	N0	M0
IIB	T3b	N0	M0	T3b	N0	M0
	T4a	N0	M0	T4a	N0	M0
IIC	T4b	N0	M0	T4b	N0	M0
III[c]	Any T	N1	M0	—	—	—
		N2				
		N3				
IIIA	—	—	—	T1–4a	N1a	M0
				T1–4a	N2a	M0
IIIB	—	—	—	T1–4b	N1a	M0
				T1–4b	N2a	M0
				T1–4a	N1b	M0
				T1–4a	N2b	M0
				T1–4a/b	N2c	M0
IIIC	—	—	—	T1–4b	N1b	M0
				T1–4b	N2b	M0
				Any T	N3	M0
IV	Any T	Any N	M1	Any T	Any N	M1

[a]Clinical staging includes microstaging of the primary melanoma and clinical and/or radiologic evaluation for metastases. By convention, it should be used after complete excision of the primary melanoma with clinical assessment for regional and distant metastases.

[b]Pathological staging includes microstaging of the primary melanoma and pathological information about the regional lymph nodes gained after partial (i.e., sentinel node biopsy) or complete lymphadenectomy. Pathological stages 0 and 1A are the exceptions; patients with this stage of disease do not require pathological evaluation of the lymph nodes.

[c]There are no stage III subgroups for clinical staging.

Adapted from Balch CM, Gershenwald JE, Soong SJ, et al. Final version of 2009 AJCC melanoma staging and classification. *J Clin Oncol.* 2009;27(36):6199–6206.

T Classification

Breslow tumor thickness and tumor ulceration serve as the dominant prognostic factors in the T classification. A third prognostic factor—mitotic rate—is important for staging among patients with thin (T1) primary lesions.

Breslow tumor thickness, measured in millimeters, is determined by using an ocular micrometer to measure the total vertical height of the melanoma from the granular layer to the area of deepest penetration. Clark level of invasion is determined by assessing the extent of penetration into the dermis. Consistent and uniform data now support the conclusion that measurement of Breslow tumor thickness is more reproducible than measurement of Clark level of invasion and that Breslow tumor thickness is the more accurate predictor of outcome. Moreover, the AJCC Melanoma Task Force has adopted the Breslow depth values of 1, 2, and 4 mm as cut-offs for the T categories (Table 3.1). Although the importance of mitotic rate (an indicator of proliferation of the primary melanoma) was first suggested in 1953, contemporary evidence-based analyses have refined this understanding. In the current 7th edition of the AJCC staging system, based on a large database analysis that includes mitotic rate (considered at a cut-point of $1/mm^2$), this factor (defined as the number of mitoses per mm^2) has replaced level of invasion as a key prognostic factor in staging for T1 melanoma. More recently, mitotic rate has not only been found to correlate with tumor thickness but it has also been found to be the second most important negative prognostic factor (after tumor thickness) in Stage I and II melanomas. For the T1 category of melanomas, one or more mitoses per mm^2 lead to the designation T1b. Several studies have emphasized the importance of standardizing the reporting of mitotic rate. The current recommendation is to use the "hot spot" method, in which the mitotic activity in the microscopy field with the greatest number of mitoses is measured first, and then other fields are subsequently measured until a total of 1 mm^2 is assessed. The "hot spot" strategy allows for acceptable reproducibility (Table 3.1).

Primary tumor ulceration is histopathologically defined as the absence of an intact epidermis overlying a portion of the primary tumor. Importantly, ulcerated melanomas are associated with a significantly worse prognosis than non-ulcerated melanomas of the same thickness. In the T category of the AJCC staging system, ulcerated tumors are always designated by *b* following the numerical T (Fig. 3.1A and B).

N Classification

The N classification refers to melanoma metastases to regional lymph node basins and other intralymphatic manifestations of tumor dissemination (e.g., in-transit and satellite metastases). In the AJCC staging system, regional nodal tumor burden is the most important predictor of survival in patients without distant disease.

Both the actual number of lymph nodes and the tumor burden (microscopic vs. macroscopic) within the node are assessed. Patients who have clinically negative lymph nodes but pathologically documented nodal metastases are defined as having "microscopic" or "clinically occult" nodal metastases (designated by the letter *a* in the N category of the staging system). In contrast, patients with clinical evidence of nodal metastases that is confirmed on pathological examination are defined as having "macroscopic" or "clinically apparent" nodal metastases (designated by the letter *b* in the N category of the staging system). Survival rates for patients with macroscopic nodal disease are significantly worse than rates for patients with microscopic nodal disease. Data from the World Health Organization (WHO) Melanoma Program showed that patients who underwent wide local excision and concomitant elective regional lymph node dissection and were found on pathological review to have microscopic nodal disease fared significantly better than patients who underwent wide local excision followed by therapeutic lymphadenectomy performed after nodal disease became clinically evident (5-year survival rates, 48.2% vs. 26.6%, $P = 0.04$).

Multiple studies have demonstrated that the number of pathologically involved lymph nodes is a dominant and independent predictor of outcome in patients with melanoma. In the analysis on which the 7th edition AJCC staging system is based, the best prognostic grouping of positive nodes was 1 versus 2 to 3 versus 4 or more. These cut-offs for number of positive nodes have therefore been incorporated into the N classification of the AJCC staging system.

Interestingly, the presence of tumor ulceration, a dominant prognostic factor within the T classification system, has also been shown to be an independent adverse prognostic factor in patients with regional nodal disease. In fact, ulceration

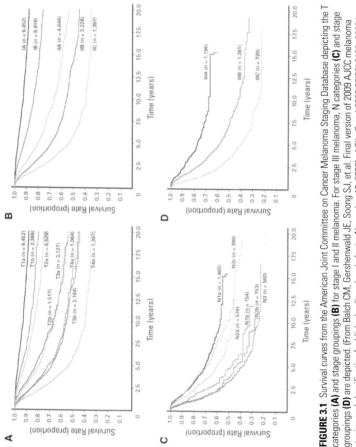

FIGURE 3.1 Survival curves from the American Joint Committee on Cancer Melanoma Staging Database depicting the T categories **(A)** and stage groupings **(B)** for stage I and II melanoma. For stage III melanoma, N categories **(C)** and stage groupings **(D)** are depicted. (From Balch CM, Gershenwald JE, Soong SJ, et al. Final version of 2009 AJCC melanoma staging and classification [published online ahead of print November 16, 2009]. *J Clin Oncol.* 2009;27(36):6199–6206.)

| | Five-Year Survival for Stage III Melanoma Based Upon Number of Metastatic Nodes, Primary Tumor Ulceration, and Nodal Tumor Burden (Microscopic Vs. Macroscopic Disease) |

Primary Tumor Ulceration	No. of Nodal Micrometastases, % ± SE ($n = 1,872$)			No. of Nodal Macrometastases, % ± SE ($n = 441$)		
	1	2–3	≥4	1	2–3	≥4
Absent	81.5 ± 1.9 (777)	73.2 ± 3.7 (246)	38.0 ± 8.5 (46)	51.6 ± 7.2 (75)	46.6 ± 7.9 (67)	45.4 ± 9.1 (50)
Present	56.6 ± 2.9 (531)	53.9 ± 4.2 (223)	34.0 ± 8.3 (49)	49.4 ± 6.2 (88)	37.7 ± 6.2 (93)	29.2 ± 6.7 (68)

(From Balch CM, Gershenwald JE, Soong SJ, et al. Multivariate analysis of prognostic factors among 2,313 patients with stage III melanoma: comparison of nodal micrometastases versus macrometastases [published online ahead of print April 5, 2010]. *J Clin Oncol.* 2010;28(14):2452–2459.

of the primary tumor was the only primary tumor prognostic feature that independently predicted survival in patients with nodal metastases. As such, patients with an ulcerated primary lesion are upstaged within the N category (as well as the T category) compared with patients with similar nodal tumor burden with a nonulcerated primary lesion (Table 3.3 and Fig. 3.1C and D).

The presence of clinically or microscopically detectable satellite metastases (classically defined as skin or subcutaneous lesions within 2 cm of the primary tumor) or in-transit metastases (skin or subcutaneous metastases more than 2 cm from the primary lesion but not beyond the regional nodal basin) are types of regional metastasis and, together with regional lymph nodes, are included in the N classification. Satellites and in-transit metastases are assigned a separate classification, N2c. (See the Management of In-transit Metastases section.) Because patients who have both satellites or in-transit metastases and concomitant lymph node metastases have a worse outcome than patients with either disease feature alone, patients with lymph node metastases and microsatellites or in-transit metastases are classified as N3, regardless of the number of synchronous metastatic lymph nodes.

M Classification

The M classification refers to melanoma metastases to distant sites and is classified as stage IV. Within the M classification there is only one stage, M1, but there are three subcategories. The subcategories reflect survival differences among patients with metastatic disease, depending on the anatomical sites of metastases. Distant metastases to the skin, subcutaneous tissue, or distant lymph nodes are designated M1a; they are associated with a better prognosis than metastases at any other anatomical site. Metastases to the lungs are associated with an intermediate prognosis and are designated M1b. Visceral metastases are associated with the worst prognosis and are designated M1c.

Serum lactate dehydrogenase (LDH) level is also included in the M category because in the analysis on which the 7th edition AJCC melanoma staging system was based, serum LDH level was an important predictor of poor prognosis in patients with metastatic disease. Patients with distant metastases who have an elevated serum LDH level at the time of staging are assigned to category M1c, regardless of the site(s) of their distant metastases.

EXTENT OF DISEASE EVALUATION

In addition to physical examination, several adjuncts are used to determine the extent of disease. The National Comprehensive Cancer Network (NCCN) provides guidelines to evaluate for possible metastatic melanoma with imaging. For melanoma in situ, imaging studies are not recommended. For stages IA, IB, and IC melanoma, imaging is recommended only if there are specific signs or symptoms that need evaluation. For stage III melanoma, baseline imaging with a chest x-ray, computed tomographic scan, PET/CT, and magnetic resonance imaging (MRI) of the brain can be considered. Ultrasonography with fine-needle aspiration of the associated lymph node basins may be useful in detecting metastatic disease in lymph nodes. Staging, however, is generally not necessary prior to definitive surgical intervention. Patients who present with suspected stage IV are generally staged with computed tomography (CT) of the chest, abdomen, and pelvis +/− positron emission tomography (PET) as well as MRI of the brain. In addition, image-guided percutaneous biopsy of concerning lesions can be used to confirm disease; excisional biopsy of suspected metastatic lesions is rarely indicated for diagnostic purposes.

MANAGEMENT OF LOCAL DISEASE

Local control of a primary melanoma requires wide excision of the tumor or biopsy site—down to but generally not including the deep fascia—with a margin of normal-appearing skin (Fig. 3.2). The risk of local recurrence correlates more with tumor thickness than with margins of surgical excision. Thus, it is rational to vary surgical margins according to tumor thickness.

Margin Width

Historically, even thin melanomas were excised with wide margins (3 to 5 cm). Studies have demonstrated, however, that narrower margins are often associated with the same recurrence rates as wider margins.

The first randomized study involving surgical margins for melanomas less than 2 mm thick was reported by the WHO Melanoma Group. In an update of the study including 612 patients randomly assigned to a 1-cm or 3-cm margin of excision, there were no local recurrences among patients with primary melanomas thinner than 1 mm. There were four local recurrences among the 100 patients with melanomas 1 to 2 mm thick, and all four occurred in patients with 1-cm margins. There was no significant difference in survival between the 1- and 3-cm surgical margin groups. These results demonstrate that a 1-cm excision margin is safe for thin (<1 mm thick) melanomas. A multi-institutional prospective randomized trial from France compared 2- and 5-cm excisional margins in 362 patients with melanomas less than 2 mm thick. There were no differences in local recurrence rate or survival between the two groups. Similarly, a randomized trial from Sweden compared 989 melanomas patients with lesions less than 2 mm thick excised with 2- and 5-cm margins. The results were similar. With regard to thicker lesions, a randomized clinical trial from the United Kingdom, the United Kingdom Melanoma Study Group (UKMSG) Trial, compared 1- and 3-cm excisional margins in 900 patients with melanomas at least 2 mm thick. With a median follow-up time of 60 months, a 1-cm margin was associated with a significantly increased risk of locoregional recurrence (37% vs. 32% for 3-cm margins); however, overall survival was similar in the two groups. For intermediate thickness lesions, a randomized prospective study conducted by the Intergroup Melanoma Committee compared 2- and 4-cm radial margins of excision for 1- to 4-mm thickness melanomas. There was no difference in local recurrence rate between the two groups. Forty-six percent of patients in the 4-cm group required skin grafts, whereas only 11% of

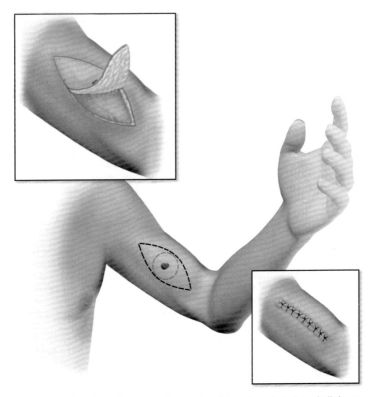

FIGURE 3.2 Wide excision of melanoma. Appropriate radial margin marked schematically (center, purple line) along with properly axially oriented elliptical incision to facilitate primary closure (inset, bottom right) after wide excision (inset, top left.) (Courtesy of Jeffrey Gershenwald, MD, Houston, TX. Copyright retained by Dr. Gershenwald and the University of Texas MD Anderson Cancer Center).

patients in the 2-cm group did ($P < 0.001$). Of note, however, a trend for improved 10-year disease-specific survival was seen in 4-cm margins (77%) versus 2-cm margins (70%). A clinical trial directly comparing 1-cm and 2-cm margins for 1–2 mm melanomas has not been performed. Based upon data from the WHO trial and the Intergroup Melanoma Trial, 2-cm margins are recommended when the anatomic location is favorable and primary closure can be achieved. Since there is no demonstrable survival advantage for a 2-cm margin over a 1-cm margin in 1–2 mm melanomas, a 1-cm margin can be justified in cases in which a 2-cm margin is not easily achievable.

The optimal margin width for thick melanomas (>4 mm) is still unknown. A retrospective review of 278 patients with thick primary melanomas from MD Anderson Cancer Center and Moffitt Cancer Center demonstrated that the width of the excision margin (≤2 cm vs. >2 cm) did not significantly affect local recurrence, disease-free survival, or overall survival rates after a median follow-up of 27 months.

TABLE 3.4	Summary of Recommendations for Excision Margins

Tumor Thickness	Excision Margin
<1 mm	1 cm
1–2 mm	1–2 cm
2–4 mm	2 cm
>4 mm	2 cm[a]

[a]No randomized prospective trials have specifically addressed this cohort.
Ross MI, Gershenwald JE. Evidence-based treatment of early-stage melanoma. *J Surg Oncol.* 2011;104(4):341–353.

In addition, based upon data from the UKMSG Trial (investigators concluded that a 3-cm margin is better than 1-cm margin for melanomas that are 2–4 mm thick) and the Intergroup Melanoma Trial (4-cm margin is not superior to a 2-cm margin for same tumor thickness), a margin greater than 2 cm is not necessary for these thick melanomas.

Based in large part on the data from randomized, prospective trials, several recommendations can be made for margins of excision (Table 3.4). Patient with melanoma in situ, a 0.5-cm to 1-cm margin is adequate. Patients with invasive melanoma less than 1 mm thick can be treated with a 1-cm margin of excision. For patients with melanoma 1 to 2 mm thick, a simple recommendation is difficult because this patient population has been studied in several trials evaluating a range of excision margins. In general, a 2-cm margin is preferred if anatomically and functionally feasible, and in regions of anatomical constraint (e.g., the face), a 1-cm margin is sufficient. This recommendation is based on the fact that overall survival was similar for patients with 1- and 3-cm margins in the WHO trial. Patients with melanoma 2 to 4 mm thick can be treated with a 2-cm margin. In patients with melanoma thicker than 4 mm, a 2-cm margin is probably safe, although no prospective randomized trials have specifically addressed this thickness group.

Wound Closure

If there is any question about the ability to achieve suitable wound closure, a plastic or reconstructive surgeon should be consulted. Options for closure include primary closure, skin grafting, and local and distant flaps.

Primary closure is the method of choice for most lesions, but it should be avoided when it will distort the appearance of a mobile facial feature or interfere with function. Many defects can be closed using an advancement flap, undermining the skin and subcutaneous tissues to permit primary closure. Primary closure usually requires that the longitudinal axis of an elliptical incision be at least three times the length of the short axis. The skin and subcutaneous tissue are removed down to but not including the fascia. The incision may be oriented in a "lazy S" pattern so as to allow primary closure. Closure of the wound edges is usually performed in two layers—a dermal layer of 3-0 or 4-0 undyed absorbable sutures and either interrupted skin closure using 3-0 or 4-0 nonabsorbable sutures or a running subcuticular skin closure using 4-0 monofilament absorbable sutures. Three layers are sometimes used, particularly for primary melanomas of the back. After removal, the specimen should be oriented for accurate assessment of histologic margins.

Application of a skin graft is one of the simplest reconstructive methods used for wound closure. Split-thickness skin grafts are used most commonly. For lower-extremity primary lesions, split-thickness grafts should be harvested from the extremity opposite the melanoma. In general, skin grafts should be harvested from an area remote from the primary melanoma and outside the zone of potential in-transit metastasis. A full-thickness skin graft can provide a result that is both more durable and of higher aesthetic quality than a split-thickness graft. Full-thickness grafts have most commonly been used on the face, where aesthetic considerations are most significant. Donor sites for full-thickness skin graft to the face should be chosen from locations that are likely to match the color of the face, such as the postauricular or preauricular skin or the supraclavicular portion of the neck.

Local flaps offer numerous advantages for repair of defects that cannot be closed primarily, especially on the distal extremities and on the head and neck. Color match is excellent, durability of the skin is essentially normal, and normal sensation is usually preserved. Transposition flaps and rotation flaps of many varieties have been used successfully.

Distant flaps should be used when sufficient tissue for a local flap is not available and when a skin graft would not provide adequate wound coverage. Myocutaneous flaps and free flaps can be used. Discussion of such complex methods is beyond the scope of this chapter, but these techniques are familiar to plastic and reconstructive surgeons and are discussed in greater detail in Chapter 24.

Special Anatomical Sites

Fingers and Toes

More than three-fourths of subungual melanomas involve either the great toe or the thumb. A melanoma located on the skin of a digit or beneath the nail should be removed by a digital amputation, with as much of the digit saved as possible. In general, amputations are performed at the middle interphalangeal joint of the fingers or proximal to the distal joint of the thumb. More proximal amputations are not associated with improved survival. For a melanoma located on a toe, an amputation of the entire digit at the metatarsal–phalangeal joint is generally indicated; for melanomas of the great toe, the amputation can be performed proximal to the interphalangeal joint. Lesions arising between two digits can be treated with soft tissue excision with the defect being reconstructed with a flap or skin graft. Sometimes, however, amputation of both digits may be needed.

Sole of the Foot

Excision of a melanoma on the plantar surface of the foot often produces a sizable defect in a weight-bearing area. If possible, a portion of the heel or ball of the plantar surface should be retained to bear the greatest burden of pressure. When oncologically possible, deep fascia over the extensor tendons should be preserved as a base for skin graft coverage. A plantar flap, which can be raised either laterally or medially, can provide well-vascularized local tissue for weight-bearing areas, while also providing some sensation. Staged closure of some plantar melanomas, particularly of the heel, has been performed with initial use of a vacuum-assisted closure device to stimulate granulation tissue followed by staged skin graft application. Such an approach may obviate complex reconstruction and has essentially eliminated the need for extensive flap reconstruction of the heel.

Face

Because of numerous functional and cosmetic considerations, facial lesions usually cannot be excised with more than a 1-cm margin. The tumor diameter, the tumor thickness, and the tumor's exact location on the face must all be considered when margin width is planned. Radiation therapy can be considered as an adjunct when margins are closer than desired. Mohs microsurgery has been proposed by some dermatologic surgeons as a means to remove melanoma with a minimal surgical margin. With this technique, resection occurs with serial histologic evaluations until the entire lesion is removed. Formal comparison between Mohs microsurgery and standard surgical margins is still lacking.

Breast

Wide excision with primary closure is the treatment of choice for melanoma on the skin of the breast; mastectomy is not generally recommended.

Umbilicus

Melanomas near or in the umbilicus may require resection of the umbilicus. In these cases, rotational flaps can often be used to reconstruct the umbilicus.

Mucosal Melanoma

Patients with true mucosal melanoma—including melanoma of the mucosa of the respiratory tract, vagina, and anal canal—generally have a poor prognosis. Because of their relative scarcity, few clinical trials have evaluated treatment options. We usually do not recommend an aggressive surgical approach to patients with clinically localized disease. In particular, we generally recommend local excision of anal melanomas rather than abdominoperineal resection. Abdominoperineal resection is associated with greater morbidity, leaves the patient with a permanent colostomy, offers no survival advantage, and does not treat at-risk inguinal nodes unless the procedure is combined with groin dissection. Adjuvant radiation therapy may be administered to patients with mucosal melanoma in an attempt to decrease the risk of locoregional recurrence.

MANAGEMENT OF REGIONAL LYMPH NODES

Regional lymph nodes are the most common site of melanoma metastasis. Lymph node involvement is categorized as microscopic (found only on histologic examination after removal of clinically uninvolved nodes) or macroscopic (clinically evident). Effective palliation and sometimes cure can be achieved in patients with regional metastases. Fine-needle aspiration or core biopsy can usually yield a diagnosis in patients who develop clinically enlarged regional nodes. Open biopsy is rarely warranted.

The management of clinically negative regional lymph nodes has been the focus of a long and sometimes contentious debate. Historically, some surgeons preferred to perform lymphadenectomy only for clinically demonstrable nodal metastases. This type of excision has been termed *delayed* or *therapeutic lymph node dissection* (TLND). Other surgeons have chosen to excise the nodes even when they appeared normal in patients who are at increased risk of developing nodal metastases. This excision has been termed *immediate, prophylactic,* or *elective lymph node dissection* (ELND). More recently, many surgeons have adopted a selective approach to regional lymph node dissection—the technique of intraoperative lymphatic mapping and sentinel lymph node (SLN) identification originally developed by Morton et al.

Therapeutic Lymph Node Dissection

With TLND, only patients with known metastases undergo a major lymphadenectomy; this reduces the number of potentially unnecessary lymphadenectomies. The disadvantage of TLND is that delaying treatment until lymph node metastases are clinically evident may result in many patients having distant micrometastases at the time of lymphadenectomy. Chances for cure may therefore be diminished.

Elective Lymph Node Dissection

ELND has the theoretical advantage of treating melanoma nodal metastases at a relatively early stage in the natural history of the disease. The disadvantage of ELND is that many patients undergo surgery when they do not have nodal metastasis. Advocates of ELND argued that patients with clinically negative, histologically positive lymph nodes at ELND had a better chance for survival (50% to 60%) than did patients in whom the regional lymph nodes were not dissected, and clinically apparent metastases developed in the regional lymph nodes during follow-up (15% to 35%). None of four randomized, prospective studies assessing ELND have demonstrated an overall survival advantage for this technique. Two trials, one from the WHO and another from the Mayo Clinic, were ultimately criticized because the study populations were at low risk for occult nodal disease, and patients were therefore unlikely to benefit from the proposed surgical treatment.

Although ELND did not offer a survival benefit to all patients, two prospective randomized trials that targeted higher-risk, clinically node-negative patients suggested that ELND may have some survival benefit in certain patient subgroups. In the WHO ELND Trial, patients with truncal melanoma at least 1.5 mm thick were randomized to wide local excision and ELND versus wide local excision and observation. Updated results from this trial demonstrated that patients in the ELND treatment arm who were found to have microscopic nodal disease at ELND had better overall survival than did patients in whom palpable adenopathy developed after wide excision alone. The long-term results of the Intergroup Melanoma Trial are similar. In this trial, patients with intermediate-thickness melanomas (1.0 to 4.0 mm) who underwent wide excision and ELND were compared with a similar group of patients who underwent wide excision alone followed by observation of the regional nodal basin. Although this trial did not demonstrate a difference in overall 10-year survival rates, four prospectively selected subgroups were found to have significantly better 10-year survival with ELND than with nodal observation: patients whose primary tumors were without ulceration (84% vs. 77%, $P = 0.03$); patients with primary tumor thickness between 1.0 and 2.0 mm (vs. thicker) (86% vs. 80%, $P = 0.03$); patients with extremity (vs. truncal) melanoma (84% vs. 78%, $P = 0.05$); and patients younger than 60 years (81% vs. 74%, $P = 0.03$). The results of a multicenter trial from Germany also demonstrated an absolute survival advantage, of at least 13%, for patients with positive nodes detected on sentinel lymph node biopsy (SLNB) compared with patients with positive nodes detected during observation of the nodal basin. Although this analysis was retrospective, the results were consistent with the findings of the WHO study.

Taken together, these data called into question recommendations to delay lymphadenectomy until palpable nodal disease develops; the data also supported the use of alternative approaches to permit earlier identification of occult nodal disease. A more rational, selective approach, lymphatic mapping and SLNB, has now been widely adopted. This technique satisfies many proponents of both ELND and TLND.

Intraoperative Lymphatic Mapping and Sentinel Lymph Node Biopsy

Several investigators have proposed intraoperative lymphatic mapping and SLNB as a minimally invasive procedure for identifying the approximately 20% of patients who harbor occult microscopic disease. This approach is sometimes termed *selective lymphadenectomy.*

Several studies have demonstrated that the SLNs are the first nodes to contain metastases, if metastases are present, and thus the pathological status of the SLNs reflects that of the entire regional nodal basin. If the SLN lacks metastasis, the remainder of the regional lymph nodes are unlikely to contain disease, and a completion lymphadenectomy need not be performed. Multiple studies have demonstrated that the immediate false-negative rate for SLNB is less than 5%. Other studies have confirmed the validity of the SLN concept and the accuracy of SLNB as a staging procedure. It is imperative, however, that the surgeon employing SLNB have adequate pathology and nuclear medicine support.

Sentinel Lymph Node Biopsy Technique

Lymphatic mapping and SLNB is performed at the time of wide excision of the primary tumor or biopsy site. If the wide local excision has already been performed, the SLNB can still generally be performed with equivalent accuracy. Since the introduction of lymphatic mapping and SLNB, the technique has undergone several refinements that have resulted in improved detection of SLNs.

Use of a vital blue dye (isosulfan blue 1%) to help identify SLNs has been part of the lymphatic mapping and SLNB procedure since its introduction. The blue dye is injected into the patient intradermally around the intact tumor or biopsy site. The blue dye is taken up by the lymphatic system and carried via afferent lymphatics to the SLN. The draining nodal basin is explored, and the afferent lymphatic channels and first draining lymph nodes (the SLNs) are identified by the uptake of the blue dye. With the use of blue dye alone, a SLN is identified in approximately 85% of cases. Although this initial approach was promising, it left 15% of patients unable to benefit from SLNB because no SLN was identified.

Subsequently, additional techniques have been incorporated that have significantly improved SLN localization: (a) preoperative lymphoscintigraphy and (b) intraoperative injection of technetium-99 (^{99}Tc)-labeled sulfur colloid accompanied by intraoperative use of a handheld gamma probe. Preoperative lymphoscintigraphy using ^{99}Tc-labeled sulfur colloid permits the identification of patients with multiple draining nodal basins and patients with lymphatic drainage to SLNs located outside standard nodal basins, including epitrochlear, popliteal, and ectopic sites (Fig. 3.3). In patients with melanomas that drain to multiple regional nodal basins, the histologic status of one draining basin does not predict the status of other basins. In one study, among 54 patients who underwent SLNB of an unexpected nodal site, 7 (13%) had lymph node metastases in that location. In four of the seven patients, the only positive SLN was from the unusual site. Therefore, it is particularly important to identify and assess all at-risk regional nodal basins to properly stage the disease. An advance from traditional nuclear imaging is the use of single photon emission computed tomography (SPECT) imaging merged with CT. SPECT/CT facilitates localization of SLNs by overlaying radiotracer uptake activity onto the CT image and is particularly helpful in the head and neck region. In up to 30% of cases, the surgical approach has been revised on the basis of results of SPECT/CT imaging.

Probably the most important development in the SLNB technique has been the introduction of intraoperative lymphatic mapping using a handheld gamma probe. In this approach, 0.5 to 1.0 mCi of ^{99}Tc-labeled sulfur colloid is injected intradermally 1 to 4 hours before surgery. During surgery, a handheld gamma probe is used to transcutaneously identify SLNs that will be removed. The use of both blue dye and radiocolloid increases the surgeon's ability to identify the SLN (greater than 96% to 99% accuracy) compared with the use of blue dye alone (84% accuracy). Although most clinicians use this combined modality approach, some favor the single-agent strategy of ^{99}Tc-labeled sulfur colloid alone, and they have reported similarly excellent results.

Incidence and Predictors of Positive Sentinel Lymph Nodes

Knowledge of the factors predictive of a positive SLN is useful for counseling patients regarding treatment options. In most studies, the incidence of positive

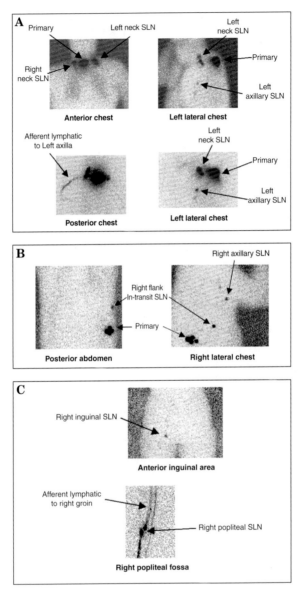

FIGURE 3.3 Preoperative lymphoscintigraphy. After injection of ^{99}Tc-labeled sulfur colloid at the primary cutaneous melanoma site (upper midline back), preoperative lymphoscintigraphy revealed **(A)** drainage to multiple nodal basins (bilateral neck and left axilla), **(B)** "in-transit"/ectopic sentinel lymph nodes (SLNs) in the right flank region and right axilla from a primary tumor of the right lateral back, and **(C)** SLNs in a right lower-extremity popliteal fossa lymph node basin and a right inguinal lymph node basin from a primary tumor of the heel. (Photos courtesy of Jeffrey E. Gershenwald, MD. Copyright retained by Dr. Gershenwald and the University of Texas MD Anderson Cancer Center).

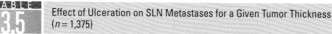

Effect of Ulceration on SLN Metastases for a Given Tumor Thickness (n = 1,375)

Tumor Thickness (mm)	Total Patients (%)	Positive SLN					
			Not Ulcerated		Ulcerated		P Value[a] Ulcerated vs. Not
		All (%)	(%)	AJCC Stage[b]	(%)	AJCC Stage[b]	
≤1.00	28	4	3	IA	16	IB	0.026
1.01–2.00	38	12	11	IB	22	IIA	0.007
2.01–4.00	23	28	25	IIA	34	IIB	0.115
>4.00	11	44	33	IIB	53	IIC	0.021
All Patients	100	17	12		35		<0.0001

[a]Fisher exact test for each tumor thickness group.
[b]Stage groupings calculated using tumor thickness and ulceration data only.
SLN, sentinel lymph node; AJCC, American Joint Committee on Cancer.
Reprinted from Rousseau DL Jr, Ross MI, Johnson MM, et al. Revised American Joint Committee on Cancer staging criteria accurately predict sentinel lymph node positivity in clinically node-negative melanoma patients. *Ann Surg Oncol.* 2003;10(5):569–574, with permission.

SLNs in patients undergoing SLNB ranges from 15% to 20%. However, multivariate analyses have revealed several factors that increase the risk of positive SLNs: increased tumor thickness, ulceration, high mitotic rate, young age, and axial tumor location. In one report, the incidence of positive SLN was 4% among patients with melanomas 1.0 mm or thinner and 44% among patients with melanomas thicker than 4.00 mm (Table 3.5). In the same report, patients with ulcerated primary tumors had a higher incidence of SLN metastases compared with those with nonulcerated lesions (35% vs. 12%, respectively). The incidence of SLN metastases by AJCC stage is shown in Figure 3.4. The incidences of positive SLNs for stages IA, IB, IIA, IIB, and IIC were 2%, 9%, 24%, 34%, and 53%, respectively.

Prognostic Value of Sentinel Lymph Node Status

The prognostic significance of the pathological status of the SLNs has been convincingly demonstrated. Data from the MD Anderson Cancer Center demonstrated that SLN status was the most significant clinicopathological prognostic factor with respect to survival in patients with melanoma. In an analysis of 1,487 patients who underwent SLNB (median tumor thickness, 1.5 mm), the 5-year survival rate for patients with positive SLNs was 73.3%, compared with 96.8% for patients with negative SLNs (Fig. 3.5). Several other multivariate regression analyses have shown that regional lymph node status is the most powerful predictor of recurrence (both regional and distant) and survival, even among patients with thick melanomas. Taken together with patients who have clinical regional disease, according to analysis of the AJCC database, 5-year survival rates for patients with stage III disease range from 81% for patients with only one microscopically positive lymph node and a nonulcerated primary melanoma to 29% for patients with clinically evident nodal disease with more than three pathologically involved nodes (Table 3.3).

The prognostic importance of distinguishing between microscopically and macroscopically positive lymph nodes has been emphasized by incorporation of this criterion into the AJCC melanoma staging system. The concept of tumor

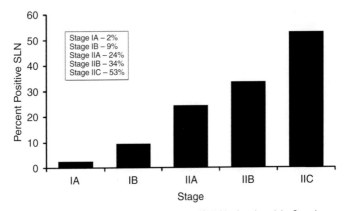

FIGURE 3.4 Incidence of positive sentinel lymph nodes (SLNs) by American Joint Committee on Cancer disease stage ($n = 1,375$). The difference between each stage is statistically significant. The *inset* shows the percentage of patients with a positive SLN within each category. (Reprinted from Rousseau DL, Jr, Ross MI, Johnson MM, et al. Revised American Joint Committee on Cancer staging criteria accurately predict sentinel lymph node positivity in clinically node-negative melanoma patients. *Ann Surg Oncol.* 2003;10:569–574, with permission.)

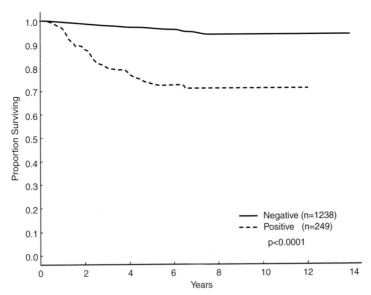

FIGURE 3.5 Disease-specific survival by sentinel lymph node (SLN) status in 1,487 patients. SLN status was the most significant clinicopathological prognostic factor with respect to survival. The 5-year disease-specific survival rate was 73.3% for patients with positive SLNs, compared with 96.8% for patients with negative SLNs.

burden will likely be important in the era of SLNB as accurate microscopic staging of SLNs becomes even more widespread and patients are better stratified on the basis of microscopic tumor burden into similar risk subgroups. In fact, several studies have shown that the diameter of the largest lymph node tumor nodule and the total lymph node tumor volume are significant predictors of recurrence and survival. In one study, a tumor deposit diameter of 3 mm was identified as a significant cut-off point. The 3-year survival probability was 86% for patients with a largest tumor deposit diameter of 3 mm or less and 27% for patients with a largest deposit diameter greater than 3 mm. In the future, as our understanding of the significance of microscopic nodal tumor burden is refined, clinical decisions regarding the need for and extent of further surgery or adjuvant therapy may also be based on the extent of microscopic nodal tumor burden.

The Multicenter Selective Lymphadenectomy Trial-I (MSLT-1) was designed to assess whether a selective approach to regional lymphadenectomy—limiting complete nodal dissection to patients with microscopic disease in SLNs—confers a survival benefit compared with wide local excision of the primary melanoma and observation of the regional nodal basin. Patients with primary cutaneous melanomas at least 1 mm thick or with Clark level IV or V tumors with any Breslow thickness were eligible for the trial. Patients were randomly assigned to wide excision alone plus observation or wide excision plus lymphatic mapping and SLNB, with subsequent completion lymphadenectomy if SLNs were positive. At the third interim analysis published in 2006, there was no significant difference between the observation group and the SLNB group in the primary end point of melanoma-specific survival at 5 years (86.6% vs. 87.1%; hazard ratio, 0.92; 95% confidence interval [CI], 0.67 to 1.25; $P = 0.58$). Nonetheless, in a prespecified analysis, patients in the observation group in whom clinical nodal recurrence developed (and also underwent delayed lymph node dissection) had significantly poorer melanoma-specific survival at 5 years than did those in the SLNB group whose nodes were positive (and had early lymphadenectomy) (52.4% vs. 72.3%; hazard ratio, 0.51; 95% CI, 0.32 to 0.81; $P = 0.007$). The validity of this comparison is based on the assumption that all SLNB-detected micrometastases seen on examination of the sentinel-node–biopsy specimen would have progressed to palpable disease if left untreated. Of note, the final analysis of MSLT-I has not yet been published.

Pathological Evaluation of Sentinel Lymph Nodes

Pathologists have traditionally examined the multitude of lymph nodes obtained from a lymphadenectomy by examining one hematoxylin-eosin–stained section from each paraffin block. This conventional approach, however, can miss disease in SLNs, primarily because of sampling error. In one study, 8 of 10 patients who underwent SLNB and subsequently developed regional nodal failure in nodal basins that were negative for disease according to conventional histologic examination of SLNs had microscopic disease detected when the SLNs were reassessed using specialized pathological techniques. Data from this and other studies suggest that failure to use specialized techniques, rather than failure to correctly identify SLNs, accounts for many cases of false-negative findings on SLNB.

With the SLNB technique, fewer lymph nodes are submitted for analysis than are submitted with complete lymphadenectomy, and the pathologist can therefore focus on only those nodes—the SLNs—that are at the highest risk. Currently, the combination of hematoxylin–eosin assessment of several levels and immunohistochemical analysis is generally considered a standard practice in assessing SLNs. Several antibodies directed against melanoma-associated antigens (S-100, HMB-45, tyrosinase, MAGE3, and MART-1) are routinely used for immunohistochemical evaluation. Because certain antibodies have low specificity (S-100) and others have low sensitivity (HMB-45, MAGE3, and tyrosinase), a panel of antibodies is commonly used. At MD Anderson Cancer Center, this panel includes HMB-45 and MART-1.

The use of frozen section for immediate evaluation of SLNs is highly controversial in melanoma. Frozen sections usually provide suboptimal morphology and may lack the subcapsular region of the lymph node (the area most likely involved in small metastases). Also, processing of the frozen tissue requires additional sectioning and micrometastases may be lost in the discarded unexamined sections. Therefore, for SLNs from patients with melanoma, most protocols consider the examination of routinely processed material (formalin-fixed, paraffin-embedded) as the gold standard. A possible alternative is touch preparation/cytologic analysis of specimens; these approaches seem to provide accurate and cost-effective SLN assessment in some specialized centers. We feel strongly that the use of frozen section risks a lower accuracy of detection of metastatic lesions. In general, this approach is employed only if a grossly suspicious SLN is identified and if a formal preoperative discussion of possible concomitant completion lymphadenectomy has occurred.

Because even the combination of histologic and immunohistochemical examination of SLNs may fail to identify isolated melanoma cells or oligocellular deposits, some have suggested a molecular-based approach to examination of SLNs. With use of the reverse transcriptase–polymerase chain reaction (RT-PCR), it is estimated that one melanoma cell in a background of 1×10^6 to 1×10^7 normal cells can be identified. Some investigators have proposed, however, that this level of diagnostic sensitivity may actually overestimate clinically relevant disease. Some studies show that the prognosis of patients with an SLN that is positive by RT-PCR but negative by histologic or immunohistochemical analysis is worse than that of patients who have SLNs negative by both techniques. Although preliminary results have been intriguing, the true clinical significance of positive RT-PCR findings in a histologically negative SLN is still unknown, in part because many studies that have addressed this question to date had short follow-up times and did not compare RT-PCR with current standard histologic techniques. It therefore remains difficult to draw final conclusions about the prognostic significance of SLNs that are positive by RT-PCR but negative by current conventional histologic analysis. Importantly, a few studies suggest that patients with submicroscopic disease detected by tyrosinase RT-PCR do not have a higher recurrence risk than patients with RT-PCR–negative SLNs. The relative clinical importance of conventional histologic examination, serial sectioning, immunohistochemical analysis, and molecular staging in patients undergoing lymphatic mapping and SLNB is still being evaluated.

Identifying Additional Disease in Nonsentinel Nodes
Currently, patients who have a melanoma-positive SLN identified on SLNB subsequently undergo completion lymphadenectomy. When the non-SLNs are excised and evaluated by hematoxylin–eosin staining and immunohistochemistry, however, only 12% to 25% of completion lymphadenectomy specimens contain additional nodes with metastatic disease. Because more than two-thirds of patients have metastatic disease identified only in SLNs, there has been interest in identifying patients who, despite having a positive SLN, have a low probability of metastatic disease in non-SLNs.

In an analysis of primary tumor and SLN characteristics, the number of SLNs harvested, the Breslow thickness of the primary tumor, and SLN burden (largest focus of metastasis, total area of metastases, number of metastatic foci, and extracapsular extension) most accurately predicted the presence of tumor in non-SLNs. These features alone and in combination predicted the presence of tumor in non-SLNs with high accuracy. Although these results are intriguing and warrant further study, decisions regarding completion lymphadenectomy cannot yet be made strictly on the basis of primary tumor or SLN characteristics. Completion lymphadenectomy following identification of a positive SLN remains the current standard of care. The Multicenter Selective Lymphadenectomy Trial II (MSLT-II) seeks to answer this question by randomizing patients to nodal observation or completion lymphadenectomy after a positive SLN.

Current Practice Guidelines for the Use of Sentinel Lymph Node Biopsy
Candidates for SLN biopsy include patients with newly diagnosed clinically node-negative primary melanoma who are predicted to be at intermediate or high risk of harboring occult regional nodal disease based on primary tumor characteristics. Although uniform risk thresholds have not been completely resolved, a tumor thickness threshold of at least 1 mm has gained wide acceptance. While routine use of SLN biopsy in patients with thin (<1 mm) melanoma is not indicated because of the overall low risk of nodal involvement in this group, a selective approach to SLN biopsy for patients with thin melanoma has evolved in many centers on the basis of the presence of at least one of the following adverse risk factors of the primary melanoma: ulceration, ≥ 1 mitosis per mm^2, lymphovascular invasion, invasion of the reticular dermis (Clark IV) or subcutaneous tissue (Clark V), or a thickness of at least 0.75 mm. The use of the Clark level IV and V as an indication for SLNB is an area of controversy as is the presence of regression in the primary specimen. In addition, a positive deep margin on review of the biopsy specimen should be part of the consideration to perform a SLN since a biopsy with a positive deep margin may lead to underestimation of the thickness of the primary melanoma. The National Comprehensive Cancer Network (NCCN) guidelines recommend performing SLNB on patients who are stage IB (≤ 1.00 mm thick with ulceration or a mitotic rate ≥ 1 mitosis per mm^2, or 1.01 to 2.00 mm thick without ulceration) or stage II (1.01 to 2.00 mm thick with ulceration, or >2.00 mm thick). In addition, while acknowledging that there is no consensus, the guidelines recommend considering SLNBs in Stage IA patients who have concerning characteristics like Breslow thickness of 0.75 mm, positive deep margins, lymphovascular invasion or Clark level IV or V. The NCCN does not recommend SLNB in low-risk patients such as those who have a Breslow thickness of <0.5 mm and <2 mitoses per mm^2 unless there are specific clinical indications (NCCN version 4.2011).

The presence of clinically evident lymphadenopathy at the time of diagnosis obviates the need for SLNB, as these patients will generally receive TLNDs in the absence of synchronous distant metastasis.

When the SLNs are negative, no further surgery is performed, and the remaining regional lymph nodes are left intact. When the SLNs show evidence of metastatic disease, completion lymphadenectomy of the affected nodal basin is the current standard of care. Pathological evaluation of completion lymphadenectomy specimens often reveals no additional disease. However, it is important to remember that completion lymphadenectomy specimens are routinely assessed with standard histologic techniques rather than the more rigorous examination reserved for SLNB specimens. As a result, there may actually be additional disease in the completion nodal specimen that goes undetected. This disease would, in theory, represent a potential source of subsequent recurrence if it were not removed. Because such recurrences are difficult to treat surgically and may contribute to significant morbidity, completion lymphadenectomy performed for microscopic disease provides the potential for improved regional control. In addition, identifying patients with minimal disease burden by using the SLN approach may help identify the group of patients who may derive an improved survival benefit from early TLND. Furthermore, knowledge of the pathological status of the

SLNs allows proper staging and thus facilitates decision-making regarding adjuvant treatment. (See also MSLT-II trial earlier.)

Morbidity of Lymph Node Surgery

Complications associated with SLNB for melanoma were evaluated in 2,120 patients in an analysis of data from the Sunbelt Melanoma Trial. Overall, 96 (4.6%) of the patients developed major or minor complications associated with SLNB, whereas 103 (23.3%) of 444 patients experienced complications associated with SLNB plus completion lymph node dissection. The authors concluded that SLNB alone is associated with significantly less morbidity compared with SLNB plus completion lymph node dissection. Similar to the Sunbelt Melanoma Trial, in MSLT-1, SLNB did not significantly add much to the morbidity of melanoma surgery as compared with wide excision of the primary melanoma alone. However, SLNs cannot always be identified.

Formal lymphadenectomy is associated with higher complications rates, particularly in the inguinal region. Cormier et al., prospectively followed 53 patients at MD Anderson Cancer who underwent inguinal lymphadenectomy for melanoma and found the acute wound complication rate to be 77.4% with a wound infection rate of 54.7% and a wound dehiscence rate of 52.8%. In multivariate analysis, only body mass index was found to be associated with an increase in complications. The infection rate reported after lymphadenectomy in MSLT-1 was 12%.

The study also noted that lymphedema varied significantly depending on the lymph nodes basins that were dissected (i.e., 9.0% for axillary lymphadenectomy vs. 26.6% for inguinal lymphadenectomy.) Lymphedema is among the most serious long-term complications of formal lymphadenectomy. Inguinal lymphadenectomy–associated lymphedema was not altered significantly by the addition of a deep groin dissection. In addition, the number of lymph nodes removed did not appear to alter the lymphedema rate significantly. In the study by Cormier et al., the lymphedema rate at 3-months was 85% using qualitative measures and 45% by quantitative measures for patients who underwent inguinal lymphadenectomy. Three series have shown that the incidence of lower extremity edema after groin dissection can be decreased by preventive measures, including perioperative antibiotics, elastic stockings, leg elevation exercises, and diuretics. Even with preventive measures, lymphedema can still develop. Prophylactic measures are important because reversing the progression of edema is difficult.

The complication rate for axillary lymph node dissections is lower in comparison to inguinal dissections. The most frequent complication is wound seroma that varies from 3% to 23%. Other common complications include cellulitis and lymphedema (approximately 10%). For all types of lymph node dissections, skin flap problems can occur. Expectant management of ischemic edges may result in full-thickness necrosis and prolonged hospitalization. Therefore, if skin flap edges are of questionable viability, the patient may be returned to the operating room early for flap revision.

Technical Considerations

Axillary Dissection

General. Axillary dissection must be complete and include levels I, II, and III lymph nodes (Fig. 3.6). The arm, shoulder, and chest are prepared and included in the surgical field.

Incision. We use a horizontal, slightly S-shaped incision beginning anteriorly along the superior portion of the pectoralis major muscle, traversing the axilla over the fourth rib, and extending inferiorly along the anterior border of the latissimus dorsi muscle. The incision should be constructed so that previous scars are removed with the specimen.

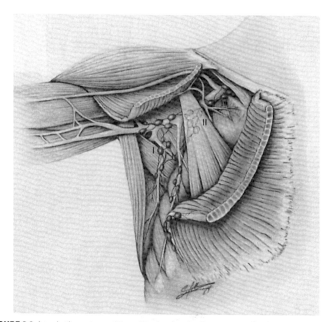

FIGURE 3.6 Lymphatic anatomy of the axilla showing the three groups of axillary lymph nodes defined by their relationship to the pectoralis minor muscle. The highest axillary nodes (level III) medial to the pectoralis minor muscle should be included in an axillary lymph node dissection for melanoma. (From Balch CM, Milton GW, Shaw HM, et al., eds. *Cutaneous Melanoma.* Philadelphia, PA: Lippincott; 1985, with permission.)

Skin Flaps. Skin flaps are raised anteriorly to the midclavicular line, inferiorly to the sixth rib, posteriorly to the anterior border of the latissimus dorsi muscle, and superiorly to just below the pectoralis major insertion. The medial side of the latissimus dorsi muscle is dissected free from the specimen, exposing the thoracodorsal vessels and nerve. The lateral edge of the dissection then proceeds cephalad beneath the axillary vein. These maneuvers allow the remainder of the dissection to proceed from medial to lateral. The fatty and lymphatic tissue over the pectoralis major muscle is dissected free around to its undersurface, where the pectoralis minor muscle is encountered. The interpectoral groove is exposed.

Lymph Node Dissection. The medial pectoral nerve is preserved. The interpectoral nodes are dissected free. The upper axilla is exposed by bringing the patient's arm over the chest by adduction and internal rotation. If nodes are bulky, the pectoralis minor muscle may be divided to facilitate exposure. Dissection proceeds from the apex of the axilla inferolaterally. Dissection of the upper axillary lymph nodes should be sufficiently complete that the thoracic outlet beneath the clavicle, Halsted's ligament, and subclavius muscle are seen (Fig. 3.7). Fatty and lymphatic tissues are dissected downward over the axillary vein. The apex of the dissected specimen may be tagged. Dissection then continues until the thoracodorsal vessels and the long thoracic and thoracodorsal nerves are identified. The fatty tissue between the two nerves is separated from the subscapularis muscle. The specimen

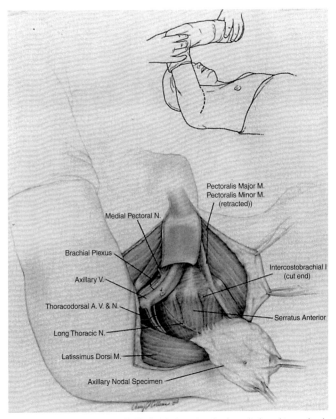

FIGURE 3.7 Access to the upper axilla. The arm is draped so that it can be brought over the chest wall during the operation. This facilitates retraction of the pectoralis muscles upward to reveal the level III axillary lymph nodes. (From Balch CM, Milton GW, Shaw HM, et al., eds. *Cutaneous Melanoma*. Philadelphia, PA: Lippincott; 1985, with permission.)

is removed from the lateral chest wall. Intercostobrachial nerves traversing the specimen are sacrificed. The specimen is swept off the latissimus dorsi and serratus anterior muscles.

Wound Closure. One 15 F closed-suction catheter is placed percutaneously through the inferior flap into the axilla. An additional catheter may be inserted through the inferior flap and placed over the pectoralis major muscle. The skin is closed with interrupted 3-0 undyed absorbable sutures and running 4-0 subcuticular undyed absorbable sutures.

Postoperative Management. Suction drainage is continued until output is less than 30 mL per day for two consecutive days. By approximately 3–4 weeks, the suction catheters are removed, regardless of the amount of drainage, to avoid infection. Any subsequent collections of serum are removed by needle aspiration. Mobilization of the arm is discouraged during the first 7 to 10 days after surgery. Over the ensuing 4 weeks, gradual mobilization of the arm is encouraged.

Superficial Groin Dissection

General. For groin dissection, the patient is placed in a slight frog-leg position with hip externally rotated and the knee flexed.

Incision. A reverse lazy-S incision is made from superomedial to the anterior superior iliac spine, vertically down to the inguinal crease, obliquely across the crease, and then vertically down to the apex of the femoral triangle. Previous SLNB sites should be excised with the specimen.

Skin Flaps. The limits of the skin flaps are medially to the pubic tubercle and the midbody of the adductor magnus muscle, laterally to the lateral edge of the sartorius muscle, superiorly to above the inguinal ligament, and inferiorly to the apex of the femoral triangle.

Lymph Node Dissection. Dissection is carried down to the muscular fascia superiorly (Fig. 3.8). All fatty, node-bearing tissue is swept down to the inguinal ligament and

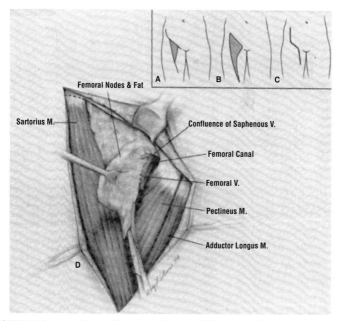

FIGURE 3.8 Technique of inguinal lymph node dissection. **(A)** The borders of the femoral triangle are the inguinal ligament superiorly, the sartorius laterally, and, the adductor longus medially. **(B)** The lymphatic contents removed during a superficial inguinal lymphadenectomy include the lymphatic contents of the femoral triangle as well as nodal tissue that lies superficial to the external oblique superior to the inguinal ligament. **(C)** The lazy S incision used for an inguinal lymphadenectomy. **(D)** The anatomy visualized during an inguinal lymphadenectomy. (From Balch CM, Milton GW, Shaw HM, et al., eds. *Cutaneous Melanoma.* Philadelphia, PA: Lippincott; 1985, with permission.)

off the external oblique fascia. Medially, the spermatic cord or round ligament is exposed, and nodal tissue is swept laterally. Nodal tissue is swept off the adductor fascia to the femoral vein. At the apex of the femoral triangle, the saphenous vein is identified. If the saphenous vein can be preserved, nodal tissue is removed from the vessel circumferentially: otherwise, it is sacrificed. Laterally, nodal tissue is dissected off the sartorius muscle and the femoral nerve. With dissection in the plane of the femoral vessels, the nodal tissue is elevated up to the level of the fossa ovalis, where the saphenous vein is suture-ligated at the saphenofemoral junction if it is sacrificed. The specimen is dissected to beneath the inguinal ligament, where it is divided. Cloquet's node (the lowest iliac node) is sent as a separate specimen for frozen-section examination (Fig. 3.9).

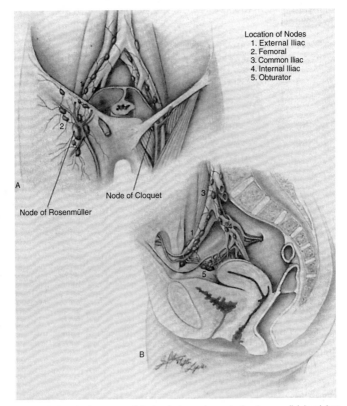

Location of Nodes
1. External Iliac
2. Femoral
3. Common Iliac
4. Internal Iliac
5. Obturator

Node of Cloquet

Node of Rosenmüller

FIGURE 3.9 A: Lymphatic anatomy of the inguinal area demonstrating the superficial and deep lymphatic chains. Cloquet's node lies at the transition between the superficial and deep inguinal nodes. It is located beneath the inguinal ligament in the femoral canal. **B:** The iliac nodes include those on the common and superficial iliac vessels and the obturator nodes. Obturator nodes should be excised as part of an iliac nodal dissection. (From Balch CM, Milton GW, Shaw HM, et al., eds. *Cutaneous Melanoma.* Philadelphia, PA: Lippincott; 1985, with permission.)

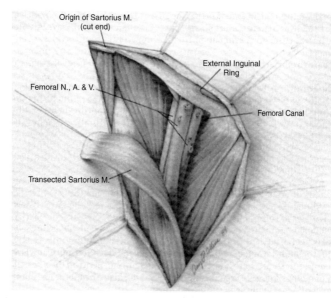

FIGURE 3.10 Transection of the sartorius muscle at its origin on the anterior superior iliac spine in preparation for transposition over the femoral vessels and nerves. (From Balch CM, Milton GW, Shaw HM, et al., eds. *Cutaneous Melanoma.* Philadelphia, PA: Lippincott; 1985, with permission.)

Sartorius Muscle Transposition. The sartorius muscle is divided at its origin on the anterior superior iliac spine (Fig. 3.10). The lateral femoral cutaneous nerve is preserved. The proximal two or three neurovascular bundles going to the sartorius muscle are divided to facilitate transposition. The muscle is placed over the femoral vessels and tacked to the inguinal ligament, fascia of the adductor, and vastus muscle groups.

Wound Closure. The skin edges are examined for viability and trimmed back to healthy skin, if necessary. Intravenous administration of fluorescein followed by examination using a Wood lamp may be used to identify poorly perfused skin edges. Two closed-suction drains are placed through separate small incisions inferiorly. One is laid medially and the other is laid laterally within the operative wound. The wound is closed with interrupted 3-0 undyed absorbable sutures in the dermis and followed by skin staples.

Postoperative Management. The patient begins ambulating the day following surgery; a custom-fit elastic stocking may be used during the day for 6 months. After this period, the stocking may be discontinued if no leg swelling occurs. Suction drainage is continued until output is less than 30 mL per day for two consecutive days. By approximately 3 to 4 weeks, the suction catheters are removed, regardless of the amount of drainage, to avoid infection.

Dissection of the Iliac and Obturator Nodes

General. We generally perform deep dissection—dissection of the iliac and obturator nodes—for the following indications: (a) known involvement of the nodes revealed by preoperative imaging studies, (b) more than three grossly positive nodes in the superficial lymph node dissection specimen, or (c) metastatic disease in Cloquet's node by frozen-section examination.

Incision. To gain access to the deep nodes, we extend the skin incision superiorly.

Lymph Node Dissection. The external oblique muscle is split from a point superomedial to the anterior superior iliac spine to the lateral border of the rectus sheath. The internal oblique and transversus abdominis muscles are divided, and the peritoneum is retracted superiorly. An alternative approach is to split the inguinal ligament vertically, medial to the femoral vein. The ureter is exposed as it courses over the iliac artery. Dissection continues in front of the external iliac artery to separate the external iliac nodes. The inferior epigastric artery and vein are divided, if necessary. Dissection of the lymph nodes continues to the bifurcation of the common iliac artery. Nodes in front of the external iliac vein are dissected to the point at which the internal iliac vein proceeds under the internal iliac artery. The plane of the peritoneum is traced along the wall of the bladder, and the fatty tissues and lymph nodes are dissected off the perivesical fat starting at the internal iliac artery. Dissection is completed on the medial wall of the external iliac vein, and the nodal chain is further separated from the pelvic fascia until the obturator nerve is seen. Obturator nodes are located in the space between the external iliac vein and the obturator nerve (in an anteroposterior direction) and between the internal iliac artery and the obturator foramen (in a cephalad–caudad direction). The obturator artery and vein usually need not be disturbed.

Wound Closure. The transversus abdominis, internal oblique, and external oblique muscles may be closed with running sutures. The inguinal ligament, if previously divided, is approximated with interrupted nonabsorbable sutures to Cooper's ligament medially and to the iliac fascia lateral to the femoral vessels. A closed suction drain is placed in the deep pelvis space exiting through a separate small incision.

Postoperative Management. Suction drainage is continued until output is less than 30 mL per day for two consecutive days. The pelvic drain is usually removed prior to hospital discharge. Ambulation is encouraged the day after surgery. Patients are hospitalized postoperatively for expectant management of potential ileus after deep pelvic surgery and pain control.

Neck Dissection

Lymph node metastases from melanomas in the head and neck were previously believed to follow a predictable pattern. However, it is now known that lymphatic drainage from melanomas of the head and neck can be multidirectional and unpredictable. ELND or SLNB may be misdirected in as many as 59% of patients if the operation is based on classic anatomical studies without preoperative lymphoscintigraphy. These findings strongly support the use of lymphoscintigraphy in patients with melanomas in the head and neck.

At MD Anderson Cancer Center, the treatment of choice for patients with melanoma in the head and neck region and clinically involved nodes is wide local excision of the primary lesion with either modified radical neck dissection or selective neck dissection, followed by adjunctive radiation therapy.

Melanomas arising on the scalp or face anterior to the pinna of the ear and superior to the commissure of the lip can metastasize to intraparotid lymph nodes because these nodes are contiguous with the cervical nodes. When intraparotid nodes are clinically involved, it is advisable to combine neck dissection with parotid lymph node dissection and then administer radiation therapy.

SPECIAL CLINICAL SITUATIONS

Giant Congenital Nevi

A giant congenital nevus has been defined as a nevus that measures at least 15 cm in diameter or at least twice the size of the affected person's palm. Patients with giant congenital nevi have an estimated 4% to 10% lifetime risk of developing a melanoma. Half of the melanomas that develop in giant congenital nevi develop within the first 5 years of life. Decisions about the management of giant congenital nevi are difficult because such lesions are often so extensive that prophylactic surgical excision is impossible. When the location and size of a lesion permit prophylactic excision, excision should be considered before the age of 2 years. Although data are limited, potential negative prognostic indicators that may aid in decision-making include large size and the presence of satellite lesions.

Metastatic Melanoma of Unknown Primary Site

1.1% to 8.8% of patients with melanoma present with metastatic disease from melanoma of unknown primary (MUP) site. Various reasons have been proposed for the phenomenon of melanoma of unknown primary site. Anbari et al. suggested the following possibilities for primary lesions: an unrecognized melanoma, a treated melanoma that had been initially misdiagnosed, a spontaneously regressed melanoma, and malignant transformation of a melanocyte that had travelled to a metastatic location. In order for metastatic melanoma to be classified as melanoma of unknown primary site, the histologic diagnosis must be confirmed, previous excisions, if any, should be evaluated for a possible diagnosis of melanoma, and less common primary sites for melanoma must be thoroughly evaluated. The most common presentation is in the axillary lymph node basin (>50%). The next most common presentation site is the cervical lymph node basin.

Several studies have compared these patients with similar cohorts having equivalent nodal status and a known primary site for recurrence and survival. Although patients with unknown primary tumors were historically believed to have worse prognoses, several recent large studies have contradicted these earlier findings. Patients with metastatic melanoma and an unknown primary tumor must be examined carefully from scalp to toes for a potential primary tumor site. Furthermore, careful pathologic review should be performed to ensure that an unusual presentation of a primary lesion is not confused for a nodal metastasis. To study this subgroup of patients, strict criteria were established in the course of retrospective analyses to exclude patients with primary tumors that have been missed (Table 3.6).

In a study from the University of Texas MD Anderson Cancer Center, Cormier et al. conducted a retrospective analysis of consecutive patients (from 1990 to 2001) with melanoma metastatic to regional lymph nodes. Among these patients, 71 patients

---

TABLE 3.6	Metastatic Melanoma of Unknown Primary: Stringent Definition of Patient Population

Exclude patients with any of the following:

- History of having had a mole, birthmark, freckle, chronic paronychia, or skin blemish previously excised, electrodesiccated, or cauterized
- Metastatic melanoma in one of the node-bearing areas and presentation with a scar indicating previous local treatment in the skin area drained by this lymphatic basin
- No recorded physical examination of anus and genitalia
- Previous orbital enucleation or exenteration

with MUP and 466 controlled patients who had regional lymph node metastases of a similar stage with a known primary site were identified. The authors found that after they underwent lymph node dissection, patients with MUP were classified with N1b disease (47%), N2b disease (14%), or N3 disease (39%). With a median follow-up of 7.7 years, the 5-year and 10-year overall survival rates were 55% and 44%, respectively, for patients with MUP, compared with 42% and 32%, respectively, for the control group ($P = 0.04$). By multivariate analyses, age 50 years or older, male gender, and N2b or N3 disease status were identified as adverse prognostics factors, and MUP was identified as a favorable prognostic factor (hazard ratio 0.61; 95% CI, 0.42 to 0.86; $P = 0.006$) for overall survival. The authors concluded that the relatively favorable long-term survival of patients with MUP in this study has a natural history that is similar to (if not better than) the survival of many patients with stage III disease. Therefore, patients with MUP should be treated with an aggressive surgical approach with curative intent and should be considered for stage III adjuvant therapy protocols. Similar results were found at the John Wayne Cancer Center, in which Lee et al. retrospectively evaluated 1,571 patients who had palpable nodal metastases with known or unknown primaries. Five-year overall survival was approximately 55% among patients with unknown primaries versus approximately 44% for those with known primaries. Other negative prognostic determinants were age ≥60 years, male gender, and nodal tumor burden. The authors suggested that host immunologic response against the primary lesion could explain this difference.

For patients with melanoma of unknown primary site, surgical resection should be considered. Patients should have a thorough history taken and physical examination with a focus on evaluating for any history of lesions being excised or otherwise destroyed and an evaluation for melanoma that may have been unrecognized. In particular, if the metastatic lesion is to a lymph node basin, the drainage areas of that lymphatic basin should undergo particularly rigorous examination. Furthermore, patients should undergo staging evaluation with CT of the chest, abdomen, and pelvis, and MRI of the brain. Along these lines, patients with nodal disease should be staged as stage III and treated in an aggressive surgical fashion similar to other stage III patients since these patients have survival rates similar to stage III patients with known primaries.

Desmoplastic Melanoma

Desmoplastic melanoma is an uncommon histologic variant of melanoma that is characterized by unusual spindle-cell morphology and the presence of fusiform melanocytes dispersed in a prominent collagenous stroma. In fact, the rarity of the lesion makes it often misdiagnosed as benign. Classically presenting as a thick primary tumor, desmoplastic melanoma has been associated with a higher incidence of local recurrence than nondesmoplastic melanoma. Histologically, desmoplastic melanoma may display morphologic heterogeneity. Specifically, some desmoplastic melanomas are characterized by a uniform desmoplasia that is prominent throughout the entire tumor ("pure" desmoplastic melanoma), whereas other desmoplastic melanomas appear to arise in association with other histologic subtypes ("mixed" desmoplastic melanoma). Distinguishing the phenotypic heterogeneity of desmoplastic melanomas is important for stratifying patients with regard to rate of lymph node metastasis and prognosis. In 2006, Pawlik et al. published results from 1,850 patients in which those with pure desmoplastic melanoma had a much lower incidence of positive SLNs than patients with mixed desmoplastic melanoma or nondesmoplastic melanoma. Although some authors have reported a worse prognosis for patients with desmoplastic melanoma, the majority of studies have described a better prognosis for patients with desmoplastic melanoma compared with patients who have nondesmoplastic melanoma of similar stage. In a few studies in which pure desmoplastic melanoma was differentiated from mixed desmoplastic melanoma, patients with mixed desmoplastic melanoma had a greater risk of death or metastatic disease than patients with the pure form. Some desmoplastic tumors are noted to have perineural invasion, which increases their tendency for local recurrence. Adjuvant radiation can be considered in these cases.

ADJUVANT THERAPY FOR LOCOREGIONAL DISEASE

Interferon Alfa-2b

High-dose IFN alfa-2b is approved by the U.S. Food and Drug Administration as adjuvant treatment for patients with melanoma who have a high risk of recurrence. Patients with locally advanced, recurrent, nodal, in-transit, or satellite disease should be considered candidates for adjuvant high-dose IFN alfa-2b.

Approval of IFN alfa-2b was based on the results of the Eastern Cooperative Oncology Group (ECOG) E1684 prospective randomized trial, which assigned 287 patients to high-dose IFN alfa-2b or observation after wide local excision. The IFN alfa-2b dosage was 20 million units/m^2/day intravenously for 4 weeks followed by 10 million units per m^2 three times a week subcutaneously for the next 48 weeks. Both node-positive and high-risk node-negative (T4pN0) patients were included; the majority of patients had experienced recurrence of disease in the regional nodes after prior wide local excision. All patients underwent either ELND or TLND. Of the 287 patients enrolled, 89% were node positive. IFN alfa-2b improved median overall survival from 2.8 to 3.8 years and improved 5-year relapse-free survival (RFS) rates from 26% to 37% at a median follow-up of 7 years. The beneficial effect of IFN alfa-2b was most pronounced in the node-positive patients. Of note, the rate of toxic effects was high: Two patients died, 67% of patients experienced grade 3 toxic effects, and 50% of patients either stopped treatment early or required dose reduction.

A recent updated analysis of E1684, at a median follow-up of 12.6 years, showed a persistent gain in median disease-free survival (45.8 months for the IFN alfa-2b arm vs. 32 months for observation). The overall survival difference, however, was no longer statistically significant, possibly because deaths from intercurrent illness on both arms overshadowed melanoma-specific mortality.

The E1690 trial, another ECOG trial, was initiated before a significant impact on survival had been noted in E1684. In E1690, designed as a confirmation and extension of E1684, 642 patients with high-risk (stage IIb or III) melanoma were randomized in a three-arm study to receive the E1684 high-dose regimen, low-dose IFN alfa-2b (3 million units per m^2 three times a week for 2 years), or observation only. Seventy-five percent of the patients had nodal metastases (50% had recurrent disease in the regional nodes). Unlike E1684, E1690 allowed entry of patients with T4 primary tumors, regardless of whether lymph node dissection was performed, and 25% of the patients in the trial had deep primary tumors (compared with 11% in E1684).

In E1690, at a median follow-up of 52 months, high-dose IFN alfa-2b demonstrated a RFS benefit exceeding that of low-dose IFN alfa-2b or observation. The 5-year estimated RFS rates for high-dose IFN alfa-2b, low-dose IFN alfa-2b, and observation were 44%, 40%, and 35%, respectively ($P = 0.03$). The RFS benefit was equivalent for node-negative and node-positive patients. As of this writing, neither high-dose nor low-dose IFN alfa-2b has demonstrated an overall survival benefit compared with observation.

An analysis of salvage therapy for patients whose disease relapsed on E1690 demonstrated that a significantly larger proportion of patients in the observation arm than in the high-dose IFN arm received IFN alfa-containing salvage therapy, which may have confounded interpretation of the survival benefit of assigned treatments. Some of the discrepancy between the findings of E1684 and E1690 may be attributable to differences in patient demographic profiles. E1690 included patients with more favorable disease characteristics: only 75% of patients were node positive, and of these, 51% had nodal recurrence. In E1690, 25% of patients enrolled were clinical stage II; in E1684, 11% were pathological stage II. Presumably, some of the clinical stage II patients in E1690 would have been pathological stage III had lymphadenectomy been required. An updated analysis of E1690 with a median follow-up of 7.2 years has confirmed the study's original conclusions. Furthermore, pooled analysis of ECOG 1684 and ECOG 1690, demonstrated that high-dose IFN led to improved disease-free survival versus placebo, but there remained no benefit with regards to overall survival.

ECOG trial E1694 was initiated to compare the efficacy and safety of a ganglioside vaccine with the efficacy and safety of high-dose IFN alfa-2b in patients with stage IIb or stage III melanoma. The ganglioside GM2 is a serologically well-defined melanoma antigen and the most immunogenic ganglioside expressed on melanoma cells. Preliminary studies had suggested that the antibody response to GM2 was correlated with relapse-free and overall survival. In E1694, 774 eligible patients with high-risk melanoma (tumor thickness >4.0 mm or regional lymph node metastasis) were randomized to receive high-dose IFN alfa-2b or GM2 vaccine. The study was closed early by the data safety monitoring board because of the clear superiority of IFN alfa-2b in terms of both disease-free and overall survival. The estimated 2-year RFS rates were 62% in the high-dose IFN alfa-2b arm and 49% in the GM2 vaccine arm. Furthermore, analysis of the hazard of relapse and death in subgroups based on the number of lymph nodes demonstrated the superiority of IFN alfa-2b over GM2 in all nodal subsets. E1694 also showed a statistically significant benefit for IFN alfa-2b in node-negative high-risk patients.

A pooled meta-analysis of primary data from the ECOG/Intergroup trials of high-dose IFN ($n = 1,916$) revealed a clear benefit of high-dose IFN alfa-2b in terms of RFS and a more modest benefit in terms of overall survival (odds ratio = 0.9, $P = 0.05$). Data from an updated analysis of the ECOG database demonstrated that (a) the survival impact of IFN alfa-2b was confined to regimens that incorporated both high-dose induction and high-dose subcutaneous maintenance; (b) reduction of hazard was observed early; and (c) the RFS advantage was sustained off treatment, in contrast to the more limited RFS advantage reported by the low-dose trials.

Results of trials investigating low-dose IFN alfa-2b have been disappointing. The previously mentioned E1690 trial, a three-arm trial that included low-dose IFN alfa-2b as one of the treatments, demonstrated no significant improvement in RFS in patients with high-risk stage II or stage III melanoma who received low-dose IFN alfa-2b for 2 years. The modest improvement in the low-dose IFN alfa-2b arm compared with the control arm disappeared within 2 years after therapy was stopped. The European Organization for Research and Treatment of Cancer (EORTC) 18871 trial also demonstrated that a regimen of very low-dose IFN alfa-2b (1 million units per m^2) injected subcutaneously on alternate days for 1 year did not affect overall survival for patients with high-risk melanoma. Because of the lack of a demonstrable durable clinical benefit, low-dose IFN alfa-2b has not been approved as adjuvant therapy for melanoma in the United States. Similarly, intermediate dose interferon was studied with EORTC 18952. No disease-free or overall survival benefits were demonstrated.

In March 2011, the FDA approved PEG-IFN alfa-2b for the adjuvant treatment of melanoma with microscopic or gross nodal involvement. The treatment is to be started within 84 days of definitive surgical resection including complete lymphadenectomy. The medication is dosed as a once-weekly subcutaneous injection that may be self-injected. The recommended dose is 6 µg/kg/week subcutaneously for 8 doses, followed by 3 µg/kg/week subcutaneously for up to 5 years. Approval was based on EORTC 18991, an open label, multicenter trial that enrolled 1,256 patients. Patients who had adequate surgical resection of their primary cutaneous melanoma and affected regional lymph nodes were randomized to receive either PEG-IFN alfa-2b or observation for a 5-year period. Stratification factors included type of nodal involvement (microscopic vs. gross), number of positive nodes (1, 2 to 4, 5 or more, or not assessed), Breslow primary thickness (<1.5 mm, ≥1.5 to 4 mm, ≥4 mm), ulceration of primary tumor (present or absent or unknown), sex, and study center. Patients were assessed for local and regional recurrence or distant metastases every 3 months for the first 2 years of treatment and subsequently every 6 months through the end of the trial. Improved RFS was seen in the PEG-IFN alfa-2b cohort compared to the observation group (hazard ratio 0.82 [95% CI: 0.71, 0.96]; unstratified log-rank $P = 0.011$). The estimated median RFS was 34.8 months (95% CI: 26.1, 47.4) and 25.5 months (95% CI: 19.6, 30.8) in the PEG-IFN alfa2b and observation arms, respectively. However, there was no difference in overall survival seen between the two groups (hazard ratio 0.98 [95% CI: 0.82, 1.16]). A total of 33% of patients receiving PEG-IFN alfa-2b discontinued treatment due to adverse reactions. The most common adverse reactions present at the time of treatment discontinuation were fatigue, depression, anorexia, increased ALT, increased AST, myalgia, nausea, headache, and pyrexia.

Chemotherapy

No studies have demonstrated a benefit of adjuvant chemotherapy in patients with melanoma who are at high risk for relapse. On the contrary, a randomized trial of adjuvant dacarbazine versus no treatment showed a statistically significant decrease in survival in the adjuvant treatment arm. Adjuvant chemotherapy should be considered only in the context of a clinical trial.

Monoclonal Antibodies

The role of monoclonal antibodies for the treatment of melanoma is now being studied in the adjuvant setting. E1609, a phase III randomized trial, is enrolling resected high-risk patients who are being randomized to receive either ipilimumab (see below) or high-dose interferon α-2b in the adjuvant setting. The results of this study are eagerly anticipated.

MANAGEMENT OF IN-TRANSIT DISEASE

Traditionally, in-transit disease has been described as recurrent locoregional disease found in the dermis or subcutaneous tissue more than 2 cm away from the primary melanoma but before the regional lymph node basin. This pattern of recurrence is unique to melanoma and is reported to occur in 3% to 10% of melanoma cases. Although the molecular determinants and pathophysiology of in-transit disease are poorly understood, in-transit recurrences are likely an intralymphatic manifestation of melanoma metastases. Independent predictors of in-transit recurrence include age older than 50 years, a lower-extremity primary tumor, increasing tumor thickness, ulceration, and nodal involvement. Regional nodal metastases occur in about two-thirds of patients with in-transit disease and, if present, are associated with lower survival rates. Predictors of distant recurrence among patients with in-transit recurrence include positive SLN status, in-transit tumor size of at least 2 cm, and disease-free interval before in-transit recurrence of less than 12 months. Interestingly, recent data suggest that patients who present with synchronous, distant, and in-transit disease have a worse disease-specific survival compared with patients who present with only in-transit or distant disease.

Some have suggested that dissection of the regional nodal basin—by either SLNB (see section below) or complete lymphadenectomy—increases the risk of in-transit metastases. These authors hypothesize that dissection disturbs lymph flow, leading to deposition of metastatic cells in the intervening lymphatic vessels. A critical analysis of the data, however, provides compelling evidence that neither SLNB nor completion lymph node dissection in SLN-positive patients increases the incidence of in-transit metastases. In a collaborative review by MD Anderson Cancer Center and the Sydney Melanoma Unit of 3,400 patients with primary melanomas at least 1 mm thick treated over a 10-year period at the Sydney Melanoma Unit, there was no significant difference in the rate of in-transit metastases between patients treated with wide local excision alone (4.9%) and those treated with wide local excision and SLNB (4.5%). Because the two groups were similar in terms of median tumor depth, rate of ulceration, and Clark level, these data strongly support the concept that early nodal intervention has little impact on the natural history of in-transit metastases. In a separate study of 1,395 patients from The University of Texas MD Anderson Cancer Center, patients with a positive SLN had a significantly higher rate of in-transit metastases (12%) than patients with a negative SLN (3.5%). Taken together, these data indicate that biology—not surgical technique—establishes the risk of in-transit metastases.

For patients with in-transit metastases confined to a limb that are not amenable to standard surgical measures (e.g., patients with recurrent and/or multiple in-transit metastases and patients with large-burden in-transit disease), regional chemotherapy techniques such as isolated limb perfusion or, more recently, isolated limb infusion may be considered. Amputation is rarely indicated.

Hyperthermic Isolated Limb Perfusion

Hyperthermic isolated limb perfusion with melphalan has been used to treat in-transit metastases of the extremities since the mid-1950s. With this procedure, a formal lymph node dissection is performed which provides exposure to the critical vessels of interest. Subsequently, cannulae are inserted and the extremity is placed on an extracorporeal bypass circuit after a tourniquet is inflated effectively isolating the limb from systemic circulation. Melphalan is currently the most active single agent for use in hyperthermic isolated limb perfusion. Overall response rates of 7% to 80% (complete response rate, 46%; partial response rate, 34%) can be achieved, and the median response duration in patients with a complete response ranges from 9 to 19 months. Nonrandomized studies of hyperthermic limb perfusion by Lienard et al. reported a high complete response rate (90%) with a combination of melphalan, tumor necrosis factor-α (TNF-α), and interferon-γ (IFN-γ) and a somewhat lower response rate with melphalan alone (52%). The durability of these responses has not been reported. Fraker et al. reported a 100% response rate in patients treated with melphalan alone and a 90% response rate in patients treated with melphalan, IFN-γ, and TNF-α, although the latter combination resulted in a higher complete response rate (80% vs. 61%). A multicenter randomized trial sponsored by the American College of Surgeons Oncology Group comparing melphalan alone with a combination of melphalan and TNF-α for patients who have in-transit metastases was closed to accrual early because an interim analysis failed to reveal a benefit for TNF-α. As a result, TNF-α is not currently being used in the United States in isolated limb perfusion procedures.

The routine use of hyperthermic isolated limb perfusion in the adjuvant setting has marginal, if any, benefit. Although a randomized multicenter phase III trial of 86 patients (Hafstrom et al.) showed increased disease-free interval in patients with in-transit metastases and regional lymph node metastasis, this effect was transient and predominantly occurred in patients with a more favorable prognosis (tumor thickness of 1.5 to 2.99 mm). This study showed no benefit of isolated limb perfusion with respect to time to distant metastasis or survival duration.

Although hyperthermic isolated limb perfusion may be effective as primary treatment for in-transit metastases, the isolated limb perfusion technique involves a complex and invasive operative procedure entailing expensive equipment, long operating times, and considerable ancillary staff. In an attempt to achieve similar results using less complex techniques, a new regional chemotherapy technique, isolated limb infusion, has recently been developed for the management of in-transit metastases.

Isolated Limb Infusion

Isolated limb infusion is essentially a low-flow isolated limb perfusion performed via percutaneously inserted catheters but without oxygenation of the circuit (Fig. 3.11). Using standard radiologic techniques, catheters are inserted percutaneously into the main artery and vein of the unaffected limb (or they can be placed in the main artery and vein in the affected limb, i.e., brachial or popliteal artery and vein) and delivered intravascularly to the tumor-bearing extremity. Under general anesthesia, after a pneumatic tourniquet is inflated proximally, cytotoxic agents

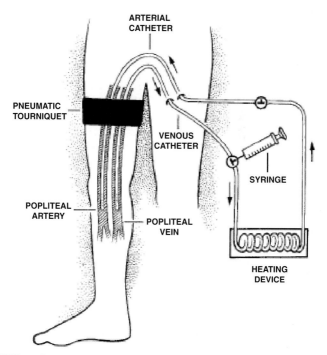

FIGURE 3.11 Schematic drawing depicting an isolated limb infusion. The catheters are typically placed percutaneously by an interventional radiologist via the contralateral extremity, with the catheter tips positioned in the tumor-bearing extremity just below the inguinal ligament in the superficial femoral artery and vein. After inflation of the tourniquet, chemotherapy is manually infused for 20 to 30 minutes, after which the limb is washed out with normal saline. (Reprinted from Lindner P, Doubrovsky A, Kam PC, et al. Prognostic factors after isolated limb infusion with cytotoxic agents for melanoma. *Ann Surg Oncol.* 2002;9:127–136, with permission.)

(generally melphalan and actinomycin-D) are infused through the arterial catheter and "hand-circulated" with a syringe technique for 20 to 30 minutes. Progressive hypoxia occurs because, in contrast to isolated limb perfusion, no oxygenator is used. The hypoxia and acidosis associated with isolated limb infusion are therapeutically attractive because numerous cytotoxic agents, including melphalan, appear to damage tumor cells more effectively under hypoxic conditions. In fact, hypoxia and acidosis have been reported to increase the cytotoxic effects of melphalan in experimental models by a factor of 3.

At the completion of the drug exposure, the limb vasculature is flushed with a crystalloid solution via the arterial catheter, and the effluent is discarded. Although the limb tissues are exposed to the cytotoxic agent for only a short period (up to 30 minutes), there appears to be adequate cellular uptake for tumor cell killing. Isolated limb infusion has been shown to yield response rates similar to those observed after conventional hyperthermic isolated limb perfusion; overall response rates of 85% (complete response rate, 41%; partial response rate, 44%) have been achieved in at least one study. A recent multi-institutional study (Beasley et al.) revealed a 31% complete response rate and a 33% partial response rate. Because of the simplicity of the isolated infusion technique, it may be a more attractive option for patients with prohibitive comorbidities or the elderly.

Toxicity and Morbidity

Hyperthermic isolated limb perfusion and isolated limb infusion can be associated with potentially significant regional adverse effects, including myonecrosis, nerve injury, compartment syndrome, and arterial thrombosis, sometimes necessitating fasciotomy or even major amputation. Following isolated limb infusion, regional adverse effects appear to be similar to those reported after conventional hyperthermic isolated limb perfusion, with 41% of patients experiencing grade II toxic effects and 53% experiencing grade III toxic effects. Systemic toxic effects, including hypotension and adult respiratory distress syndrome, have sometimes been seen with the addition of TNF-α to the perfusion or infusion regimen. To avoid renal injury secondary to high creatine phosphokinase levels, the rate of fluid resuscitation may need to be increased and alkalinizing the urine has theoretical benefits. Steroids have been used empirically to reduce the amount of muscle injury. Of note, the peak creatine phosphokinase level is generally on postoperative day #1 for isolated limb perfusion versus day #4 for isolated limb infusion leading patients in the latter group to have longer hospital stays. Because both limb perfusion and infusion require a high degree of technical expertise and are associated with a significant risk of complications, the procedures should be performed only in centers that have experience with the technique. At present, there is little evidence to justify the use of prophylactic perfusion or infusion, except as part of a clinical trial.

MANAGEMENT OF LOCAL RECURRENCE

True local recurrence is defined as recurrence at the site of the primary tumor, within or continuous with the scar, and is most likely the result of incomplete excision of the primary tumor; it represents a relatively rare pattern of recurrence. In many cases, such "local recurrences" may more appropriately be considered persistence of the primary tumor. A local recurrence consisting of a single lesion in a patient whose primary melanoma had favorable prognostic features may be appropriately treated with wide local excision similar to a primary melanoma lesion. Patients with local recurrences consisting of multiple, small, and superficial lesions may be treated in a fashion similar to that used to treat patients with in-transit disease (see previous section).

MANAGEMENT OF DISTANT METASTATIC DISEASE

Common sites of distant metastasis in melanoma patients are, in order of decreasing frequency, skin and subcutaneous tissues (40%), lungs (12% to 36%), liver, and brain. Patients with systemic metastases have a poor prognosis, with a historical median survival ranging from 6 to 12 months. General guidelines for choosing treatment modalities follow. Recently, and for the first time in over a decade, treatment for distant metastatic melanoma has been proven to prolong survival (see Targeted Therapy section later). Nonetheless, experimental treatments (i.e., clinical trials) remain a robust option for most patients in whom distant metastases are diagnosed.

Surgery

Complete metastasectomy should be considered in patients in whom it is an option. In stage IV patients who underwent complete metastasectomy as part of an adjuvant stage IV clinical trial (Canvaxin phase III trial), 5-year survival was a remarkable 40%. Several nonrandomized trials have demonstrated similar results after complete resection of all evident metastases. Patient selection is critical for the strategy of complete surgical metastasectomy. Of more than 4,229 patients at John Wayne Cancer Center with stage IV melanoma, only 33.6% underwent surgical resection. The 5-year overall survival for this group was 16%, versus 7% for those who did not undergo resection. To aid in proper patient selection, a thorough imaging evaluation is suggested, including MRI of the brain and CT or PET/CT of the chest, abdomen, and pelvis. Patient factors also play a role in selection. Patients should not have comorbidities that would preclude a possible full recovery from surgery within 4 to 8 weeks so as to allow for the initiation of adjuvant or systemic therapies. Finally, the biology of the malignancy itself should be considered: patients whose distant metastasis developed following a longer disease-free interval or who present with isolated or oligometastatic disease are, in general, more likely to be considered for surgical resection.

Surgery is also a very effective palliative treatment for isolated accessible distant metastases. Examples of accessible lesions include isolated visceral metastases, isolated brain metastases, and occasionally isolated lung metastases. Palliative strategies may improve functional status and render patients more likely to tolerate systemic treatments.

Lesions Causing Gastrointestinal Tract Obstruction

Gastrointestinal tract obstruction from metastatic melanoma is usually due to large polypoid lesions that mechanically obstruct the bowel or act as a lead point for intussusceptions. These submucosal lesions are generally removed by bowel resection. Multiple lesions often have to be removed and may include nearby structures. Patients should also be prepared for the possibility of an ileostomy or colostomy.

Pulmonary Metastases

After subcutaneous metastases, the lungs are the next most common site of distant melanoma metastases. The 1-year survival in these patients is 53%. The value of pulmonary resection for melanoma metastases is controversial. In a study examining 65 pulmonary resections performed for histologically proven pulmonary metastases discovered after treatment of the primary melanoma, the post-thoracotomy actuarial survival rate was 25% at 5 years (median interval from pulmonary resection to death, 18 months). Survival was not affected by the location, histologic subtype, Breslow thickness, or Clark level of the primary tumor, or by the type of resection. Patients without regional nodal metastases before thoracotomy had a median survival of 30 months, compared with 16 months for all other patients. The authors concluded that patients with isolated pulmonary metastases from melanoma may benefit from resection of those metastases. However, many patients with stage IV disease are not resectable at the time of stage IV diagnosis. A study of patients who presented with melanoma pulmonary metastasis found that only 21% were resectable at diagnosis. A retrospective evaluation of the International Registry of Lung Metastases, however, found that melanoma patients who underwent complete pulmonary metastasectomy had a 5-year survival rate of 22%.

Liver Metastases
Approximately 15% to 20% of patients with distant metastatic melanoma have liver metastases. Historically, the median survival of patients with liver metastases has ranged from 2 to 7 months. Chemotherapy is generally of limited efficacy against liver metastases. Some investigators have suggested that resection of hepatic metastasis is not warranted because of the associated dismal prognosis. Other investigators have suggested that resection may be appropriate only in patients with an ocular primary tumor because their clinical course is better than that of patients with liver metastases from cutaneous primary tumors. In a retrospective multicenter series of 40 patients who underwent resection of liver metastases from melanoma, 75% of the patients developed a subsequent recurrence. Patients with cutaneous melanoma were significantly more likely to have a subsequent recurrence outside the liver, suggesting that the disease is systemic at the time of hepatic resection. No patient with cutaneous melanoma metastatic to the liver was alive at 5 years. Thus, selection of patients for resection of hepatic metastases must be individualized and include an extensive evaluation of the extent of the disease. In a study from the John Wayne Cancer Institute and the Sydney Melanoma Unit ($N = 1,750$ melanoma patients with hepatic disease), only 2% were candidates for hepatic resection. The 5-year survival in the resected group (complete or incomplete) was 29% versus 4% for those who did not undergo surgery. Similarly, a multi-institutional study that included MD Anderson Cancer Center, Duke University Medical Center, and centers in France and Italy revealed a median survival of 23.6 months in these highly selected patients who underwent resection. As with other sites of metastases, resection should be performed as part of a multidisciplinary approach.

Brain Metastases
Melanoma ranks behind only small-cell carcinoma of the lungs as the most common tumor that metastasizes to the brain. An unusual feature of brain metastases is their propensity for hemorrhage, which occurs much more frequently with melanoma than other primary tumors. Hemorrhage occurs in 33% to 50% of patients with brain metastases from melanoma. Prognosis worsens with an increasing number of lesions and the presence of neurologic symptoms; median survival has been reported to be 3 to 4 months.

Surgical excision (followed in selected cases by cranial irradiation) is the treatment of choice in the case of a solitary, surgically accessible brain metastasis. Tumor excision is relatively safe, alleviates symptoms in most patients, and prevents further neurologic damage. Although long-term disease-free survival is uncommon, a rare patient may live more than 5 years after surgery. Radiation therapy is preferred when the lesions are numerous or are located in areas that preclude a safe operation. Stereotactic radiosurgery is also an option for patients with small to medium brain metastases who have a reasonable life expectancy and no signs of increased intracranial pressure. For patients with multiple metastases that are not amenable to resection, whole brain radiation may assist in slowing the growth of metastases.

Recurrent Distant Metastases

Unfortunately, many patients undergoing complete surgical resection of distant metastatic melanoma (stage IV) develop recurrent disease. A recent study examined whether a second metastasectomy could prolong the survival of patients with recurrent stage IV melanoma. In this study, the recurrent disease affected soft tissue, pulmonary, gastrointestinal, cerebral, skeletal, and gynecologic sites. Median survival following treatment for recurrent stage IV melanoma was 18.2 months after complete metastasectomy, compared with 12.5 months after a palliative surgical procedure and 5.9 months after nonsurgical management. The 5-year survival rate was 20% for patients in the complete metastasectomy group, compared with 7% for those in the palliative surgery group and 2% for those in the nonsurgical group. By multivariate analysis, the two most important prognostic factors for survival following diagnosis of recurrent stage IV melanoma were a prolonged disease-free interval before recurrence and complete surgical removal of the recurrent disease. These findings indicate that in a very highly select patient population, metastasectomy can prolong the survival of patients with recurrent stage IV melanoma and should be considered if all clinically evident tumors can be resected.

Targeted Therapy

BRAF Inhibitors

Recently, attention has turned to leveraging our improved understanding of the underlying molecular biology of melanoma by using such information to develop potential pathway-specific targeted therapeutics as a potential treatment for patients with metastatic melanoma. An important example of this approach is the development of novel therapeutics that target mutant BRAF (V600E). The BRAF gene encodes for production of B-RAF, a protein involved in cell signaling and growth. BRAF mutations have been found in approximately 50% of invasive cutaneous melanomas. BRIM 3 is a randomized, open-label, controlled, multicenter, phase III study that compared a BRAF inhibitor, PLX4032 (vemurafenib), to dacarbazine for treatment of previously untreated, unresectable, stage IIIC or stage IV melanoma in patients harboring a BRAF mutation. The inhibitor targets the common V600E BRAF mutation. Interim analysis of 675 patients (presented at ASCO, 2011 and simultaneously published by Chapman et al. in the New England Journal of Medicine) revealed superiority in overall survival and progression-free survival for vemurafenib. The response rate of patients on vemurafenib was 48.4% compared with 5.5% for patients receiving dacarbazine. While such a response rate for single modality therapy is essentially unprecedented in the treatment of metastatic melanoma, enthusiasm has been tempered, at least to some extent, by the observation that disease recurrence has been observed in the majority of patients 6 to 8 months following initiation of therapy. Identification of mechanisms of resistance comprises a very active component of contemporary melanoma research, a goal of which is to identify potential combinatorial approaches that may reduce resistance pathways and promote longer-term response. Also important is the observation that up to 25% of patients who receive BRAF inhibitors develop squamous carcinoma of the skin, often in the form of keratoacanthomas.

KIT Inhibitors

KIT mutations have been another recent therapeutic target for patients with metastatic melanoma. Several case reports had previously demonstrated a benefit for individual patients who were treated with a KIT inhibitor. More recently, Carvajal et al. published the results of a phase II study of 28 patients with unresectable metastatic melanoma who had KIT mutations and were treated with imatinib mesylate. In this study, 16% of patients had durable responses that lasted more than a year. Certain mutations in KIT were identified to be more responsive to treatment.

Chemotherapy

Single-agent chemotherapy has historically been a standard of care for systemic chemotherapy in patients with metastatic melanoma, but response rates remain quite poor. Dacarbazine is the drug of choice, with a response rate of 16%. Other drugs, including cisplatin, paclitaxel, docetaxel, and the dacarbazine analog, temozolomide, have also shown activity in this disease.

On the basis of the observed single-agent activity, several combination regimens have been investigated. The Dartmouth regimen (dacarbazine, cisplatin, carmustine, and tamoxifen) was initially reported to have an overall response rate of 55% and complete response rate of 20%. However, subsequent multicenter trials have failed to corroborate these favorable results. In fact, in randomized phase III trials, the two most active combination chemotherapy regimens, the Dartmouth regimen and cisplatin, vinblastine, and dacarbazine, have not proven to be superior to single-agent dacarbazine in terms of overall survival. Other combinations, such as temozolomide and cisplatin, have not been shown to have clear benefits in terms of response rates but may be associated with a higher incidence of grade 3 or grade 4 emesis. If no objective response is observed after two or three courses of a particular chemotherapy regimen, it is usually prudent to discontinue that regimen and consider other approaches. In general, even when metastatic melanoma responds to systemic chemotherapy, the duration of the response is usually short, in the range of 3 to 6 months (see also Biochemotherapy later).

Immunotherapy and Biological Therapy

Immunotherapy with either interleukin (IL)-2 or IFN has demonstrated response rates of 10% to 15% in appropriately selected patients. In patients who have a complete response, responses can be of greater durability than those with chemotherapy. IL-2 promotes the proliferation, differentiation, and recruitment of T, B, and NK cells and initiates cytolytic activity in a subset of lymphocytes. In patients who had a complete response to IL-2, the majority (86%) remained in ongoing complete remission from 39 to more than 148 months. In patients with a partial response, median response duration has been 36 to 45 months. Although the overall response rate is low (10% to 15%), the durability of the responses led the U.S. Food and Drug Administration to approve high-dose IL-2 for metastatic melanoma in 1998. However, IL-2 and IFN administration is associated with multiple side effects; therefore, these agents should be administered only by physicians experienced in the management of such therapies. One major systemic toxic effect with high-dose IL-2 administration is "capillary leak syndrome." This toxic effect is, fortunately, uncommon, but it can be life-threatening.

Morton et al. demonstrated that intralesional injection of viable bacillus Calmette–Guérin (BCG) organisms could lead to the regression of intradermal melanoma metastasis. Even more significantly, uninjected lesions occasionally regressed following BCG therapy. This finding demonstrated the ability of the body's immune system to destroy melanoma when properly stimulated, leading to investigations of BCG as a potential therapy for melanoma. Although several nonrandomized trials using historical controls and two small randomized trials of intralesional or intralymphatic BCG showed a statistically significant overall survival benefit in favor of BCG, multiple other randomized trials failed to substantiate these findings. Nonetheless, interest in modulating the immune system to treat melanoma has persisted.

Monoclonal Antibodies

Monoclonal antibody therapy is generally well tolerated and has shown activity in phase I trials in patients with metastatic melanoma. Monoclonal antibodies have been used to target radiation and potent toxins to tumors, and anti-idiotype antibodies have been used to stimulate immune responses. Ipilimumab is a humanized monoclonal antibody that blocks CTLA-4, a key regulatory molecule of the immune system. In a phase III, randomized prospective trial Hodi et al. evaluated a total of 676 patients who received ipilimumab, ipilimumab plus a vaccine, and the peptide vaccine alone. Overall response and disease control were seen to be highest in the ipilimumab alone cohort. Median overall survival was 10.1 months for this cohort and overall response was 10.9%. Disease control was 28.5% with 60% of the ipilimumab cohort having a significant response at 2 years.

In March 2011, the Food and Drug Administration approved ipilimumab as a second-line treatment for metastatic melanoma. A more recent study has demonstrated the benefit of ipilimumab in the first-line setting. In a phase III, double-blinded study of 502 metastatic melanoma patients randomized to ipilimumab plus dacarbazine versus placebo plus dacarbazine by Robert et al., the ipilimumab arm had a significantly higher overall survival (11.2 months vs. 9.2 months) and durable response (19.3 months vs. 8.3 months).

Tumor Vaccines

Tumor vaccines have been used in the treatment of advanced melanoma and as adjuvant therapy for patients with high-risk melanoma. These vaccines may contain (a) irradiated tumor cells, usually obtained from the patient (b) partially or completely purified melanoma antigens or (c) tumor cell membranes from melanoma cells infected with virus (viral oncolysates). Synthetic vaccines containing genes that encode for tumor antigens and the peptide antigens themselves are also being evaluated, as are vaccines containing genes encoding for immune costimulatory signal proteins.

Allogeneic tumor cell vaccines, generally prepared from cultured cell lines or lysates thereof, offer several potential important advantages over autologous tumor cell vaccines: Allogeneic vaccines are readily available and can be standardized, preserved, and distributed in a manner akin to any other therapeutic agent. To date, the majority of studies involving allogeneic tumor vaccines have been small, single-institution studies. None of these have demonstrated an unequivocal benefit for immunotherapy with allogeneic tumor cells administered in conjunction with BCG compared with no treatment or treatment with BCG alone. Two randomized studies (Hoon et al. [1990] and Oratz et al. [1991]) have been conducted in which allogeneic melanoma vaccines were administered with or without cyclophosphamide given for 3 days prior to vaccination. The results of these studies have been conflicting, with one suggesting a decrease in suppressor cell activity and one suggesting an increase in suppressor cell activity and augmented antibody response.

Novel vaccine strategies under investigation include administration of synthetic peptides based on known melanoma T-cell antigens, genetic vaccines, and combinations of vaccines with cytokines or costimulatory molecules. Morton et al. conducted nonrandomized studies of a polyvalent melanoma vaccine (Canvaxin) in patients with stage III or stage IV disease. Matched-pair analyses of data from extensive phase 2 trials demonstrated a consistent overall survival benefit for Canvaxin therapy in stage III melanoma (5-year overall survival rate: 49% for Canvaxin vs. 37% for no vaccine; $P = 0.0001$) and stage IV melanoma (5-year overall survival rate: 39% for Canvaxin vs. 20% for no vaccine; $P = 0.0009$). Vaccine-induced immune responses have correlated with improved survival after resection of local, regional, and distant disease. Two separate randomized phase 3 clinical trials of Canvaxin in patients with stage III or IV melanoma, however, were discontinued in 2005 based on the recommendation of the data safety monitoring board after an interim analysis of the study data. The monitoring board found that the data were unlikely to provide significant evidence of a survival benefit for Canvaxin versus placebo in patients with stage III or stage IV melanoma.

In 2002, the Southwest Oncology Group published the results of a large, randomized trial (S9035) comparing coadministration of an allogeneic melanoma cell lysate (Melacine) and detoxified endotoxin/mycobacterial cell wall skeleton (DETOX) versus no treatment in patients with intermediate thickness, node-negative melanoma. The primary aim of this trial was to determine the effect of the vaccine on relapse-free survival. A secondary aim was to determine if the effectiveness of the vaccine was based on patients' HLA class I allele expression. At a median follow-up of 4.1 years, there was no difference in overall relapse-free survival between the two groups. The patients in the vaccine arm expressing at least 2 M5 alleles, however, had better disease-free survival than the corresponding patients in the observation arm. Furthermore, vaccine-arm patients expressing at least 2 M5 alleles had better disease-free survival than vaccine-arm patients expressing fewer than 2 M5 alleles.

Current vaccine trials include the gp100 DNA-based vaccine and a GM-CSF–encoding second-generation oncolytic herpes virus vaccine (OncoVex). The latter showed promise with a 26% overall response rate in a phase II trial of unresectable stages II and III disease. The phase III trial of OncoVex completed accrual in June 2011.

Cellular Therapies

Cellular therapies also exhibit some promise. Rosenberg et al. at the U.S. National Cancer Institute, and others, have reported their experiences with adoptive immunotherapy using tumor-infiltrating lymphocytes (TIL) and, more recently, dendritic cells. An overall response rate of 37% was seen in patients with stage IV disease treated with adopted immunotherapy. Ten studies have been performed to date. Key steps affecting the response rate include the effectiveness of lymphodepletion prior to T cell transfer, extranodal source of TIL, short culture duration, short TIL doubling time, greater autologous tumor lysis by TIL, and TIL secretion of granulocyte–macrophage stimulating factor. The technique, however, requires specialized expertise and an elaborate infrastructure.

Additional forms of cellular-based therapy are being developed, including effector cells from tumor vaccine-primed lymph nodes. Trials using in vitro pulsed dendritic cell infusion are ongoing. In addition, new work is examining whether preferential induction of apoptosis by sequential 5-Aza-2 deoxycytidine-depsipeptide (FR901228) treatment in melanoma cells to improve recognition of specific targets by cytolytic T lymphocytes may serve as a useful adjunct to immunotherapy.

Biochemotherapy

Multiple trials have been conducted to investigate the benefit of combining biological therapy with chemotherapy (so-called biochemotherapy). These trials indicate that biochemotherapy is associated with higher response rates and longer median survivals than chemotherapy alone. Specifically, phase I and II studies have evaluated combinations of IL-2, IFN, and chemotherapy (cisplatin, dacarbazine, or cyclophosphamide). Results from a series of small studies using combinations of IL-2, IFN alfa, and cisplatin have indicated overall response rates from 40% to 50%. A phase III trial was completed at MD Anderson Cancer Center that compared inpatient sequential biochemotherapy with traditional outpatient chemotherapy with respect to response, time to progression, overall survival rate, and toxicity. All patients had either stage IV or inoperable stage III disease, an ECOG performance status of 0 to 3, no symptomatic brain metastases, no prior chemotherapy, and adequate cardiac, hematologic, and renal reserves. The response rate was 48% with biochemotherapy and 25% with standard chemotherapy ($P = 0.0001$). The time to progression was 4.6 months with biochemotherapy and 2.4 months with standard chemotherapy ($P = 0.0007$). The median survival was 11.8 months with biochemotherapy and 9.5 months with standard chemotherapy ($P = 0.055$). Biochemotherapy did induce severe constitutional toxic effects—myelosuppression, infections, and hypotension—but all of these were found to be manageable on the general ward. In a more recent phase II trial by the same group, the addition of IFN alfa-2a to IL-2 was examined. Although the response rate for this regimen was low, durable responses with median survival durations of 30+ months were seen in selected patients. The phase III trial, however, failed to show biochemotherapy to be superior to interferon, so the study was closed early. The most recent meta-analysis of chemotherapy versus biochemotherapy was performed in 2007 (Ives et al.). The study concluded that there was no advantage in either arm for duration of response or overall survival. Biochemotherapy, however, was superior in delaying disease progression, in partial response, and in complete response.

RADIATION THERAPY

Wide excision is the standard treatment for primary melanoma, but radiation treatment has been attempted in patients who have been deemed inoperable for various reasons (e.g., severe medical comorbidities). In one study of 95 invasive melanomas treated with high-dose radiation, the 5-year survival was 70%. In cases in which the local recurrence rate is unacceptably high (inability to obtain wide margins, satellitosis, desmoplastic melanoma), adjuvant radiation to the primary site is a consideration.

The role of adjuvant radiation to regional lymph node basins has been more clearly defined. Several retrospective studies have demonstrated that lymph node basins with multiple positive nodes, one or more metastatic lymph nodes larger than 3 cm in diameter, extracapsular extension, or recurrent regional disease may benefit from adjuvant radiation. Regional control after modified radical neck dissection for palpable cervical disease can lead to 90% regional control. The treatment, however, is associated with a 10% 5-year complication rate. A randomized controlled trial from Australia examined 234 patients at high risk for regional recurrence after lymphadenectomy. These patients were stratified to either observation or 48Gy of radiation. The observation group had a 26.8% recurrence rate versus 20% for the adjuvant radiation group. Overall survival, however, was not found to be different. The importance of local control in reducing morbidity, however, should not be underestimated, and future research goals may include randomized clinical trials to further define the role of adjuvant radiation therapy alone or in combination with systemic therapy. In general, patients with multiple involved or matted regional nodes or with extracapsular extension of regional lymphatic metastases should be considered for adjuvant radiation therapy.

External-beam radiation therapy can provide long-term local control and effective palliation. Symptomatic bone metastases from melanoma also frequently respond to external-beam radiation therapy. In addition, recurrent subcutaneous and nodal disease can also sometimes be treated in this fashion. Please see the Brain Metastases section (earlier) for discussion of whole brain radiation and stereotactic brain radiation.

FOLLOW-UP AND SURVEILLANCE

Melanoma has a more variable and unpredictable clinical course than almost any other human cancer. At MD Anderson Cancer Center, the schedule of follow-up evaluations for patients with melanoma varies according to the risk of recurrence. In general, patients with early-stage melanoma (in situ or <1.0 mm thick, nonulcerated, lymph-node negative) have follow-up visits every 6 months for 2 years and then annually. Patients with thicker and ulcerated melanomas and those with positive lymph nodes generally return for follow-up visits more frequently—every 3 to 4 months up to 3 years, every 6 months during Years 3 and 4, and annually thereafter. At each visit, the patient undergoes a physical examination concentrating on lymph node basins, skin survey, and measurement of LDH (omitted in melanoma in situ and thin melanomas.) Abnormal findings may prompt further workup. Particular attention should be paid to signs or symptoms of central nervous system involvement which may require brain MRI. Extensive radiographic evaluation of asymptomatic patients with AJCC stage I or stage II melanoma who are clinically free of disease rarely reveals metastases and thus is not routinely performed. Radiographic evaluation is generally performed for patients with microscopic stage III disease prior to adjuvant therapy, and selectively prior to completion lymphadenectomy for a positive SLN. Chest x-ray is generally performed as part of follow-up, except for patients with in situ and thin melanoma. CT or PET/CT should be considered every 6 to 12 months to evaluate for recurrent or new metastatic disease in patients with stage III or IV disease. MRI of the brain is also often performed for surveillance in patients who are stage IIIC or IV. The role of ultrasound of regional lymph nodes has been studied for surveillance of patients with stages I to III disease, but its role is not well defined.

Recommended Readings

Albertini JJ, Cruse CW, Rapaport D, et al. Intraoperative radio-lymph-scintigraphy improves sentinel lymph node identification for patients with melanoma. *Ann Surg.* 1996;223:217–224.

Aloia TA, Gershenwald JE. Management of early-stage cutaneous melanoma. *Curr Prob Surg.* 2005;42:468–534.

Aloia TA, Gershenwald JE. Utility of computed tomography and magnetic resonance imaging staging before completion lymphadenectomy in patients with sentinel lymph node-positive melanoma. *J Clin Oncology.* 2006;24(28):2858–2865.

Anbari KK, Schucter LM, Bucky LP, et al. Melanoma of unknown primary site: presentation, treatment, and prognosis—a single institution study. University of Pennsylvania Pigmented Lesion Study Group. *Cancer.* 1997;79:1816–1821.

Andtbacka RH, Gershenwald JE. Role of sentinel lymph node biopsy in patients with thin melanoma. *J Natl Compr Canc Netw.* 2009;7(3):308–317.

Ang KK, Peters LJ, Weber RS, et al. Postoperative radiotherapy for cutaneous melanoma of the head and neck region. *Int J Radiat Oncol Biol Phys.* 1994;30:795–798.

Bafaloukos D, Tsoutsos D, Kalofonos H, et al. Temozolomide and cisplatin versus temozolomide in patients with advanced melanoma: a randomized phase II study

of the Hellenic Cooperative Oncology Group. *Ann Oncol.* 2005;16:950–957.

Balch CM. The role of elective lymph node dissection in melanoma: rationale, results, and controversies. *J Clin Oncol.* 1988;6:163–172.

Balch CM, Gershenwald JE, Soong SJ, et al. Final version of 2009 AJCC melanoma staging and classification [published online ahead of print November 16, 2009]. *J Clin Oncol.* 2009;27(36):6199–6206.

Balch CM, Gershenwald JE, Soong SJ, et al. Multivariate analysis of prognostic factors among 2,313 patients with stage III melanoma: comparison of nodal micrometastases versus macrometastases [published online ahead of print April 5, 2010]. *J Clin Oncol.* 2010;28(14):2452–2459.

Balch CM, Morton DL, Gershenwald JE, et al. Sentinel node biopsy and standard of care for melanoma. *J Am Acad Dermatol.* 2009;60(5):872–875.

Balch CM, Soong SJ, Bartoluccci AA, et al. Efficacy of an elective regional lymph node dissection of 1 to 4 mm thick melanomas for patients 60 years of age and younger. *Ann Surg.* 1996;224:255–266.

Balch CM, Soong SJ, Ross MI, et al. Long-term results of a multi-institutional randomized trial comparing prognostic factors and surgical results for intermediate thickness melanomas (1.0 to 4.0 mm). Intergroup Melanoma Surgical Trial. *Ann Surg Oncol.* 2000;7:87–97.

Ballo MT, Ang KK. Radiotherapy for cutaneous malignant melanoma: rationale and indications. *Oncology (Huntingt).* 2004;18:99–107, discussion 107–110, 113–114.

Ballo MT, Garden AS, Myers JN, et al. Melanoma metastatic to cervical lymph nodes: can radiotherapy replace formal dissection after local excision of nodal disease? *Head Neck.* 2005;27:718–721.

Ballo MT, Strom EA, Zagars GK, et al. Adjuvant irradiation for axillary metastases from malignant melanoma. *Int J Radiat Oncol Biol Phys.* 2002;52:964–972.

Ballo MT, Zagars GK, Gershenwald JE, et al. A critical assessment of adjuvant radiotherapy for inguinal lymph node metastases from melanoma. *Ann Surg Oncol.* 2004;11:1079–1084.

Beasley GM, Caudle A, Peterson RP, et al. A multi-institutional experience of isolated limb perfusion: defining response and toxicity in the US. *J Am Coll Surg.* 2009;208(5):706–715.

Bedrosian I, Faries MB, Guerry DT, et al. Incidence of sentinel node metastasis in patients with thin primary melanoma (< or = 1 mm) with vertical growth phase. *Ann Surg Oncol.* 2000;7:262–267.

Bollag G, Hirth P, Tsai J, et al. Clinical efficacy of a RAF inhibitor needs broad target blockade in BRAF-mutant melanoma. *Nature.* 2010;467(7315):596–599.

Bowles TL, Xing Y, Hu CY, et al. Conditional survival estimates improve over 5 years for melanoma survivors with node-positive disease [published online ahead of print April 6, 2010]. *Ann Surg Oncol.* 2010;17(8):2015–2023.

Cannon-Albright LA, Goldgar DE, Meyer LJ, et al. Assignment of a locus for familial melanoma, MLM, to chromosome 9p13-p22. *Science.* 1992;258:1148–1152.

Carvajal RD, Antonescu CR, Wolchok JD, et al. KIT as a therapeutic target in metastatic melanoma. *JAMA.* 2011;305(22):2327–2334.

Cascinelli N, Morabito A, Santinami M, et al. Immediate or delayed dissection of regional nodes in patients with melanoma of the trunk: a randomised trial. *Lancet.* 1998;351:793–796.

Chang SB, Askew RL, Xing Y, et al. Prospective assessment of postoperative complications and associated costs following inguinal lymph node dissection (ILND) in melanoma patients [published online ahead of print March 25, 2010]. *Ann Surg Oncol.* 2010;17(10):2764–2772.

Chapman PB, Hauschild A, Robert C, et al. Improved survival with vemurafenib in melanoma with BRAF V600E mutation [published online ahead of print June 5, 2011]. *N Engl J Med.* 2011;364(26):2507–2516.

Chung MH, Gupta RK, Hsueh E, et al. Humoral immune response to a therapeutic polyvalent cancer vaccine after complete resection of thick primary melanoma and sentinel lymphadenectomy. *J Clin Oncol.* 2003;21:313–319.

Clary BM, Brady MS, Lewis JJ, et al. Sentinel lymph node biopsy in the management of patients with primary cutaneous melanoma: review of a large single-institutional experience with an emphasis on recurrence. *Ann Surg.* 2001;233:250–258.

Cochran AJ, Wen DR, Huang RR, et al. Prediction of metastatic melanoma in nonsentinel nodes and clinical outcome based on the primary melanoma and the sentinel node. *Mod Pathol.* 2004;17:747–755.

Cormier JN, Xing Y, Feng L, et al. Metastatic melanoma to lymph nodes in patients with unknown primary sites. *Cancer.* 2006;106:2012–2020.

Curtin JA, Busam K, Pinkel D, et al. Somatic activation of KIT in distinct subtypes of melanoma [published online ahead of print August 2006]. *J Clin Oncol.* 2006; 24(26):4340–4346.

Curtin JA, Fridlyand J, Kageshita T, et al. Distinct sets of genetic alterations in melanoma. *N Engl J Med.* 2005;353(20):2135–2147.

Davies MA, Gershenwald JE. Targeted therapy for melanoma: a primer. *Surg Oncol Clin N Am.* 2011;20(1):165–180.

Dickson PV, Gershenwald JE. Staging and prognosis of cutaneous melanoma. *Surg Oncol Clin N Am.* 2011;20(1):1–17.

Dudley ME, Wunderlich JR, Robbins PF, et al. Cancer regression and autoimmunity in patients after clonal repopulation with antitumor lymphocytes. *Science.* 2002;298: 850–854.

Dudley ME, Wunderlich JR, Yang JC, et al. Adoptive cell transfer therapy following non-myeloablative but lymphodepleting chemotherapy for the treatment of patients with refractory metastatic melanoma. *J Clin Oncol.* 2005;23:2346–2357.

Eton O, Legha SS, Bedikian AY, et al. Sequential biochemotherapy versus chemotherapy for metastatic melanoma: results from a phase III randomized trial. *J Clin Oncol.* 2002;20:2045–2052.

Evans GR, Friedman J, Shenaq J, et al. Plantar flap reconstruction for acral lentiginous melanoma. *Ann Surg Oncol.* 1997;4:575–578.

Faries MB, Thompson JF, Cochran A, et al. The impact on morbidity and length of stay of early versus delayed complete lymphadenectomy in melanoma: results of the Multicenter Selective Lymphadenectomy Trial (I) [published online ahead of print July 8, 2010]. *Ann Surg Oncol.* 2010;17(12):3324–3329.

Flaherty KT, Puzanov I, Kim KB, et al. Inhibition of mutated, activated BRAF in metastatic melanoma. *N Engl J Med.* 2010;363(9):809–819.

Fraker DL, Alexander HR, Andrich M, et al. Treatment of patients with melanoma of the extremity using hyperthermic isolated limb perfusion with melphalan, tumor necrosis factor, and interferon gamma: results of a tumor necrosis factor dose-escalation study. *J Clin Oncol.* 1996;14:479–489.

Gannon CJ, Rousseau DL Jr, Ross MI, et al. Accuracy of lymphatic mapping and sentinel lymph node biopsy after previous wide local excision in patients with primary melanoma. *Cancer.* 2006;107(11):2647–2652.

Gershenwald JE, Andtbacka RH, Prieto VG, et al. Microscopic tumor burden in sentinel lymph nodes predicts synchronous nonsentinel lymph node involvement in patients with melanoma. *J Clin Oncol.* 2008;26(26):4296–4303.

Gershenwald JE, Berman RS, Porter G, et al. Regional nodal basin control is not compromised by previous sentinel lymph node biopsy in patients with melanoma. *Ann Surg Oncol.* 2000;7:226–231.

Gershenwald JE, Colome MI, Lee JE, et al. Patterns of recurrence following a negative sentinel lymph node biopsy in 243 patients with stage I or II melanoma. *J Clin Oncol.* 1998;16:2253–2260.

Gershenwald JE, Mansfield PF, Lee JE, et al. Role for lymphatic mapping and sentinel lymph node biopsy in patients with thick (> or = 4 mm) primary melanoma. *Ann Surg Oncol.* 2000;7:160–165.

Gershenwald JE, Prieto VG, Colome-Grimmer MI, et al. The prognostic significance of microscopic tumor burden in 945 melanoma patients undergoing sentinel lymph node biopsy. Paper presented at: 36th Annual Meeting of the American Society of Clinical Oncology; 2003; New Orleans, LA.

Gershenwald JE, Prieto VG, Johnson M. AJCC stage III (nodal) criteria accurately predict survival in sentinel node-positive melanoma patients. Paper presented at: 3rd International Sentinel Node Congress; 2002; Yokohama, Japan.

Gershenwald JE, Ross MI. Sentinel-lymph-node biopsy for cutaneous melanoma. *N Engl J Med.* 2011;364(18):1738–1745.

Gershenwald JE, Soong SJ, Balch CM. American Joint Committee on Cancer (AJCC) Melanoma Staging Committee. 2010 TNM staging system for cutaneous melanoma . . . and beyond. *Ann Surg Oncol.* 2010;17(6):1475–1477.

Gershenwald JE, Thompson W, Mansfield PF, et al. Multi-institutional melanoma lymphatic mapping experience: the prognostic value of sentinel lymph node status in 612 stage I or II melanoma patients. *J Clin Oncol.* 1999;17:976–983.

Gershenwald JE, Tseng CH, Thompson W, et al. Improved sentinel lymph node localization in patients with primary melanoma with the use of radiolabeled colloid. *Surgery.* 1998;124:203–210.

Gill M, Celebi JT. B-RAF and melanocytic neoplasia. *J Am Acad Dermatol.* 2005;53:108–114.

Gray-Schopfer VC, da Rocha Dias S, Marais R. The role of B-RAF in melanoma. *Cancer Metastasis Rev.* 2005;24:165–183.

Hafstrom L, Rudenstam CM, Blomquist E, et al. Regional hyperthermic perfusion with melphalan after surgery for recurrent malignant melanoma of the extremities. Swedish Melanoma Study Group. *J Clin Oncol.* 1991;9:2091–2094.

Hawkins WG, Busam KJ, Ben-Porat L, et al. Desmoplastic melanoma: a pathologically and clinically distinct form of cutaneous melanoma. *Ann Surg Oncol.* 2005;12:207–213.

Hayward N. New developments in melanoma genetics. *Curr Oncol Rep.* 2000;2:300–306.

Heaton KM, Sussman JJ, Gershenwald JE, et al. Surgical margins and prognostic factors in patients with thick (>4 mm) primary melanoma. *Ann Surg Oncol.* 1998;5:322–328.

Hodi FS, O'Day SJ, McDermott DF, et al. Improved survival with ipilimumab in patients with metastatic melanoma [published online ahead of print June 5, 2010]. *N Engl J Med.* 2010;363(8):711–723. Erratum in: *N Engl J Med.* 2010;363(13):1290.

Holly EA, Aston DA, Cress RD, et al. Cutaneous melanoma in women. I. Exposure to sunlight, ability to tan, and other risk factors related to ultraviolet light. *Am J Epidemiol.* 1995;141:923–933.

Holly EA, Cress RD, Ahn DK. Cutaneous melanoma in women. III. Reproductive factors and oral contraceptive use. *Am J Epidemiol.* 1995;141:943–950.

Homsi J, Grimm JC, Hwu P. Immunotherapy of melanoma: an update. *Surg Oncol Clin N Am.* 2011;20(1):145–163.

Hoon DS, Foshaq AJ, Nizzie AS, et al. Suppressor cell activity in a randomized trial of patient receiving active specific immunotherapy with melanoma cell vaccine and low dosages of cyclophosphamide. *Cancer Res.* 1990;50(17):5358–5364.

Hsueh EC, Essner R, Foshag LJ, et al. Prolonged survival after complete resection of disseminated melanoma and active immunotherapy with a therapeutic cancer vaccine. *J Clin Oncol.* 2002;20:4549–4554.

Ivan D, Prieto VG. An update on reporting histopathologic prognostic factors in melanoma. *Arch Pathol Lab Med.* 2011; 135(7):825–829.

Ives NJ, Stowe RL, Lorigan P, Wheatley K. Chemotherapy compared with biochemotherapy for the treatment of metastatic melanoma: a meta-analysis of 18 trials involving 2,621 patients. *J Clin Oncol.* 2007;27(34):5426–5434.

Jemal A, Devesa SS, Fears TR, et al. Cancer surveillance series: changing patterns of cutaneous malignant melanoma mortality rates among whites in the United States. *J Natl Cancer Inst.* 2000;92:811–818.

Jemal A, Siegel R, Xu J, et al. Cancer statistics, 2010. *CA Cancer J Clin.* 2010;60(5):277–300.

Kammula US, Ghossein R, Bhattacharya S, et al. Serial follow-up and the prognostic significance of reverse transcriptase-polymerase chain reaction—staged sentinel lymph nodes from melanoma patients. *J Clin Oncol.* 2004;22:3989–3996.

Kang JC, Wanek LA, Essner R, et al. Sentinel lymphadenectomy does not increase the incidence of in-transit metastases in primary melanoma. *J Clin Oncol.* 2005; 23:4764–4770.

Kim KB, Legha SS, Gonzalez R, et al. A randomized phase III trial of biochemotherapy versus interferon-alpha-2b for adjuvant therapy in patients at high risk for melanoma recurrence. *Melanoma Res.* 2009;19(1):42–49.

Kirkwood JM, Ibrahim JG, Sondak VK, et al. High- and low-dose interferon alfa-2b in high-risk melanoma: first analysis of intergroup trial E1690/S9111/C9190. *J Clin Oncol.* 2000;18:2444–2458.

Kirkwood JM, Ibrahim JG, Sosman JA, et al. High-dose interferon alfa-2b significantly prolongs relapse-free and overall survival compared with the GM2-KLH/QS-21 vaccine in patients with resected stage IIB–III melanoma: results of intergroup trial E1694/S9512/C509801. *J Clin Oncol.* 2001;19:2370–2380.

Kirkwood JM, Manola J, Ibrahim J, et al. A pooled analysis of Eastern Cooperative Oncology Group and intergroup trials of adjuvant high-dose interferon for melanoma. *Clin Cancer Res.* 2004;10:1670–1677.

Kirkwood JM, Strawderman MH, Ernstoff MS, et al. Interferon alfa-2b adjuvant therapy of high-risk resected cutaneous melanoma: the Eastern Cooperative Oncology Group Trial EST 1684. *J Clin Oncol.* 1996;14:7–17.

Koops HS, Vaglini M, Suciu S, et al. Prophylactic isolated limb perfusion for localized, high-risk limb melanoma: results of a multicenter randomized phase III trial. European Organization for Research and Treatment of Cancer Malignant Melanoma Cooperative Group Protocol 18832, the World Health Organization Melanoma Program Trial 15, and the North American Perfusion Group Southwest Oncology Group-8593. *J Clin Oncol.* 1998;16:2906–2912.

Kroon HM, Moncrieff M, Kam PC, et al. Outcomes following isolated limb infusion for melanoma. A 14-year experience [published online ahead of print May 29, 2008]. *Ann Surg Oncol.* 2008;15(11):3003–3013.

Kroon HM, Thompson JF. Isolated limb infusion: a review. *J Surg Oncol.* 2009; 100(2):169–177.

Lazovich D, Vogel RI, Berwick M, et al. Indoor tanning and risk of melanoma: a case-control study in a highly-exposed population [published online ahead of print]. *Cancer Epidemiol Biomarkers Prev.* 2010;19(6):1557–1568.

Lee CC, Faries MB, Wanek LA, et al. Improved survival after lymphadenectomy for nodal metastases from an unknown primary melanoma. *J Clin Oncol.* 2008; 26(4):535–541.

Lienard D, Ewalenko P, Delmotte JJ, et al. High-dose recombinant tumor necrosis factor alpha in combination with interferon gamma and melphalan in isolation perfusion of the limbs for melanoma and sarcoma. *J Clin Oncol.* 1992;10:52–60.

Lindner P, Doubrovsky A, Kam PC, et al. Prognostic factors after isolated limb infusion with cytotoxic agents for melanoma. *Ann Surg Oncol.* 2002;9:127–136.

Long GV, Menzies AM, Nagrial AM, et al. Prognostic and clinicopathologic associations of oncogenic BRAF in metastatic melanoma [published online ahead of print February 22, 2011]. *J Clin Oncol.* 2011;29(10):1239–1246.

McMasters KM. The Sunbelt Melanoma Trial. *Ann Surg Oncol.* 2001;8:41S–43S.

McMasters KM, Reintgen DS, Ross MI, et al. Sentinel lymph node biopsy for melanoma: how many radioactive nodes should be removed? *Ann Surg Oncol.* 2001;8:192–197.

Moore-Olufemi S, Herzog C, Warneke C, et al. Outcomes in pediatric melanoma: comparing prepubertal to adolescent pediatric patients. *Ann Surg.* 2011;253(6):1211–1215.

Morton DL. Immune response to postsurgical adjuvant active immunotherapy with Canvaxin polyvalent cancer vaccine: correlations with clinical course of patients with metastatic melanoma. *Dev Biol (Basel).* 2004;116:209–217, discussion 229–236.

Morton DL, Cochran AJ, Thompson JF. The rationale for sentinel-node biopsy in primary melanoma. *Nat Clin Pract Oncol.* 2008;5(9):510–511.

Morton DL, Cochran AJ, Thompson JF, et al. Sentinel node biopsy for early-stage melanoma: accuracy and morbidity in MSLT-I, an international multicenter trial. *Ann Surg.* 2005;242(3):302–311; discussion 311–313.

Morton D, Mozzilo N, Thompson J, et al. An international, randomized, double-blind, phase 3 study of the specific active immunotherapy agent, onamelatucel-L (Canvaxin), compared to placebo as a post-surgical adjuvant in AJCC stage IV melanoma [abstract 12]. Presented at the Society of Surgical Oncology Cancer Symposium, 59th Annual Meeting; March 23–26, 2006; San Diego, CA.

Morton DL, Thompson JF, Cochran AJ, et al. Sentinel-node biopsy or nodal observation in melanoma. *N Engl J Med.* 2006;355(13):1307–1317. Erratum in: *N Engl J Med.* 2006;355(18):1944.

Morton DL, Wen DR, Wong JH, et al. Technical details of intraoperative lymphatic mapping for early stage melanoma. *Arch Surg.* 1992;127:392–399.

Murali R, Desilva C, Thompson JF, et al. Factors predicting recurrence and survival in sentinel lymph node-positive melanoma patients. *Ann Surg.* 2011;253(6):1155–1164.

Murali R, Desilva C, Thompson JF, et al. Non-Sentinel Node Risk Score (N-SNORE): a scoring system for accurately stratifying risk of non-sentinel node positivity in patients with cutaneous melanoma with positive sentinel lymph nodes [published

online ahead of print September 7, 2010]. *J Clin Oncol.* 2010;28(29):4441–4449.

O'Meara AT, Cress R, Xing G, et al. Malignant melanoma in pregnancy. A population-based evaluation. *Cancer.* 2005;103:1217–1226.

Oratz R, Dugan M, Roses DF, et al. Lack of effect of cyclophosphamide on the immunogenicity of melanoma antigen vaccine. *Cancer Res.* 1991;51(14):3643–3647.

Patnana M, Bronstein Y, Szklaruk J, et al. Multimethod imaging, staging, and spectrum of manifestations of metastatic melanoma [published online ahead of print January 9, 2011]. *Clin Radiol.* 2011;66(3):224–236. Review.

Pawlik TM, Ross MI, Gershenwald JE. Lymphatic mapping in the molecular era. *Ann Surg Oncol.* 2004;11:362–374.

Pawlik TM, Ross MI, Johnson MM, et al. Predictors and natural history of in-transit melanoma after sentinel lymphadenectomy. *Ann Surg Oncol.* 2005;12:587–596.

Pawlik TM, Ross MI, Thompson JF, et al. The risk of in-transit melanoma metastasis depends on tumor biology and not the surgical approach to regional lymph nodes. *J Clin Oncol.* 2005;23:4588–4590.

Pawlik TM, Ross MI, Prieto VG, et al. Assessment of the role of sentinel lymph node biopsy for primary cutaneous desmoplastic melanoma. *Cancer.* 2006;106(4):900–906.

Pawlik TM, Zorzi D, Abdalla EK, et al. Hepatic resection for metastatic melanoma: distinct patterns of recurrence and prognosis for ocular versus cutaneous disease [published online ahead of print March 14, 2006]. *Ann Surg Oncol.* 2006;13(5):712–720.

Porter GA, Ross MI, Berman RS, et al. How many lymph nodes are enough during sentinel lymphadenectomy for primary melanoma? *Surgery.* 2000;128:306–311.

Porter GA, Ross MI, Berman RS, et al. Significance of multiple nodal basin drainage in truncal melanoma patients undergoing sentinel lymph node biopsy. *Ann Surg Oncol.* 2000;7:256–261.

Poulikakos PI, Rosen N. Mutant BRAF melanomas–dependence and resistance. *Cancer Cell.* 2011;19(1):11–15.

Prieto VG. Sentinel lymph nodes in cutaneous melanoma. *Clin Lab Med.* 2011;31(2):301–310.

Ranieri JM, Wagner JD, Azuaje R, et al. Prognostic importance of lymph node tumor burden in melanoma patients staged by sentinel node biopsy. *Ann Surg Oncol.* 2002;9:975–981.

Ribas A, Flaherty KT. BRAF targeted therapy changes the treatment paradigm in melanoma. *Nat Rev Clin Oncol.* 2011;8(7):426–433.

Rigel DS, Russak J, Friedman R. The evolution of melanoma diagnosis: 25 years beyond the ABCDs [published online ahead of print July 29, 2010]. *CA Cancer J Clin.* 2010;60(5):301–316.

Robert C, Thomas L, Bondarenko I, et al. Ipilimumab plus dacarbazine for previously untreated metastatic melanoma. *N Engl J Med.* 2011;364(26):2517–2526.

Romano E, Scordo M, Dusza SW, et al. Site and timing of first relapse in stage III melanoma patients: implications for follow-up guidelines [published online ahead of print May 17, 2010]. *J Clin Oncol.* 2010;28(18):3042–3047.

Rosenberg SA, Yannelli JR, Yang JC, et al. Treatment of patients with metastatic melanoma with autologous tumor-infiltrating lymphocytes and interleukin 2. *J Natl Cancer Inst.* 1994;86:1159–1166.

Ross MI, Gershewald JE. How should we view the results of the Multicenter Selective Lymphadenectomy Trial-1 (MSLT-1). *Ann Surg Oncol.* 2008;15(3):670–673.

Ross MI, Gershenwald JE. Evidence-based treatment of early-stage melanoma. *J Surg Oncol.* 2011;104(4):341–353.

Ross MI, Thompson JF, Gershenwald JE. Sentinel lymph node biopsy for melanoma: critical assessment at its twentieth anniversary. *Surg Oncol Clin N Am.* 2011; 20(1):57–78.

Rousseau DL Jr, Ross MI, Johnson MM, et al. Revised American Joint Committee on Cancer staging criteria accurately predict sentinel lymph node positivity in clinically node-negative melanoma patients. *Ann Surg Oncol.* 2003;10:569–574.

Scolyer RA, Long GV, Thompson JF. Evolving concepts in melanoma classification and their relevance to multidisciplinary melanoma patient care [published online ahead of print March 21, 2011]. *Mol Oncol.* 2011;5(2):124–136.

Scolyer RA, Prieto VG. Melanoma pathology: important issues for clinicians involved in the multidisciplinary care of melanoma patients. *Surg Oncol Clin N Am.* 2011;20(1):19–37.

Scolyer RA, Thompson JF, McCarthy SW. Intraoperative frozen-section evaluation can reduce accuracy of pathologic assessment of sentinel nodes in melanoma patients. *J Am Coll Surg.* 2005; 201(5):821–823.

Sim FH, Taylor WF, Pritchard DJ, et al. Lymphadenectomy in the management of stage I malignant melanoma: a prospective randomized study. *Mayo Clin Proc.* 1986;61:697–705.

Smith MA, Fine JA, Barnhill RL, et al. Hormonal and reproductive influences and risk of melanoma in women. *Int J Epidemiol.* 1998;27:751–757.

Sondak VK, Liu PY, Tuthill RJ, et al. Adjuvant immunotherapy of resected, intermediate-thickness, node-negative melanoma with an allogeneic tumor vaccine: overall results of a randomized trial of the Southwest Oncology Group. *J Clin Oncol.* 2002;20:2058–2066.

Soong SJ, Ding S, Coit D, et al. AJCC Melanoma Task Force. Predicting survival outcome of localized melanoma: an electronic prediction tool based on the AJCC Melanoma Database [published online ahead of print April 9, 2010]. *Ann Surg Oncol.* 2010;17(8):2006–2014.

Sosman JA, Unger JM, Liu PY, et al. Adjuvant immunotherapy of resected, intermediate-thickness, node-negative melanoma with an allogeneic tumor vaccine: impact of HLA class I antigen expression on outcome. *J Clin Oncol.* 2002;20:2067–2075.

Sumner WE III, Ross MI, Mansfield PF, et al. Implications of lymphatic drainage to unusual sentinel lymph node sites in patients with primary cutaneous melanoma. *Cancer.* 2002;95:354–360.

Thompson JF, Kam PC. Isolated limb infusion for melanoma: a simple but effective alternative to isolated limb perfusion. *J Surg Oncol.* 2004;88:1–3.

Thompson JF, McCarthy WH, Bosch CM, et al. Sentinel lymph node status as an indicator of the presence of metastatic melanoma in regional lymph nodes. *Melanoma Res.* 1995;5:255–260.

Thompson JF, Soong SJ, Balch CM, et al. Prognostic significance of mitotic rate in localized primary cutaneous melanoma: an analysis of patients in the multi-institutional American Joint Committee on Cancer melanoma staging database [published online ahead of print April 25, 2011]. *J Clin Oncol.* 2011;29(16):2199–2205.

Turley RS, Raymond AK, Tyler DS. Regional treatment strategies for in-transit melanoma metastasis. *Surg Oncol Clin N Am.* 2011;20(1):79–103.

Uren RF. SPECT/CT lymphoscintigraphy to locate the sentinel lymph nodes in melanoma. *Ann Surg Oncol.* 2009;16:1459–1460.

van Poll D, Thompson JF, Colman MH, et al. A sentinel node biopsy does not increase the incidence of in-transit metastasis in patients with primary cutaneous melanoma. *Ann Surg Oncol.* 2005;12:597–608.

Veronesi U, Adamus J, Bandiera DC, et al. Delayed regional lymph node dissection in stage I melanoma of the skin of the lower extremities. *Cancer.* 1982;49:2420–2430.

Veronesi U, Adamus J, Bandiera DC, et al. Inefficacy of immediate node dissection in stage 1 melanoma of the limbs. *N Engl J Med.* 1977;297:627–630.

Veronesi U, Cascinelli N, Adamus J, et al. Thin stage I primary cutaneous malignant melanoma. Comparison of excision with margins of 1 or 3 cm. *N Engl J Med.* 1988;318:1159–1162.

Weber J, Atkins M, Hwu P, et al. Immunotherapy Task Force of the NCI Investigational Drug Steering Committee. White paper on adoptive cell therapy for cancer with tumor-infiltrating lymphocytes: a report of the CTEP subcommittee on adoptive cell therapy [published online ahead of print February 15, 2011]. *Clin Cancer Res.* 2001;17(7):1664–1673.

Wrightson WR, Wong SL, Edwards MJ, et al. Complications associated with sentinel lymph node biopsy for melanoma. *Ann Surg Oncol.* 2003;10:676–680.

Xing Y, Badgwell BD, Ross MI, et al. Lymph node ratio predicts disease-specific survival in melanoma patients. *Cancer.* 2009;115(11):2505–2513.

Xing Y, Bronstein Y, Ross MI, et al. Contemporary diagnostic imaging modalities for the staging and surveillance of melanoma patients: a meta-analysis [published online ahead of print November 16, 2010]. *J Natl Cancer Inst.* 2011; 103(2):129–142.

Xing Y, Chang GJ, Hu CY, et al. Conditional survival estimates improve over time for patients with advanced melanoma: results from a population-based analysis. *Cancer.* 2010;116(9):2234–2241.

Nonmelanoma Skin Cancer

Melinda M. Mortenson, Kelly Herne, Sharon R. Hymes, and Janice N. Cormier

EPIDEMIOLOGY AND ETIOLOGY

Basal cell carcinoma (BCC) and squamous cell carcinoma (SCC) constitute the majority of nonmelanoma skin cancers (NMSC), and it is estimated that together they are responsible for greater than 1 million cases annually. While BCC is 4 to 5 times more common than SCC, the incidence of both tumor types continues to rise despite growing awareness of the risk factors for these skin cancers. The overall incidence increases with age and is known to be higher in men than in women.

Development of NMSC is multifactorial and is related to various genotypic, phenotypic, and environmental risk factors. Ultraviolet (UV) solar radiation is considered to be the dominant risk factor for the development of both BCC and SCC, supported by the fact that most of these tumors tend to present on sun-exposed areas of the body. The development of BCC is thought to arise from intense intermittent sun exposure leading to burns, whereas SCC appears to be linked to the cumulative dose of UV solar radiation over time. Sun exposure earlier in life appears to be more influential in skin cancer development than that received later in life. Markers of UV sensitivity (e.g., fair-skin, light eyes, blond or red hair) and intensity of exposure (i.e., increased incidence for individuals living in proximity to the equator) are associated with increased NMSC risk as is additional UV exposure from recreational tanning booths and UV light therapy. One case-controlled study showed that use of tanning devices was associated with an estimated twofold risk for both SCC (odds ratio = 2.5) and BCC (odds ratio = 1.5). Another prospective study showed that treatment of psoriasis with oral psoralen in combination with light treatment (PUVA therapy) resulted in an increased adjusted relative risk of 8.6 for SCC; the risk for BCC was much lower.

Another important risk factor for both BCC and SCC is immunosuppression. Long-term, repeated immunosuppression therapy such as that used for solid organ transplant has been shown to increase the risk of SCC 40- to 250-fold, and for BCC, over 10-fold. NMSC in immunosuppressed patients tend to be multiple and behave more aggressively with a higher risk of recurrence and metastases (5% to 8%). Patients with acquired immunodeficiency syndrome also have an increased incidence of NMSC, and factors such as human papilloma virus (HPV) infection may act synergistically with UV exposure to increase risk. Moreover, HPV infection, especially HPV 16 and 18, has been implicated in the development of anogenital SCC.

Exposure to ionizing radiation increases the risk of NMSC threefold and often presents decades after initial exposure. This risk has been shown to be dose-dependent. Chemical exposures such as arsenic, tar, soot, tobacco, asphalt, and mineral oil have all been associated with an increased risk of SCC. SCC can also arise from areas of chronic inflammation and healing such as from scars, burn sites, or ulcers; this type of SCC is also known as Marjolin ulcer.

Patients with genetic syndromes including xeroderma pigmentosum, albinism, Muir–Torre syndrome, dystrophic epidermolysis bullosa, Fanconi anemia, Werner syndrome, nevoid basal cell syndrome, and Li-Fraumeni syndrome have an increased incidence of NMSC. Xeroderma pigmentosum is a rare autosomal recessive disease characterized by photophobia, severe sun sensitivity, and advanced sun damage. Affected individuals have defective DNA excision repair, and when exposed to UV radiation, develop malignancies of the skin and eyes at a rate 1,000 times that of the general population. Aggressive sun protection in the form of full-body sun suits and regular skin examinations are critical for patients with xeroderma pigmentosum. Ideally, these patients should only go outside at night. Nevoid basal cell syndrome is an autosomal dominant disorder characterized by the development of multiple BCCs. BCCs in patients with nevoid basal cell syndrome are often quite small but can number in the hundreds on any given skin surface. These patients are exquisitely sensitive to radiation and should avoid excessive sun exposure and radiation therapy. Regular follow-up is important, as such tumors are difficult to monitor and treat.

Similar to other tumor types, a previous diagnosis of cutaneous carcinoma increases the risk of future NMSCs to as high as 35% at 3 years and 50% at 5 years.

DIFFERENTIAL DIAGNOSIS

Several epidermal tumors common to the skin can resemble or are precursors to NMSC. Recognition of these tumors is important for both tumor surveillance and cancer prevention.

Seborrheic keratoses are benign proliferations of epidermis that can appear on any part of the skin, except mucous membranes, and usually appear after the age of 30 years. They are not related to sun exposure but are common on the face, neck, and trunk, often in large numbers. They initially appear as flat brown macules, eventually becoming larger, "stuck-on" brown plaques with dull crumbly surfaces (Fig. 4.1A). Seborrheic keratoses can sometimes be confused with melanoma, and biopsy of these lesions is prudent if any sudden changes in size or color occur.

Actinic keratoses (AKs) are premalignant lesions with the potential to develop into SCCs. They are found mainly on sun-exposed areas of light-skinned individuals. These lesions most commonly present as skin-colored, erythematous, or brown ill-defined patches with adherent scales (Fig. 4.1B). These lesions are extremely common on the face, scalp, ears, and lips and can often be better appreciated by palpation rather than by inspection with the naked eye.

Keratoacanthoma is a tumor that often occurs on older, sun-damaged skin and is most commonly found on the neck and face. These tumors originate in pilosebaceous glands and may grow rapidly as a red- or skin-colored dome-shaped nodule with a central crater. Maximum size may be attained at 6 to 8 weeks with slow regression over a period of months leaving a residual scar. These tumors can be confused both clinically and histologically with SCC, and there are reports of progression of keratoacanthomas to invasive or metastatic carcinoma. Classification of these tumors as a well-differentiated variant of invasive SCC has been proposed. Surgical excision of keratoacanthomas with 3 to 5 mm margins is recommended, and Mohs surgery may be employed in cosmetically sensitive areas. These tumors are radiation sensitive if surgery is not an option.

A cutaneous horn is the clinical description for a growth that appears as a dense cone of epithelium resembling a horn (Fig. 4.1C). They range in size from several millimeters to over a centimeter and are generally white or yellowish in color; they also tend to appear on sun-exposed skin of older individuals. Histologically, cutaneous horns can develop from benign lesions such as warts or seborrheic keratoses, from premalignant lesions such as AKs and SCC in situ or from malignant lesions such as SCCs. Up to 15% of cutaneous horns demonstrate invasive SCC at the base, and excision of these tumors is always indicated.

Nevus sebaceous is a benign tumor of the scalp that appears at or soon after birth as a yellowish-orange, well-demarcated plaque. Initially, the surface has a

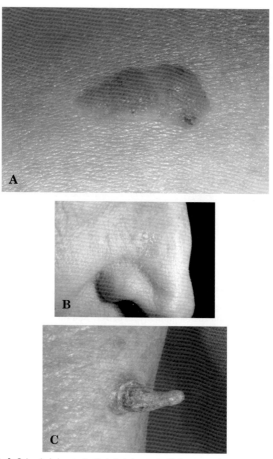

FIGURE 4.1 A: Seborrheic keratosis. **B:** Actinic keratosis. **C:** Cutaneous horn.

smooth or waxy appearance that gradually becomes more warty or verrucous during puberty. In adulthood, approximately 10% of these lesions develop into BCC. It is therefore recommended that these lesions be excised or closely monitored for the life of the patient.

BASAL CELL CARCINOMA

BCC is the most common cancer in humans and the most common type of skin cancer. BCCs are believed to arise from hair follicle cells and are therefore found almost exclusively on hair-bearing skin. Most lesions are found on sun-exposed areas such as the head and neck, but non-sun-exposed areas are also at risk. These tumors tend to grow slowly, but when untreated can lead to invasion of local structures including muscle, cartilage, and bone. Although the biological behavior of

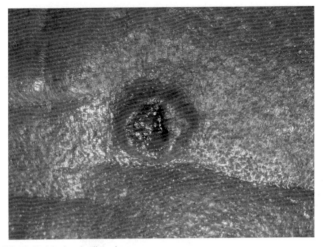

FIGURE 4.2 Nodular basal cell carcinoma.

BCC is characterized by local and sometimes disfiguring invasiveness, metastasis is rare, occurring in less than 0.05% of cases.

There are multiple histologic subtypes of BCC, and subtype is predictive of its behavior. Less aggressive subtypes include nodular or superficial BCC, while higher risk subtypes include sclerosing, infiltrating, micronodular, and basosquamous carcinoma. The higher risk subtypes tend to have subclinical extension exceeding the visible borders of the lesion making treatment more difficult.

Nodular BCC is the classic lesion of this type of NMSC. It appears as a pink translucent nodule with rolled edges and is often described as "pearly." In dark-skinned individuals, these tumors are often pigmented and can resemble melanoma. Overlying telangiectasias and ulceration are common (Fig. 4.2). They occur predominantly on the face.

Superficial BCC is a variant that is more common on the limbs and trunk and on other areas with little or no sun exposure. It presents as a slow-growing, scaly pink plaque and can easily be confused with psoriasis, superficial SCC or SCC in situ (Bowen disease). Gentle traction on the periphery of the lesion often demonstrates a shiny translucent surface characteristic of BCC which can assist with diagnosis.

The sclerosing or morpheaform type represents the rarest form of BCC and is often difficult to recognize. It presents as a poorly defined indurated or sclerotic plaque which can be mistaken for a scar. In addition, this type of BCC frequently is found to be larger histopathologically than is clinically evident. Therefore, both diagnosis and treatment remain a challenge.

Basosquamous carcinomas have features of both BCC and SCC. These are aggressive tumors with potential to metastasize.

SQUAMOUS CELL CARCINOMA

SCC is the second most common cutaneous carcinoma and accounts for roughly 20% of all NMSCs. In addition, SCC is responsible for the majority of deaths from NMSC. SCC develops from keratinocytes of the epidermis and has many clinical

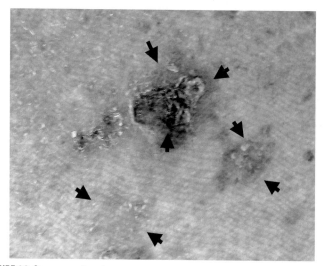

FIGURE 4.3 Squamous cell carcinoma.

variants. As stated previously, it can arise from precursor lesions such as AK or can develop at the base of a cutaneous horn. Uncommonly, SCC presents de novo as a single lesion on otherwise normal appearing skin. The most common lesion is found on sun-damaged skin, especially on the head, neck, or arms. The lesions are usually red, poorly defined plaques or nodules with an ulcerated, friable surface (Fig. 4.3). Bowen disease, or SCC in situ, is characterized by a well-demarcated pink plaque with a raised border and uniform scaling throughout.

SCC has a higher metastatic potential than BCC, with an overall 5-year metastatic risk of 5%. However, many factors affect the metastatic potential of any given tumor, and there are subgroups with higher risk (Table 4.1). Regional lymph nodes are the most common metastatic site, with distant sites such as bone, brain, and lungs occasionally reported. For tumors of the head and neck, the parotid gland is a common site for metastases. In general, features that indicate high risk for metastasis also predict risk for recurrence.

WORK-UP/BIOPSY TECHNIQUES

Work-up of any NMSC should include a thorough history, including reported duration, rate of growth, associated symptoms, previous treatment, and risk factors for NMSC. Changes noted by the patient may be quite subtle and include itching, tenderness, bleeding, or changes in size, color, or texture. A detailed head-to-toe skin examination should be performed with careful inspection and palpation of suspicious lesions. In patients suspected of having SCC, the draining lymph node basins should be evaluated for nodal metastases by palpation. In general, radiologic studies are not necessary for the evaluation of patients with SCC, however, if high-risk features are present a magnetic resonance imaging can be obtained to evaluate the extent of local involvement as can an ultrasound for the evaluation of regional nodal basin.

Any cutaneous lesion suspicious for malignancy should be biopsied for pathological assessment. Biopsy of suspicious pigmented lesions should be limited to punch or excisional biopsy techniques in which the full thickness of the dermis can

TABLE 4.1	Risk Factors for Recurrence and Metastases in Squamous Cell Carcinoma	
	Low-Risk Feature	**High-Risk Feature**
Clinical Factors		
Tumor size	<2 cm	>2 cm
Location	Trunk, extremities	Lip, ear, genitalia
Borders	Well defined	Ill defined
Arising from scar, inflammation	No	Yes
Prior radiation	No	Yes
History of immunosuppression	No	Yes
Primary versus recurrent	Primary	Recurrent
Histology		
Differentiation	Well differentiated	Poorly differentiated
Perineural invasion	No	Yes
Depth of invasion	<4 mm or < Clark level IV	≥4 mm or Clark level IV/V
Subtype	—	Adenoid (acantholytic) adenosquamous, desmoplastic
Excision	Complete	Incomplete

be evaluated. A punch biopsy usually ranges in size from 2 to 8 mm and involves removing a cylinder of tissue, ideally to the level of the subcutaneous fat. Often, entire lesions can be removed for pathological examination; if not, the most suspicious aspect of the tumor may be sampled.

Shave biopsy is an excellent technique for superficial lesions or nonpigmented lesions suspicious for BCC or SCC. It is also a good biopsy technique for cutaneous horns or keratoacanthomas provided the base of the tumor is included in the specimen. A shave biopsy involves injecting local anesthesia into the epidermis and upper dermis and then performing a tangential sample at the base of the wheal. A sterile flexible razor blade or a 15 blade is recommended so that the mid-dermis is included in the biopsy specimen. If performed too superficially, invasion into the dermis cannot be evaluated and rebiopsy may be required.

Excisional biopsy involves removal of the entire lesion with a margin of clinically clear tissue and is generally used for classic lesions such as superficial SCCs or nodular and superficial BCCs. Margins can be evaluated in the specimen, and further treatment is often unnecessary.

STAGING

The 7th edition of the American Joint Committee on Cancer (AJCC) *Cancer Staging Manual* has improved the staging of cutaneous SCC. Most notably, high-risk features including histologic grade (poorly differentiated or undifferentiated), anatomic site (ear or nonglabrous lip), Clark level ≥4, depth >2 mm, and perineural invasion are now included. A T1 tumor is ≤2 cm with less than two high-risk features, while a T2 tumor is >2 cm or can be any size when two or more high-risk features are present. Recognizing that increased nodal burden correlates with decreased survival, nodal staging has also been updated and is now characterized as N0 to N3 based on the size and number of involved nodes rather than the previous 6th edition characterization as either present (N1) or absent (N0) (Table 4.2).

TABLE 4.2	American Joint Committee on Cancer Staging of Cutaneous Squamous Cell Carcinoma and Other Cutaneous Carcinoma

TNM Staging System[a]

Cutaneous Squamous Cell Carcinoma and Other Cutaneous Carcinoma[b]

Tumor

T1	Tumor <2 cm in greatest dimension with less than two high-risk features[c]
T2	Tumor >2 cm in greatest dimension OR tumor any size with two or more high-risk features
T3	Tumor with invasion of maxilla, mandible, orbit, or temporal bone
T4	Tumor with invasion of skeleton or perineural invasion of skull base

Nodes

N0	No regional lymph node metastasis
N1	Metastasis in a single ipsilateral lymph node, ≤3 cm in greatest dimension
N2	Metastasis in a single ipsilateral lymph node, >3 cm but <6 cm in greatest dimension; or in bilateral or contralateral lymph nodes, none >6 cm in greatest dimension
N3	Metastasis in a lymph node, >6 cm in greatest dimension

Metastasis

M0	No distant metastases
M1	Distant metastases

Stage Groupings

Stage	T	N	M
Stage I	T1	N0	M0
Stage II	T2	N0	M0
Stage III	T3	N0	M0
	T1–3	N1	M1
Stage IV	T1–3	N2	M0
	T Any	N3	M0
	T4	N Any	M0
	T Any	N Any	M1

[a]Adapted from the 7th edition of the *AJCC Cancer Staging Manual*.
[b]Does not include Merkel cell carcinoma.
[c]High-risk features for the primary tumor (T) staging: >2 mm thickness, Clark level ≥IV, perineural invasion, primary site ear or non-hair-bearing lip, poorly differentiated or undifferentiated.

TREATMENT

The treatment of NMSC requires careful evaluation of tumor size, pathological characteristics, anatomical location, age, overall health of the patient, cost to the patient, and cosmesis. Treatment modalities can be divided into surgical and nonsurgical therapies although surgical intervention is often the mainstay of treatment.

Surgical Techniques

Primary surgical excision with a margin of clinically normal tissue allows subsequent evaluation of the entire specimen for clear margins. Predetermined margins of 4 mm to 10 mm should be performed along Langer lines to achieve the best cosmetic result. For low-risk lesions a 4 to 6 mm margin should be adequate, and for high-risk lesions a 10-mm margin should be used. Recurrent BCC is associated with a poor cure rate, and a 10-mm excision margin is recommended. For incompletely excised lesions, re-excision is recommended if possible.

Mohs micrographic surgery involves removal of the clinical margins of the tumor under local anesthesia with immediate evaluation of the margins with frozen sections. Small incremental sections are removed until the margins are clear. This technique allows for the best cosmetic results by preserving normal tissue, while ensuring that larger lesions with subclinical extension are entirely removed. Mohs micrographic surgery of primary and recurrent NMSC of the head and neck has a cure rate (negative histologic margin) of 99%, the reconstructive choices after Mohs surgery are similar to those available after traditional excision. Although Mohs micrographic surgery is time-consuming and requires skilled practitioners, the benefits of superior cosmesis and excellent cure rates make it the treatment of choice for many patients. Indications for Mohs procedure are centrofacially located tumors, large tumors, poorly defined tumor margins, recurrent lesions, lesions with perineural or perivascular involvement, tumors at a site of prior radiation therapy, tumors in the setting of immunosuppression, and patients with high-risk histological subtypes of BCC.

There has been considerable interest in performing sentinel lymph node (SLN) biopsy in selected patients with high-risk SCC in hopes that detection and treatment of subclinical nodal metastases will lead to improved outcomes for these patients. In a pooled evaluation of 83 high-risk SCC patients, all patients with a positive SLN had lesions >2 cm in diameter. Among patients with tumors <2 cm, 2.1 to 3 cm, and >3 cm in diameter, the proportions of patients with a positive SLN were 0%, 15.8%, and 30.4%, respectively. While the available data suggest SLN biopsy can accurately identify micrometastatic nodal disease in patients with SCC, studies to date are limited by small sample size, limited follow-up, and lack of uniform criteria. Additional studies will be needed before definitive guidelines can be established with respect to SLN biopsy.

Destructive Techniques

Destructive techniques for superficial BCC and SCC include curettage, cryotherapy, and laser ablation. Curettage involves debulking the tumor under local anesthesia with a sharp curette until firm underlying dermis is reached. The base is hyfrecated, and the process is repeated two or three times. This technique is reserved for small (<1 cm), primary, low risk, or superficial tumors in non-hair-bearing areas, and as such is not suitable for recurrent or ill-defined tumors. The technique is based on the ability of the sharp curette to differentiate friable tumor tissue from normal dermis. If subcutaneous fat is reached during this technique, it is necessary to convert to surgical excision, as the curette will no longer be able to distinguish soft fat tissue from tumor.

Cryotherapy is a destructive method primarily reserved for the treatment of precancerous lesions such as AKs and occasionally for small, superficial, low-risk, primary BCCs or SCCs. Liquid nitrogen is either sprayed with a cryogen or is directly applied to the lesion with cotton-tipped applicators for a period of time such that the visible thawing of the lesions takes at least 15 seconds (30 seconds for superficial SCC or BCC). Ablation with a carbon dioxide laser may be considered for precancerous lesions or low-risk BCC. However, follicular involvement may be difficult to treat and lead to recurrence.

Nonsurgical Therapies

Radiation therapy is often reserved for patients unable or unwilling to undergo surgical treatment of primary lesions or when clear margins cannot be obtained by

Mohs or more extensive surgery. It is also considered for the adjuvant treatment of recurrent or histologically aggressive tumors (e.g., those exhibiting perineural invasion). For high-grade SCC with perineural involvement or invasion into bone, radiation therapy is generally recommended in conjunction with surgical excision. Radiation therapy can be further used as adjuvant or palliative treatment for lymph node metastases. Disadvantages of radiation therapy include acute and chronic radiation changes (dyspigmentation, telangiectasia, radiodystrophy), higher recurrence rates in BCC, lack of margin control, and increased number of treatment sessions. As radiation therapy can result in NMSC decades after exposure, it should be used cautiously in young patients. It is also contraindicated in nevoid BCC.

Topical therapies for superficial NMSC and AKs include 5% fluorouracil (5-FU) and imiquimod creams. 5-FU is an antineoplastic antimetabolite. Imiquimod is a synthetic immune response modifier that enhances cell-mediated immune response via the induction of proinflammatory cytokines. These topical therapies are most commonly used for AKs as well as for superficial BCCs and SCCs in situ when surgery or other treatment techniques are contraindicated or impractical. Topical 5-FU is not appropriate for nodular BCC and is not recommended for SCC due to high recurrence rates. Treatment regimens for AKs with 5-FU vary widely; in general, 5-FU is applied to the affected area once or twice daily for a period ranging from 2 to 6 weeks. Re-treatment several months later, either with cryotherapy or other modalities, may be necessary. For the treatment of superficial BCC, 5-FU can be applied daily to the tumor and several millimeters of surrounding skin for a period of at least 4 weeks. After a 2- to 3-week respite, the area is then evaluated clinically for residual tumor. Biopsy is often indicated to ensure adequate therapy. Significant erythema, stinging, oozing, and crusting are often reported, especially with more aggressive treatment regimens. 5-FU can be applied to an entire region, such as the face, chest, arms, or hands.

Imiquimod therapy is approved for the treatment of AKs and superficial BCC but should not be used for SCC. In general, less local skin reaction is reported compared to 5-FU. For AKs the cream is applied 2 nonconsecutive days a week for 16 weeks. For superficial BCC, the cream should be applied 5 nights a week for at least 6 weeks. After a 2- to 3-month respite, the lesion is evaluated either clinically or histologically (rebiopsy) to confirm adequate therapy. While imiquimod can also be used for nodular BCC the treatment duration requires 12 weeks and the response is lower (76%) compared to a greater than 85% success rate for superficial BCC. Imiquimod is often well tolerated, causes minimal or no scarring, and is particularly useful for multiple lesions concentrated in one area.

Photodynamic therapy (PDT) is another noninvasive method used for the treatment of AKs and superficial BCC. A photosensitizer (most commonly, aminolevulinic acid) is applied to the skin and activated with a light source. The tumor cells retain the photosensitizer for longer periods of time than normal cells, resulting in preferential killing. Cure rates for AKs are reported to be as high as 90%; however, recurrence rates at 5 years for superficial and nodular BCC have been reported to be as high as 14% to 22%, respectively. Side effects include burning or stinging pain during the treatment and posttreatment periods, erythema, swelling, and temporary hyper- or hypopigmentation, but overall the cosmetic results are superior in comparison to surgery or cryotherapy. Systemic PDT has also been tested as a treatment for BCC and may be appropriate for individuals presenting with multiple lesions or nevoid BCC syndrome.

Chemoprevention with low-dose oral retinoids has shown some promise in the prevention of SCC for chronically immunosuppressed patients who have undergone organ transplantation. However, long-term therapy is needed, as beneficial effects are often lost when these drugs are discontinued.

SCREENING, PREVENTION, AND FOLLOW-UP

Aggressive screening of patients at risk for skin cancer is essential to minimize the morbidity and mortality of NMSC. Patients at risk include those with light skin types, immunosuppression, and a family or personal history of skin cancer. Exposure to UV radiation should be limited in children with regular use of sunscreen from an early age. Appropriate SPF level and application techniques should be emphasized for all patients, especially regarding applications to the face and neck.

Regular examination of the skin by a dermatologist is recommended for all patients at risk for skin cancer on at least an yearly basis. A complete skin examination includes examination of the entire skin surface, including the scalp, with particular attention to previous areas of skin cancer. For patients with a history of AKs or NMSCs, regular follow-up with a dermatologist is recommended. For patients with SCC, most recurrences or metastases will occur within 2 years, and almost all will occur within 5 years. In addition, patients with a history of SCC should undergo a thorough examination of all regional lymph node basins to evaluate for metastases.

Recommended Readings

Alam M, Ratner D. Cutaneous squamous-cell carcinoma. *N Engl J Med.* 2001;344(13): 975–983.

American Cancer Society. *Cancer Facts & Figures 2009.* Atlanta: American Cancer Society; 2009.

American Joint Committee on Cancer. *AJCC Cancer Staging Manual.* 7th ed. New York, NY: Springer; 2010.

Basset-Seguin N, Ibbotson SH, Emtestam L, et al. Topical methyl aminolaevulinate photodynamic therapy versus cryotherapy for superficial basal cell carcinoma: a 5 year randomized trial. *Eur J Dermatol.* 2008;18:547–553.

Harwood CA, Leedham-Green M, Leigh IM, et al. Low-dose retinoids in the prevention of cutaneous squamous cell carcinomas in organ transplant recipients: a 16-year retrospective study. *Arch Dermatol.* 2005;141(4):456–464.

Karagas MR, Stannard VA, Mott LA, et al. Use of tanning devices and risk of basal cell and squamous cell skin cancers. *J Natl Cancer Inst.* 2002;94(3):224–226.

Lansbury L, Leonardi-Bee J, Perkins W, et al. Interventions for non-metastatic squamous cell carcinoma of the skin. *Cochrane Database Syst Rev.* 2010;4: CD007869.

Lee DA, Miller SJ. Nonmelanoma skin cancer. *Facial Plast Surg Clin North Am.* 2009; 17(3):309–324.

Madan V, Lear JT, Szeimies RM. Non-melanoma skin cancer. *Lancet.* 2010;375 (9715):673–685.

Mosterd K, Arits AH, Thissen MR, et al. Histology-based treatment of basal cell carcinoma. *Acta Derm Venereol.* 2009;89(5): 454–458. Review. Erratum in: *Acta Derm Venereol.* 2009;89(6):667.

Renzi C, Caggiati A, Mannooranparampil TJ, et al. Sentinel lymph node biopsy for high risk cutaneous squamous cell carcinoma: case series and review of the literature. *Eur J Surg Oncol.* 2007;33(3): 364–369.

Smoller BR. Squamous cell carcinoma: from precursor lesions to high-risk variants. *Mod Pathol.* 2006;19:S88–S92.

Stern RS, Liebman EJ, Vakeva L. Oral psoralen and ultraviolet-A light (PUVA) treatment of psoriasis and persistent risk of nonmelanoma skin cancer. PUVA Follow-up Study. *J Natl Cancer Inst.* 1998;90:1278–1284.

Soft-tissue and Bone Sarcoma

Abigail S. Caudle, Keith A. Delman, and Janice N. Cormier

EPIDEMIOLOGY

Sarcomas are rare tumors that account for less than 1% of all newly diagnosed adult cancers and 7% of all newly diagnosed cancers in children. In 2008, an estimated 10,390 new cases of soft-tissue sarcoma were diagnosed in the United States, with 5,150 patients expected to die of the disease. To complicate matters, the broad designation of "sarcoma" actually encompasses a wide variety of more than 50 histologic subtypes such as soft-tissue sarcomas, bone sarcomas (osteosarcomas/chondrosarcomas), Ewing's sarcomas, and peripheral primitive neuroectodermal tumors.

Soft-tissue sarcomas can occur anywhere in the body. The majority of primary lesions originate in an extremity (59%), with the next most frequent anatomical site of origin being the trunk (19%), followed by the retroperitoneum (13%) and the head/neck region (9%). The most common histologic types of soft-tissue sarcoma in adults (excluding Kaposi sarcoma) are malignant fibrous histiocytoma (24%), leiomyosarcoma (21%), liposarcoma (19%), synovial sarcoma (12%), and malignant peripheral nerve sheath tumors (6%). Rhabdomyosarcoma is the most common soft-tissue sarcoma of childhood and accounts for approximately 250 cases annually.

During the past 25 years, a multimodality treatment approach has been successfully applied to patients with extremity sarcomas, and this has led to improvements in both survival and quality of life. However, patients with abdominal sarcomas continue to have high rates of recurrence and poor overall survival. The overall 5-year survival rate for patients with all stages of soft-tissue sarcoma is 50% to 60%. Of the patients who die of sarcoma, most will succumb to metastatic disease, which 80% of the time occurs within 2 to 3 years of the initial diagnosis.

ETIOLOGY

Numerous factors have been associated with an increased risk of soft-tissue sarcoma. These factors are discussed in the following sections.

Trauma

Although patients with sarcoma frequently report a history of trauma in the tumor area, a causal relationship has not been established. More often, a minor injury calls attention to a pre-existing tumor that may be accentuated by edema or a hematoma.

Occupational Chemicals

Exposure to some herbicides such as phenoxyacetic acids and wood preservatives containing chlorophenols has been linked to an increased risk for soft-tissue sarcoma. Several chemical carcinogens, including Thorotrast (thorium oxide), vinyl chloride, and arsenic, have been associated with hepatic angiosarcoma. Exposure to asbestos has been associated with mesothelioma.

Previous Radiation Exposure

External radiation therapy is a rare but well-established cause of soft-tissue sarcoma. An 8- to 50-fold increase in the incidence of sarcomas has been noted for patients treated for cancers of the breast, cervix, ovary, testes, and lymphatic system. In addition, the risk for sarcomas after radiation therapy increases with higher dosage. The interval between irradiation and the development of sarcoma is usually at least 10 years. In a review of 160 patients with postirradiation sarcomas, the most common histologic types were osteogenic sarcoma, malignant fibrous histiocytoma, angiosarcoma, and lymphangiosarcoma. Postirradiation sarcomas are often diagnosed at a more advanced stage and are therefore associated with a poorer prognosis compared with other sarcomas.

Chronic Lymphedema
In 1948, Stewart and Treves were the first to describe the association of chronic lymphedema following axillary dissection with subsequent lymphangiosarcoma. Lymphangiosarcoma has also been observed in patients following filarial infections and in the lower extremities of patients with congenital primary lymphedema.

Genetic Predisposition
Specific inherited genetic alterations have been associated with an increased risk of bone and soft-tissue sarcomas. For example, patients with Gardner syndrome (familial polyposis) have a higher than normal incidence of desmoids, patients with germ-line mutations in the tumor suppressor gene *p53* (Li-Fraumeni syndrome) have a high incidence of sarcomas, and patients with von Recklinghausen disease who have abnormalities in the neurofibromatosis type 1 gene have an increased risk of neurofibrosarcomas. Soft-tissue sarcomas can also occur in patients with hereditary retinoblastoma as a second primary malignancy.

Oncogene Activation
Oncogenes are genes that are capable of inducing malignant transformation and tend to drive cells toward proliferation. Several oncogenes have been identified in association with soft-tissue sarcomas, including *MDM2*, *N-myc*, *c-erB2*, and members of the *ras* family. Amplification of these genes has been shown to correlate with an adverse outcome in patients with various soft-tissue sarcomas. Activating point mutations in *c-KIT* are seen in approximately 85% to 95% of patients with gastrointestinal stromal tumors (GISTs) and have important implications for the management of these patients.

Cytogenetic analysis of soft-tissue tumors has led to the identification of distinct chromosomal translocations in oncogenes that are associated with certain histologic subtypes. These include the TLS–CHOP fusion, which is observed in myxoid liposarcoma, and the EWS–ATF1 fusion, which is observed in clear cell sarcoma, among others. The gene rearrangements best characterized to date are those found in Ewing's sarcoma, clear cell sarcoma, myxoid liposarcoma, alveolar rhabdomyosarcoma, desmoplastic small round cell tumors, and synovial sarcoma.

Tumor Suppressor Genes
Tumor suppressor genes play a critical role in suppressing tumor cell growth. However, these genes can be inactivated as a result of hereditary or sporadic mechanisms. Two genes that have shown the greatest relevance to soft-tissue tumors are the retinoblastoma (*Rb*) tumor suppressor gene and the *p53* tumor suppressor gene. Mutations or deletions in *Rb* can lead to the development of retinoblastoma, as well as sarcomas of soft tissue and bone. Mutations in the *p53* tumor suppressor gene are the most common mutations in human solid tumors and have been observed in 30% to 60% of cases of soft-tissue sarcomas.

PATHOLOGY

Sarcomas are a heterogeneous group of tumors that not only arise predominantly from the embryonic mesoderm, but can also arise from the ectoderm (e.g., peripheral nervous sheath tumors). Mesodermal cells give rise to the connective tissues distributed throughout the body, including pericardium, pleura, blood vessel endothelium, smooth and striated muscle, bone, cartilage, and synovium. These are the cells from which nearly all sarcomas originate. Consequently, sarcomas develop in a wide variety of anatomical sites.

Despite the various histologic subtypes, sarcomas have many common clinical and pathological features. The overall clinical behavior of most types of sarcoma is similar and determined by anatomical location (depth, specifically related to fascial boundaries), grade, and size. The dominant route of metastasis is hematogenous. Tumor grade has been firmly established to have prognostic significance and has therefore been incorporated into the staging of soft-tissue sarcomas. However, some experts have suggested that the pathological classification is far more important than grade when other pretreatment variables are taken into account. Table 5.1 shows a breakdown of the histologic types of tumors by their aggressiveness. Tumors with little or no metastatic potential include desmoids, atypical lipomatous tumors (also called well-differentiated liposarcoma), dermatofibrosarcoma protuberans (DFSPs), and hemangiopericytomas. Those subtypes with an intermediate risk of metastatic spread include myxoid liposarcoma, myxoid malignant fibrous histiocytoma, and extraskeletal chondrosarcoma. Highly aggressive tumors that have a substantial metastatic potential include angiosarcoma, clear cell sarcoma, pleomorphic

T A B L E **5.1**	Breakdown of Sarcoma Histologic Type by Tumor Aggressiveness

Low Metastatic Potential
Desmoid tumor
Atypical lipomatous tumor
Dermatofibrosarcoma protuberans
Hemangiopericytoma

Intermediate Metastatic Potential
Myxoid liposarcoma
Myxoid malignant fibrous histiocytoma
Extraskeletal chondrosarcoma

High Metastatic Potential
Alveolar soft part sarcoma
Angiosarcoma
Clear cell sarcoma ("melanoma of soft parts")
Epithelioid sarcoma
Extraskeletal Ewing's sarcoma
Extraskeletal osteosarcoma
Malignant fibrous histiocytoma
Liposarcoma (pleomorphic and dedifferentiated)
Leiomyosarcoma
Neurogenic sarcoma (malignant schwannoma)
Rhabdomyosarcoma
Synovial sarcoma

and dedifferentiated liposarcoma, leiomyosarcoma, rhabdomyosarcoma, and synovial sarcoma. Approximately 15% of all soft-tissue sarcomas occur in the retroperitoneum. Approximately 80% are malignant, with liposarcoma, fibrosarcoma, leiomyosarcoma, and malignant fibrous histiocytoma accounting for the vast majority of the histologic types.

In as many as 25% to 40% of cases, expert sarcoma pathologists may disagree about specific histologic diagnoses or criteria for defining tumor grade. This low concordance rate may stem from the fact that few pathologists have the opportunity to study many of these rare tumors during their careers. It also emphasizes the need for more objective molecular and biochemical markers to improve the accuracy of conventional histologic assessment.

STAGING

The staging criteria for soft-tissue sarcomas in the current version of the American Joint Committee on Cancer (AJCC) staging guidelines consist of the histopathological grade (G), tumor size and depth (T), and the presence of metastases (distant [M] or nodal [N]). Several revisions were added to the 7th edition AJCC sarcoma staging system which recently went into place, reflecting our evolving understanding of the biology of sarcoma, specifically the influence of histopathologic subtype on prognosis. For instance, GISTs are now classified separately from the other sarcomas. Desmoid tumors, Kaposi's sarcomas, and infantile fibrosarcomas are also now excluded from the system while angiosarcoma, extraskeletal Ewing's sarcoma, and DFSP have been added to the list of histologic types. Grading has been reformatted to a three-grade system instead of the previous four-grade protocol. Lastly, N1 disease has been reclassified as stage III disease. The new staging system for GIST and soft-tissue sarcoma is shown in Table 5.2.

Histopathological Grade
Histopathological grade remains the most important prognostic factor for determining disease-free and overall survival rate which is reflected in the staging system as low-grade tumors are classified as stage I regardless of tumor size or depth. To accurately determine tumor grade, an adequate tissue sample must be well fixed, well stained, and reviewed by an experienced sarcoma pathologist. The pathological features that define grade include cellularity, differentiation, pleomorphism, necrosis, and the number of mitoses.

Tumor Size
Tumor size at presentation is also an important determinant of outcome. Sarcomas have classically been stratified into two groups based on size: T1 lesions (≤5 cm) and T2 lesions (>5 cm). The 2009 AJCC staging system continues to use depth (i.e., superficial or deep) to define prognosis. Extremity soft-tissue sarcomas that are superficial to the investing muscular fascia are designated *a* lesions in the T score (Ta), whereas tumors deep to the fascia and all retroperitoneal and visceral lesions are designated *b* (Tb).

Nodal Metastases
Lymph node metastases are rare, with less than 5% of soft-tissue sarcomas metastasizing to the nodes. Nodal metastases are associated with a poor prognosis and are currently classified as stage III disease. A few histologic subtypes, such as epithelioid sarcoma, rhabdomyosarcoma, clear cell sarcoma, angiosarcoma, and malignant fibrous histiocytoma, have been found to be associated with a higher incidence of nodal involvement (10% to 20%).

New Staging System for GIST and Soft-tissue Sarcoma

7th Edition AJCC Soft-tissue Sarcoma Staging System

Primary Tumor (T)

TX	Primary tumor cannot be assessed
T0	No evidence of primary tumor
T1	Tumor ≤5 cm in greatest dimension
	T1a Tumor above superficial fascia
	T1b Tumor invading or deep to superficial fascia
T2	Tumor >5 cm in greatest dimension
	T2a Tumor above superficial fascia
	T2b Tumor invading or deep to superficial fascia

Regional Lymph Nodes (N)

NX	Regional lymph nodes cannot be assessed
N0	No regional lymph node metastasis
N1	Regional lymph node metastasis

Distant Metastasis (M)

MX	Distant metastasis cannot be assessed
M0	No distant metastasis
M1	Distant metastasis

Histopathological Grade (G)

GX	Grade cannot be assessed
G1	Grade 1
G2	Grade 2
G3	Grade 3

Stage Grouping

Stage I		
	A	T1a N0 M0 G1, Gx
		T1b N0 M0 G1, Gx
	B	T2a N0 M0 G1, Gx
		T2b N0 M0 G1, Gx
Stage II		
	A	T1a N0 M0 G2, G3
		T1b N0 M0 G2, G3
	B	T2a N0 M0 G2
		T2b N0 M0 G2
Stage III		T2a, T2b N0 M0 G3
		Any T N1 M0 Any G
Stage IV		Any T Any N M1 Any G

7th Edition AJCC GIST Staging System

Primary Tumor (T)

Tx	Primary tumor cannot be assessed
T0	No evidence of primary tumor
T1	Tumor ≤2 cm
T2	Tumor >2 cm but ≤5 cm
T3	Tumor >5 cm but ≤10 cm
T4	Tumor >10 cm

(*continued*)

TABLE 5.2	New Staging System for GIST and Soft-tissue Sarcoma (*continued*)

7th Edition AJCC GIST Staging System (*continued*)

Regional Lymph Nodes (N)	
Nx	Regional lymph nodes cannot be assessed
N0	No regional lymph node metastasis
N1	Regional lymph node metastasis
Distant Metastasis (M)	
M0	No distant metastasis
M1	Distant metastasis
Stage Grouping—*Gastric GIST*	
Stage I	
A	T1 or T2 N0 M0 Low mitotic rate
B	T3 N0 M0 Low mitotic rate
Stage II	T1, T2 N0 M0 High mitotic rate
	T4 N0 M0 Low mitotic rate
Stage III	
A	T3 N0 M0 High mitotic rate
B	T4 N0 M0 High mitotic rate
Stage IV	Any T N1 M0 Any Rate
	Any T Any N M1 Any Rate
Stage Grouping—*Small Intestinal GIST*	
Stage I	T1 or T2 N0 M0 Low mitotic rate
Stage II	T3 N0 M0 Low mitotic rate
Stage III	
A	T1 N0 M0 High mitotic rate
	T4 N0 M0 Low mitotic rate
B	T2, T3, T4 N0 M0 High mitotic rate
Stage IV	Any T N1 M0 Any rate
	Any T Any N M1 Any rate

Adapted from Edge SB, Bird DR, Compton CC, et al., eds. *Cancer Staging Manual.* 7th ed. Philadelphia, PA: Lippincott-Raven; 2009.

Distant Metastasis
Distant metastases occur most frequently in the lung. Resection of the pulmonary lesions in selected patients with isolated lung metastases may offer up to a 30% 5-year survival rate. Other potential sites of metastasis include bone, brain, and liver. Visceral and retroperitoneal sarcomas have a propensity to metastasize to the liver and peritoneum.

General Principles
While this represents a heterogeneous group of patients, there are some general principles of evaluation, treatment, and follow-up that are applicable to all sarcoma patients.

Radiographic Evaluation
The goals of pretreatment radiologic imaging are to accurately define the local extent of a tumor and to look for metastatic disease. Magnetic resonance imaging (MRI) has supplanted computed tomography (CT) as the imaging technique of choice in the evaluation of soft-tissue sarcomas of the extremity, except in patients

who do not have access to MRI or who have a contraindication to MRI. MRI accurately delineates muscle groups and distinguishes between bone, vascular structures, and tumor. In addition, sagittal and coronal views allow three-dimensional evaluation of anatomical compartments.

CT remains the imaging technique of choice for evaluating retroperitoneal sarcomas. A CT scan of the abdomen and pelvis should also be obtained when the histologic assessment of an extremity sarcoma reveals myxoid liposarcoma, because this histologic subtype is known to metastasize to the abdomen and retroperitoneum. Chest CT is used most often in patients with high-grade lesions to evaluate for the presence of metastatic disease. Searches for bone and brain metastases are rarely indicated, unless a patient has symptoms of metastases to these sites. The power of CT as a diagnostic tool is growing rapidly; in addition to giving invaluable information about anatomic considerations, the radiologic subtleties between different histologic types have been increasingly appreciated. In one study from the MD Anderson Cancer Center (MDACC), differences between well-differentiated and dedifferentiated retroperitoneal liposarcomas were accurately predicted in 100% of patients by CT scan. This additional information may be helpful in patients for whom pathologic diagnosis is equivocal or questioned because of sampling error. Future advances may even make it possible to avoid the need for pathologic diagnosis in selected patients before initiation of therapy.

Pathologic Evaluation

Accurate preoperative histologic diagnosis is a critical step in determining the primary treatment of a soft-tissue sarcoma. The biopsy should yield enough tissue so that a pathological diagnosis can be made without increasing the risk of complications. Core-needle biopsy and fine-needle aspiration have been demonstrated to be reliable means of obtaining enough material for an accurate pathological diagnosis particularly when the pathological findings correlate closely with clinical and imaging findings. Biopsy performed under ultrasound or CT guidance can improve the positive yield rate by helping pathologists more accurately locate the needle in the tumor, particularly in patients with deep extremity or retroperitoneal tumors.

Treatment

The treatment of sarcoma requires a multidisciplinary team that is in constant communication with each other. At MDACC, sarcoma cases are discussed regularly at multidisciplinary conferences that include radiologists, pathologists, surgical oncologists, medical oncologists, as well as radiation oncologists. Often neoadjuvant chemotherapy or radiotherapy is helpful in selected patients. Specific management schema will be addressed later as it pertains to each sarcoma subtype. The overall principles include maximal locoregional control with complete surgical resection when possible, adjunct radiotherapy and chemotherapy, as well as constant surveillance for distant metastasis and appropriate systemic chemotherapy or even surgical metastasectomy in carefully selected patients.

Follow-up

The rationale behind follow-up strategies to detect the recurrence of any type of cancer is that the early recognition and treatment of recurrent, local, or distant disease can prolong survival. The ideal follow-up strategy should therefore be easy to implement, accurate, and cost-effective.

The development of metastases is the primary determinant of survival in patients with soft-tissue sarcoma. The site of recurrence is related to the anatomical site of the primary tumor. Extremity sarcomas generally recur in the form of distant pulmonary metastases, whereas retroperitoneal or intra-abdominal sarcomas tend to recur as frequently locally as they do in the lungs.

Whether the early detection of recurrence can improve overall survival depends on the availability of effective therapeutic interventions. A few reports involving small numbers of patients have shown that it is possible to salvage patients with recurrent local disease with radical re-excision with or without radiation therapy. Similarly, several groups have reported on patients who have experienced prolonged survival following the resection of pulmonary metastases. These limited data form the impetus for the aggressive surveillance strategies taken in patients with soft-tissue sarcomas.

The majority of soft-tissue sarcomas that recur do so within the first 2 years after the completion of therapy. Patients should therefore be evaluated with a complete history and physical examination every 3 months with a chest radiograph and tumor site imaging during this high-risk period. If the chest radiograph reveals a suspicious nodule, a CT scan of the chest should be obtained for further assessment. Most experts recommend that the tumor site be evaluated with either MRI for an extremity tumor or CT for intra-abdominal or retroperitoneal tumors. In some circumstances, ultrasonography can be used to look for the recurrence of an extremity tumor either locally or at a distant site. Follow-up intervals may be lengthened to every 6 months, with annual imaging during years 2 through 5 after the completion of therapy. After 5 years, patients should be assessed annually and a chest radiograph should be obtained.

EXTREMITY SOFT-TISSUE SARCOMAS

More than 50% of soft-tissue sarcomas originate in an extremity. The most common histologic subtypes that occur in the extremity include malignant fibrous histiocytoma, liposarcoma, synovial sarcoma, and fibrosarcoma, although various other histologic types are also seen in the extremities.

Clinical Presentation

Most extremity soft-tissue sarcomas present as an asymptomatic mass, but the size at presentation usually depends on the anatomical site of the tumor. For example, although a 2- to 3-cm tumor may become readily apparent on the back of the hand, a tumor in the thigh may grow to 10 to 15 cm in diameter before it becomes apparent. Frequently, trauma to the affected area will call attention to the pre-existing lesion. Small lesions that on the basis of the clinical history remain unchanged for several years may be closely observed without biopsy. However, all other tumors should be biopsied.

Surgery

The type of surgical resection performed in patients with extremity soft-tissue sarcomas is determined by a number of factors, including tumor location, tumor size, the depth of invasion, the involvement of nearby structures, the need for skin grafting or autogenous tissue reconstruction, and the patient's performance status. In the 1970s, 50% of patients with extremity sarcomas were treated with amputation for local control of their tumors. However, despite a local recurrence rate of less than 10% following radical surgery, large numbers of patients continued to die from metastatic disease. This realization led to the development and adoption of other methods of local therapy that combined conservative surgical excision with postoperative radiation therapy, with resultant local control rates of 78% to 91%.

Wide local excision is the primary treatment for patients with extremity sarcomas. It is important, when planning surgery and radiotherapy, to remember that there is generally a zone of compressed reactive tissue that forms a pseudocapsule around the tumors and that tumors may extend beyond this pseudocapsule. The inexperienced surgeon may mistakenly use this to guide resection. The goal of local therapy is to resect the tumor with at least a 2-cm margin of surrounding normal soft tissue. In some anatomical areas, however, these margins are not attainable because of the proximity of vital structures. When possible, the biopsy site or tract should also be included en bloc with the resected specimen.

Elective regional lymphadenectomy is rarely indicated in patients with soft-tissue sarcomas. However, in patients with rhabdomyosarcoma or epithelioid sarcoma with suspicious clinical or radiologic findings, fine-needle aspiration of the lymph nodes should be performed preoperatively. In these rare cases, a lymph node dissection may be indicated for regional control of the disease. There are scattered single institution reports of sentinel lymph node biopsy in these subgroups; however, the numbers are too small to critically assess its role in the management of these patients. A prospective trial is currently under way to evaluate the role of lymphatic mapping and sentinel lymph node biopsy in pediatric patients with extremity rhabdomyosarcomas.

There have been several studies that have shown favorable local control rates for patients with extremity tumors treated with conservative resection combined with radiation therapy. For example, in a small study from the National Cancer Institute, there was no difference in survival among patients treated with conservative surgery plus radiation therapy compared with patients treated with amputation. In 1985, on the basis of the limited data available, the National Institutes of Health developed a consensus statement recommending limb-sparing surgery for the majority of patients with high-grade extremity sarcomas. However, amputation remains the treatment of choice for patients whose tumor cannot be grossly resected with a limb-sparing procedure that preserves function (<5% of cases).

Radiation Therapy

The primary goal of radiation therapy is to optimize local tumor control. The evidence for adjunctive radiation therapy in patients eligible for conservative surgical resection comes from two randomized trials and a number of large single-institution reports. In one of these randomized trials, conducted by the National Cancer Institute, 91 patients with high-grade extremity tumors were treated with limb-sparing surgery followed by chemotherapy alone or radiation therapy plus adjuvant chemotherapy. A second group of 50 patients with low-grade tumors were treated with resection alone versus resection with radiation therapy. The 10-year local control rate for all patients receiving radiation therapy was 98% compared with 70% for those not receiving radiation therapy.

In the second randomized trial, which was performed at the Memorial Sloan-Kettering Cancer Center, 164 patients were randomized to observation or brachytherapy following conservative surgery. The 5-year local control rate for patients with high-grade tumors was 66% in the observation group and 89% in the group treated with brachytherapy. There was no significant difference between the groups of patients with low-grade tumors.

At the M. D. Anderson Cancer Center, radiation therapy is used as an adjunct to surgery for patients with intermediate- and high-grade tumors of any size. However, because T1 tumors are less frequently associated with local recurrences, radiation therapy for these patients is currently considered on an individual basis because it may not confer a significant clinical benefit, especially in patients who have had optimal surgical management with microscopically negative margins. Recent studies have failed to demonstrate an improvement in the 5-year recurrence or survival rates in patients with small sarcomas who received postoperative radiation therapy.

Preoperative Versus Postoperative External-beam Radiation Therapy

The optimal timing of external-beam radiation therapy for sarcomas located either in an extremity or in the retroperitoneum remains a focus of active investigation. Currently, the only randomized trial comparing preoperative and postoperative radiation therapy is a multicenter trial performed in Canada. In this trial, from October 1994 to December 1997, patients were randomized to receive either 50 Gy of external-beam radiation therapy preoperatively or 66 Gy of external-beam radiation therapy postoperatively. One hundred ninety patients were entered into the study. With a median follow-up of 3.3 years, the recurrence- and progression-free survival rates were similar between the groups, with the only statistically significant difference being in the rates of wound complications. That is, the incidence of wound complications was 35% in the patients who received preoperative therapy, but only 17% in the patients who received postoperative radiation therapy.

At MDACC, despite the potential for increased wound problems, radiation therapy is preferentially given preoperatively for several reasons. First, this enables multidisciplinary planning with the radiation oncologist, medical oncologist, and surgeon to occur early in the course of therapy while the tumor is in place. Also, preoperative radiation therapy allows lower doses of radiation to be delivered to an undisturbed tissue bed that is potentially better oxygenated. In addition, the size of the preoperative radiation fields and the number of joints included in the fields is significantly smaller than those of postoperative radiation fields, which may result in an improved functional outcome.

Critics of preoperative radiation therapy cite the difficulty with the pathological assessment of margins and the increased incidence of wound complications as deterrents to preoperative radiation therapy. However, plastic surgery techniques that include advanced tissue transfer procedures are being used more frequently in patients with such high-risk wounds. The outcomes in patients treated in this fashion have been encouraging, with a high success rate (>90%) of healed wounds from a single-stage operation.

Brachytherapy
Brachytherapy, which involves the placement of multiple catheters in the tumor resection bed at the time of surgery, has been reported to achieve local control rates comparable to those achieved with external-beam radiation therapy. Guidelines have been established that recommend placing the afterloading catheters at 1-cm intervals with a 2-cm margin around the surgical bed. Usually, after the fifth postoperative day, the catheters are then loaded with radioactive wires (iridium 192) that deliver 42 to 45 Gy to the tumor bed over 4 to 6 days. The frequency of wound complications associated with brachytherapy is similar to that seen for postoperative radiation therapy (approximately 10%).

The primary benefit of brachytherapy is the shorter overall treatment time of 4 to 6 days, compared with the 4 to 6 weeks generally required by preoperative or postoperative regimens. Brachytherapy also produces less radiation scatter in critical anatomical regions (e.g., gonads, joints), with improved function a potential clinical benefit. Cost-analysis comparisons of brachytherapy versus external-beam radiation therapy have further shown that the charges for adjuvant irradiation with brachytherapy are lower than those for external-beam radiation therapy.

Systemic Chemotherapy
Despite improvements in the local control rate, metastasis and death remain significant problems for patients with high-risk soft-tissue sarcomas. This high-risk group includes localized sarcomas that are in nonextremity sites, tumors which show an intermediate- or high-grade histology, or large (T2) tumors. The treatment regimen for patients with high-risk localized disease, metastatic disease, or both, usually includes chemotherapy.

As a group, sarcomas include histologic subtypes that are very responsive to cytotoxic chemotherapy as well as subtypes that are universally resistant to current agents. Only three drugs, doxorubicin, dacarbazine, and ifosfamide, have consistently achieved response rates of at least 20% as single-agent treatments in patients with advanced soft-tissue sarcomas. The majority of active chemotherapeutic trials have included doxorubicin as part of the treatment regimen. The response rate to ifosfamide has been found to vary from 20% to 60% in single-institution series in which higher-dose regimens have been used or in which it has been given in combination with doxorubicin.

Adjuvant (Postoperative) Chemotherapy

Individual randomized trials of adjuvant chemotherapy have failed to demonstrate an improvement in disease-free and overall survival in patients with soft-tissue sarcomas. However, there are several criticisms of these individual trials that may explain why they failed to demonstrate improvement in survival. First, the chemotherapy regimens used were suboptimal, in that single-agent drugs (most commonly doxorubicin) were studied and dosing schedules were less intensive. Second, the sample sizes in these trials were not large enough to allow the detection of clinically significant differences in survival. Third, the majority of patients who did not respond to the initial treatment regimen were started on other chemotherapeutic regimens that potentially affected disease-free and overall survival. Finally, most studies included patients at low risk for metastasis and death, that is, those with small (<5 cm) and low-grade tumors.

Hence, adjuvant chemotherapy for patients with soft-tissue sarcomas remains controversial. To help settle this issue, a formal meta-analysis called the Sarcoma Meta-Analysis Collaboration was conducted in 1997. This group analyzed the data on 1,568 patients from 14 trials of doxorubicin-based adjuvant chemotherapy to determine the effect of adjuvant chemotherapy on localized, resectable soft-tissue sarcomas. With a median follow-up of 9.4 years, doxorubicin-based chemotherapy was found to have significantly lengthened the time to local and distant recurrence and the overall recurrence-free survival. However, the absolute improvement in the overall survival rate for the entire group was only 4%, which was not statistically significant. When subsets of patients were examined, there was a 7% increase in the survival rate in those patients with extremity tumors.

Neoadjuvant (Preoperative) Chemotherapy

The rationale for neoadjuvant/preoperative chemotherapy for soft-tissue sarcomas is that, given that only 30% to 50% of patients will respond to standard chemotherapeutic regimens, it enables the oncologist to identify those select patients in whom specific regimens are effective, as shown by measuring the primary tumor in situ. Patients whose tumors shrink after two or four courses of chemotherapy subsequently undergo local treatment with surgery and/or radiation therapy, followed by postoperative chemotherapy with the same agents that were administered preoperatively. At the same time, patients who do not respond to short courses of preoperative chemotherapy are spared the toxic effects of prolonged postoperative chemotherapy with agents to which the tumor is insensitive.

In an effort to better assess the role of chemotherapy, a cohort analysis of the combined databases from both the M. D. Anderson Cancer Center and the Memorial Sloan-Kettering Cancer Center was recently performed. The data on 674 patients with stage III extremity sarcoma who received either preoperative or postoperative doxorubicin-based chemotherapy were reviewed to determine their outcomes (5-year disease-specific survival, as well as 5-year local and distant recurrence rates). The 5-year disease-specific survival rate was 61%, and the probability of local and distant recurrences at 5 years was 83% and 56%, respectively.

An important conclusion from this study was that the clinical benefits of doxorubicin-based chemotherapy in patients with high-risk extremity sarcomas were not sustained beyond 1 year after therapy. The investigators then went on to compare their study with the Sarcoma Meta-Analysis Collaboration and made the following observations. First, the patient population of the Sarcoma Meta-Analysis Collaboration was more heterogeneous than that of the cohort study, in that it included patients with both primary and recurrent extremity and nonextremity sarcomas. Second, there were also fewer uncontrolled variables in the cohort study. On the basis of these findings, the authors urged caution when reviewing studies of chemotherapeutic regimens with a short-term follow-up and concluded that there remains no consensus regarding the role of chemotherapy in patients with localized high-risk soft-tissue sarcomas.

Isolated Limb Perfusion/Infusion
While limb salvage has become possible for the majority of patients with soft-tissue sarcomas, it is not feasible in approximately 10% of patients. Since amputation does not improve survival in these patients, new therapies to increase limb salvage rates are currently being investigated. One of the most promising regional chemotherapy techniques is isolated limb perfusion (ILP) and, more recently, isolated limb infusion (ILI).

The technique of ILP involves isolation of the main artery and vein of the involved limb from the systemic circulation; external iliac vessels are used for thigh tumors, femoral or popliteal vessels for calf tumors, and axillary vessels for upper-extremity tumors. The vessels are then cannulated and connected to a pump oxygenator similar to that used in cardiopulmonary bypass. A tourniquet or Esmarch bandage is applied to the limb to achieve complete vascular isolation. The limb is then heated using both external heating and warming of the perfusates, and chemotherapeutic agents are added to the perfusion circuit and recirculated for 90 minutes. At the end of the procedure, the drugs are washed out of the limb, the cannulas are removed, and the blood vessels repaired.

Recently, interest has developed in the less invasive technique of ILI. This technique has also been termed *minimally invasive isolated limb perfusion*. Instead of open cannulation of the vessels, infusion catheters are placed by interventional radiologists. The patient is then transferred to the operating room with the catheters in place. A tourniquet is applied and chemotherapy is administered via a non-oxygenated bypass circuit creating ischemic conditions in the limb. Ischemic conditions are believed to enhance the efficacy of the chemotherapeutic agents. As with ILP, after isolated chemotherapy infusions, the limb is washed out, and the catheters and tourniquets are removed.

As expected, it is difficult at this stage to interpret results for this technique since the data available represent a small population with heterogeneous histologies in which a variety of chemotherapeutic agents and conditions have been used. One of the largest series from the Netherlands used ILP with tumor necrosis factor-α and melphalan in 217 patients with soft-tissue sarcomas. They report a response rate of 75% and a limb salvage rate of 87%. From early reports, it seems that ILI is equally as efficacious. For instance, the Sydney Melanoma Unit reported a response rate of 90% in 21 patients using ILI; however, the recurrence rate in this study was 42%. While this technique is still offered only at a handful of institutions, early results are promising for these patients in which amputation is their only other option.

Management of Local Recurrence
Disease can recur in up to 20% of patients with extremity sarcoma, but patients with microscopically positive surgical margins are the ones in whom the risk of

local recurrence is greatest. It remains a matter of controversy, however, as to what the impact of local failures is on survival and distant disease-free survival. Many believe recurrence represents a harbinger of distant metastatic disease. Regardless, the adequacy of the surgical resection clearly plays a role in determining whether disease recurs locally.

An isolated local recurrence should be treated aggressively with margin-negative re-resection (possibly amputation) plus radiation therapy. Patients previously treated with external-beam radiation therapy may be considered for brachytherapy or intraoperative radiation therapy. Several small studies have shown that patients with isolated local recurrences may be successfully retreated, with local recurrence-free survival rates approaching 72%.

Management of Distant Disease

Distant metastases occur in 40% to 50% of patients with intermediate- and high-grade extremity sarcomas, compared with only 5% of patients with low-grade sarcomas. Most metastases to distant sites occur within 2 years of the initial diagnosis. The predominant site of distant metastases from primary extremity sarcomas is the lung (73% of cases).

Lung metastases should be resected if there are no extra pulmonary metastases, the patient is medically fit enough to withstand a thoracotomy, and the lesions are amenable to resection. Large series have revealed 3-year survival rates of 40% to 50% in patients with completely resected pulmonary metastases. A disease-free interval of more than 12 months, the ability to resect all metastatic disease, age younger than 50 years, and absence of preceding local recurrence were found to be independent prognostic factors in a multivariate analysis of patients who underwent resection of pulmonary metastases.

General Recommendations

General recommendations for the management of extremity soft-tissue sarcomas are as follows:

1. Soft-tissue tumors that are enlarging or greater than 3 cm in diameter should be evaluated with radiologic imaging (ultrasonography or CT), and a tissue diagnosis made on the basis of fine-needle aspiration or core-needle biopsy findings.
2. Evaluate for metastatic disease once a sarcoma diagnosis is established: chest radiography for low- or intermediate-grade lesions and T1 tumors, and chest CT for high-grade or T2 tumors.
3. A wide local excision with 2-cm margins is adequate therapy for low-grade lesions and T1 tumors.
4. Radiation therapy plays a critical role in the management of T2 tumors.
5. Patients with recurrent high-grade sarcomas or distant metastatic disease should be considered for preoperative (neoadjuvant) or postoperative (adjuvant) chemotherapy.
6. An aggressive surgical approach should be taken in the treatment of patients with an isolated local recurrence or resectable distant metastases.

RETROPERITONEAL SARCOMAS

Fifteen percent of soft-tissue sarcomas in adults occur in the retroperitoneum. Most retroperitoneal tumors are malignant, and approximately one-third are soft-tissue sarcomas. The differential diagnosis in a patient presenting with a retroperitoneal tumor includes lymphoma, germ cell tumors, and undifferentiated carcinomas. The most common retroperitoneal sarcomas (RPS) are liposarcomas, malignant fibrous histiocytomas, and leiomyosarcomas. Histology is a key component to overall prognosis in RPS. A recent analysis of the MDACC database of 1,118 patients with RPS specifically addressed this question. This study stratified patients into three histologic subgroups based on overall survival: atypical lipomatous tumors (ALT), non-ALT liposarcoma, and all other subtypes. The 5-year overall survival for patients presenting with a primary tumor showed dramatic differences among the three subgroups with rates of 95% in ALT, 40% in non-ALT liposarcoma, and 48% in all others. This difference was also seen in 5-year overall survival for recurrent tumors: 86% for ALT versus 25% in non-ALT liposarcoma, and 43% in others ($P < 0.0001$).

Although significant advances in our understanding of extremity soft-tissue sarcomas have resulted in improved treatments and outcomes, similar progress has not been achieved in our understanding and treatment of retroperitoneal soft-tissue sarcomas. For several reasons, patients with retroperitoneal soft-tissue sarcomas generally have a worse prognosis than those with extremity sarcomas. One reason is that retroperitoneal soft-tissue sarcomas commonly grow to large sizes before they become clinically apparent, by which time they often involve important vital structures, which precludes surgical resection. A second reason is that the surgical margins that can be obtained around these sarcomas are often inadequate because of anatomical constraints.

Clinical Presentation
Retroperitoneal sarcomas generally present as large masses; nearly 50% are larger than 20 cm at the time of diagnosis. They typically do not produce symptoms until they grow large enough to compress or invade contiguous structures. On occasion, patients may present with neurologic symptoms, resulting from the compression of lumbar or pelvic nerves, or obstructive gastrointestinal symptoms, resulting from the displacement or direct tumor involvement of an intestinal organ.

Evaluation
The workup in a patient with a retroperitoneal mass begins with an accurate history that should exclude signs and symptoms of lymphoma (e.g., fever, night sweats). A complete physical examination with particular attention to all nodal basins and a testicular examination in males are critically important. Laboratory assessment can be helpful; an increased lactate dehydrogenase level can be suggestive of lymphoma, whereas an increased β-human chorionic gonadotropin level, alpha-fetoprotein level, or both can indicate a germ cell tumor.

The radiologic assessment should include a CT scan of the abdomen and pelvis to define the extent of the tumor and its relationship to surrounding structures, particularly vascular structures. Imaging should include the liver in a search for metastases and discontinuous abdominal disease. The kidneys should also be evaluated to assess bilateral renal function. Thoracic CT is indicated to look for lung metastases. A CT-guided core-needle biopsy is appropriate for obtaining a tissue diagnosis in patients presenting with an equivocal history, an unusual-appearing mass, an unresectable tumor, or distant metastasis and in patients who are potentially eligible for a neoadjuvant protocol.

Management
Complete surgical resection is the most effective treatment for primary or recurrent retroperitoneal sarcomas, but it is frequently not possible. For example, in several retrospective assessments of patients with retroperitoneal sarcoma, complete surgical excision was achieved in only 40% to 60% of patients. The effects of an incomplete surgical resection on outcome are significant. First, incomplete resection

increases the chance of local recurrence. This is vital since local recurrence is often the cause of mortality in RPS. This has been shown by MDACC in a study of 83 patients treated with surgery and radiotherapy. Five-year local recurrence-free survival was 33% after an incomplete resection versus 62% after a complete resection ($P = 0.01$). This study further highlights the importance of local recurrence in that of the 38 patients dying of disease, local recurrence was the sole site of disease in 16 (42%) patients and was a component of progression in an additional 11 (29%). Second, incomplete resection has also been associated with a risk of developing distant metastasis that is almost four times higher than those who undergo complete resection. Finally, it has an important impact on survival. In an analysis of 500 patients with RPS treated at the Memorial Sloan-Kettering Cancer Center, the median survival duration of patients who underwent complete resection was 103 months versus 18 months for patients who underwent incomplete resection, which was no different than the survival seen in patients treated with observation without resection thus demonstrating that there is no survival benefit from debulking procedures.

Careful preoperative planning is of paramount importance when considering surgical resection in these patients. Because of anatomic location, multiorgan resection is often required to achieve a complete resection. In one study from Milan, 53% of RPS resections involved resection of at least one organ with almost half of those requiring removal of more than one organ. Organs commonly requiring resection include kidney, bowel, stomach, and pancreas. Often, vessels must be resected requiring reconstruction. Thus, multidisciplinary surgical teams must sometimes be utilized in order to achieve a complete resection. Also, special consideration must be given to the tumors relation to major vessels and nerves as this is often the limiting factor in achieving a complete resection.

That said, palliative surgical procedures may be performed to reduce the symptoms of intestinal obstruction or bleeding. In particular, patients with atypical lipomatous tumors, also termed *well-differentiated liposarcomas,* may benefit symptomatically from repeated tumor debulking.

Adjuvant Therapy

Chemotherapy has not been shown to be an effective treatment for retroperitoneal sarcomas. Several centers have ongoing protocols to determine the role of preoperative chemotherapy and radiation therapy for these tumors, but the findings from these studies have not yet been released. A trial sponsored by the American College of Surgeon's Oncology Group evaluating the benefit of preoperative radiation in patients with retroperitoneal sarcomas recently closed for failure to meet accrual targets.

Management of Recurrent Disease

Retroperitoneal sarcomas recur in two-thirds of patients. In addition to recurring locally in the tumor bed and metastasizing to the lungs, retroperitoneal leiomyosarcomas frequently spread to the liver. Retroperitoneal sarcomas can also recur diffusely throughout the peritoneal cavity (sarcomatosis). The approach to resectable recurrent disease after the treatment of a retroperitoneal sarcoma is similar to the approach taken after the recurrence of an extremity sarcoma. However, the ability to resect a recurrent retroperitoneal sarcoma declines precipitously with each recurrence. In a large series of patients treated at the Memorial Sloan-Kettering Cancer Center, the authors were able to resect recurrent tumors in 57% of patients with a first recurrence, but in only 20% of patients after a second recurrence and 10% after a third recurrence. Isolated liver metastases, if stable over several months, may be amenable to resection, radiofrequency ablation, or chemoembolization.

Not only does each local recurrence affect surgical therapy, it can also be associated with a change in the biology of the disease. For example, in as many as 25% of patients, well-differentiated liposarcoma may recur in a poorly differentiated form or develop areas of dedifferentiation. Dedifferentiated retroperitoneal liposarcoma is more aggressive with a greater propensity for distant metastasis than its well-differentiated precursor.

GASTROINTESTINAL STROMAL TUMORS

GISTs constitute the majority of mesenchymal tumors involving the gastrointestinal tract. It is estimated that there are 2,500 to 6,000 cases per year in the United States. Although the clinical presentation of these tumors varies depending on the tumor size and anatomical location, most tumors are found incidentally at the time of endoscopy or radiologic imaging. GISTs arise most frequently in the stomach (60% to 70%), followed by the small intestine (20% to 25%), colon and rectum (5%), and esophagus (<5%). Most GISTs are sporadic and, in 95% of cases, solitary. Most patients with GISTs present in the fifth to the seventh decades of life, and these tumors are equally distributed between the genders. Symptoms of these lesions include pain and gastrointestinal bleeding, with abdominal mass a frequent finding.

Since the late 1990s, it has been recognized that GISTs have distinctive immunohistochemical and genetic features. GISTs originate from the intestinal pacemaker cells (the interstitial cells of Cajal), which express CD117, a transmembrane tyrosine kinase receptor that is the product of the c-KIT proto-oncogene. The expression of CD117 has emerged as an important defining feature of GISTs, being found in at least 95% of cases. The pathogenesis of these tumors is related to mutations in the *c-KIT* gene. Exploitation of this genetic characteristic has led to significant inroads into the development of successful therapy for these tumors.

Treatment

GIST tumors are an example of the power of targeted therapy in cancer therapeutics. In the past, surgical resection was the main treatment for GIST. While surgery remains the standard treatment for resectable tumors, the addition of systemic therapy has markedly improved outcomes. The goal of surgery should be resection with a 1 to 2 cm margin if possible. For tumors located in the stomach, a wedge resection can often accomplish this goal. Minimally invasive techniques using laparoscopy are increasingly being used in the management of GISTs. Total gastrectomy is rarely required, although may be necessary in some cases depending on location and size of the tumor. In these cases, neoadjuvant therapy is very helpful to decrease tumor size and to decrease tumor friability. However, despite complete surgical resection, a large proportion of patients (76% in one study from the Memorial Sloan-Kettering Cancer Center) develop local recurrence. Factors such as large tumor size, tumor location in the duodenum or rectum, incomplete resection, high mitotic count, and mutation status (such as deletion in KIT exon 11) are associated with an increased risk of recurrence. Salvage surgery for these recurrences is associated with a 15-month median survival.

The development of imatinib mesylate (Gleevec, formerly known as STI571; Novartis), has made a dramatic impact on the survival of patients with GIST. Gleevec is a selective tyrosine kinase inhibitor of *c-KIT* and platelet-derived growth factor receptor alpha (PDGFR-α). In February 2002, imatinib mesylate was approved by the U.S. Food and Drug Administration for use in the treatment of GISTs on the basis of the results of trials conducted in patients with metastatic and locally advanced disease (Table 5.3). Overall response rates are seen in 48% to 71% of patients. Overall median survival in patients with advanced GIST who are treated with imatinib is 57 months compared to only 9 months in historical controls.

TABLE 5.3 Summary of Clinical Trials of Imatinib Mesylate in Patients with Advanced Gastrointestinal Stromal Tumor

Study, Year	Phase	No. of Patients	Overall Response	CR	PR	2-y Overall Survival	Progression-free Survival
Van Oosterom et al., 2001	I	36	53%	0%	53%	—	—
Demetri et al., 2002	II	147	54%	0%	54%	—	—
Verwiej et al., 2003	II	27	71%	4%	67%	—	73% (1 y)
Rankin et al., 2004	III	746					
– 400 mg daily			48%	3%	45%	78%	50% (2 y)
– 800 mg daily			48%	3%	45%	73%	53% (2 y)
Verweij et al., 2004	III	946					
– 400 mg daily			50%	5%	45%	69%	44% (2 y)
– 800 mg daily			54%	6%	48%	74%	55% (2 y)

CR, complete response; PR, partial response.

The genotype of the *c-KIT* mutation is important: patients with mutations in exon 11 have higher response rates than those with exon 9 mutations, although both groups respond better than those without a mutation. Its benefit in the adjuvant setting was shown in the randomized, placebo-controlled ACOSOG Z9001 trial which enrolled 713 GIST patients with KIT mutations after complete surgical resection. Patients received 1 year of therapy with either 400 mg of Gleevac daily versus a placebo. Adjuvant imatinib improved 1 year relapse free survival rates to 98% versus 83% in the placebo group ($P < 0.0001$).

Given the success of Gleevec, it is increasingly used as a neoadjuvant adjunct in locally advanced tumors. The RTOG S-0132/ACRIN 6665 trial is currently ongoing assessing the effectiveness of preoperative imatinib therapy. The 5-year results will be available in 2011. Maximal tumor response is usually seen after 6 to 12 months at which point surgery can safely be performed. PET scan is a useful tool in evaluating tumor response in these patients. Patients who do not show an early response can be switched to another targeted therapy or can be referred directly for surgery.

However, even in patients who harbor the KIT mutation, 5% show primary resistance to imatinib and 14% develop resistance. Sunitinib malate ("Sutent," Pfizer) is a tyrosine kinase inhibitor with multiple targets including KIT, PDGFR, and VEGFR with different binding characteristics than imatinib. In a randomized, placebo-blinded trial in imatinib-refractory patients, median time to progression was 27.3 weeks in the sunitinib group versus 6.4 weeks in the placebo group ($P < 0.0001$).

OTHER SOFT-TISSUE LESIONS

Sarcoma of the Breast

Sarcomas of the breast are rare tumors, accounting for less than 1% of all breast malignancies and less than 5% of all soft-tissue sarcomas. Various histologic subtypes have been reported to occur within the breast, including angiosarcoma, stromal sarcoma, fibrosarcoma, and malignant fibrous histiocytoma. Cystosarcoma phyllodes is generally considered to be a separate entity from other soft-tissue sarcomas because these tumors are believed to originate from hormonally responsive stromal cells of the breast and the majority are benign.

As with sarcomas at other anatomical sites, the histopathological grade and size of the tumor are important prognostic factors. Likewise, the likelihood of local recurrences increases as the tumor size increases; tumors smaller than 5 cm are associated with better overall survival. Local and distant recurrences are more common in patients with high-grade lesions. Complete excision with negative margins is the primary therapy. Simple mastectomy carries no additional benefit if complete excision can be accomplished by segmental mastectomy. Because of low rates of regional lymphatic spread, axillary dissection is not routinely indicated. Neoadjuvant chemotherapy or radiation therapy may be considered for patients with large, high-risk tumors.

Desmoids
Desmoid tumors do not metastasize and are considered low-grade sarcomas. Approximately half of these tumors arise in the extremity, with the remaining lesions located on the trunk or in the retroperitoneum. Abdominal wall desmoids are associated with pregnancy and are believed to arise as the result of hormonal influences. Patients with Gardner syndrome may have retroperitoneal desmoids as an extracolonic manifestation of the disease. Surgical resection with wide local excision should be the primary therapy for desmoid tumors. Local recurrence may occur in up to one-third of patients. Adjuvant radiation therapy has been associated with a reduced incidence of local recurrence. Radiation therapy can also control tumor growth for an extended period of time in tumors that are surgically unresectable, or in patients that are not considered to be surgical candidates.

Dermatofibrosarcoma Protuberans
DFSP is a neoplasm arising in the dermis that may occur anywhere in the body. Approximately 40% arise on the trunk, with most of the remaining tumors distributed between the head and neck and extremities. The lesion presents as a nodular, cutaneous mass that shows slow and persistent growth. Satellite lesions may be found in patients with larger tumors. Wide local excision is recommended, although recurrence rates can be as high as 30% to 50%. In genetic analysis, a COL1A1–PDGF-B fusion protein is often expressed in DFSPs. This has clinical relevance in that patients with metastatic DFSP have shown responses to imatinib, which is a tyrosine kinase inhibitor of PDGF.

BONE SARCOMAS
Epidemiology
Malignant tumors of the musculoskeletal system constitute 10% of newly diagnosed cancers in the population younger than 30 years of age, with 1,000 cases diagnosed annually in the United States. However, malignant tumors arising from the skeletal systems represent only 0.2% of all primary cancers. Osteosarcoma and Ewing's sarcoma are the two most common malignant conditions of bone. Osteosarcoma has a peak frequency during adolescent growth, whereas Ewing's sarcoma occurs most frequently in the second decade of life.

Clinical Presentation
The most common presentation of bone sarcomas (Ewing's sarcoma or osteosarcoma) is pain or swelling in a bone or joint. As with soft-tissue sarcomas in adults, often a traumatic event draws attention to the swelling and can throw off the correct diagnosis. Osteosarcoma most commonly involves the metaphysis of long

bones, especially the distal femur, proximal tibia, or humerus. Ewing's sarcoma may involve flat bones or the diaphysis of tubular bones such as the femur, pelvis, tibia, and fibula. Ewing's sarcoma may also occur in soft tissues. Chondrosarcoma occurs most commonly in the pelvis, proximal femur, and shoulder girdle.

Up to 25% of patients presenting with osteosarcoma or Ewing's sarcoma have metastatic disease at presentation. The most frequent metastatic sites for osteosarcoma include the lung (90% of cases) and the bone (10%), whereas Ewing's sarcoma metastases occur in the lung (50%), bone (25%), and bone marrow (25%).

Staging
As with soft-tissue sarcomas, histopathological grade is a crucial component of the staging of bone sarcomas. The surgical staging system for musculoskeletal sarcoma is based on the system by Enneking and includes prognostic variables such as histopathological grade (G), the location of the tumor (T), and the presence or absence of metastases (M). The three stages are stage I, low grade (G1); stage II, high grade (G2); and stage III, G1 or G2 with the presence of metastases (M1). Each stage is then designated *a* if the lesion is anatomically confined within well-delineated surgical compartments (T1) and *b* if the lesion is located beyond such compartments in ill-defined fascial planes and spaces (T2).

Diagnosis
The evaluation of patients with a suspected bone tumor should include a thorough history and physical examination, plain radiographs, and MRI of the entire affected bone. Bone scanning and CT of the chest are also necessary.

On plain radiographs, malignant bone tumors show irregular borders, and there is often evidence of bone destruction and a periosteal reaction. Soft-tissue extension is also frequently seen.

Biopsy
A core-needle biopsy is the diagnostic procedure of choice in a patient suspected of harboring an osteosarcoma. A core-needle biopsy performed under radiographic guidance should yield diagnostic findings in almost all cases of osteosarcoma.

Treatment
Effective multimodality therapy for childhood musculoskeletal tumors has dramatically improved the 5-year survival rates from 10% to 20% in 1970 to the current 60% to 70%. Limb salvage is the standard treatment for most patients with osteosarcoma.

Surgery
Whenever feasible, limb salvage is the standard surgical approach to bone sarcomas. Successful limb-sparing surgery consists of three phases: tumor resection, bone reconstruction, and soft-tissue coverage. Complete surgical extirpation of the primary tumor and any metastases is essential in patients with osteosarcoma because this tumor is relatively resistant to radiation therapy.

It is also desirable to resect Ewing's sarcoma, if this can be done. If surgical removal with a wide surgical margin can be achieved, the prognosis is favorable (12-year relapse-free survival of 60%). However, Ewing's sarcoma most typically involves the pelvis with an extensive soft-tissue mass that invades the pelvic cavity, which makes it difficult to carry out radical surgery.

Surgical resection is usually the only treatment indicated for the management of chondrosarcomas because this type of tumor is unresponsive to existing systemic therapies.

Chemotherapy

Chemotherapy has revolutionized the treatment of most bone sarcomas and is considered standard care for osteosarcoma and Ewing's sarcoma. The bleak 15% to 20% survival rate achieved with surgery alone during the 1960s has improved to 55% to 80% through the addition of chemotherapy to surgical resection. The timing of chemotherapy, the mode of delivery, and the drug combinations continue to be studied in multi-institutional trials, so further improvements in the clinical outcome are anticipated. Effective agents include doxorubicin, cisplatin, methotrexate, ifosfamide, and cyclophosphamide. Randomized clinical trials of patients with osteosarcoma have shown that the use of combination chemotherapy in addition to surgery results in cure rates of 58% to 76%. Preoperative chemotherapy is an attractive option because it can lead to the downstaging of tumors, which then enables the maximal application of limb-sparing surgery. In addition, tumor necrosis following preoperative chemotherapy has been shown to be the most important prognostic variable determining survival.

Multiagent chemotherapy has also been demonstrated to be essential in the treatment of Ewing's sarcoma. Trials spanning more than 20 years performed by the Intergroup Study of Ewing's sarcoma have established the efficacy of multidrug regimens (i.e., regimens that involve combinations of vincristine, doxorubicin, cyclophosphamide, ifosfamide, and etoposide) in increasing the 5-year relapse-free survival rates to up to 70% in patients with nonmetastatic disease. Agents currently being investigated as treatments for osteosarcoma include trastuzumab, inhaled granulocyte–macrophage colony-stimulating factor, and imatinib mesylate, among others.

Radiation Therapy

Because osteosarcomas are generally radiation resistant, radiation therapy is predominantly used for the palliation of large, unresectable tumors. In contrast, radiation therapy is the primary mode of treatment for most localized Ewing's sarcomas. Preoperative irradiation may also be considered to reduce tumor volume before surgical resection is attempted.

Recurrent Disease

Bone tumors disseminate through the bloodstream and commonly metastasize to the lungs and bony skeleton. In the past, only 10% to 30% of patients presenting with detectable metastatic osteosarcoma became long-term disease-free survivors. More recent studies have shown that combined modality approaches consisting of surgical resection of the primary tumor and metastatic deposits in conjunction with multiagent chemotherapy can improve 5-year disease-free survival rates to up to 47%.

Ewing's sarcoma may recur in the form of distant disease as long as 15 years after the initial diagnosis. In a retrospective analysis of 241 patients with Ewing's sarcoma of the pelvis, tumor volume, responsiveness to chemotherapy, and adequate surgical margins were found to be the major factors that influenced prognosis.

Patients with suspected tumor recurrence should undergo a complete evaluation to determine the extent of the disease. The resection of pulmonary metastases has become the mainstay of treatment for patients with osteosarcoma. Prognosis can generally be determined by the response to previous therapy, duration of remission, and extent of metastases. Multimodality therapy, including chemotherapeutic agents not previously used, is the general recommendation for treatment.

Sacrococcygeal Chordoma

The notochord remnant is the site of origin of this rare tumor. Chordomas are locally aggressive tumors that have a high propensity to recur. Because symptoms can be vague, diagnosis can be delayed. Surgical resection should involve a multidisciplinary team that includes the surgical oncologist, neurosurgeon, and reconstructive plastic surgeon. A two-stage procedure is frequently used at the M. D. Anderson Cancer Center. At the first stage, the blood supply to the tumor arising from the iliac vessels is controlled through an anterior approach. Several days later, the tumor is resected via a posterior approach. Radiation therapy should be considered because of high rates of local recurrence.

Recommended Readings

American Joint Committee on Cancer. *AJCC Cancer Staging Manual*. 6th ed. Philadelphia, PA: Lippincott-Raven; 2002.

Anaya DA, Lahat G, Wang X, et al. Establishing prognosis in retroperitoneal sarcoma: a new histology-based paradigm. *Ann Surg Oncol*. 2009;16:667–675.

Arndt CA, Crist WM. Common musculoskeletal tumors of childhood and adolescence. *N Engl J Med*. 1999;341:342.

Ayala AG, Ro JY, Fanning CV, et al. Core needle biopsy and fine-needle aspiration in the diagnosis of bone and soft tissue lesions. *Hematol Oncol Clin North Am*. 1995;9:633.

Baldini EH, Goldberg J, Jenner C, et al. Long-term outcomes after function-sparing surgery without radiotherapy for soft tissue sarcoma of the extremities and trunk. *J Clin Oncol*. 1999;17:3252.

Ballo MT, Zagars GK, Pollock RE, et al. Retroperitoneal soft tissue sarcoma: an analysis of radiation and surgical treatment. *Int J Radiat Oncol Biol Phys*. 2007;67(1): 158–163.

Barkley HT, Martin RG, Romsdahl MM, et al. Treatment of soft tissue sarcomas by preoperative irradiation and conservative surgical resection. *Int J Radiat Oncol Biol Phys*. 1988;14:693.

Billingsley KG, Burt ME, Jara E, et al. Pulmonary metastases from soft tissue sarcoma: analysis of patterns of disease and postmetastasis survival. *Ann Surg*. 1999;229:602.

Billingsley KG, Lewis JJ, Leung DH, et al. Multifactorial analysis of the survival of patients with distant metastasis arising from primary extremity sarcoma. *Cancer*. 1999;85:389.

Brady MS, Gaynor JJ, Brennan MF. Radiation-associated sarcoma of bone and soft tissue. *Arch Surg*. 1992;127:1379.

Brennan MF, Casper ES, Harrison LB, et al. The role of multimodality therapy in soft tissue sarcoma. *Ann Surg*. 1991;214:328.

Casson AG, Putnam JB, Natarajan G, et al. Five year survival after pulmonary metastasectomy for adult soft tissue sarcoma. *Cancer*. 1992;69:662.

Chang AE, Kinsella T, Glatstein E, et al. Adjuvant chemotherapy for patients with high-grade soft tissue sarcomas of the extremity. *J Clin Oncol*. 1988;6:1491.

Chang AE, Matory YL, Dwyer AJ, et al. Magnetic resonance imaging versus computed tomography in the evaluation of soft tissue tumors of the extremities. *Ann Surg*. 1997;205:340.

Cormier JN, Huang X, Xing Y, et al. Cohort analysis of patients with localized, high-risk, extremity sarcoma treated at two cancer centers: chemotherapy-associated outcomes. *J Clin Oncol*. 2004;22:4567.

Davis AM, Bell RS, Goodwin PJ. Prognostic factors in osteosarcoma: a critical review. *J Clin Oncol*. 1994;12:423.

Dematteo RP, Ballman KV, Antonescu CR, et al. Adjuvant imatinib mesylate after resection of localized, primary gastrointestinal stromal tumor: a randomized, double-blind, placebo-controlled trial. *Lancet*. 2009;272(9688):1058–1060.

Demetri GD, von Mehren M, Blanke CD, et al. Efficacy and safety of imatinib mesulate in advanced gastrointestinal stromal tumors. *N Engl J Med*. 2002;347(7):472–480.

Demetri GD, van Oosterom AT, Garrett CR, et al. Efficacy and safety of sunitinib in patients with advanced gastrointestinal stromal tumor after failure of imatinib: a randomized controlled trial. *Lancet*. 2006;368:1329–1338.

Eggermont AM, Schrafford T, Koops H, et al. Isolated limb perfusion with tumor necrosis factor and melphalan for limb salvage in 186 patients with locally advanced soft tissue extremity sarcoma. The cumulative multicenter European experience. *Ann Surg*. 1996;224:756.

Eilber FR, Eckardt J. Surgical management of soft tissue sarcomas. *Semin Oncol*. 1997;24:526.

Fong Y, Coit DG, Woodruff JM, Brennan MF. Lymph node metastasis from soft tissue sarcoma in adults. Analysis of data from a prospective database of 1772 sarcoma patients. *Ann Surg*. 1993;217:72.

Geer RJ, Woodruff J, Casper ES, et al. Management of small soft tissue sarcomas of the extremity in adults. *Arch Surg*. 1992; 127:1285.

Glenn J, Sindelar WF, Kinsella T, et al. Results of multimodality therapy of resectable soft tissue sarcomas of the retroperitoneum. *Surgery*. 1985;97:316.

Gronchi A, Casali PG, Fiore M, et al. Retroperitoneal soft tissue sarcomas: patterns of recurrence in 167 patients treated at a single institution. *Cancer*. 2004;100:2448–2455.

Grunhagen DJ, de Witt JHW, Graveland WJ, et al. Outcome and prognostic factor analysis of 217 consecutive isolated limb perfusions with tumor necrosis factor-α and melphalan for limb-threatening soft tissue sarcoma. *Cancer*. 2006;106(8): 1775–1784.

Gutman H, Pollock RE, Benjamin RS, et al. Sarcoma of the breast: implications for extent of therapy. The M. D. Anderson experience. *Surgery*. 1994;116:505.

Heslin MJ, Smith JK. Imaging of soft tissue sarcomas. *Surg Oncol Clin North Am*. 1999;8:91.

Hoffmann C, Ahrens S, Dunst J, et al. Pelvic Ewing sarcoma: a retrospective analysis of 241 cases. *Cancer*. 1999;85:869.

Huth JF, Eilber FR. Patterns of metastatic spread following resection of extremity soft tissue sarcomas and strategies for treatment. *Semin Surg Oncol*. 1988;4:20.

Jaques DP, Coit DG, Hajdu SI, et al. Management of primary and recurrent soft tissue sarcoma of the retroperitoneum. *Ann Surg*. 1990;212:51.

Karakousis CP, Proimakis C, Rao U, et al. Local recurrence and survival in soft tissue sarcomas. *Ann Surg Oncol*. 1996; 3:255.

Lahat G, Madewell JE, Anaya DA, et al. Computed tomography scan-driven selection of treatment for retroperitoneal liposarcoma histologic subtypes. *Cancer*. 2009; 115(5):1081–1090.

Lawrence W Jr, Donegan WL, Natarajan N, et al. Adult soft tissue sarcomas. A pattern of care survey of the American College of Surgeons. *Ann Surg*. 1987;205: 349.

Levine EA. Prognostic factors in soft tissue sarcoma. *Semin Surg Oncol*. 1999;17:23.

Lewis JJ, Leung D, Woodruff JM, Brennan MF. Retroperitoneal soft tissue sarcoma: analysis of 500 patients treated and followed at a single institution. *Ann Surg*. 1998;228:355.

Lienard D, Ewalenko P, Delmotte JJ, et al. High-dose recombinant tumor necrosis factor alpha in combination with interferon gamma and melphalan in isolation perfusion of the limbs for melanoma and sarcoma. *J Clin Oncol*. 1992;10:52.

Limb-sparing treatment of adult soft-tissue sarcomas and osteosarcomas. National Institutes of Health Consensus Development Conference Statement. *Natl Inst Health Consens Dev Conf Consens Statement*. 1985;5(6): 18 p.

Lindberg RD, Martin RG, Romsdahl MM, et al. Conservative surgery and postoperative radiotherapy in 300 adults with soft tissue sarcomas. *Cancer*. 1981;47:2391.

Localio AS, Eng K, Ranson JHC. Abdominosacral approach for retrorectal tumors. *Am Surg*. 1980;179:555.

Mazanet R, Antman KH. Adjuvant therapy for sarcomas. *Semin Oncol*. 1991;18:603.

Midis GP, Pollock RE, Chen NP, et al. Locally recurrent soft tissue sarcoma of the extremities. *Surgery*. 1998;123:666.

Moncrieff MD, Kroon HM, Kam PC, et al. Isolated limb infusion for advanced soft tissue sarcoma of the extremity. *Ann Surg Oncol*. 2008;15(10):2749–2756.

Patel SR, Benjamin RS. New chemotherapeutic strategies for soft tissue sarcomas. *Semin Surg Oncol*. 1999;17:47.

Pezzi CM, Pollock RE, Evans HL, et al. Preoperative chemotherapy for soft tissue sarcoma of the extremities. *Ann Surg*. 1990;211:476.

Pisters PW, Harrison LB, Leung DH, et al. Long-term results of a prospective randomized trial of adjuvant brachytherapy in soft tissue sarcoma. *J Clin Oncol*. 1996;14:859.

Pisters PWT, Harrison LB, Woodruff JM, et al. A prospective randomized trial of adjuvant brachytherapy in the management of low grade soft tissue sarcomas of the extremity and superficial trunk. *J Clin Oncol*. 1994;12:1150.

Pisters PW, Leung DH, Woodruff J, et al. Analysis of prognostic factors in 1,041 patients with localized soft tissue sarcomas of the extremities. *J Clin Oncol*. 1996;14:1679.

Pollock RE, Karnell LH, Menck HR, et al. The National Cancer Data Base report on soft tissue sarcoma. *Cancer*. 1996;78:2247.

Potter DA, Kinsella T, Glatstein E, et al. High-grade soft tissue sarcomas of the extremities. *Cancer*. 1986;58:190.

Ramanathan RC, A'Hern R, Fisher C, et al. Modified staging system for extremity soft tissue sarcomas. *Ann Surg Oncol*. 1999;5:57.

Rankin C, von Mehren M, Blanke C, et al. Continued prolongation of survival by imatinib in patients with metastatic GIST. Update of results from North American Intergroup phase III study

S0033. *Proc Am Soc Clin Oncol.* 2004: Abstr 9005.

Razek A, Perez C, Tefft M, et al. Intergroup Ewing's sarcoma study: local control related to radiation dose, volume and site of primary lesion in Ewing's sarcoma. *Cancer.* 1980;46:516.

Rosenberg SA, Tepper J, Glatstein E, et al. The treatment of soft tissue sarcomas of the extremities: prospective randomized evaluations of (1) limb-sparing surgery plus radiation therapy compared with amputation and (2) the role of adjuvant chemotherapy. *Ann Surg.* 1982;196:305.

Sarcoma Meta-analysis Collaboration. Adjuvant chemotherapy for localized resectable soft tissue sarcoma of adults: meta-analysis of individual data. *Lancet.* 1997;350:1647.

Singer S. New diagnostic modalities in soft tissue sarcoma. *Semin Surg Oncol.* 1999;17:11.

Singer S, Corson JM, Demetri GD, et al. Prognostic factors predictive of survival for truncal and retroperitoneal soft tissue sarcoma. *Ann Surg.* 1995;221:185.

Storm FK, Mahvi DM. Diagnosis and management of retroperitoneal soft tissue sarcoma. *Ann Surg.* 1991;214:2.

Suit HD, Mankin HJ, Wood WC, et al. Treatment of the patient with stage M0 soft tissue sarcoma. *J Clin Oncol.* 1988;6:854.

Tanabe KK, Pollock RE, Ellis LM, et al. Influence of surgical margins on outcome in patients with preoperatively irradiated extremity soft tissue sarcomas. *Cancer.* 1994;73:1652.

Van Geel AN, Pastorino U, Jauch KW, et al. Surgical treatment of lung metastases: the European Organization for Research and Treatment of Cancer-soft tissue and bone sarcoma group study of 255 patients. *Cancer.* 1996;77:675.

Van Oosterom AT, Judson IR, Verweij J, et al. Safety and efficacy of imatinib (STI571) in metastatic gastrointestinal stromal tumours: a phase I study. *Lancet.* 2001; 358(9291):1421–1423.

Varma DG. Optimal radiologic imaging of soft tissue sarcomas. *Semin Surg Oncol.* 1999;17:2.

Verweij J, Casali PG, Zalcberg J, et al. Progression-free survival in gastrointestinal stromal tumours with high-dose imatinib: randomized trail. *Lancet.* 2004;364(9440): 1127–1134.

Verweij J, van Oosterom A, Blay JY, et al. Imatinib mesylate (STI-571 Glivec, Gleevec) is an active agent for gastrointestinal stromal tumours, but does not yield response in other soft-tissue sarcomas that are unselected for a molecular target. Results from an EORTC Soft Tissue and Bone Sarcoma Group phase II study. *Eur J Cancer.* 2003;39(14)2006–2011.

Verweij J, van Oosterom A, Somers R, et al. Chemotherapy in the multidisciplinary approach to soft tissue sarcomas: EORTC soft tissue and bone sarcoma group studies in perspective. *Ann Oncol.* 1992;3(suppl 2):75.

Whooley BP, Mooney MM, Gibbs JF, et al. Effective follow-up strategies in soft tissue sarcoma. *Semin Surg Oncol.* 1999;17:83.

Yang JC, Chang AE, Baker AR, et al. Randomized prospective study of the benefit of adjuvant radiation therapy in the treatment of soft tissue sarcomas of the extremity. *J Clin Oncol.* 1998;16:197.

Zahm SH, Fraumeni JR Jr. The epidemiology of soft tissue sarcoma. *Semin Oncol.* 1997;24:504.

6 Cancers of the Head and Neck

Kenneth A. Newkirk and F. Christopher Holsinger

EPIDEMIOLOGY AND PATHOGENESIS

Cancers of the head and neck represent a relatively small, albeit significant, group of cancers. The treatment of these malignancies is associated with significant functional and aesthetic morbidities that have a dramatic impact on patients' quality of life. Although the majority of cancers of the head and neck arise in the upper aerodigestive tract and salivary glands, cancers of the skin, thyroid gland, and parathyroid glands deserve special consideration and are addressed in Chapters 3, 4, and 16.

Cancers of the head and neck represent approximately 3% of all cancers in the United States (and approximately 6% worldwide in 2002), with approximately 45,000 head and neck cancers diagnosed in 2004. The majority of head and neck cancers are diagnosed in the sixth to eighth decades, with males having a 4:1 ratio. Tobacco exposure represents the most significant risk factor for cancers of the head and neck, with alcohol consumption being both a synergistic and an independent risk factor. The risk of tobacco-related head and neck cancers increases proportionately with the degree of exposure. In addition, for some patients, genetic instability (e.g., hypopharyngeal cancers associated with Plummer–Vinson syndrome), viral infections (e.g., Ebstein–Barr virus [EBV] associated with nasopharyngeal cancer, human papilloma virus associated with tonsillar cancers), and occupational (e.g., saw dust exposures and sinonasal adenocarcinomas) and environmental exposures (e.g., ultraviolet exposure and lower lip cancers, betel nut use and buccal cancers, reverse cigarette smoking and palatal cancers) have been implicated in some head and neck cancers. A small group of patients (particularly young patients with oral tongue cancers) have no identifiable risk factors and have a particularly aggressive course. Some studies suggest that the disease course may be more aggressive in African Americans than in whites, with death rates for African American males being twice than for white males with the same disease (larynx and oral cavity cancers).

PATHOLOGY

Squamous cell carcinoma (SCC) represents the most common histologic type, accounting for more than 90% of tumors. Tumors may have either an ulcerative or an exophytic growth pattern. Histologically, the tumors may be in situ or invasive. Histologic differentiation (well, moderate, and poorly differentiated) has been reported to have prognostic implications, but this has not been universally confirmed. Basaloid, spindle-shaped SCCs and verrucous carcinoma are believed to be variants of SCC, and distinguishing among the variants may have prognostic implications. Premalignant lesions, such as leukoplakia and erythroplakia, are associated with a high risk of cancer development.

CLINICAL PRESENTATION, EVALUATION, AND PROGNOSIS

The clinical signs and symptoms of cancer of the upper aerodigestive tract are site-specific. The most common presenting symptom for head and neck cancers is pain. Other symptoms that are suggestive of cancer of the upper aerodigestive tract are the presence of a nonhealing ulcer, bleeding, hoarseness, dysphagia, odynophagia, otalgia (referred pain), facial pain, neck mass, or new lesion intraorally. Symptoms can occur secondary to local destruction or involvement of adjacent structures (neural, soft tissue, or bony involvement). The clinician should be alerted to the fact that an adult, with any of these signs and symptoms that do not resolve within 2 weeks, should be referred to an experienced clinician for evaluation.

Clinical examination of the head and neck includes visual inspection and palpation (bimanual evaluation) of the scalp, external ears, ear canals, mucous membranes of the eyes, nasal passages, oral cavity, nasopharynx, oropharynx, hypopharynx, and larynx. Examination of the larynx and pharyngeal regions is performed by either mirror examination or flexible endoscopy. Care must be taken to examine the major salivary glands visually and manually. A detailed cranial nerve examination is important for documenting pretreatment function because locally aggressive cancers may cause functional deficits pretreatment and because various treatment modalities may be associated with posttreatment dysfunction. Examination of the neck for spread to cervical lymph nodes of the upper jugulodigastric chain is important prognostically. The grouping of cervical nodes of the jugulodigastric chain provides a uniform system for communicating between clinicians. Metastasis to specific nodal groups or echelons can be predictive of the location of the primary site when patients present with a cervical metastasis from an unknown primary.

Biopsies of suspicious lesions can be performed in either the clinic or the operating room. Biopsies are performed with either a scalpel or punch biopsy forceps of the primary lesion or fine-needle aspiration (FNA) of suspicious lymph nodes. FNA of neck masses is as accurate as open biopsy in experienced cytopathologist's hands and is preferred over open biopsy to reduce the risk of tumor spillage and seeding of the neck. Intraoperative panendoscopy (direct laryngoscopy, esophagoscopy, nasal endoscopy, and bronchoscopy) is performed to provide adequate tissue for diagnosis from areas inaccessible in the clinic, to allow for better hemostasis, and to detail the extent of the disease for treatment planning. Improvements in fiber-optic technology (e.g., transnasal esophagoscopy) are expanding the scope of what can be evaluated and successfully biopsied in the clinical setting.

Radiographic imaging includes plain x-rays, computed tomography (CT) scans, magnetic resonance imaging (MRI) scans, ultrasound, and positron emission tomography scanning. Chest x-rays help determine the presence of distant metastasis (approximately 15% of patients) or second primaries (5% to 10%). Panorex films help determine whether mandible involvement is present. CT scans from the skull base to the clavicles provide detailed information on the extent of local soft tissue and bony involvement of upper aerodigestive tract tumors and the presence of regionally metastatic disease to the upper cervical jugulodigastric chain.

In general, prognosis for upper aerodigestive tract cancers is determined by the size of the primary, as well as the presence of regional (cervical) nodal metastasis and distant metastasis, with bulkier disease being associated with a worse prognosis. The presence of nodal metastasis decreases survival by 50% and is associated with an increased risk of distant metastasis. Staging for head and neck cancer is based on the American Joint Committee on Cancer classification and is outlined in Table 6.1. The T stage defines the size and extent of the primary; the N stage defines the size, number, and location of nodal spread; and the M stage refers to the presence or absence of distant metastasis. Approximately 15% of head and neck cancer patients will develop distant metastasis.

In addition to the traditional prognostic markers, depth of invasion, perineural invasion and perivascular invasion at the primary tumor site, and lymph node extracapsular spread are associated with worse prognosis. Survival for early-stage disease (stages I and II) across sites falls in the 80% to 90% range, but drops to 3% to 40% for stage III and IV disease. Much research is currently being done to identify more selective biological and molecular predictive and prognostic markers, such as the expression of mutated p53 and epidermal growth factor receptor expression.

TABLE 6.1	American Joint Committee on Cancer Staging System for Head and Neck Cancers

Stage Grouping

Stage I	T1, N0, M0
Stage II	T2, N0, M0
Stage III	T3, N0, M0
	T1–T3, N1, M0
Stage IV	T4, N0 or N1, M0
	Any T, N2 or N3, M0
	Any T, any N, M1

Primary Tumor (T) Dependent on Anatomic Location

Regional Lymph Nodes (N)

N0	No regional lymph node metastasis
N2a	Metastasis in single ipsilateral lymph node >3 cm but <6 cm
N2b	Metastasis in multiple ipsilateral lymph nodes, none >6 cm
N2c	Metastasis in bilateral or contralateral lymph nodes, none >6 cm
N3	Metastasis in a lymph node >6 cm

Metastatic Disease

M0	No evidence of distant metastasis
M1	Evidence of distant metastasis

Adapted from Greene FL, Page DL, Fleming ID, et al., eds. *AJCC Cancer Staging Manual.* 6th ed. New York, NY: Springer-Verlag; 2002, with permission.

The mainstay for treatment of early-stage head and neck cancer is single modality therapy, either surgery or radiation therapy. More advanced disease is more appropriately treated with multimodality therapy. Chemotherapy has played an increasing role in the primary treatment of advanced head and neck cancer, in addition to maintaining its traditional role in treating recurrent or unresectable disease.

For most sites (oral cavity, sinonasal, salivary glands), surgery is the treatment of choice for early-stage disease and provides the best chance for cure if an adequate margin of resection is obtained. Limiting factors may be the potential functional deficit or cosmetic deformity to an organ system or the accessibility of the tumor to complete surgical extirpation. Advances in surgical reconstructive techniques and prosthetics have expanded the envelope of what is appropriate surgical removal.

For early-stage disease at some sites (larynx, pharynx), radiation therapy is as effective a treatment modality as surgery, with the benefit of preserving anatomical structures. For more advanced disease, radiation is an important adjunct preoperatively and postoperatively in controlling local and regional disease and in sterilizing microscopic disease. Indications for postoperative radiation therapy are positive surgical resection margins, perineural or perivascular invasion, extracapsular spread, locally aggressive poorly differentiated tumors, tumor spillage during resection, and advanced-stage disease. Although it provides the benefit of potential "organ preservation," radiation is not without significant functional deficits. Mucositis may be severe with an acute onset. It may also be very painful, leading to dysphagia. Xerostomia (dry mouth) and dysphagia are often underappreciated but debilitating long-term sequelae. In addition to salivary gland dysfunction, thyroid dysfunction and fibrosis and scarring of soft tissues are potential long-term sequelae of radiation therapy. Multimodality therapy is the mainstay of therapy for advanced (stage II and IV) disease.

An important part of treatment is preservation of function posttreatment. Organ-specific system rehabilitation is particularly important in maintaining adequate voice and swallowing function.

Follow-up for cancers of the head and neck is important because most recurrences will occur within 2 years of treatment. At The University of Texas M. D. Anderson Cancer Center, follow-up of patients occurs every 3 months for the first 2 years postoperatively, every 6 months for the next 3 years, and yearly thereafter until 5 years. A chest x-ray and liver function studies are performed yearly.

NECK DISSECTION

Nodal metastases are associated with a 50% decrease in survival. Disease of the neck can be treated effectively with surgery and/or radiation. Limited disease (single node) with no extracapsular spread may be treated with single modality therapy, while more advanced disease may require combination therapy.

Traditionally, surgery of the neck consists of one of the following types of neck dissections: *radical neck dissection* (RND), *modified radical neck dissection* (MRND), and *selective neck dissection*. The RND consists of removal of all cervical lymph nodes in levels I to V, the sternocleidomastoid muscle, the internal jugular vein, and the spinal accessory nerve. The limits of the dissection are the inferior border of the mandible superiorly, the clavicle inferiorly, the trapezius posteriorly, the lateral border of the sternohyoid muscle anteriorly, and the deep cervical fascia overlying the levator scapulae and the scalene muscles deeply. In an attempt to decrease postoperative morbidity, the MRND was designed. It is similar to the RND but involves preservation of the spinal accessory nerve, internal jugular vein, and/or the sternocleidomastoid muscle.

A selective neck dissection involves removal of limited cervical lymph node groups (levels I–III [a *supraomohyoid neck dissection*], levels II–IV [a *lateral neck dissection*], levels II–V, VII, and postoccipital and retroauricular nodes [a *posterolateral neck dissection*]), along with preservation of the spinal accessory nerve, internal jugular vein, and sternocleidomastoid muscle. The type of selective neck dissection performed depends on the site and histology of the primary tumor and the most common routes of lymphatic spread. A supraomohyoid neck dissection is performed for clinically limited (nonpalpable) spread from oral cavity cancers, a lateral neck dissection for clinically limited (nonpalpable) spread from larynx cancers, and a posterolateral neck dissection for skin cancers (e.g., melanoma, SCC) of the scalp. Of note, a level VI or *anterior compartment neck dissection* is used in the management of thyroid cancer, along with a lateral neck dissection. More extensive disease encountered at surgery may warrant a more involved neck dissection. All patients undergoing dissection of the spinal accessory nerve will have some degree of neuropraxia and should undergo postsurgical physical therapy rehabilitation.

In patients treated with surgery of the primary and neck dissection preradiation at M. D. Anderson, a selective neck dissection (e.g., supraomohyoid neck dissection for oral cavity cancers, lateral neck dissection for laryngeal cancers) is the procedure most commonly used for clinically occult disease. Clinical nodal disease is treated by a MRND. For postradiation patients, selective neck dissection (levels II and III) is the procedure of choice for persistent adenopathy and is associated with good local-regional control and functional outcomes.

CARCINOMA OF THE ORAL CAVITY

The oral cavity is the portion of the aerodigestive tract from the vermillion border of the lips to the junction of the hard and soft palate and the circumvallate papillae of the tongue. This region anatomically includes the lips, buccal mucosa, gingiva,

TABLE 6.2	Staging System for Oral Cavity Tumors

Tis	Carcinoma in situ
T1	Tumor ≥2 cm at greatest dimension
T2	Tumor >2 cm but not 4 cm at greatest dimension
T3	Tumor >4 cm at greatest dimension
T4	Tumor invades adjacent structures (e.g., cortical bone, deep extrinsic muscle of tongue, maxillary sinus, or skin)

Adapted from Greene FL, Page DL, Fleming ID, et al., eds. *AJCC Cancer Staging Manual*. 6th ed. New York, NY: Springer-Verlag; 2002, with permission.

floor of mouth, anterior floor of mouth, anterior two-thirds of the tongue, hard palate, and retromolar trigone region. Oral cavity cancer accounts for approximately 3% of cancers in the United States, is the sixth most common cancer worldwide, and comprises 30% of all head and neck cancers. In 2005, in the United States alone, an estimated 20,000 cancers occurred in the oral cavity, and approximately 5,000 deaths were attributable to oral cavity cancers. Men are more commonly affected than women (3–4:1), and the mean age of occurrence is in the sixth to seventh decades.

Staging of the primary is based on the TNM stage, with size of the primary tumor determining the T stage. T1 lesions measure less than 2 cm, T2 measure from 2 to 4 cm, T3 measure 4 cm, and T4 measure greater than 4 cm or involve extension to local tissues (Table 6.2).

Surgical excision is the mainstay of therapy for oral cavity cancers. An adequate margin of normal tissue (at least 1 to 1.5 cm) is taken to ensure proper resection. Surgical defects can be left to heal by secondary intention or are repaired by primary closure, split-thickness skin grafting, local rotational or advancement flap reconstruction, or free flap reconstruction for large defects. Neck dissections are done for clinically evident nodal disease and electively for large primary tumors or tumors with a depth of invasion greater than 4 mm or other poor prognostic factors as listed previously. The traditional neck dissection for oral cavity lesions is a supra-omohyoid neck dissection (levels I–III), although some data exist for including level IV lymph nodes due to the possibility of skip metastasis. Primary tumors close to the midline may require bilateral neck dissections because the risk of spread to the contralateral neck may be greater than 20%.

Radiation therapy is given in the form of external-beam therapy or brachytherapy implants (primary interstitial brachytherapy implants are used for small lesions of the anterior commissure of the lip, oral tongue, and floor of mouth [T1 lesions]). Radiation therapy is only rarely used as the primary therapy and is reserved for postoperative treatment of patients at high risk for local-regional recurrence (i.e., large primary tumors [T3 or T4], primary tumors with close or positive margins, evidence of perineural or lymphovascular invasion, tumors with a depth of invasion greater than 4 mm, nodal metastasis with evidence of extracapsular spread, or multiple positive nodes).

The prognosis for early lesions (T1 and T2) of the oral cavity is good, with a 5-year survival of 80% to 90%. Survival for advanced lesions (T3 and T4) can range from 30% to 60%, depending on the factors that affect prognosis as outlined previously.

LIP

Cancer of the lip accounts for approximately 25% to 30% of oral cavity cancers, with greater than 90% being SCC and greater than 90% occurring on the lower lip. Smoking and sun exposure are major risk factors. Surgery is the treatment of choice for small lesions, with the exception of commissure lesions, which may be better treated with radiation. Cure rates approaching 90% are achievable for early lesions, with more advanced lesions having a 5-year survival of less than 50%. Nodal metastases are associated with large primary tumors; tumors of the upper lip and commissure, as well as perineural spread along the mental nerve, portend a poorer prognosis.

BUCCAL MUCOSA

Buccal mucosa cancers represent 5% of oral cavity cancers. Tobacco smoking, alcohol use, smokeless tobacco use, and betel nut use have been associated with buccal cancers. The region near the lower third molar is a common site for buccal cancers, and patients may present with trismus due to involvement of the pterygoid muscles. Cervical metastases may be common (50%) and are associated with a poor prognosis. Wide local excision is the treatment of choice, and a possible marginal mandibulectomy may be necessary to obtain clear margins. Early-stage disease may be associated with cure rates in the 60% to 70% range, while advanced tumors have survival of approximately 40%. Local-regional recurrence is a significant problem. Survival may be improved with postoperative radiation. The surgical defect may be reconstructed with local advancement flaps (e.g., tongue) or may require free flap reconstruction.

FLOOR OF MOUTH

Approximately 10% to 15% of oral cavity cancers occur in the floor of the mouth. Approximately 50% of patients will present with cervical metastasis, which, as with other oral cavity sites, is a predictor of poor prognosis. Deep tongue muscle and mandible involvement is frequently seen, requiring partial glossectomy and marginal or segmental mandibulectomy with free flap reconstruction to obtain clean margins. Bilateral cervical metastasis is not uncommon. Overall 5-year survival rates range from 30% to 70%, with stages I and II approaching 70% to 80% and stage IV disease being less than 50%.

ORAL TONGUE

Oral tongue (anterior two-thirds of the tongue) carcinoma accounts for approximately 37% of estimated new oral cavity cancers in 2005. Partial glossectomy with healing by secondary intention, primary closure, skin grafting, or free flap reconstruction is the accepted treatment. In addition to the size of the primary and histologic grade, tumor thickness also has prognostic significance for local-regional recurrence, with lesions greater than 4 mm having a 40% to 50% incidence of nodal metastasis. For tumors of 4 mm or greater thickness, an ipsilateral supraomohyoid neck dissection (levels I–III) is recommended for management of the neck. There are some data that suggest that a level IV dissection may be warranted due to the presence of skip metastasis; however, this is usually done for patients' metastasis in levels I to III. Early-stage tumors have a good prognosis (70% to 80% 3-year survival for stages I and II and 40% to 50% for stage III and IV disease), while advanced lesions require combined modality treatment. A small subset of oral tongue cancers occurs in patients younger than 40 years of age with no known risk factors; these cancers appear to be more aggressive and therefore warrant more aggressive therapy. Speech and swallowing rehabilitation are essential for good postoperative function. SCC of the base of the tongue behaves differently and is reviewed in the Cancer of the Oropharynx, Nasopharynx, and Hypopharynx section later in this chapter.

HARD PALATE

Hard palate SCCs represent approximately 0.5% of all oral cavity cancers in the United States. Cancers of the hard palate and gingiva are treated with wide local excision. Tumors within close proximity to or involving bone and large tumors may require partial palatectomy or maxillectomy to obtain clear margins. Bony defects are best reconstructed with a palatal prosthesis or obturator. Five-year cure rates approach 40% to 70% in patients without nodal disease.

CANCER OF THE LARYNX

In the United States, larynx cancers will have an estimated incidence of 10,000 new cases in 2005. Cancers occur in the sixth to eighth decades with a male-to-female ratio of 4:1. Tobacco and alcohol abuse are the most common risk factors associated with development of laryngeal cancer. The larynx is divided into three subsites—the *supraglottis*, *glottis*, and *subglottis*—that have implications for behavior, treatment, and prognosis.

The *supraglottis* is the portion of the larynx above the laryngeal ventricle and below the laryngeal surface of the epiglottis. The supraglottis contains the epiglottis, arytenoids, aryepiglottic folds, false cords, and ventricles. The lymphatic drainage is into the upper and mid-jugulodigastric chain via the pyriform sinuses and is bilateral, which makes addressing both sides of the neck for a supraglottic cancer a necessity. Sensation is via the internal branch of the superior laryngeal nerve. Cancers of the supraglottis account for 35% of laryngeal cancers. The *glottis* is the portion of the larynx that comprises the true vocal folds. The lymphatic drainage is minimal due to the close adherence of the mucosa to the underlying vocal ligament. Sensation is via the superior laryngeal nerve. Glottic cancers comprise 65% of laryngeal cancers. The *subglottis* extends from the inferior portion of the true vocal folds to the inferior border of the cricoid cartilage. Lymphatic drainage is via efferents that enter into the deep cervical jugulodigastric nodes and the paratracheal and pretracheal lymph nodes bilaterally. Subglottic cancers comprise less than 5% of laryngeal cancers. Subsite division is important for diagnosis and treatment of early tumors; however, in advanced stages, laryngeal cancers may have extensive *paraglottic* (submucosal spread around the laryngeal framework) and *transglottic* (extension across subsites) spread. Staging for laryngeal cancers varies and is listed in Table 6.3.

Presenting symptoms for laryngeal cancers include hoarseness, pain, dysphagia, and respiratory distress. Evaluation of the larynx is essential for staging of laryngeal cancers. Impaired vocal fold mobility and subsite extension portend a more advanced cancer and poorer prognosis. Cancers that affect the true vocal fold usually present early due to the impairment in function (voice and respiration). Supraglottic cancers usually present late, with submucosal and local spread, and symptoms are due to invasion of local tissues causing hoarseness, dysphagia, odynophagia, otalgia (referred pain), and respiratory distress. Imaging of the larynx (CT scanning) is important in determining local extension of the primary disease, laryngeal cartilage destruction, and the presence of clinically occult disease.

Treatment

Because glottic cancers are the most common laryngeal cancers seen, these are discussed in detail. The goal of treatment of laryngeal cancer is eradication of the disease, as well as preservation of function and anatomy when possible. Both surgery and radiation provide excellent control rates for T1 and T2 glottic lesions. Estimated 5-year survival for all cancers of the larynx is 65%. Local control rates in

TABLE 6.3	Staging System for Cancers of the Larynx

Supraglottis

T1	Tumor confined to the site of origin
T2	Tumor involving adjacent supraglottic sites, without glottic fixation
T3	Tumor limited to the larynx, with fixation and/or extension to the postcricoid medial wall of the pyriform sinus or pre-epiglottic space
T4	Massive tumor extending beyond the larynx to involve the oropharynx, soft tissues of the neck, or destruction of thyroid cartilage

Glottis

T1	Tumor confined to vocal folds, with normal vocal cord mobility
T1a	Limited to one vocal fold
T1b	Involves both vocal folds
T2	Tumor extension to supraglottis and/or subglottis with normal or impaired vocal cord mobility
T3	Tumor confined to larynx, with fixation of the vocal cords
T4	Massive tumor, with thyroid cartilage destruction and/or extension beyond the confines of the larynx

Adapted from Greene FL, Page DL, Fleming ID, et al., eds. *AJCC Cancer Staging Manual.* 6th ed. New York, NY: Springer-Verlag; 2002, with permission.

the literature for both treatment modalities range from 70% to 100%, which improves with salvage laryngectomy. T3 and T4 tumors have control rates in the 80% to 85% and 60% to 70% range, respectively. Five-year survival for T1 and T2 lesions is 80% to 90%, and for T3 and T4 disease, 50% to 60%. More advanced laryngeal cancers require combined modality therapy with total laryngectomy (or a modification thereof) and postoperative radiation therapy.

Surgery

Early-stage glottic disease may be treated effectively with surgery or radiation therapy. Surgical options for early glottic disease include vocal cord stripping, transoral laser microsurgery, hemilaryngectomy, subtotal laryngectomy (supracricoid partial laryngectomy [SCPL]), and total laryngectomy. The advantages of surgery are complete extirpation of the disease and reservation of other treatments (e.g., radiation) for future recurrences. Both vocal cord stripping and laser microsurgery may leave the cord with scarring that can make it difficult to evaluate for recurrence. A *vertical partial laryngectomy* (or *hemilaryngectomy*) involves removal of half of the larynx vertically, as well as preservation of half of the larynx vertically to maintain voice and function. Patients with small volume disease after radiation are good candidates for this procedure. For early-stage supraglottic cancers (T1 and T2), a *supraglottic or horizontal laryngectomy* may be performed. The cricoid and at least one arytenoid is preserved and sutured onto the base of the tongue, again in an attempt to preserve adequate respiration, voice, and swallowing function. Candidates for this procedure require adequate pulmonary reserve and cardiac function to prevent aspiration pneumonia.

The SCPL is an extended horizontal partial laryngectomy technique that preserves the patient's native voice and permits near-total laryngectomy without permanent tracheostoma. SCPL can include removal of the false and true vocal cords, the entire thyroid cartilage including the entire paraglottic spaces, and a portion or all of the supraglottis and pre-epiglottic space. In selected cases, one arytenoid may be resected. Phonatory function and deglutition is maintained by the movement of the spared arytenoid(s) against the tongue base. It represents a dramatic advance because it uses the patient's laryngeal framework to preserve the patient's native voice, while providing a true en bloc tumor resection.

Total laryngectomy is reserved for more advanced disease (T3 and T4) or patients who have failed previous therapy and who are likely to have poor functional outcomes (voice and swallowing) with voice-sparing surgical procedures. A bilateral lateral neck dissection can be performed at the same time for more extensive disease (a wide-field laryngectomy), and hemi- or total thyroidectomy is performed for disease that destroys cartilage or involves the pyriform sinuses, subglottis, or paratracheal nodes. In cases with significant hypopharyngeal or cervical esophageal extension, a laryngopharyngectomy can be performed and repaired with a free tissue transfer microvascular reconstruction. Postoperative radiation is typically given in advanced disease. Speech pathology consultation is essential preoperatively for adequate voice and swallowing rehabilitation postoperatively. Voice rehabilitation with an electrolarynx, tracheoesophageal puncture, or esophageal speech can lead to good voice quality. In addition to being monitored for recurrence, patients also need to be followed for potential hypothyroidism (either from surgery or radiation).

Radiation Therapy

Given the good rates of local-regional control, radiation therapy has been advocated as the treatment of choice for early-stage disease. The advantages of radiation are sparing of the anatomy with preservation of voice. The disadvantages are postradiation sequelae (e.g., xerostomia, potential radionecrosis of the laryngeal framework) and the inability to use radiation again in the event of a recurrence. Postoperative radiation therapy is typically given to patients with extensive primary disease (submucosal spread, subsite extension [i.e., supra- or subglottic, extralaryngeal extension]), disease with positive margins, multiple positive lymph nodes, or lymph nodes with extracapsular spread, and patients requiring prelaryngectomy tracheotomy (who have a higher risk of stomal recurrence).

Typical doses of primary radiation for early laryngeal disease are in the 65 to 70 Gy range. For glottic cancers, the radiation can be focused on the primary site due to the low incidence of nodal metastasis. For supraglottic cancers with a higher propensity of cervical metastasis at the time of diagnosis, fields should encompass the primary nodal drainage basins (levels II–V), with doses in the 50 to 60 Gy ranges.

CANCER OF THE OROPHARYNX, NASOPHARYNX, AND HYPOPHARYNX

The pharynx is a tubular structure that contains the larynx. The pharynx can be divided into three anatomical subsites: the nasopharynx, the oropharynx, and the hypopharynx. The anatomical boundaries of the oropharynx are the anterior tonsillar pillar, uvula and base of tongue, and the vallecular surface of the epiglottis inferiorly. Included in this subsite are the pharyngeal tonsils and the base of tongue. The nasopharynx is separated from the oropharynx by the soft palate. The boundaries of the hypopharynx are the laryngeal surface of the epiglottis, the pyriform sinuses, the posterior pharyngeal wall, and the postcricoid area above the cricopharyngeus muscle. Lymphatic drainage for the nasopharynx is the retropharyngeal lymph node basin, the parapharyngeal lymph nodes, and the upper and posterior jugulodigastric nodes. Lymphatics for the oropharynx are in the deep, upper jugulodigastric chain, while the hypopharynx drains into the mid- and lower deep jugulodigastric chain. Bilateral cervical metastases are not uncommon. The parapharyngeal space is a potential space located outside the pharynx proper. It is pyramidal in shape and extends from the skull base to the hyoid bone. Most tumors of this region are benign; the most common tumors arise from the deep lobe of the parotid gland and include unusual histologic variants such as pleomorphic adenomas, paragangliomas, and neurogenic tumors (schwannomas and neurofibromas), rather than the common squamous tumors of the upper aerodigestive tract.

The most common presenting symptoms are pain, dysphagia, referred otalgia, and a neck mass. In an attempt to cure disease with decreased morbidity and to preserve function (swallowing), external-beam radiation (tonsil, hypopharynx, base of tongue) has become the treatment of choice for oropharyngeal and hypopharyngeal cancers. Survival rates have been in the 70% to 80% range for stage I and II disease and 50% for stage II disease. Surgery is reserved for small lesions and recurrent disease, due to the increased morbidity associated with surgery. Brachytherapy is also used in some centers for base of tongue tumors.

Nasopharyngeal cancers are malignancies that arise from or near the fossa of Rosenmüller in the nasopharynx. These cancers are most commonly seen in regions of China and Africa, where there is a strong association with EBV. Indeed, EBV viral capsid IgA antigen (VC) and early antigen IgA (EA) titers serve as a tumor marker for recurrence. The average age at presentation is in the fifth and sixth decades. Most patients present with a painless neck mass, nasal obstruction, unilateral serous otitis media, or epistaxis. Cranial neuropathy (particularly involving cranial nerves II, IV, V, and VI) may occur as a result of skull base invasion, which may be seen in as many as 25% of patients. An irregular mass is seen on nasopharyngoscopy. Tumors are classified according to the World Health Organization classification (type I being well-differentiated keratinizing SCC, type II being nonkeratinizing carcinoma, and type III being poorly differentiated [undifferentiated] carcinoma, which includes lymphoepitheliomas and anaplastic carcinomas).

The mainstay of therapy is cisplatin-based chemotherapy and radiation therapy to the nasopharyngeal bed and primary draining lymph node echelons. Tumors are staged based on extent of disease with stage I tumors limited to the nasopharynx; stage II disease involving extension into the oropharynx, nasal fossa, and parapharyngeal space; stage III disease involving extension into the skull base fossa and paranasal sinuses; and stage IV disease involving the infratemporal fossa, orbit, and hypopharynx, or with intracranial extension and/or cervical adenopathy. Five-year survival for nasopharyngeal carcinoma is less than 20% for type I tumors and approaches 50% for type II and III tumors. Surgery may be used for limited early-stage disease, but it is associated with significant morbidity. Neck dissections are performed for residual disease after chemoradiotherapy.

Cancers of the hypopharynx usually present at advanced stages (greater than 60% are stage III and IV) and are associated with poor local control and survival. The majority of cancers occur in the pyriform sinus (70% to 80%), and nodal disease at the time of presentation is common (70% to 80%). Chemoradiation is the mainstay of therapy, although total laryngectomy or laryngopharyngectomy may be suitable for some patients. Five-year survival for hypopharyngeal cancers is dismal, ranging from 20% to 40%.

CANCER OF THE NASAL CAVITY AND PARANASAL SINUSES

The nasal cavity extends from the external nasal dorsum and pyriform aperture to the choana and the nasopharynx, and from the nasal floor (which is comprised of the maxilla anteriorly and the palatine bone posteriorly) to the nasal roof (which houses the olfactory bulbs and cranial nerve I). The nasal septum, which is composed of cartilage anteriorly and the vomer and perpendicular plate of the ethmoid bones posteriorly, separates the nose into halves. The lateral nasal walls house the ostia for the paranasal sinuses; the nasofrontal duct; and the inferior, middle, and superior turbinates. The nasal cavity and paranasal sinuses are lined by respiratory epithelium (pseudostratified ciliated columnar epithelium), except at the nasal vestibule, which is lined by keratinizing squamous epithelium. The sensory innervation to the nasal and paranasal mucosa is from branches of the trigeminal nerve (V1 and V2). The blood supply is from the external carotid (superior labial, angular, and internal maxillary arteries) and internal carotid (anterior and posterior ethmoidal arteries) arteries.

There are four paired paranasal sinuses: the maxillary, frontal, ethmoid, and sphenoid sinuses. The sinuses communicate with the nasal cavity through their ostia. The ostium of the maxillary sinus drains underneath the middle turbinate at the osteomeatal complex, as do the ostia of the anterior and middle ethmoid sinuses. The frontal sinus drains through the nasofrontal duct located at the anterior aspect of the nose. The ostia of the sphenoid sinuses are located above and medial to the superior turbinate on the face of the sinus. Lymphatic drainage of the paranasal sinuses occurs via the retropharyngeal, parapharyngeal, and deep upper jugulodigastric lymph nodes.

The most common presenting symptoms for sinonasal tumors are unilateral nasal obstruction, facial pain, facial numbness, and epistaxis. Patients may also present with unilateral serous otitis media (due to obstruction of the eustachian tube orifice), epiphora, or excessive tearing (due to obstruction of the nasolacrimal duct, which drains underneath the inferior turbinate). Nodal metastases are uncommon in sinonasal malignancies. Occupational exposures are associated with certain sinonasal malignancies (e.g., wood dust with adenocarcinomas, smoking nickel and heavy metal exposures with SCCs).

Evaluation of the nose and paranasal sinuses includes external and endoscopic inspection. Biopsies of nasal and paranasal tumors should be done cautiously because of the risk of bleeding and cerebrospinal fluid leak due to intracranial extension and may warrant imaging prior to biopsy. Imaging (both CT scan and MRI scan) is important in determining the extent of the disease (i.e., extension beyond the nose and paranasal sinuses into the brain, orbit, skull base, and infratemporal fossa). Contrast CT scan is used to determine the presence of bony destruction and the vascularity of the lesion. MRI scanning is helpful in delineating the extent of soft-tissue destruction (intracranial and intraorbital involvement) and distinguishing tumor from inspissated fluid on T2-weighted images.

Benign tumors of the nasal cavity include nasal papillomas and angiofibromas. Nasal papillomas are divided into squamous and Schneiderian papillomas (the most common). Schneiderian papillomas usually present with unilateral nasal obstruction, epistaxis, and rhinorrhea. There are three subtypes of Schneiderian papillomas: cylindrical, septal, and inverting, the latter two being the most common. Septal papillomas account for 50% of Schneiderian papillomas. They arise from the nasal septum, are exophytic in nature, and occur most commonly in males in the third to sixth decades of life. Inverting papillomas most commonly arise from the lateral nasal wall, are polypoid in nature, occur most commonly in males (fifth to eighth decades), and, as the name implies, push the stroma inward (hence, the term inverting papilloma). Up to 15% of tumors may harbor SCC, and there is a risk (10%) of squamous degeneration. Surgical excision is the treatment of choice; this involves a medial maxillectomy or an open or endoscopic resection of the lateral nasal wall.

Angiofibromas are benign locally destructive vascular tumors. They are seen most commonly in young males (second to fourth decades) who present with a history of unilateral nasal obstruction and recurrent, refractory epistaxis. It is a smooth lobulated mass arising in the posterior lateral nose near the sphenopalatine foramen (derives its blood supply from the sphenopalatine artery). Contrast CT scan or MRI is diagnostic (anterior bowing of the posterior maxillary sinus wall [Holman–Miller sign]). Office biopsy should not be performed due to the risk of bleeding. Surgery following embolization (within 48 hours) is the treatment of choice.

Sinonasal malignancies are rare, accounting for less than 5% of head and neck malignancies. The differential for sinonasal malignancies include mucosal melanomas, sarcomas, SCCs, sinonasal undifferentiated carcinomas, lymphomas (angiocentric T-cell lymphoma), esthesioneuroblastomas (also called olfactory neuroblastomas), extramedullary plasmacytomas, adenocarcinomas, and adenoid cystic carcinomas. Hematoxylin and eosin staining may only reveal small blue cells, making the diagnosis difficult. Immunohistochemical analysis is important in establishing the diagnosis.

The most common type of sinonasal tumor is SCC, occurring predominantly in males in the sixth to eighth decades. Histologically, they are similar to SCCs elsewhere in the head and neck. Mucosal melanomas are rare (1% to 2% of all melanomas), with a fairly equal male-to-female ratio. Up to one-third may be amelanotic, and immunohistochemical staining is important in establishing the diagnosis. Survival is poor, with less than 30% of patients alive at 5 years. Esthesioneuroblastoma is a rare tumor arising from the olfactory neuroepithelium with intranasal extension. Epistaxis, anosmia, pain, and nasal obstruction are common presenting symptoms. Combined nasal and intracranial surgery (craniofacial resection) followed by radiation is the preferred treatment. Five-year survival approaches 70% for resectable disease, although there is a high incidence of local recurrence. Angiocentric T-cell lymphoma is a non-Hodgkin lymphoma that may present with nasal obstruction, epistaxis, and local tissue destruction of the midline midface (septum). The tissues are friable and necrotic on endoscopy. Multiple biopsies may be needed to confirm the diagnosis. Radiation is the treatment of choice. Sinonasal sarcomas are rare and associated with a poor prognosis. Treatment usually involves some combination of surgery and radiation. Chemotherapy may be used, based on the histologic subtype. Sinonasal undifferentiated carcinoma is also rare and associated with a poor prognosis. Local extension is common (intracranial and intraorbital). Craniofacial resection with postoperative radiation is the treatment of choice. Extramedullary plasmacytoma is the most common type of localized plasma cell neoplasm in the head and neck; yet, it accounts for less than 1% of all head and neck neoplasms. Males are more commonly affected than females (3:1), and up to 70% occur in the head and neck. Nasal obstruction and epistaxis are common. CT and MRI are nondiagnostic, and biopsy is important in establishing the diagnosis. Staining for lambda and kappa light chains confirms the diagnosis. Systemic workup for multiple myeloma is important because these tumors may progress to multiple myeloma in up to 30% of cases. Radiation is the treatment of choice with local control rates of 70% to 80% and 5-year survival of 60% to 70%. Adenocarcinomas and adenoid cystic carcinomas are commonly seen in sinus malignancies and are associated with local extension and perineural spread.

Surgery followed by radiation has been the accepted treatment for these disorders. Small tumors are amenable to surgical extirpation via open or endoscopic approaches. Small squamous cell tumors of the nasal vestibule respond well to brachytherapy. However, due to the late presentation of many sinonasal tumors and local extension to the skull base and orbit, surgery may be associated with high morbidity (e.g., neurologic sequelae and sacrifice of the orbit). Surgery may entail a partial or total rhinectomy, partial or total maxillectomy and adjacent sinuses (ethmoid and frontal), orbital exenteration, and combined approaches with neurosurgery for intracranial extension (craniofacial resection). Neck dissection is reserved

for clinically gross disease. There are some data that suggest that preoperative chemotherapy may be beneficial in minimizing the extent of surgery, but this remains
investigational. Prognosis for sinonasal malignancies is poor, with overall 5-year
survival rates of 20% to 30%. Survival for early-stage disease (60% to 70% for T1) is
better than for latter stages (10% to 20% for T4).

UNKNOWN PRIMARY WITH CERVICAL METASTASIS

Approximately 2% to 9% of patients who present with SCC metastatic to the neck
will have an undiagnosed or unknown primary at the time of presentation. However, after careful evaluation and workup, approximately 90% of these patients will
have a primary diagnosis. Thus, only approximately 10% of patients have an
unknown primary tumor. Although persistent adenopathy can be associated with
numerous inflammatory or infectious conditions (e.g., cat scratch disease, atypical
mycobacterium), malignant cervical adenopathy should be suspected in patients
with adenopathy that persists for more than 2 weeks after appropriate medical
(antibiotic) therapy. The most common pathology seen is ACC, although lymphoma, melanoma metastasis from the skin, and metastatic thyroid, lung, and
breast cancer may rarely present with persistent adenopathy in the head and neck.

A thorough history and physical examination, which should include endoscopy to rule out the primary, should be performed on all patients. Random biopsies
of potential sites are not recommended. However, goal-directed biopsies of suspicious areas and bilateral tonsillectomy are indicated, depending on the site of the
nodal metastasis, because as many as 25% of tonsils may harbor an occult primary.
The site of nodal metastasis may indicate the site of the primary. For example, cystic or level II adenopathy may suggest an oropharyngeal primary (base of tongue or
tonsil), while level V adenopathy may be suggestive of a nasopharyngeal or thyroid
primary and a supraclavicular node may suggest a lung or gastrointestinal primary.
Common occult upper aerodigestive tract sites for primary disease are the tonsil,
base of tongue, pyriform sinus, and nasopharynx. If FNA suggests a primary other
than SCC, then an appropriate, systemic metastatic workup needs to be performed.
Directed diagnostic imaging of the head and neck, such as CT or MRI scanning, is
important. The role of positron emission tomography scans has not been established in head and neck cancers, but data are promising in the setting of known and
unknown primary disease, depending on the volume of disease present.

Treatment for true unknown cervical primaries is surgery (neck dissection),
radiation, or surgery followed by postoperative radiation, either to the nodal basin
alone or with elective irradiation of the most common mucosal sites (i.e., the nasopharynx, oropharynx, hypopharynx, and supraglottis). Data suggest that there may
be a decrease in the occurrence of an occult primary with the latter approach. Some
authors view this as controversial and recommend reserving radiation to the elective sites until a primary develops to reduce the morbidity associated with radiation.

Surgery for squamous cell primaries usually entails a selective or MRND. If
there is single nodal disease with no poor prognostic criteria (e.g., extracapsular
spread, multiple nodes, less than 3 cm), then surgery alone or radiation alone may
result in a good outcome. For bulkier, more aggressive disease, surgery (e.g., MRND,
RND) and radiation (usually postoperative, but sometimes preoperative) is the
treatment of choice. Surgery is also indicated for the diagnosis of metastatic well-
differentiated thyroid cancer, which would entail a total thyroidectomy and neck
dissection (lateral and anterior compartment).

Surgery for tumors of infraclavicular origin (e.g., breast or gastrointestinal)
must be carefully considered in light of the high risk of systemic metastasis elsewhere in the body. If the tumor is limited to the neck with no other distant metastasis, then surgery and postoperative radiation may improve local control. For

poorly differentiated tumors suggestive of nasopharyngeal origin, the preferred treatment is radiation.

Five-year survival for treatment of unknown squamous cervical metastases approaches 40% to 60% in many studies, whether using surgery alone or surgery and radiation. Close follow-up is important because the primary will declare itself in as many as 20% of patients. Prognosis for metastatic disease from an infraclavicular primary is poor, being less than 10% in most studies.

CANCERS OF THE EAR AND TEMPORAL BONES

The ear is composed of the external ear (pinna, auricle, and external canal), the middle ear, and the inner ear. The epithelium over the external ear is squamous with adjacent adnexal and glandular (sebaceous) structures while ciliated epithelium and glands line the middle ear. The framework of the auricle and outer third of the external canal is comprised of elastic cartilage, while the inner third of the external canal and middle ear is made up of the temporal bone.

Cancers of the ear and temporal bones are rare and account for less than 1% of all head and neck cancers. Although cutaneous malignancies of the pinna and auricle are common, cancers of the temporal bone are rare. The majority of tumors of the ear involve the auricle (>80%), followed by the ear canal and middle ear and mastoid. Males are more commonly affected, and sun exposure is a major risk factor. SCC is the most common histologic cancer of the outer ear, followed by basal cell carcinomas. Rhabdomyosarcomas and adenocarcinomas can occur in the middle ear. Pain, aural fullness, conductive hearing loss, ulceration, and chronic otorrhea are common presenting symptoms. Extension toward the middle ear may be associated with cranial neuropathies such as facial paralysis and sensorineural hearing loss in up to one-third of patients.

Surgery is often the preferred therapy for SCC and basal cell carcinomas, although radiation therapy may play a role in highly selected cases. Small lesions of the outer ear are treated effectively by partial or total auriculectomy. Early external canal lesions can be effectively treated by sleeve resection. Lateral temporal bone resection is reserved for large tumors with medial extension, which may include parotidectomy for parotid nodal metastasis.

Survival for cancers of the outer ear approaches 90% for cancers confined to the auricle, with decreasing prognosis for those with medial extension and middle ear extension to less than 30%. Temporal bone malignancies have a survival rate of 20% to 30% at 5 years.

NEOPLASMS OF THE SALIVARY GLAND

Salivary gland tissue in the upper aerodigestive tract consists of three pairs of major salivary glands—parotid glands, submandibular or submaxillary glands, and sublingual glands—and thousands of minor salivary glands that exist in the mucosa of the lips, buccal mucosa, hard and soft palate, and oropharynx. The parotid glands lie lateral and posterior to the mandible and can be divided into a superficial and a deep lobe by the course of the facial nerve. The deep lobe of the parotid gland abuts the prestyloid, parapharyngeal space, and deep lobe parotid tumors (e.g., pleomorphic adenomas) are the most common tumors in this region. The duct of the parotid gland (Stensen's duct) drains intraorally near the second maxillary molar. Lymph nodes are present in the substance of the gland, and the nodal basin for the parotid gland is the preauricular and upper jugulodigastric nodes. Of note, the parotid gland and associated lymph nodes are a primary nodal drainage basin for scalp and auricular malignancies, and a parotidectomy should be included in any comprehensive treatment of these malignancies. The submandibular glands are located beneath the mandible and their ducts (Wharton ducts) and drain near the frenulum of the tongue in the floor of the mouth. The marginal mandibular branch of the facial nerve overlies the gland superficially, the facial vessels (and associated lymph nodes) are intimately associated with gland, and the lingual and hypoglossal nerves are closely associated with the deep surface of the gland. The sublingual glands are located deep to the mucosa of the floor of the mouth on top of the mylohyoid muscle.

Tumors of the salivary glands can occur in both major and minor salivary glands, with the majority occurring in the major salivary glands. The majority of tumors occur in the parotid glands (90%), and the majority of these are benign (80%). As the size of the gland decreases, the risk of malignancy increases, with 50% of submandibular gland tumors being malignant and 80% of sublingual gland tumors being malignant. Some tumors are associated with previous radiation exposure or smoking (e.g., Warthin tumors). However, the majority of salivary gland tumors have no identifiable risk factors.

Most salivary gland tumors present as a painless mass, although rapid growth and pain may be seen but are not always suggestive of more ominous or aggressive disease because inflammatory or infectious diseases can present with similar symptoms (e.g., parotitis or collagen vascular diseases such as Sjögren syndrome or Wegner granulomatosis). Facial paralysis, nodal metastasis, and local tissue invasion may be indicative of a more aggressive disease. Of note, Bell's palsy (idiopathic facial nerve paralysis) is a diagnosis of exclusion, and the patient with a sudden facial nerve paralysis should have a parotid malignancy (either primary or metastatic from a skin primary) ruled out.

FNA is helpful in establishing the diagnosis but is highly dependent on the skill of the cytopathologist (accuracy ranges from 60% to 90%). If an FNA cannot establish the diagnosis, then an open, excisional biopsy should be performed. In the case of the parotid gland, an excisional biopsy would entail performing a *superficial parotidectomy* to identify and preserve the facial nerve. Incisional biopsy should be avoided to prevent tumor violation, tumor spillage, and, in the case of the parotid gland, facial nerve injury. CT and MRI scans are helpful in detailing the extent of disease (e.g., parapharyngeal space extension of deep lobe parotid tumors or skull base involvement).

The majority of tumors in the salivary glands are benign, with pleomorphic adenomas being the most common. Other benign tumors include Warthin tumors (which are associated with smoking and are bilateral in 10% of cases), monomorphic adenomas, and oncocytomas. Malignant tumors include mucoepidermoid carcinomas, adenoid cystic carcinomas, adenocarcinomas, and SCCs.

Treatment

Surgery is the mainstay of therapy for all parotid tumors. For benign tumors, superficial parotidectomy and submandibular gland excision are both diagnostic and curative. Because of the intimate relationship of the parotid gland and submandibular glands to the facial nerve and its branches, as well as the morbidity associated with facial nerve paralysis, only gross involvement of the nerve by tumor is an indication for sacrifice. Pleomorphic adenomas are the most common benign tumors of the salivary glands. Care must be taken to remove a rim of normal tissue around the tumor, as well as to avoid rupture of the pseudocapsule and tumor spillage, to reduce the risk of recurrence.

Malignant tumors of the salivary glands typically require surgery and radiation. The exceptions are low-grade neoplasms (e.g., low-grade mucoepidermoid carcinomas and polymorphous low-grade adenocarcinomas), which may be treated with surgery alone. Superficial parotidectomy is indicated for small lesions. For parotid tumors with deep lobe extension, total parotidectomy with facial nerve preservation is the treatment of choice. Gross involvement of the facial nerve by tumor is an indication for sacrifice of the nerve. In such cases, the nerve should be traced proximally (as far back as the brainstem, if necessary) until tumor is cleared. This is especially true of adenoid cystic carcinomas, which are neurotropic tumors. Sacrifice of the facial nerve should be repaired immediately either by interpositional nerve grafting (using the sural nerve from the leg or medial antebrachial cutaneous nerve from the arm) or a cranial nerve XII to VII grafting. Parotid tumors with local extension (skin or external canal involvement) may require a mastoidectomy (to trace the nerve proximally) and removal of the lateral part of the temporal bone. Excision of the submandibular gland and adjacent facial lymph nodes is the treatment for submandibular tumors. As with the parotid, only gross involvement with tumor is an indication for nerve sacrifice (e.g., lingual and hypoglossal nerves), and local extension to surrounding tissues (e.g., floor of mouth musculature, tongue) necessitates more radical surgery. Neck dissection (selective) is reserved for clinically apparent neck disease.

Radiation is reserved for primary treatment of malignant tumors in patients who are poor surgical candidates or who do not want to undergo surgery, as well as for the postoperative treatment of high-grade or recurrent disease. Adenoid cystic carcinomas, high-grade mucoepidermoid carcinomas, high-grade adenocarcinomas, SCCs, and metastatic disease to the neck are typically irradiated. In addition, patients with pleomorphic adenomas that are recurrent or involve gross tumor spillage may be candidates for postoperative radiation. Doses to the primary tumor bed are in the range of 50 to 70 Gy.

Five-year survival for benign tumors approaches 100%, with the greatest risk of recurrence occurring in patients who have had inadequate initial operations. For malignant tumors, 5-year survival is 70% to 90% for low-grade tumors and 20% to 30% for high-grade malignancies. Regional and distant recurrences range from 15% to 20% and are common in tumors with perineural invasion (e.g., adenoid cystic carcinomas). Adenoid cystic carcinomas have a propensity to spread along nerves and metastasize to the lung; therefore, surveillance should entail imaging (i.e., MRI scans and chest X-rays) to exclude recurrence.

Recommended Readings

Al-Sarraf M, LeBlanc M, Giri PG, et al. Chemoradiotherapy versus radiotherapy in patients with advanced nasopharyngeal cancer: phase III randomized intergroup study 0099. *J Clin Oncol*. 1998;16(4):1310–1317.

Ang KK, Jiang GL, Frankenthaler RA, et al. Carcinoma of the nasal cavity. *Radiother Oncol*. 1992;24:163–168.

Benner SE, Pajak TF, Lippman SM, et al. Prevention of second primary tumors with isotretinoin in patients with squamous cell carcinoma of the head and neck: long-term follow-up. *J Natl Cancer Inst*. 1994;84:140–141.

Byers RM, Clayman GL, McGill D, et al. Selective neck dissections for squamous carcinoma of the upper aerodigestive tract: patterns of regional failure. *Head Neck*. 1999;21:499–505.

Byers RM, Wolf PF, Ballantyne AJ. Rationale for elective modified neck dissection. *Head Neck Surg*. 1988;10:160–167.

Carrau RL, Segas J, Nuss DW, et al. Squamous cell carcinoma of the sinonasal tract invading the orbit. *Laryngoscope*. 1999;109:230–235.

Clayman GL, Johnson CJ II, Morrison W, et al. The role of neck dissection after chemoradiotherapy for oropharyngeal cancer with advanced nodal disease. *Arch Otolaryngol Head Neck Surg*. 2001;172(2):135–139.

Colletier PJ, Garden AS, Morrison WH, et al. Postoperative radiation for squamous cell carcinoma metastatic to cervical lymph nodes from an unknown primary site: outcomes and patterns of failure. *Head Neck*. 1998;20(8):674–681.

Diaz EM Jr, Holsinger FC, Zuniga ER, et al. Squamous cell carcinoma of the buccal mucosa: one institution's experience with

119 previously untreated patients. *Head Neck.* 2003;25(4):267–273.

Disa JJ, Hu QY, Hidalgo DA. Retrospective review of 400 consecutive free flap reconstructions for oncologic surgical defects. *Ann Surg Oncol.* 1997;4(8):663–669.

Eden BV, Debo RF, Larner JM, et al. Esthesioneuroblastoma. Long-term outcome and patterns of failure—the University of Virginia experience. *Cancer.* 1994;73:2556–2562.

Fagan JJ, Collins B, Barnes L, et al. Perineural invasion in squamous cell carcinoma of the head and neck. *Arch Otolaryngol Head Neck Surg.* 1998;124:637–640.

Fee WE, Roberson JB, Goffinet DR. Long-term survival after surgical resection of recurrent nasopharyngeal cancer after radiotherapy failure. *Arch Otolaryngol Head Neck Surg.* 1991;117(11):1233–1236.

Forastiere A, Koch W, Trotti A, et al. Head and neck cancer [review]. *N Engl J Med.* 2001;345(26):1890–1900.

Fordice J, Kershaw C, El Naggar A, et al. Adenoid cystic carcinoma of the head and neck: predictors of morbidity and mortality. *Arch Otolaryngol Head Neck Surg.* 1999;125:149–152.

Frankenthaler RA, Byers RM, Luna MA, et al. Predicting occult lymph node metastasis in parotid cancer. *Arch Otolaryngol Head Neck Surg.* 1993;119:517–520.

Frankenthaler RA, Luna MA, Lee SS, et al. Prognostic variables in parotid gland cancer. *Arch Otolaryngol Head Neck Surg.* 1991;117:1251–1256.

Garden AS, Morrison WH, Clayman GL, et al. Early squamous cell carcinoma of the hypopharynx: outcomes of treatment with radiation alone to the primary disease. *Head Neck.* 1996;18:317–322.

Garden AS, Weber RS, Ang KK, et al. Postoperative radiation therapy for malignant tumors of minor salivary glands. *Cancer.* 1994;73(10):2563–2569.

Greenberg JS, Fowler R, Gomez J, et al. Extent of extracapsular spread: a critical prognosticator in oral tongue cancer. *Cancer.* 2003;97(6):1464–1470.

Gwozdz JT, Morrison WH, Garden AS, et al. Concomitant boost radiotherapy for squamous carcinoma of the tonsillar fossa. *Int J Radiat Oncol.* 1997;39(1):127–135.

Harrison LB, Zelefsky MJ, Sessions RB, et al. Base of tongue cancer treated with external beam irradiation plus brachytherapy: oncologic and functional outcome. *Radiology.* 1992;184:267–270.

Hong WK, Endicott J, Itri LM, et al. 13-cis Retinoic acid in the treatment of oral leukoplakia. *N Engl J Med.* 1986;315:1501–1505.

Induction chemotherapy plus radiation compared with surgery plus radiation in patients with advanced laryngeal cancer. The Department of Veterans Affairs Laryngeal Cancer Study Group. *N Engl J Med.* 1991;324(24):1685–1690.

Johnson JT, Myers EN, Hao SP, et al. Outcome of open surgical therapy for glottic carcinoma. *Ann Otol Rhinol Laryngol.* 1993; 102:752–755.

Jungehulsing M, Scheidhauer K, Damm M, et al. 2[F]-Fluoro2-deoxy-D-glucose positron emission tomography is a sensitive tool for the detection of occult primary cancer (carcinoma of unknown primary syndrome) with head and neck lymph node manifestation. *Otolaryngol Head Neck Surg.* 2000;123:294–301.

Khuri FR, Lippman SM, Spitz MR, et al. Molecular epidemiology and retinoid chemoprevention of head and neck cancer. *J Natl Cancer Inst.* 1997;89:199.

Kirchner JA, Cornog JL, Holmes RE. Transglottic cancer. *Arch Otolaryngol.* 1974;99 :247–251.

Kraus DH, Dubner S, Harrison LB, et al. Prognostic factors for recurrence and survival in head and neck soft tissue sarcomas. *Cancer.* 1994;74:697–702.

Kraus DH, Zelefsky MJ, Brock HA, et al. Combined surgery and radiation therapy for squamous cell carcinoma of the hypopharynx. *Otolaryngol Head Neck Surg.* 1997;116:637–641.

Laccourreye H, Laccourreye O, Weinstein G, et al. Supracricoid laryngectomy with cricohyoidoepiglottopexy: a partial laryngeal procedure for glottic carcinoma. *Ann Otol Rhinol Laryngol.* 1990; 99(6 pt 1):421–426.

Laccourreye H, Laccourreye O, Weinstein G, et al. Supracricoid laryngectomy with cricohyoidopexy: a partial laryngeal procedure for selected supraglottic and transglottic carcinomas. *Laryngoscope.* 1990;100(7):735–741.

Machtay M, Rosenthal DI, Hershock D, et al. Organ preservation therapy using induction plus concurrent chemoradiation for advanced resectable oropharyngeal carcinoma: a University of Pennsylvania phase II trial. *J Clin Oncol.* 2002;20(19):3964–3971.

Mendenhall WM, Parsons JT, Stringer SP, et al. Management of Tis, T1, and T2 squamous cell carcinoma of the glottic larynx. *Am J Otolaryngol.* 1994;15(4):250–257.

Myers EN, Alvi A. Management of carcinoma of the supraglottic larynx: evolution, current concepts and future trends. *Laryngoscope.* 1996;106:559–567.

Myers EN, Suen JC, eds. *Cancer of the Head and Neck.* Philadelphia, PA: WB Saunders; 1996.

Papadimitrakopoulou VA, Clayman GL, Shin DM, et al. Biochemoprevention for dysplastic lesions of the upper aerodigestive tract. *Arch Otolaryngol Head Neck Surg.* 1999;125:1083–1089.

Spiro RH. Salivary neoplasms: overview of a 35-year experience with 2807 patients. *Head Neck Surg.* 1986;8:177–184.

Spiro RH, DeRose G, Strong EW. Cervical node metastasis of occult origin. *Am J Surg.* 1983;146:441–446.

Spiro RH, Huvos AG, Wong GY, et al. Predictive value of tumor thickness in squamous carcinoma confined to the tongue and floor of the mouth. *Am J Surg.* 1986;152:345–350.

Steiner W. Results of curative laser microsurgery of laryngeal carcinomas. *Am J Otolaryngol.* 1993;14:116–121.

Stern SJ, Goepfert H, Clayman G, et al. Orbital preservation in maxillectomy. *Otolaryngol Head Neck Surg.* 1993;109:111–115.

Stern SJ, Goepfert H, Clayman G, et al. Squamous cell carcinoma of the maxillary sinus. *Arch Otolaryngol Head Neck Surg.* 1993;119(9):964–969.

Sturgis EM, Potter BO. Sarcomas of the head and neck region. *Curr Opin Oncol.* 2003;15(3):239–252.

Urken ML, Weinberg H, Buchbinder D, et al. Microvascular free flaps in head and neck reconstruction. *Arch Otolaryngol Head Neck Surg.* 1994;120:633–640.

Wanebo HJ, Koness RJ, MacFarlane JK, et al. Head and neck sarcoma: report of the Head and Neck Sarcoma Registry. Society of Head and Neck Surgeons Committee on Research. *Head Neck.* 1992;14:1–7.

Weber RS, Benjamin RS, Peters LJ, et al. Soft tissue sarcomas of the head and neck in adolescents and adults. *Am J Surg.* 1986;152(4):386–392.

Weber RS, Berkey BA, Forastiere A, et al. Outcome of salvage total laryngectomy following organ preservation therapy: the Radiation Therapy Oncology Group trial 91–11. *Arch Otolaryngol Head Neck Surg.* 2003;129(1):44–49.

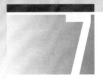

Thoracic Malignancies

Shanda H. Blackmon and Ara A. Vaporciyan

PRIMARY NEOPLASMS OF THE LUNG

In 2009, lung cancer accounted for an estimated 159,390 deaths and 219,440 new cases of cancer in the United States. With approximately 30% of all cancer deaths attributable to lung cancer, it is the most common cause of cancer-related death in both men and women, killing more people than breast, prostate, and colon cancer combined. However, as seen in Figure 7.1, the overall age-adjusted death rates for lung cancer have begun to level off. This leveling off is attributable to an overall decrease in the number of males who smoke and no further increase in the number of women who smoke. Unfortunately, this good news is countered by a disturbing increase in smoking among certain minority and adolescent age groups. The overall 5-year survival rate for lung cancer is only 15%, primarily because the disease is usually advanced at presentation; but if the disease is diagnosed and treated at an early stage, the 5-year survival rate approaches 60% to 70%.

Epidemiology

Smoking is the primary etiology in more than 80% of lung cancers, and secondhand smoke increases the risk of lung cancer by 30%. Despite the strong association of lung cancer with smoking, such cancers develop in only 15% of heavy smokers. Giant bullous emphysema and airway obstructive disease can act synergistically with smoking to induce lung cancer, perhaps because of poor clearance and trapping of carcinogens. Industrial and environmental carcinogens have been implicated, including residential radon gas, asbestos, uranium, cadmium, arsenic, and terpenes.

Pathology

Lung cancer can be broadly separated into two groups: non–small-cell lung cancers (NSCLCs) and small-cell lung cancers (SCLCs). This is a popular division because, for the most part, NSCLC is often managed with surgery when the tumor is localized, whereas SCLC is almost always managed nonsurgically with chemotherapy and radiation therapy. The three major types of NSCLC are adenocarcinoma, squamous cell carcinoma, and large-cell carcinoma (Table 7.1).

Non–small-cell Lung Carcinoma

Adenocarcinoma is the most common type of NSCLC and accounts for more than 40% of cases. It is the most common lung cancer found in nonsmokers and women. The lesions tend to be located in the periphery of the lung and are more likely to develop systemic metastases, even in the face of small primary tumors.

Bronchoalveolar cell carcinoma is a subset of adenocarcinoma, whose incidence appears to be increasing. This tumor is more frequent in women and nonsmokers, and can present as a single mass, multiple nodules, or an infiltrate. The clinical course can vary from indolent progression to rapid diffuse dissemination.

Squamous cell carcinoma accounts for approximately 25% of all lung cancers. Most (66%) present as central lesions. Cavitation is found in 7% to 10% of cases. Unlike adenocarcinoma, the tumor often remains localized, tending to spread initially to regional lymph nodes rather than systemically.

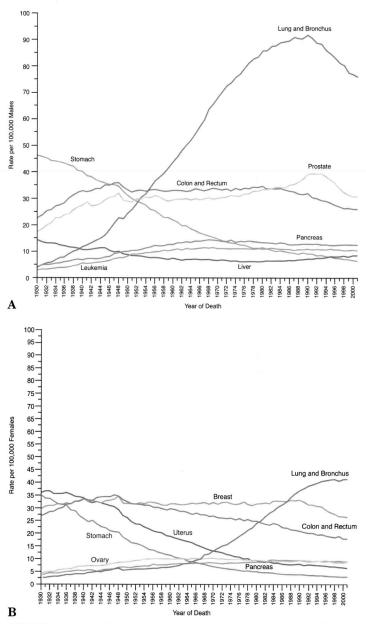

FIGURE 7.1 Annual age-adjusted cancer death rates for selected cancer types in males (**A**) and females (**B**), United States, 1930 to 2001.

TABLE 7.1   Frequency of Histologic Subtypes of Primary Lung Cancer

Cell Type	Estimated Frequency (%)
Non–small-cell Lung Cancer	
Adenocarcinoma	40
Bronchoalveolar	2
Squamous cell carcinoma	25
Large-cell carcinoma	7
Small-cell Lung Cancer	
Small-cell carcinoma	20
Neuroendocrine, well differentiated	1
Carcinoids	5

Large-cell carcinoma accounts for approximately 7% to 10% of all lung cancers. Clinically, large-cell carcinomas behave aggressively, with early metastases to the regional nodes in the mediastinum and distant sites such as the brain.

Small-cell Lung Carcinoma

Small-cell carcinoma is associated with neuroendocrine carcinoma because of ultrastructural and immunohistochemical similarities. Some pathologists think small-cell carcinomas represent a spectrum of disease beginning with the well-differentiated, benign carcinoid tumor (Kulchitsky I), including the less differentiated atypical carcinoids (Kulchitsky II) or neuroendocrine carcinomas, and ending with the undifferentiated small-cell carcinomas (Kulchitsky III). Small-cell carcinomas tend to present with metastatic and regional spread, and are usually treated with chemotherapy with or without radiation therapy. Surgery is only used to remove the occasional localized peripheral nodule.

Carcinoids tend to arise from major bronchi and as such are frequently central tumors that often present with hemoptysis. Metastases are rare and surgery is frequently curative. Immunohistochemically, carcinoids express neuron-specific enolase, chromogranin, and synaptophysin virtually without exception.

Neuroendocrine carcinomas or *atypical carcinoids* occur more peripherally than carcinoids and have a more aggressive course, although surgery should still be considered according to clinical stage. Without appropriate immunostaining, they may inadvertently be classified as large-cell carcinomas.

Diagnosis

Signs and symptoms occur in 90% to 95% of patients at the time of diagnosis. Intraparenchymal tumors cause cough, hemoptysis, dyspnea, wheezing, and fever (often due to infection from proximal bronchial tumor obstruction). Regional spread of the tumor within the thorax can lead to pleural effusions or chest wall pain. Less common symptoms are superior vena cava syndrome, Pancoast syndrome (shoulder and arm pain, Horner syndrome, and weakness or atrophy of the hand muscles), and involvement of the recurrent laryngeal nerve, the phrenic nerve, the vagus nerve, or the esophagus. Paraneoplastic syndromes are found in 10% of patients with lung cancer, most commonly those with SCLC. These syndromes are numerous and can affect endocrine, neurologic, skeletal, hematologic, and cutaneous systems.

A standard chest radiograph (CXR) is the initial diagnostic study for the evaluation of suspected lung cancer, followed routinely by computed tomography (CT).

CT should include imaging of the liver and adrenal glands to rule out two common sites for intra-abdominal metastases. CT helps assess local extension to other thoracic structures and the presence of mediastinal adenopathy. At present, magnetic resonance imaging (MRI) adds little to the information gained by CT imaging. Positron emission tomography (PET), especially integrated PET–CT, has become a frequent method of distinguishing benign from malignant pulmonary nodules. Although the accuracy of PET scanning in evaluating a pulmonary nodule can exceed 90% in some studies, clinicians should be aware that false-negative PET scans occur in patients with neoplasms having low metabolic activity (carcinoid and bronchioalveolar neoplasms). Even with advances in imaging, histologic confirmation will frequently be required to distinguish benign from malignant disease and to determine the histologic type of cancer. For a solitary lesion with a high index of suspicion (using Fleischner criteria based on size, growth, and risk category of the patient), histologic confirmation can be obtained at the time of surgery (thoracotomy or video-assisted thoracic surgery [VATS]) using frozen sectioning of a wedge resection or a needle biopsy. If immediate surgery is not appropriate, then tissue can be obtained by sputum cytology, bronchoscopy, and biopsy (for central lesions), by electromagnetic bronchial navigation-guided biopsy or fine-needle aspiration (for more peripheral lesions), or by CT-guided core-needle biopsy or fine-needle aspiration. Patients with benign lesions should be followed for interval growth over a period of at least 2 years.

Staging

The primary goal of pretreatment staging is to determine the extent of disease so prognosis and treatment can be determined. In SCLC, most patients present with metastatic or advanced locoregional disease. A simple two-stage system classifies the SCLC as limited or extensive disease. Limited disease is confined to one hemithorax, ipsilateral or contralateral hilar or mediastinal nodes, and ipsilateral supraclavicular lymph nodes. Extensive disease has spread to the contralateral supraclavicular nodes or distant sites such as the contralateral lung, liver, brain, or bone marrow. Staging for SCLC requires a bone scan, bone marrow biopsy, and CT scans of the abdomen, brain, and chest.

The staging of NSCLC was initially proposed in 1985: the International Lung Cancer Staging System or International Staging System (ISS). This system is based on TNM (Tumor, Node, Metastasis) classifications as shown in Table 7.2. Survival rates for patients with NSCLC by stage of disease are shown in Figure 7.2. Because of heterogeneity within groups, further modifications to the ISS have been recently adopted. T1 tumors are now classified as T1a and T1b depending on size less than or equal to 2 cm (T1a) or greater than 2 cm but less than 3 cm (T1b). T2 tumors are now classified as T2a and T2b depending on size greater than 3 cm but less than or equal to 5 cm (T2a) and greater than 5 cm but less than or equal to 7 cm (T1b). Tumors greater than 7 cm (formally T2) are now classified as T3 as are tumors with additional nodules identified in the same lobe (formally T4). Tumors with additional nodules in a different lobe of the ipsilateral lung are now classified as T4 (formally M1). Finally, pleural dissemination is now classified as M1 (formally T4).

Staging of NSCLC involves a thorough history and physical examination, CXR, and CT scans of the chest and upper abdomen, with the adjunctive use of PET–CT scanning when available. Unfortunately, CT cannot definitively predict mediastinal nodal involvement because not all malignant lymph nodes are enlarged, and many enlarged nodes are simply larger because of proximal infection. Lymph nodes larger than 1 cm on short axis have a 30% chance of being benign, whereas lymph nodes smaller than 1 cm still have a 15% chance of containing tumor. PET–CT has a higher negative predictive value in the evaluation of mediastinal N2 disease (96%),

TABLE 7.2	TNM Descriptors and Staging for NSCLC

Primary Tumor (T)

Tx	Primary tumor cannot be assessed or tumor proven by the presence of malignant cells in sputum or bronchial washings but not visualized by imaging or bronchoscopy
T0	No evidence of primary tumor
Tis	Carcinoma in situ
T1	Tumor ≤3 cm in greatest dimension, surrounded by lung or visceral pleura, without bronchoscopic evidence of invasion more proximal than the lobar bronchus[a] (i.e., not in the main bronchus)
T1a	Tumor ≤2 cm in greatest dimension
T1b	Tumor >2 cm but ≤3 cm in greatest dimension
T2	Tumor >3 cm but ≤7 cm or tumor with any of the following features: T2 tumors with these features are classified as T2a if ≤5 cm Involves main bronchus, >2 cm distal to the carina Invades visceral pleura (PL1 or PL2) Associated with atelectasis or obstructive pneumonitis that extends to the hilar region but does not involve the entire lung
T2a	Tumor >3 cm but ≤5 cm in greatest dimension
T2b	Tumor >5 cm but ≤7 cm in greatest dimension
T3	Tumor >7 cm or one that directly invades any of the following: Parietal pleural (PL3) chest wall (including superior sulcus tumors), diaphragm, phrenic nerve, mediastinal pleura, parietal pericardium; or tumor in the main bronchus (<2 cm distal to the carina[b] but without involvement of the carina; or associated atelectasis or obstructive pneumonitis of the entire lung or separate tumor nodule(s) in the same lobe
T4	Tumor of any size that invades any of the following: Mediastinum, heart, great vessels, trachea, recurrent laryngeal nerve, esophagus, vertebral body, carina, separate tumor nodule(s) in a different ipsilateral lobe

Regional Lymph Nodes (N)

Nx	Regional lymph nodes cannot be assessed
N0	No regional lymph node metastasis
N1	Metastasis to ipsilateral peribronchial and/or ipsilateral hilar lymph nodes, and intrapulmonary nodes involved by direct extension of the primary tumor
N2	Metastasis to ipsilateral mediastinal and/or subcarinal lymph nodes(s)
N3	Metastasis to contralateral mediastinal, contralateral hilar, ipsilateral or contralateral scalene, or supraclavicular lymph node(s)

Distant Metastasis (M)

M0	No distant metastasis (no pathologic M0; use clinical M to complete stage group)
M1	Distant metastasis present
M1a	Separate tumor nodule(s) in a contralateral lobe; tumor with pleural nodules or malignant pleural (or pericardial) effusion
M1b	Distant metastasis

Stage Classification

CLINICAL is denoted with c, Pathologic is denoted with p, and y descriptor is used for patients after neoadjuvant therapy

(*continued*)

TABLE 7.2	TNM Descriptors and Staging for NSCLC (*continued*)		
Group	**T**	**N**	**M**
Occult	TX	N0	M0
0	Tis	N0	M0
IA	T1a	N0	M0
	T1b	N0	M0
IB	T2a	N0	M0
IIA	T2b	N0	M0
	T1a	N1	M0
	T1b	N1	M0
	T2a	N1	M0
IIB	T2b	N1	M0
	T3	N0	M0
IIIA	T1a	N2	M0
	T1b	N2	M0
	T2a	N2	M0
	T2b	N2	M0
	T3	N1	M0
	T3	N2	M0
	T4	N0	M0
	T4	N1	M0
IIIB	T1a	N3	M0
	T1b	N3	M0
	T2a	N3	M0
	T2b	N3	M0
	T3	N3	M0
	T4	N2	M0
	T4	N3	M0
IV	Any T	Any N	M1a
	Any T	Any N	M1b

Additional Descriptors:
Histologic grade (G)
(*AKA overall grade*)

Grading System	**Grade**
2 grade system	Grade I or 1
3 grade system	Grade II or 2
4 grade system	Grade III or 3
Not available	Grade IV or 4

Additional Descriptors:

Lymph-Vascular Invasion (LVI)
LVI (absent)/Not identified
LVI Present/Identified
Not applicable
Unknown/Indeterminate

(*continued*)

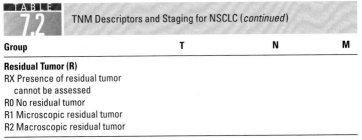

Group	T	N	M
Residual Tumor (R)			
RX Presence of residual tumor cannot be assessed			
R0 No residual tumor			
R1 Microscopic residual tumor			
R2 Macroscopic residual tumor			

[a]The uncommon superficial spreading tumor of any size with its invasive component limited to the bronchial wall, which may extend proximally to the main bronchus, is also classified as T1a.

[b]Most pleural (and pericardial) effusions with lung cancer are due to tumor. In a few patients, however, multiple cytopathologic examinations of pleural (pericardial) fluid are negative for tumor, and the fluid is nonbloody and is not an exudate. Where these elements and clinical judgment dictate that the effusion is not related to the tumor, the effusion should be excluded as a staging element and the patient should be classified as M0.

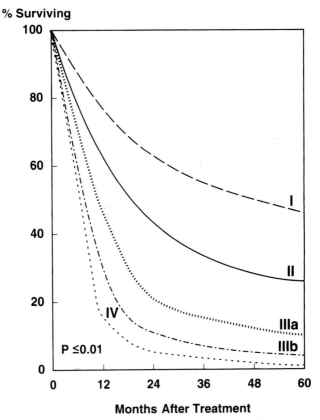

FIGURE 7.2 Cumulative survival according to clinical stage of non–small-cell lung cancer.

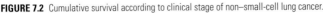

although false positives can occur in patients with granulomatous disease, inflammatory processes, and rheumatoid nodules. In patients with obvious metastatic disease, there is little role for PET imaging. Patients with subtle signs of possible distant metastases need to be investigated more carefully, and PET represents an ideal test in this situation. A solitary site of possible metastasis by PET requires a biopsy of the site in question. Patients with clinical stage III tumors by CT should undergo a PET. Patients with discrete nodal enlargement on CT should undergo tissue confirmation of these nodes regardless of the PET findings. Most investigators agree that a biopsy is required for confirmation of PET-positive mediastinal disease and/or suspected metastases. Conversely, most investigators also agree that patients with early-stage (T1N0) lung cancer who have a PET–CT negative mediastinum do not necessarily need a mediastinoscopy to prove the mediastinum is free of disease, as the addition of mediastinoscopy only achieves a 1.1% positive detection of N2 nodes in such a circumstance. If a PET or PET–CT is unavailable and the mediastinal lymph nodes are normal on CT (<1 cm), routine mediastinoscopy is recommended because it reduces N2 prevalence from 19% to 8%. Because of the low yield in asymptomatic early-stage patients (T1N0), a bone scan, or imaging of the brain should only be obtained when metastatic disease to these sites is suspected by history.

Treatment

Pretreatment Assessment

Once a patient has been staged clinically with noninvasive tests, a physiological assessment should be performed to determine the patient's ability to tolerate different therapeutic modalities. In addition to a general evaluation of the patient's overall medical status, specific attention should be paid to the cardiovascular and respiratory systems. Cardiovascular screening should include a history and physical examination, as well as a CXR and electrocardiography. Patients with signs and symptoms of significant cardiac disease should undergo further noninvasive testing, including either exercise testing, echocardiography, or nuclear perfusion scans. Significant reversible cardiac problems should be addressed before therapy (i.e., chemotherapy, radiation therapy, or surgery).

The pulmonary reserve of patients with lung cancer is commonly diminished as a result of tobacco abuse. Simple spirometry is an excellent initial screening test to quantify a patient's pulmonary reserve and ability to tolerate surgical resection. A predicted postoperative forced expiratory volume in 1 second (FEV_1) of less than 0.8 L or less than 35% of predicted postoperative FEV_1 is associated with an increased risk of perioperative complications, respiratory insufficiency, and death. The predicted postoperative FEV_1 is estimated by subtracting the contribution of the lung to be resected from the preoperative FEV_1. In certain instances, the lung to be resected does not contribute much to the preoperative FEV_1 because of tumor, atelectasis, or pneumonitis. Thus, more accurate determination of predicted postoperative FEV_1 can be obtained by performing a ventilation–perfusion scan and subtracting the exact contribution of the lung to be resected. In good performance patients with borderline spirometry criteria, oxygen consumption studies can be obtained that measure both respiratory and cardiac capacity. A maximum oxygen consumption (VO_2 max) of greater than 15 mL min^{-1} kg^{-1} indicates low risk, whereas a VO_2 max of less than 10 mL min^{-1} kg^{-1} is associated with high risk (a mortality rate of more than 30% in some series). Additional risk factors for lung resection include a predicted postoperative diffusing capacity (DLCO) or maximum ventilatory ventilation (MVV) of less than 40% and hypercarbia (>45 mm CO_2) or hypoxemia (<60 mm O_2) on preoperative arterial blood gases. For a summary of risk classification, refer to Table 7.3. In conjunction with clinical assessment (6-minute

TABLE 7.3 Pulmonary Assessment and Risk for Thoracic Resection

Average Risk	High Risk	Prohibitive Risk
ppoFEV1% > 40	ppoFEV1% 20–40	ppoFEV1% < 20
ppoDLCO% > 40	ppoDLCO% 20–40	ppoDLCO% < 20
$pO_2 > 60$	pO_2 45–60	$pO_2 < 45$
$pCO_2 < 45$	pCO_2 45–60	$pCO_2 > 60$
VO_2 max > 15	VO_2 max 10–15	VO_2 max < 10

walk and number of flights of stairs climbed), these tests can help identify those patients at high risk for complications during and after surgical resection.

Preoperative training with an incentive spirometer, initiation of bronchodilators, weight reduction, good nutrition, and cessation of smoking for at least 2 weeks before surgery can help minimize complications and improve performance on spirometry for patients with marginal pulmonary reserve.

Non–small-cell Lung Carcinoma

In early-stage NSCLC, surgery is a critical part of treatment. Unfortunately, more than 50% to 70% of NSCLC patients present with advanced disease for which surgery alone is not an option. An algorithm for treatment based on clinical stage is presented in Figure 7.3. Physiologically fit patients with early-stage lesions (stage I or II) are treated with surgery. Lesser resections like segmentectomy, wedge resection, or nonsurgical treatment (like stereotactic radiation therapy) is indicated if lobectomy cannot be tolerated. Five-year survival rates of 60% to 70% and 39% to 43% can be achieved for patients with stage I and II disease, respectively. Chest wall involvement without nodal spread (T3N0) was formally considered stage IIIa, but

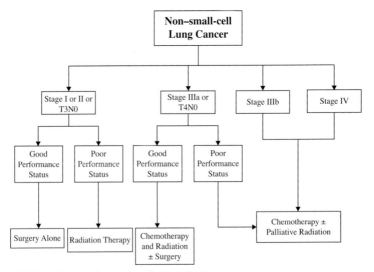

FIGURE 7.3 Algorithm for treatment of non–small-cell lung cancer.

because survival rates of 33% to 60% have been achieved with surgery, they are now considered as early-stage lesion (stage IIa). If these patients cannot tolerate surgery because of poor medical status, definitive radiation can result in survival rates of 15% to 35%.

The remainder of patients with stage IIIa disease (N2 disease or chest wall with nodal involvement) classically has a poor response to surgery, with 5-year survival rates of less than 15%. Induction therapy is favored over postoperative adjuvant therapy for NSCLC with N2 nodal involvement. When unsuspected N2 nodal disease is encountered during planned lung resection (outside of Level 5 and 6 nodes which have a better prognosis than traditional N2 nodes), the operation should be aborted to allow for neoadjuvant therapy. Induction therapy is recommended for all patients with clinical stage IIIa disease who are thought to be resection candidates. Patients who still require a pneumonectomy after induction therapy may be better served with definitive chemotherapy, although this practice varies in other countries. The standard treatment for those with stage IIIb or IV disease includes chemotherapy (platinum-based doublets) and definitive radiation therapy for local palliation. Improved survival is obtained when chemotherapy is combined with radiation therapy, although the complication rate is increased.

A small subset of stage IIIb tumors can be approached surgically. These tumors are considered stage IIIb because of local extension (T4N0) into adjacent structures rather than systemic spread (nodes, hematogenous metastases) and may benefit from aggressive surgical resection of the atrium, carina, or vertebrae. Survival rates of up to 30% have been reported. Metastatic disease is only treated surgically in the unusual circumstance of an isolated brain or adrenal metastasis with a node-negative lung primary. Several reports have documented better local control (in the brain and lung) with surgery and a subset of long-term survivors. The presence of mediastinal nodes, however, contraindicates surgical resection and mandates radiation therapy for the lung primary.

SURGERY

Pneumonectomy. The removal of the whole lung was previously the most commonly performed operation for NSCLC; it now accounts for less than 20% of all resections. Although a more complete resection is accomplished using pneumonectomy versus parenchyma-conserving techniques (lobectomy), it comes at the cost of higher mortality (4% to 10%) and morbidity without clear survival benefits.

Lobectomy. The similar survival of patients treated by lobectomy versus pneumonectomy, along with the lower morbidity and mortality (1% to 3%) associated with lobectomy, make lobectomy the preferred method of resection. Sleeve lobectomies and bronchoplasty procedures in which portions of the main bronchus are removed without loss of the distal lung have further decreased the need for pneumonectomies.

Lesser Resections. Segmentectomies and nonanatomical wedge resections are associated with increased local recurrence when compared with lobectomy. The general consensus remains that these procedures should be performed only in high-risk patients with minimal pulmonary reserve who cannot tolerate a lobectomy. The advent of CT screening for lung cancer has identified more subcentimeter cancers. The use of lesser resections is currently being reassessed for these types of cancers.

Video-assisted Thoracoscopic Surgery. During VATS lobectomy, the lung, nodes, vessels, and bronchi are not directly visualized with the naked eye but are visualized solely with a thoracoscope. VATS lobectomies are typically performed on patients with clinical stage I lung cancer, and can be performed safely with equivalent morbidity and complication rates to open lobectomy. This procedure is typically associated with less pain and equivalent survival when compared to open lobectomy. The procedure is usually reserved for tumors less than 5 to 6 cm in maximum diameter. Current relative contraindications to performing this procedure include chest wall involvement, central tumors, significant hilar adenopathy, or the presence of calcified hilar lymph nodes. Prior thoracotomy is not an absolute contraindication since the degree of adhesions and the ability to mobilize the lung adequately will vary among patients. The degree of emphysema, comorbidities, and age are not contraindications, and patients so affected are not managed differently than patients undergoing standard thoracotomy.

Extended Operations. Recent improvements in surgery and critical care have allowed certain tumors, previously considered unresectable, to be removed with acceptable morbidity and mortality. Carinal resections, sleeve resections, and extended resections for superior sulcus tumors with hemivertebrectomy and instrumentation of the spine can now be performed in a small subset of patients whose tumors were previously considered surgically unresectable. These procedures should only be performed in patients without mediastinal nodal involvement because 5-year survival rates are less than 5% for patients with extended resections in the presence of nodal involvement. Experienced multidisciplinary care is critical when addressing such advanced disease.

Mediastinal Lymph Node Dissection. Complete mediastinal lymph node dissection improves the accuracy of lung cancer staging, improves indications for subsequent adjuvant therapy, may decrease locoregional recurrence, but has not been shown to improve survival. There is no increase in morbidity associated with the addition of a complete nodal dissection compared to nodal sampling (removal of 1 or 2 nodes only from each accessible nodal station) in experienced hands.

Radiofrequency Ablation and Targeted Radiation Therapy. According to the RAPTURE study, percutaneous radiofrequency ablation yielded high proportions of sustained complete responses in carefully selected patients with pulmonary malignancies with acceptable morbidity. However, randomized trials with long-term survival data are not yet available for any of these newer techniques.

CHEMOTHERAPY

Almost 50% of patients present with extrathoracic spread, and an additional 15% are unresectable because of locally advanced tumor or inadequate pulmonary reserve. In addition, the long-term survival for completely resected stage II and IIIa tumors remains below 50% and 30%, respectively. Therefore, the use of adjuvant chemotherapy to treat patients with unresectable tumors and improve the results of resectable tumors is an area of intense investigation. A meta-analysis of these studies demonstrated a survival advantage using platinum-based therapy, although this did not reach statistical significance. These data spawned numerous large adjuvant trials in Europe and America. The first positive study to be reported was the International Adjuvant Lung Cancer Trial which enrolled nearly 1,900 completely resected stage I, II, and IIIA patients. The group that received cisplatinum-based doublet therapy had a 4.1% improvement in overall survival ($P < 0.03$), but a later analysis (7.5 years later) of the same population showed only a small but statistically insignificant improvement in overall survival. Since this initial publication, two additional positive trials (NCIC BR10 and CALGB 9633) have been presented, and with a median of 9.3-year follow-up have improvement in overall survival of 11% compared with observation. The survival benefit was strongest in patients with stage II NSCLC. These studies have required a significant shift in the postoperative management of completely resected early-stage lung cancers. Although the risk associated with adjuvant chemotherapy is small, it must be considered before initiating therapy. Therefore, we now have all patients with completely resected IB (tumor larger than 4 cm) or higher stage cancers evaluated by an oncologist for possible adjuvant chemotherapy with potential molecular staging and correlation with in vitro drug-resistance testing.

Molecular and pharmacogenetic profiles of individual tumors as well as evaluation of proteins in the serum of patients have thus far shown promising results. For example, the IALT Bio study has assisted in the selection of chemotherapeutic agents for patients with NSCLC by identifying the lack of expression of the DNA repair protein ERCC-1 as a possible predictor of increased survival after cisplatin-based chemotherapy. Tumors lacking ERCC-1 expression had a significant survival benefit from adjuvant cisplatin-based therapy whereas ERCC-1-positive tumor patients did not. Furthermore, patients who progress after standard chemotherapy are typically offered a drug that targets epidermal growth factor receptor (erlotinib) to prolong their survival. Patients with the EML4-ALK inversion mutation (who are also less likely to test positive for EGFR mutation) may also benefit from ALK-inhibitor-based therapy. Lung cancer vaccines are now also under investigation to determine if patients with poor prognostic markers (e.g., MAGE-A3) have less recurrence after treatment with a targeted vaccine. A lung metagene model also successfully predicted which patients are at a higher risk for recurrence and may aid in the selection of patients who benefit from adjuvant treatment. For a more complete list of biological or genetic markers and their prognostic value, refer to Table 7.4.

Studies examining the role of neoadjuvant chemotherapy, common in the late 1990s, have been difficult to complete due to the data regarding adjuvant treatment. Although multimodality therapy has achieved a strong foothold, the optimum timing of chemotherapy, adjuvant versus neoadjuvant, remains to be determined.

TABLE 7.4 Biological or Genetic Markers and Their Prognostic Value

Biological Variable	Prognostic Factor	Reference
bcl-2	Favorable	Martin et al., 2003
TTF1	Adverse	Berghmans et al., 2006
Cox2	Adverse	Mascaux et al., 2006
EGFR overexpression	Adverse	Nakamura et al., 2006
		Meert et al., 2002
Ras	Adverse	Mascaux et al., 2006
		Hunckarek et al., 1999
Ki67	Adverse	Martin et al., 2004
HER2	Adverse	Meert et al., 2004
		Nakamura et al., 2005
VEGF	Adverse	Delmotte et al., 2002
Microvascular density	Adverse	Meert et al., 2002
p53	Adverse	Steels et al., 2001
		Mitsudomi et al., 2000
		Huncharek et al., 2000
Aneuploidy	Adverse	Choma et al., 2001

Surveillance

The few treatment options for tumor recurrence in NSCLC have limited the cost-effectiveness of aggressive radiologic surveillance following surgical resection. Nevertheless, there is an increased incidence of second primary lung cancers (2% per year), and annual or semiannual CXR may help detect these lesions. Any patient who experiences symptoms in the interim should also be evaluated aggressively for recurrence or a new primary. The advent of low-dose helical CT scanning may change this standard, and its role in the surveillance of resected lung cancer patients is currently being evaluated. The lung, brain, bone, adrenals, and liver are the most common sites of metastases. Patients with isolated lung metastases can achieve survival rates of 25% to 40% if complete surgical resection is obtained. Because metastases can recur, resection involves limited resections (wedge or segmentectomy) to preserve lung parenchyma.

Small-cell Lung Carcinoma

Unlike NSCLC, SCLC tends to be disseminated at presentation and is therefore not amenable to cure with surgery or thoracic radiation therapy alone. Without treatment, the disease is rapidly fatal, with few patients surviving more than 6 months. Fortunately, SCLC is very sensitive to chemotherapy, and more than two-thirds of patients achieve a partial response after systemic therapy with multidrug regimens. Treatment of SCLC therefore revolves around systemic chemotherapy. An algorithm based on the extent of disease is presented in Figure 7.4. Complete response is seen in as many as 20% to 50% of patients with limited disease, but these responses are not durable, and the 5-year survival rate is still less than 10%.

Chemotherapeutic regimens for SCLC most commonly include combinations of cyclophosphamide, cisplatin, etoposide, doxorubicin, and vincristine. Thoracic radiation therapy has been shown to improve local control of the primary tumor and is often included as part of the treatment for limited SCLC. In addition, because brain metastases are noted in 80% of patients with SCLC during the course of their disease,

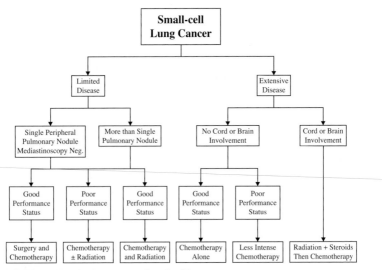

FIGURE 7.4 Algorithm for treatment of small-cell lung cancer.

patients who show no evidence of brain metastases on CT scans and who achieve a good response from therapy should be treated with prophylactic cranial irradiation to minimize the chances of developing this morbid site of treatment failure.

An infrequent but beneficial role for surgical resection of SCLC does exist. Solitary peripheral pulmonary nodules with no evidence of metastatic disease after evaluation with CT of the abdomen and chest, MRI of the brain, PET–CT, and mediastinoscopy can be treated with lobectomy and postoperative chemotherapy. In these selected patients, a 5-year survival rate of 50% has been achieved for peripheral T1N0 and T2N0. Surgery for more central lesions, however, has not been demonstrated to improve survival over that achieved with chemotherapy and radiation therapy alone.

METASTATIC NEOPLASMS TO THE LUNG

Pathology
The biology of the underlying primary malignancy determines the behavior of its metastases. Metastases may occur via hematogenous, lymphatic, direct, or aerogenous routes.

Diagnosis
Because of their predominantly peripheral localization, most pulmonary metastases remain asymptomatic, with fewer than 5% showing symptoms at presentation. Diagnosis is commonly made during radiographic follow-up after treatment of the primary malignancy.

Routine CXR during surveillance after cancer treatment is an effective means of screening patients for pulmonary metastases. Indeed, several studies have demonstrated the increased sensitivity of CT over standard CXR. However, the cost-effectiveness of CT for screening remains low, and no data as yet suggest that early detection with CT leads to improved survival. Planning of surgical interventions, however, should be based on CT findings, even though CT scanning still misses approximately 30% to 50% of the nodules found at surgery.

When multiple new pulmonary nodules are present in patients with a known previous malignancy, the likelihood of metastatic disease approaches 100%. New solitary lesions, however, can represent new primary lung cancers because many of the risk factors are similar.

Staging
No valid staging system exists for pulmonary metastases. The International Registry of Lung Metastases has identified three parameters of prognostic significance: resectability, disease-free interval, and number of metastases. The present criteria for resectability include technically resectable pulmonary nodules, control of the primary tumor, adequate predicted postoperative pulmonary reserve, and no extrathoracic metastases. This final criterion has been recently challenged as selected patients with resectable extrathoracic disease (e.g., liver and lung metastases from colon cancer) have achieved durable results with combined resections. Patients who meet these criteria should be offered metastasectomy. Favorable histologies for long-term survival following resection include sarcoma, breast, colon, and genitourinary metastases. Unfavorable histologies include melanomas, esophageal, pancreatic, and gastric cancers.

Treatment

Surgery
Preoperative evaluation for resection of pulmonary metastases is similar to that of any other pulmonary resection. Because of the increased risk of recurrent metastases and need for future thoracotomies, parenchyma-conserving procedures are

performed whenever possible (wedge resection, laser, or cautery excision). A variety of surgical approaches can be used.

Median sternotomy allows bilateral exploration with one incision. Lesions located near the posterior hilum can be difficult to reach, and exposure of the left lower lobe—especially in patients with obesity, cardiomegaly, or an elevated left hemidiaphragm—is poor.

Bilateral anterothoracosternotomy (clamshell procedure) allows excellent exposure of both hemithoraces, including the left lower lobe, although some surgeons think the incision increases postoperative pain.

Posterolateral thoracotomy allows excellent visualization of one hemithorax. However, this approach necessitates a second-stage operation when treating bilateral metastases, usually performed about 2 to 4 weeks following the first surgery.

VATS resection allows visualization of both hemithoraces during the same anesthetic. Pleural-based lesions are therefore easily visualized and excised. Unfortunately, the ability to carefully evaluate the parenchyma for deeper or smaller nonvisualized lesions is poor, and some reports suggest an increased risk of local recurrence with thoracoscopy.

At surgery, wedge resections with a 1-cm margin are preferred. Using staplers that allow the specimen side to be staple-free enhances the pathologist's ability to adequately examine the true parenchymal margin. If multiple nodules reside within one segment, lobe, or lung preclude resection with multiple wedges, then laser or cautery resections ("lumpectomy") can be performed. Anatomical resection can be used when central lesions are resected but should be applied carefully since the likelihood of recurrence is high; every effort should be made to preserve lung parenchyma.

Adjuvant Therapy

The role of radiation therapy in the treatment of pulmonary metastases is limited to the palliation of symptoms of advanced lesions with extensive pleural, bony, or neural involvement. The value of chemotherapy preoperatively or postoperatively in these clinical situations remains controversial. There are many isolated reports of the benefit of chemotherapy, especially when the primary tumor is known to be chemo-sensitive (e.g., osteosarcoma, malignant teratoma, other germ cell tumors). However, improvements in survival are more difficult to achieve with other chemo-resistant primary tumors.

Surveillance

The frequency and intensity of follow-up after resection are determined by the primary tumor but usually involve CT scans.

NEOPLASMS OF THE MEDIASTINUM

The mediastinal compartment can harbor numerous lesions of congenital, infectious, developmental, traumatic, or neoplastic origin. Earlier recommendations advocated a direct surgical approach to all mediastinal tumors, with biopsy or debulking of unresectable lesions. However, recent advances in imaging and noninvasive diagnostic techniques, as well as improvements in chemotherapy and radiation therapy, have led to a more thoughtful, multidisciplinary approach, with management decisions based on thorough preoperative evaluation.

Pathology

A study combining nine previous series was performed to better approximate the true incidence of mediastinal lesions (Table 7.5). In adults, neurogenic and thymic tumors contribute 23% and 19%, respectively, to the overall incidence, whereas in

TABLE 7.5	Overall Incidence of Mediastinal Tumors
Thymic	19 (3)[a]
Neurogenic	23 (39)[a]
Lymphoma	12
Germ cell	12
Cysts	18
Mesenchymal	8
Miscellaneous	8

[a]Numbers in parentheses represent incidence in children.

children they contribute 39% and 3%, respectively. This section does not attempt to describe the myriad cystic and other rare miscellaneous lesions but instead concentrates on the more common diagnoses.

Neurogenic tumors include schwannoma, neurofibroma, ganglioneuroblastoma, neuroblastoma, pheochromocytoma, and paraganglioma. They are the most common tumors arising in the posterior compartment.

Thymoma arises from thymic epithelium, although its microscopic appearance is a mixture of lymphocytes and epithelial cells. Thymomas are classified as lymphocytic (30% of cases), epithelial (16%), mixed (30%), and spindle cell (24%). Histologic evidence of malignancy is difficult to obtain because benign and malignant lesions can have similar histologic and cytologic features. Surgical evidence of invasion at the time of resection is the most reliable method of differentiating between malignant and benign thymomas. Completeness of resection is the best predictor of survival, and when complete resection cannot be performed, adjuvant radiation therapy is used.

Lymphomas comprise approximately 50% of childhood and 20% of adult anterior mediastinal malignancies. They are treated nonsurgically but may require surgery to secure a diagnosis.

Germ cell tumors comprise teratomas, seminomas, and nonseminomatous germ cell tumors. Teratomas are the most common and are mostly benign. Malignant teratomas are very rare and often widely metastatic at the time of diagnosis. Seminomas progress in a locally aggressive fashion. Nonseminomatous malignant tumors include embryonal carcinoma and choriocarcinoma, both of which carry a poor prognosis, and the more favorable endodermal sinus tumor.

Miscellaneous cysts and mesenchymal tumors include thyroid goiters, thyroid malignancies, mediastinal parathyroid adenomas, bronchogenic cysts, pericardial cysts, duplications, diverticula, and aneurysms.

Diagnosis

Mediastinal lesions are most commonly asymptomatic. When symptoms do occur, they result from compression of adjacent structures or systemic endocrine or autoimmune effects of the tumors. Children, with their smaller chest cavities, tend to have symptoms at presentation (two-thirds of children vs. only one-third of adults) and more commonly have malignant lesions (greater than 50%). Symptoms can include cough, stridor, and dyspnea (more common in children), as well as symptoms of local invasion such as chest pain, pleural effusion, hoarseness, Horner syndrome, upper-extremity and back pain, paraplegia, and diaphragmatic paralysis. Most symptoms are nonspecific with regard to the tumor histology with the exception of myasthenia gravis, which is strongly suggestive of thymoma.

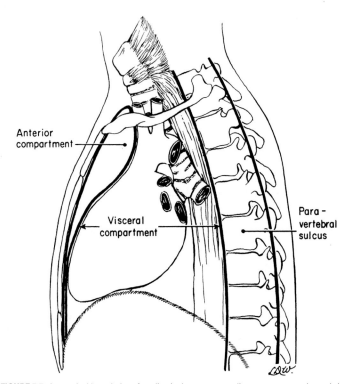

FIGURE 7.5 Anatomical boundaries of mediastinal masses according to one commonly used classification.

Fifty percent of lesions are diagnosed by CXR. The position of the tumor within the mediastinum on lateral projection can help tailor the differential diagnosis (Fig. 7.5, Table 7.6). The standard for further assessment of the lesion is CT, specifically with contrast enhancement. Certain tumors and benign conditions can be diagnosed or strongly suggested by their appearance on CT scans. Angiography or MRI may be required if a major resective procedure is planned and vascular involvement suspected. Nuclear imaging such as thyroid and parathyroid scanning, gallium scanning for lymphoma, and metaiodobenzylguanidine scanning for pheochromocytomas may also be indicated. The use of serum markers can be of some assistance in the diagnosis of some germ cell and neuroendocrine tumors.

Because many mediastinal tumors are treated without surgery, a determined effort should be made to achieve a tissue diagnosis noninvasively. Fine needle aspiration (FNA) and a transthoracic core biopsy are ideal for most tumors, although the diagnosis of lymphoma can be difficult via these methods because only a limited number of cells are retrieved. Bronchoscopy and esophagoscopy can also be useful if symptoms or imaging studies suggest tumor involvement.

If these procedures cannot achieve a diagnosis, then a mediastinoscopy to access paratracheal lesions can be performed. Although the risk of vascular or tracheobronchial injury is present, the incidence of complications is very low in experienced hands.

TABLE 7.6	Usual Location of Common Primary Tumors and Cysts of Mediastinum	
Anterior Compartment	**Visceral Compartment**	**Paravertebral Sulci**
Thymoma	Enterogenous cyst	Neurilemoma (schwannoma)
Germ cell tumors	Lymphoma	Neurofibroma
Lymphoma	Pleuropericardial cyst	Malignant schwannoma
Lymphangioma	Mediastinal granuloma	Ganglioneuroma
Hemangioma	Lymphoid hamartoma	Ganglioneuroblastoma
Lipoma	Mesothelial cyst	Neuroblastoma
Fibroma	Neuroenteric cyst	Paraganglioma
Fibrosarcoma	Paraganglioma	Pheochromocytoma
Thymic cyst	Pheochromocytoma	Fibrosarcoma
Parathyroid adenoma	Thoracic duct cyst	Lymphoma
Aberrant thyroid		

If more invasive procedures are required to make the diagnosis, an anterior or parasternal mediastinotomy (Chamberlain procedure) or thoracoscopy can be performed. Rarely, a sternotomy or thoracotomy will be required to obtain a tissue diagnosis. If the lesion is small and strongly suggestive of a thymoma on imaging then resection can be performed as the initial procedure rather than performing these more invasive biopsies and risking spillage of the tumor into the pleural cavity.

Staging
Staging is determined by the specific histologic characteristics and its extent at the time of diagnosis.

Treatment
Therapy, like staging, is determined by the type of tumor and its histologic characteristics (Table 7.7). The primary determination to be made is whether the lesion will require resection as part of its treatment or whether chemotherapy or radiation therapy is sufficient. Thymomas should all be resected, with the possibility of postoperative radiation therapy. Benign neurogenic tumors are sometimes observed in older debilitated patients; however, if the patient is healthy or if malignant potential is suspected, then resection should be pursued. Germ cell tumors should be treated on the basis of their histologic characteristics. In particular, benign teratomas should be resected, seminomas should be treated with radiation therapy, and nonseminomatous tumors should be treated initially with chemotherapy. In the subset of nonseminomatous tumors that have a residual mass but negative markers

TABLE 7.7	Frequency and Treatment of Malignant Chest Wall Tumors	
Cell Type	**Estimated Frequency (%)**	**Standard Therapy**
Chondrosarcoma	35	Surgical resection
Plasmacytoma	25	Radiation + chemotherapy
Ewing sarcoma	15	Surgery + chemotherapy
Osteosarcoma	15	Surgery + chemotherapy
Lymphoma	10	Chemotherapy ± radiation

after chemotherapy, surgical resection should be performed to rule out residual tumor. Lymphomas should not be resected and should be treated with radiation therapy or chemotherapy on the basis of their stage and histologic appearance (i.e., Hodgkin's vs. non-Hodgkin's).

Surveillance
The frequency and intensity of follow-up after resection are determined by the primary tumor. CXR remains the mainstay of surveillance, with CT scanning reserved for evaluation subsequent to abnormal CXR findings.

NEOPLASMS OF THE CHEST WALL

Primary chest wall malignancies account for less than 1% of all tumors, and include a wide variety of bone and soft-tissue lesions. The absence of large series makes the prospective evaluation of treatment options difficult. As more patients with these tumors are treated at large referral institutions, the initiation of multi-institutional trials will help settle some of the more controversial aspects of therapy.

Pathology
Primary chest wall tumors include chondrosarcoma (20%), Ewing sarcoma (8% to 22%), osteosarcoma (10%), plasmacytoma (10% to 30%), and, infrequently, soft-tissue sarcoma. Chondrosarcomas arise from the ribs in 80% of cases and from the sternum in the remaining 20%. They are related to prior chest wall trauma in 12.5% of cases and are very resistant to radiation and chemotherapeutic agents. Ewing sarcoma is part of a spectrum of disease having primitive neuroectodermal tumors at one end and Ewing sarcoma at the other. Multimodality therapy, including both radiation therapy and chemotherapy, has been shown to be beneficial for this tumor. Osteosarcomas are best treated with neoadjuvant therapy, with prognosis being predicted by the tumor's response to chemotherapy. Plasmacytoma confined to the chest must be confirmed by evaluating the remaining skeletal system. Surgery can then be used to confirm the diagnosis. If radiation therapy is unable to achieve local control, then resection may be indicated. Soft-tissue sarcomas are rare and are primarily resected. Adjuvant therapy is based on specific histologic findings.

Diagnosis
Chest wall tumors are asymptomatic in 20% of patients, whereas the remaining 80% present with an enlarging mass. A total of 50% to 60% of these patients will have associated pain. Radiographic assessment usually includes CXR and CT; however, MRI is being used instead of CT with increasing frequency because of its ability to image in multiple planes with superior anatomical distinction. Pathological diagnosis is made by FNA (64% accuracy) or core biopsy (96% accuracy). Incisional biopsies should be avoided if possible because they may interfere with subsequent surgical treatment and reconstruction.

Staging
Chest wall lesions are staged according to the primary tumor identified. Most progress to pulmonary or hepatic metastases without lymphatic involvement.

Treatment
As outlined previously, the treatment of chest wall lesions is determined by the diagnosis. Most, with few exceptions, require resection as part of the treatment. Posterior lesions reaching deep to the scapula or that require resection of less than two ribs do not require reconstruction of the chest wall. However, all other lesions require some form of stable reconstructive technique. A simple mesh closure using

Marlex or Prolene mesh is acceptable as long as the material is secured in position under tension. Some surgeons believe there is a loss of tensile strength over time. A more rigid prosthesis is methyl methacrylate sandwiched between two layers of Marlex mesh. Sternal and rib plating systems exist to enhance stabilization of a rigid repair. Long-term seroma formation or infection plague all types of repair.

If the chest wall lesion involves the overlying muscle or the skin, a large defect may be present after resection. This may require a muscle flap for final reconstruction, especially if postoperative radiation therapy is considered. Although a detailed description of the techniques available for this clinical situation is beyond the scope of this manual, a combination of muscle flap with primary skin closure, muscle flap with skin grafting, or myocutaneous flap coverage can be used.

Surveillance
Once treated and in remission, chest wall tumors tend to recur either locally, or with pulmonary or hepatic metastases. Regular follow-up with careful examination and CT scanning should suffice to detect all significant sites of recurrence.

NEOPLASMS OF THE PLEURA

There are two main types of pleural neoplasms. The first, malignant pleural mesothelioma, remains an uncommon and highly lethal tumor with no adequate method of treatment. It behaves primarily as a locally aggressive tumor with locally invasive failure after therapy and only metastasizes late in its course. Its relationship with asbestos exposure was suggested in the 1940s and 1950s, and clearly established in 1960. The second, a more localized pleural tumor known as localized fibrous tumor of the pleura, can also occur; when malignant, it is frequently classified as a localized mesothelioma.

Pathology
Localized mesotheliomas and malignant localized fibrous tumors of the pleura are very rare. There is some controversy as to whether these lesions are even mesothelial at all because no epithelial component may be identifiable. More commonly, a benign localized fibrous tumor of the pleura is found. However, diffuse pleural mesothelioma is always a malignant process. There is a 20-year latency for development of this disease after exposure to asbestos. A recent surge in the incidence of this disease reflects the widespread use of asbestos in the 1940s and 1950s, and this surge should continue because mechanisms for limiting occupational asbestos exposure were not instituted until the 1970s. Mesothelioma commonly presents as an epithelial histology and less commonly as a sarcomatoid or mixed histology. It can be hard to differentiate this lesion from metastatic adenocarcinoma. Immunohistochemistry and electron microscopy, however, have aided in establishing the diagnosis.

Diagnosis
The presentation of mesothelioma is often vague and nonspecific, with dyspnea and pain common in 90% of patients. Radiographic diagnosis in the early stage is often difficult, with the findings limited to a pleural effusion in many cases. Even CT may fail to identify any other abnormalities at this stage. The classic finding of a thick, restrictive pleural rind is a late finding. Thoracentesis is diagnostic in 50% of patients, and pleural biopsy is positive in 33%. If the diagnosis remains elusive, thoracoscopy is diagnostic in 80% of patients.

Staging
A staging system for mesothelioma has been proposed by Rusch and the International Mesothelioma Interest Group (IMIG) and is shown in Table 7.8.

TABLE 7.8	Staging of Mesothelioma

T

Tx	Primary t
T0	No evidence of primary tumor can be assessed
T1	Tumor limited to the ipsilateral parietal pleura with or without mediastinal pleura and with or without diaphragmatic plural involvement
T1a	No involvement of the visceral pleura
T1b	Tumor also involving the visceral pleura
T2	Tumor involving each of the ipsilateral pleural surfaces (parietal, mediastinal, diaphragmatic, and visceral pleura) with at least one of the following features: • Involvement of diaphragmatic muscle • Confluent visceral pleural tumor (including the fissures), or extension of tumor from visceral pleura into the underlying pulmonary parenchyma
T3	Describes locally advanced but potentially resectable tumor Tumor involving all ipsilateral pleural surfaces (parietal, mediastinal, diaphragmatic, and visceral pleura) with at least one of the following features: • Involvement of the endothoracic fascia • Extension into the mediastinal fat • Solitary, completely resectable focus of tumor extending into the soft tissues of the chest wall • Nontransmural involvement of the pericardium
T4	Describes locally advanced technically unresectable tumor Tumor involving all ipsilateral pleural surfaces (parietal, mediastinal, diaphragmatic, and visceral) with at least one of the following features: • Diffuse extension or multifocal masses of tumor in the chest wall with or without associated rib destruction • Direct transdiaphragmatic extension of tumor to the peritoneum • Direct extension of tumor to the contralateral pleura • Direct extension of tumor to one or more mediastinal organs • Direct extension of tumor into the spine • Tumor extending through to the internal surface of the pericardium with or without a pericardial effusion, or tumor involving the myocardium

N | **Lymph Nodes**

NX	Regional lymph nodes cannot be assessed
N0	No regional lymph node metastases
N1	Metastases in the ipsilateral bronchopulmonary or hilar lymph nodes
N2	Metastases in the subcarinal or the ipsilateral mediastinal lymph nodes, including the ipsilateral internal mammary and peridiaphragmatic nodes
N3	Metastases in the contralateral mediastinal, contralateral internal mammary, ipsilateral, or contralateral supraclavicular lymph nodes

M | **Metastases**

M0	No distant metastasis
M1	Distant metastasis present

(*continued*)

TABLE 7.8	Staging of Mesothelioma (*continued*)

Stage	
Stage I	T1N0M0
	I_a T_{Ia} N_0 M_0
	I_b T_{Ib} N_0 M_0
Stage II	T_2 N_0 M_0
Stage III	T1, T2 N1M0
	T1, T2 N2 M0
	Any T_3 M_0
	Any N_1 M_0
	Any N_2 M_0
Stage IV	Any T_4
	Any N_3
	Any M_1

Treatment

The treatment of mesothelioma is still evolving. Attempts at radical resections, such as extrapleural pneumonectomy, have led to some improvements in local control, but only limited impact on survival at the cost of a significantly increased operative risk. The addition of adjuvant radiotherapy can increase local control and the removal of the entire lung can facilitate its delivery. Unfortunately, better local control has led to an increase in the number of patients who succumb to systemic disease. The effectiveness of chemotherapy is limited, although new agents may be on the horizon (i.e., Pemextred). By themselves, chemotherapy and radiation therapy have had only limited benefit, with even less impact on palliation.

An alternative to aggressive resection is the role of pleurectomy which can achieve similar survival when compared with the more aggressive extrapleural pneumonectomy despite the known residual tumor left behind after pleurectomy. Many investigators have avoided an extrapleural pneumonectomy whenever patients have any evidence of advanced disease, such as nodal involvement.

Surveillance

Mesotheliomas tend to recur both locally and systemically. Local control has been significantly improved with extrapleural pneumonectomy combined with whole thorax radiation; however, systemic failure is still common. CT scans are required to detect recurrences or follow residual disease. Unfortunately, treatment options are limited, but they do include radiation therapy and chemotherapy.

Recommended Readings

PET Scanning

Detterbeck FC, Vansteenkiste JF, Morris DE, Dooms CA, Khandani AH, Socinski MA. Seeking a home for a PET, part 3: emerging applications of positron emission tomography imaging in the management of patients with lung cancer. *Chest.* 2004;126(5):1656–1666.

Erasmus JJ, Connolly JE, McAdams HP, Roggli VL. Solitary pulmonary nodules: part I. Morphologic evaluation for differentiation of benign and malignant lesions. *Radiographics.* 2000;20(1):43–58.

Erasmus JJ, McAdams HP, Connolly JE. Solitary pulmonary nodules: part II.

Evaluation of the indeterminate nodule. *Radiographics.* 2000;20(1):59–66.

Gonzalez-Stawinski GV, Lemaire A, Merchant F, et al. A comparative analysis of positron emission tomography and mediastinoscopy in staging non-small cell lung cancer. *J Thorac Cardiovasc Surg.* 2003;126(6):1900–1905.

Reed CE, Harpole DH, Posther KE, et al. American College of Surgeons Oncology Group Z0050 trial. Results of the American College of Surgeons Oncology Group Z0050 trial: the utility of positron emission tomography in staging potentially operable non-small cell lung cancer. *J Thorac Cardiovasc Surg.* 2003;126(6):1943–1951.

Adjuvant Chemotherapy for Early-stage Lung Cancer

Strauss GM, Herndon J, Maddaus MA, et al. Randomized clinical trial of adjuvant chemotherapy with paclitaxel and carboplatin following resection in stage IB non-small cell lung cancer (NSCLC): report of Cancer and Leukemia Group B (CALGB) Protocol 9633 [abstract 7019]. *Proc Am Clin Oncol.* 2004;23:17b.

The International Adjuvant Lung Cancer Trial Collaborative Group. Cisplatin-based adjuvant chemotherapy in patients with completely resected NSCLC. *N Engl J Med.* 2004;350:351–360.

Alam N, Shepherd FA, Winton T, et al. Compliance with post-operative adjuvant chemotherapy in non-small cell lung cancer. An analysis of National Cancer Institute of Canada and intergroup trial JBR. 10 and a review of the literature. *Lung Cancer.* 2005;47(3):385–394. Review. Erratum in: *Lung Cancer.* 2005;50(2):283–284.

Additional References

AJCC Cancer Staging Manual. 7th ed. Springer; 2010.

Anderson BO, Burt ME. Chest wall neoplasms and their management. *Ann Thorac Surg.* 1994;58(6):1774–1781.

Dartevelle PG. Extended operations for the treatment of lung cancer. *Ann Thorac Surg.* 1997;63:12.

Ferguson MK, ed. *Difficult Decisions in Thoracic Surgery: An Evidenced-Based Approach.* Springer; 2007.

Ginsberg RJ, Rubinstein L. The comparison of limited resection to lobectomy for T1N0 non-small cell lung cancer. LCSG 821. *Chest.* 1994;106(Suppl 6):318S–319S.

Jemal A, Siegel R, Ward E, Hao Y, Xu J, Thun MJ. Cancer statistics, 2009. *CA Cancer J Clin.* 2009;59:225–249.

MacMahon H, Austin JH, Gamsu G, et al. Guidelines for the management of small pulmonary nodules detected on CT scans: a statement from the Fleischner Society. *Radiology.* 2005;237:395–400.

Mountain CF. Revisions in the international system for staging lung cancer. *Chest.* 1997;111:1710.

Nesbitt JC, Putnam JB, Walsh GL, et al. Survival in early-stage non-small cell lung cancer. *Ann Thorac Surg.* 1995;60:466.

Pastorino U, Buyse M, Friedel G, et al. Long-term results of lung metastasectomy: prognostic analyses based on 5206 cases. *J Thorac Cardiovasc Surg.* 1997;113:37.

Roth JA, Fossella F, Komaki R, et al. A randomized trial comparing perioperative chemotherapy and surgery with surgery alone in resectable stage III non-small cell lung cancer. *J Natl Cancer Inst.* 1994;86:673.

Rusch VW. The international mesothelioma interest group: a proposed new international TNM staging system for malignant pleural mesothelioma. *Chest.* 1995;108:1122–1128.

Sculier JP, et al. The IASLC Lung Cancer Staging Project. *J Thor Oncol.* 2008;3(4):457–466.

Shields TW. Primary mediastinal tumors and cysts and their diagnostic investigation In: Shields TW, ed. *Mediastinal Surgery.* Philadelphia, PA: Lea & Febiger; 1991.

Sugarbaker DJ, Jaklitsch MT, Liptay MJ. Mesothelioma and radical multimodality therapy: who benefits? *Chest.* 1995;107:3455.

Walsh GL, Morice RC, Putnam JB, et al. Resection of lung cancer is justified in high-risk patients selected by exercise oxygen consumption. *Ann Thorac Surg.* 1994;58:704.

Walsh GL, O'Connor M, Willis KM, et al. Is follow-up of lung cancer patients after resection medically indicated and cost effective? *Ann Thorac Surg.* 1995;60:1563.

8 Esophageal Carcinoma

Wayne L. Hofstetter

In the United States and other western societies, cancer of the esophagus is relatively uncommon, representing only a small percentage of newly diagnosed invasive malignancies. However, it is the eighth most common malignancy worldwide comprising approximately 4% of the newly diagnosed tumors per year. It is highly virulent and similar to other malignancies such as lung or pancreas. The yearly incidence of esophageal cancer is comparable to its yearly total of cancer-related deaths. Treatment paradigms are individualized and are primarily related to clinical stage at presentation. Although surgical resection has traditionally been the mainstay of therapy, most newly diagnosed cancers present at a late stage and are therefore precluded from curative resection. Those patients who have been fortunate to have their disease discovered at a very early stage may be candidates for esophageal sparing mucosal resections or esophagectomy. Patients with locally advanced tumors will typically undergo multimodality approaches that combine concurrent chemoradiation followed by re-evaluation for surgery. These approaches have resulted in 5-year survival rates of 40% to 75% in the subset of patients who have a complete or near complete pathologic response after preoperative therapy. Finally, patients that present with advanced disease are treated with palliative measures which include chemotherapy, radiation, mechanical devices such as stents and/or feeding tubes, and supportive care.

EPIDEMIOLOGY

According to the National Cancer Institute database for 2010, there will be an estimated 16,640 new cases of esophageal cancer diagnosed in the United States, and 14,500 will die of the disease. In the past, squamous cell carcinomas (SCC) accounted for more than 95% of cases, but in recent years, adenocarcinoma arising in the background of Barrett esophagus has become increasingly common, and it now accounts for more than 75% of the esophageal cancers at most major American centers. Esophageal carcinoma, particularly SCC, has substantial geographic variation, from 1.5 to 7 cases per 100,000 people in most parts of the world, including the United States, to 100 to 500 per 100,000 people in its endemic areas such as northern China, South Africa, Iran, Russia, and India. Males have a two to three-fold higher overall risk than females, and a seven to ten-fold higher risk for the development of adenocarcinoma. Furthermore, in the United States, SCC is approximately five times more common among African Americans than it is among whites, whereas adenocarcinoma occurs approximately three to four times more often in whites, particularly in men. The typical patient with esophageal adenocarcinoma is a middle class, overweight male in his sixties or seventies. Both major histologic types are rare in patients younger than 40 years, but the incidence increases thereafter.

ETIOLOGY AND RISK FACTORS

Several different environmental and genetic risk factors have been identified as potential causes of esophageal cancers, particularly SCC. In geographic areas where esophageal cancer is endemic, such as in China, a single causative factor for the epidemic is unknown. However, studies are ongoing that implicate strains of human papillomavirus either as a causative agent or a carcinogenic catalyst. Other risk factors may include diets that are deficient in vitamins A, C, riboflavin, and protein, and have excessive nitrates and nitrosamines. Fungal contamination of foodstuffs with the associated aflatoxin production may be another important risk factor.

A well-established risk is the combination of smoking and alcohol consumption which has a synergistic effect on the development of esophageal SCC, increasing the risk by as much as 44 times. Other risk factors or associations for esophageal SCC include SCC of the head and neck (presumably because of the risk associated with alcohol and smoking), achalasia (as high as 30 times increased risk), strictures resulting from ingestion of caustic agents such as lye, Zenker diverticulae, esophageal webs in Plummer–Vinson syndrome, prior radiation, and familial connective tissue disorders such as tylosis (50% have cancer by 45 years). For adenocarcinoma, the primary etiologic factor is obesity and Barrett esophagus, with an estimated annual incidence of malignant transformation of 0.5% to 1%, representing 125 times greater risk than that in the general population. This risk seems to be mediated through reflux disease, and similar to colon cancers, esophageal adenocarcinomas are known to progress through a metaplasia–dysplasia–cancer sequence. Gastroesophageal reflux disease results in the overexposure of the esophageal mucosa to acid and bile. Specifically, the conjugated bile salts (secondary bile acids) are believed to synergistically damage the mucosa, leading to increased DNA methylation and variations in ploidy (as well as other genetic and molecular changes) and the formation of intestinal metaplasia (Barrett mucosa) or cardiac metaplasia. Both are recognized as precursor lesions to esophageal/gastroesophageal junction cancers. Tobacco use and the eradication of *Helicobacter pylori* are also linked to the increased incidence of esophageal adenocarcinoma in the United States.

PATHOLOGY

Esophageal cancer is seen in two main histologic types: SCC and adenocarcinoma. In the United States, approximately 20% of cases of SCC involve the upper third of the esophagus, 50% involve the middle third, and the remaining 30% extend from the distal part of the esophagus to the gastroesophageal junction. SCC rarely invades the stomach, and there is usually a discrete segment of normal mucosa between the cancer and the gastric cardia. In contrast, nearly 97% of adenocarcinomas develop in the middle and distal esophagus, and many extend into the stomach if they are centered near the gastroesophageal junction. Cancers arising in Barrett esophagus are believed to comprise upward of 50% to 70% of all adenocarcinomas involving the distal esophagus and gastroesophageal junction. They can vary in length and range in contour from flat, infiltrative lesions to fungating polypoid masses. Ulceration is often present and may even be deep enough to cause perforation. Because symptoms appear late in the progress of the disease, the typical esophageal carcinoma is a circumferential, exophytic, fungating mass that is nearly or completely transmural. Access to the submucosal lymphatics allows tumors to spread freely along a submucosal plane and present with very long tumors or multiple mucosal lesions. Similarly, early metastases to lymph nodes or distant sites are common. Microscopically, adenocarcinomas can resemble cells in the gastric cardia or colon, and most are well or moderately differentiated. Signet ring differentiation may signify a gastric cardia origin, but this is not an absolute rule.

Other less common primary malignant neoplasms of the esophagus include neuroendocrine tumors, gastrointestinal stromal tumors, variants of SCC or adenocarcinomas (e.g., adenosquamous), melanomas, sarcomas, and lymphomas.

CLINICAL FEATURES

Clinical presentation is generally insidious, and typical symptoms occur late in the course of the disease, usually precluding early intervention. Most patients experience symptoms for 2 to 6 months before they seek medical attention. The most common symptom is progressive dysphagia, which occurs in as many as 80% to 90% of patients. This is usually a late sign because the esophageal lumen must be reduced to 50% to 75% of its original size before patients experience this symptom. Typically, malignant dysphagia will begin when the esophageal functional diameter approaches 12 to 13 mm, about the size of a normal adult endoscope. Weight loss is also common, with an estimated mean weight loss of 10 kg from the onset of symptom. This sign is also an independent predictor of poor outcome, as is presentation with advanced stage. Other symptoms include varying degrees of odynophagia (in approximately 50%), as well as emesis, cough, regurgitation, anemia, hematemesis, and aspiration pneumonia. Hoarseness can be due to invasion of the recurrent laryngeal nerve, and Horner syndrome indicates invasion of the sympathetic trunk. Hematemesis and melena usually indicate friability of the tumor or its invasion into major vessels. Bleeding from the tumor mass occurs in 4% to 7% of patients and may cause considerable difficulty with treatment.

DIAGNOSTIC EVALUATION

Results of the physical examination may depend in large part on the degree of weight loss and cachexia. At times difficult to detect, enlarged cervical or supraclavicular lymph nodes can be biopsied with fine-needle aspiration (FNA) and are indicative of advanced disease. In the past, there was significance placed on plain CXR, barium swallow studies, and bone scans. However, these have been all but replaced by modern imaging. Computed tomography (CT) scans of the chest and abdomen should be obtained to assess the degree of any local invasion of mediastinal structures, adenopathy, or for evidence of dissemination/distant metastasis.

In addition to a high-resolution CT scan, integrated positron emission tomography (PET) is being used with increasing frequency in the diagnostic staging algorithm and is considered standard of care at major medical centers. It has been shown to alter the treatment course in approximately 15% of patients with locally advanced tumors, which in itself has rendered it cost-efficient. This modality is helpful in determining the significance of regional adenopathy or distant lesions and may carry prognostic information in terms of the level of initial nucleotide uptake and midterm response to preoperative treatment. It is also very efficient at detecting bone-related metastases and has primarily replaced the use of bone scans. As PET–CT is not sensitive for brain evaluation, any neurologic signs or complaints (e.g., headaches, visual disturbances, and new onset weakness) should be assessed with magnetic resonance imaging (preferred) or CT scan of the brain.

Upper endoscopy is currently the most widely used technique for the diagnosis and staging of esophageal cancer. Flexible endoscopy allows magnified visual observation and histologic sampling of the esophagus, as well as visualization of the stomach; description of tumor location within the esophagus and stomach is critical to surgical and radiation treatment planning. Biopsy and brush cytology can produce diagnostic accuracy of nearly 100% with adequate sampling, and gentle endoscopic dilation of tight strictures can be performed by experienced endoscopist to allow passage of the endoscope beyond the tumor. The addition of endoscopic ultrasound (EUS) should be used to assess the T and N descriptors of the TNM stage of the lesion. EUS is most accurate in predicting the depth of invasion of the primary lesion, and this can lead to very good insight into the potential of surrounding organ or lymph node involvement. Mediastinal, paraesophageal, para-gastric, porta-hepatis, and celiac lymph nodes are routinely identified and can be biopsied via aspiration (FNA) for diagnosis. Tumors that involve the upper or middle third of the esophagus should be evaluated by flexible and/or rigid bronchoscopy to rule out tracheobronchial involvement.

STAGING

The staging system of the American Joint Committee on Cancer (AJCC) uses the TNM classification and is the most commonly used system in the United States (Table 8.1). Although CT scanning is probably the most widely used noninvasive staging modality, its accuracy is quite limited. Overall accuracy in determining resectability and T stage have been estimated at 60% to 70%, whereas accuracy in determining N stage is generally less than 60%. Accuracy in the detection of metastatic disease is somewhat better, estimated at 70% to 90% for lesions larger than 1 cm. The use of combined imaging with PET–CT has improved the accuracy of both tests. The ability to combine anatomical irregularity to areas of abnormal Flouro–Deoxy glucose uptake on a superimposed image increases the predictive value of PET alone or CT alone. Recent studies with this technique have reported overall accuracy levels of nearly 60% and 90% in the ability to detect both locoregional nodal metastases and distant disease, respectively.

EUS is probably the most accurate means currently available for T and N staging. Reported overall accuracy for T staging is 76% to 90%; overall accuracy in predicting resectability is approximately 90% to 100% for adenocarcinoma, but decreases to 75% to 80% for SCC. Studies comparing EUS and CT scanning generally agree that EUS is superior in overall T staging and assessment of regional lymph nodes (70% to 86% accuracy). The precise differentiation between benign and malignant nodes occasionally remains problematic, however, due to micrometastases that are undetectable by EUS and enlarged inflammatory lymph nodes that are incorrectly classified as metastatic. FNA can be helpful in making this diagnosis. Minimally invasive techniques such as thoracoscopy and laparoscopy may also be utilized in the staging of esophageal cancer. Thoracoscopy allows visualization of the entire thoracic esophagus and the periesophageal nodes, when performed through the right hemithorax, or the aortopulmonary and periesophageal nodes and the lower esophagus, when performed through the left chest. Lymph nodes can be sampled for histologic evaluation, the pleura can be examined, and adjacent organ invasion (T4) can be confirmed. The overall accuracy for detecting lymph node involvement has been reported to be as high as 81% to 95%. Laparoscopy and laparoscopic ultrasonography are useful in evaluating the peritoneum, liver, gastrohepatic ligament, gastric wall, diaphragm, and the perigastric and celiac lymph nodes. Biopsies and peritoneal washings can be performed to confirm nodal or metastatic disease. These modalities are especially useful in patients with gastroesophageal junction or proximal gastric tumors. In addition, a feeding jejunostomy can be placed for nutritional support before treatment begins. Studies have suggested that the overall accuracy of laparoscopy in staging and determination of resectability in esophageal cancer is as high as 90% to 100% and that invasive staging procedures may prevent unnecessary surgical resection in as many as 20% of patients. Prospective comparisons with CT and EUS have suggested that laparoscopy and laparoscopic ultrasonography have superior overall accuracy in staging, particularly for lymph nodes and metastatic disease. Mediastinoscopy can also prove helpful in assessing regional lymph nodes at the right and left paratracheal lymph node stations, along the mainstem bronchi, in the aortopulmonary window, or in the subcarinal area.

T A B L E
8.1

TNM Staging for Esophageal Cancer

Primary Tumor (T)

Tx	Primary tumor cannot be assessed
T0	No evidence of primary tumor
Tis	High-grade dysplasia
T1	Tumor invades lamina propria, muscularis mucosae, or submucosa
T1a	Tumor invades lamina propria, muscularis mucosae
T1b	Tumor invades submucosa
T2	Tumor invades muscularis propria
T3	Tumor invades adventitia
T4a	Resectable tumor invading pleura, pericardium, or diaphragm
T4b	Unresectable tumor invading other adjacent structures, such as aorta, vertebral body, and trachea

Regional Lymph Nodes (N)

Nx	Regional nodes cannot be assessed
N0	No regional node metastasis
N1	Metastasis in 1–2 regional lymph nodes
N2	Metastasis in 3–6 regional lymph nodes
N3	Metastasis in seven or more regional lymph nodes

Distant Metastasis (M)

Mx	Presence of distant metastasis cannot be assessed
M0	No distant metastases
M1	Distant metastasis

Anatomic Stage/Prognostic Groups

Stage	T	N	M	Grade	Tumor Location[a]
Squamous Cell Carcinoma					
0	Tis (HGD)	N0	M0	1, X	Any
IA	T1	N0	M0	1, X	Any
IB	T1	N0	M0	2–3	Any
	T2–3	N0	M0	1, X	Lower, X
IIA	T2–3	N0	M0	1, X	Upper, middle
	T2–3	N0	M0	2–3	Lower, X
IIB	T2–3	N0	M0	2–3	Upper, middle
	T1–2	N1	M0	Any	Any
IIIA	T1–2	N2	M0	Any	Any
	T3	N1	M0	Any	Any
	T4a	N0	M0	Any	Any

(*continued*)

TABLE 8.1	TNM Staging for Esophageal Cancer (*continued*)				
Stage	**T**	**N**	**M**	**Grade**	**Tumor Location**[a]
IIIB	T3	N2	M0	Any	Any
IIIC	T4a	N1–2	M0	Any	Any
	T4b	Any	M0	Any	Any
	Any	N3	M0	Any	Any
Adenocarcinoma					
0	Tis (HGD)	N0	M0	1, X	
IA	T1	N0	M0	1–2, X	
IB	T1	N0	M0	3	
	T2	N0	M0	1–2, X	
IIA	T2	N0	M0	3	
IIB	T3	N0	M0	Any	
	T1–2	N1	M0	Any	
IIIA	T1–2	N2	M0	Any	
	T3	N1	M0	Any	
	T4a	N0	M0	Any	
IIIB	T3	N2	M0	Any	
IIIC	T4a	N1–2	M0	Any	
	T4b	Any	M0	Any	
	Any	N3	M0	Any	
IV	Any	Any	M1	Any	

[a]Location of the primary cancer site is defined by the position of the upper (proximal) edge of the tumor in the esophagus.
Adapted from American Joint Committee on Cancer, 7th edition.

TREATMENT

Treatment options vary according to presenting stage, patient performance status, and local expertise.

Stage 0–I

Patients with in situ carcinoma (high-grade dysplasia, HGD) or tumors that are limited to the mucosa (Stage 0 and I) may be candidates for esophageal-preserving techniques of endoscopic resection and ablation. This modality is typically limited to patients with smaller lesions (~2 cm) located within the mucosa generally penetrating no more deeply than the muscularis mucosa. Favorable factors include ability to completely resect, well-moderate differentiation, and no evidence of lymphovascular invasion. Patients with disease beyond the very superficial submucosa, or those with endoscopically unresectable lesions, or with evidence of poor differentiation and LVI should be considered for resection if medically fit. Because accurate clinical staging of early stage disease is difficult, patients in whom there is a question of depth of mucosal invasion should be considered for a diagnostic endoscopic mucosal resection (EMR) at a center of expertise with high volume. Confirmation of very early stage may result in a therapeutic organ-preserving resection. Tumors found to be more deeply invasive (Stage I, T1b) are not amenable to EMR but may also have a lower risk of metastatic lymphadenopathy and should be considered for curative resection.

Stage II–III

Tumors that invade more deeply harbor a higher probability of regional lymph node involvement. In fact, there is a direct correlation of depth of invasion to lymph node involvement, where deep submucosal lesions have approximately a 30% risk of regional lymphadenopathy and transmural tumors carry risk of 80% to 100%. Because results with surgery alone in patients with regional lymph node metastasis are relatively poor, clinical studies began to focus on including multimodality treatment in conjunction with surgery. Recent randomized trials with locally advanced disease have shown a survival advantage in groups treated with neoadjuvant chemoradiation followed by surgery compared to those treated with surgery alone. However, debate continues regarding the most appropriate treatment of a clinically staged T2N0 patient. Many argue for surgery followed by chemoradiation based on both retrospective and some prospective data. However, an equally compelling argument stands with the same level of evidence that preoperative staging is inaccurate in many patients, resulting in upstaging approximately 40% of operated patients from N0 to N+ status. These groups advocate for neoadjuvant treatment at centers of excellence, where therapy including surgery can be given with very low (2% to 3%) 30-day mortality and good overall survival.

There is little debate that locally advanced adenocarcinoma, stage IIb and III disease, should be treated with concurrent neoadjuvant chemoradiation followed by re-staging and consideration for surgical resection. Squamous cancers are increasingly being treated with definitive chemotherapy and radiation, especially those located in the cervical and very proximal esophagus. Treatment for tumors located in the mid-distal esophagus is individualized. Two European trials (Bedenne and Stahl, 2002) have shown statistical survival equipoise in groups treated with definitive chemoradiation versus chemoradiation plus surgery if they responded to therapy. Therefore, in patients with SCCA of the esophagus who have had a clinical complete response to therapy there are advocates for observation rather than surgical resection; a decision our group bases on individual cases. Nonresponding patients should be considered for resection.

Stage IV

Patients who present with nonregional lymph node involvement or other distant metastatic disease are candidates for palliative chemotherapy. On occasion, patients with stage IV disease whose tumor burden is systemically controlled become candidates for consolidative local regional therapy (chemoradiation). As there is a significant morbidity and mortality incidence associated with palliative surgical resections, this procedure is generally not recommended unless a patient has uncontrolled bleeding or perforation and would otherwise be expected to have a significant life span despite metastatic or advanced esophageal cancer. Given this, there are also nonoperative methods of controlling these complications such as mechanical stents for perforation or trachea-esophageal fistula and radiation for local control of bleeding.

Operative Approaches

There are many available techniques for performing esophageal resection, and most often this choice is based on surgeon preferences or tumor location. Esophageal tumors located distally or at the gastroesophageal junction can be managed by subtotal esophagectomy, esophagogastrectomy, or segmental esophagectomy with bowel interposition. The extent of gastric and esophageal involvement, as well as the stage of the primary tumor, should guide the surgeon to an appropriate approach. A subtotal esophagectomy through a right thoracotomy and laparotomy (Ivor Lewis or Tanner–Lewis esophagectomy) allows for generous resection of the stomach because the esophageal reconstruction takes place in the chest at or above the level of the azygous vein. Locally advanced tumors with involvement of the distal esophagus and proximal stomach lend themselves to this approach because a lymphadenectomy is easily performed in two fields and negative margins can be obtained in the stomach with less worry of gastric necrosis. However, tumors with extensive involvement of the stomach and esophagus may require an esophagogastrectomy, with interposition of small or large bowel for reconstruction. Early distal tumors or short segment Barrett esophagus with HGD can be treated with segmental esophagectomy and small bowel interposition (Merendino procedure) or vagal-sparing esophagectomy with gastric or bowel interposition.

Proximally located (e.g., upper and midesophageal) tumors often require a total esophagectomy because it is difficult to achieve negative margins with segmental or subtotal resections (e.g., Ivor Lewis esophagectomy). Given the propensity for esophageal cancers to spread in the submucosal lymphatic system, it is recommended that a minimum of a 5-cm margin, and preferably a 10-cm margin, should be taken on the esophagus. This is a critical decision-making factor when formulating a treatment algorithm for an individual patient. The two most popular methods to achieve a total or near-total esophagectomy differ according to whether thoracotomy is used for esophageal mobilization. The esophagus can be mobilized using a right thoracotomy with the conduit brought either through the posterior mediastinum (preferred) or substernally to the neck for anastomosis (McKeown or three-field approach). Alternatively, a transhiatal esophagectomy can be performed with mobilization of the intrathoracic esophagus from the esophageal hiatus to the thoracic inlet without the need for thoracotomy. The advantage of the transhiatal technique is that it avoids thoracotomy while achieving a complete removal of the esophagus. The potential disadvantages of this technique include a limited periesophageal and mediastinal lymphadenectomy, the risk of causing tracheobronchial or vascular injury during blunt dissection of the esophagus, and higher locoregional recurrence rates. In addition, the use of a cervical anastomosis is associated with a higher rate of anastomotic leakage than an intrathoracic anastomosis (12% vs. 5%, respectively) although the morbidity is much less with a cervical leak than it is with a thoracic leak. Other potential downsides to a cervical anastomosis include pharyngeal reflux, nocturnal aspiration, prolonged swallowing dysfunction after surgery, and an increased incidence of recurrent laryngeal nerve palsy. This last complication is underestimated in its importance; a patient with an intrathoracic stomach and limited ability to protect his/her airway is at great danger in the immediate postoperative period and is also in chronic danger of aspiration. On the other hand, intrathoracic anastomoses are hampered by a higher reoperation incidence when there is a postoperative anastomotic leak (about 4% to 10%) and a striking incidence of recurrent esophageal metaplasia, which has been reported in one series to occur in 80% of long-term survivors.

Patients that present with cervical esophageal carcinomas have several treatment options. Advances in chemoradiotherapy have relegated resection of most localized cervical lesions to salvage procedures. Patients that have persistent locoregional, limited disease after definitive medical therapy are candidates for segmental resections with immediate or delayed reconstruction. Small bowel, neck, or musculocutaneous free flaps are well suited to esophageal reconstructions in the cervical area, with or without pharyngolaryngectomy. An alternative option for patients with early-stage disease is immediate resection and reconstruction. At the other end of the spectrum, lengthy lesions with involvement into the thoracic esophagus may require a complete esophagectomy via a three-field approach.

Extent of Lymphadenectomy

Although it is generally agreed that surgical resection has a therapeutic role in the treatment of local and locoregional disease, great controversy remains over the extent of the resection necessary and over the value and extent of lymphadenectomy. There is one group of thought that lymph node metastases are markers for systemic disease and that removal of involved nodes in most cases offers no survival benefit. This is very likely to be true when more than six lymph nodes are involved with cancer on the surgical specimen. However, many well-respected and experienced surgeons believe that some patients with affected lymph nodes can be successfully cured with an aggressive surgical approach that focuses on wide peritumoral excision and extended lymphadenectomy using a transthoracic/thoracoabdominal and cervical approach (en bloc or radical esophagectomy). There is currently no definitive evidence to support either philosophy; however, many reports that have focused on specific subsets of patients in stages IIb to III have shown that patients who have undergone complete lymphadenectomy and have less than 10% of their resected nodes involved with metastatic disease can still look forward to prolonged survival and excellent locoregional control. Proponents of radical resection have reported increased survival rates with more extensive surgical procedures and excellent locoregional control, but most of these comparisons have been actually retrospective. Furthermore, it is unclear whether more extensive dissection actually leads to improved survival or whether these superior results are a function of more accurate staging (stage migration effect). Recent prospective randomized studies in the United States and Western Europe have failed to show any significant difference in morbidity, mortality, or recurrence rates, or in the overall survival rate when comparing transhiatal esophagectomy with transthoracic or total thoracic esophagectomy or when comparing the number of lymph nodes resected. However, there is a survival trend favoring more radical transthoracic resections over a transhiatal approach, and local regional recurrence is known to be substantially higher after a transhiatal resection. Because a statistical overall survival benefit has yet to be proven, either technique is acceptable, and it is unlikely that a prospective randomized trial will ever be performed that could conclusively prove an advantage in overall survival rate with a particular type of surgery. The choice among surgical resection techniques should be individualized to the particular characteristics of the patient. Subset analyses have shown that thoracic tumors and cancers with positive but limited lymph node involvement benefit from a complete (at least two fields, including a thoracic dissection) esophagectomy rather than a transhiatal resection (Omloo et al., 2007). The salient points that emerge from historical comparisons of these procedures is that a transhiatal resection has a tendency toward higher locoregional recurrence, but a lower incidence of ICU care, and does not require thoracotomy to complete. We personally reserve a transhiatal approach for extremes in age and stage, or for patients at high risk for thoracotomy.

Minimally invasive esophagectomy is offered in many centers around the world. Patients with appropriate lesions have the option of undergoing esophageal resection with combined thoracoscopic and laparoscopic resection followed by a small neck incision with an esophagogastric anastomosis performed in the neck, or a minimally invasive Ivor Lewis resection. Complete laparoscopic (transhiatal) resections can also be accomplished, but again, this approach makes extensive en bloc resection of mediastinal lymph nodes difficult. Early results on several hundred patients resected in this manner show no difference in survival, and a formal phase I/II trial is currently underway. Disadvantages of this modality include a fairly steep learning curve, especially for surgeons with limited laparoscopic esophageal experience and prolonged anesthetic times (although very experienced surgeons can effectively resect the esophagus in a similar amount of time as open procedures).

Reconstruction After Resection

The stomach, colon, and jejunum have all been successfully used as replacement conduits after esophagectomy. The stomach is used far more frequently because of the ease of mobilization, a hearty and redundant blood supply, limited perioperative morbidity, and the need to perform only one anastomosis.

The colon is a commonly used alternative replacement conduit. However, some surgeons prefer this conduit over the stomach in younger patients who are expected to have a prolonged survival because it provides a barrier between the stomach remnant and the residual esophagus, and this may prevent significant pharyngeal reflux and future esophageal metaplasia or dysplasia within the esophageal remnant. Either the right colon or the left colon can be used, but the segment of left and transverse colon that is supplied by the ascending branch of the left colic artery, arc of Riolan, and the marginal artery is generally a better size match to the esophagus and has more reliable arterial arcades. The colonic arterial anatomy should be evaluated preoperatively by arteriography in any patient who is expected to have extensive limiting atherosclerosis or is suspected to have had a previous bowel resection. Otherwise, in patients with a naïve abdomen, evaluation of the vasculature can take place in the operating theater. Another alternative is CT or MR angiography. Colonoscopy is necessary to rule out pathological conditions, such as telangiectasia, polyposis, synchronous neoplasm, or extensive diverticulosis, which would preclude the use of colon.

Jejunal reconstruction can be performed for lesions anywhere in the esophagus. Segmental jejunal-free flaps transferred to the neck have been used successfully after resection of hypopharyngeal or upper cervical esophageal tumors. In this case, the mesenteric vessels are usually anastomosed to the external carotid artery and the internal jugular vein. Pedicled grafts are being used when segmental distal esophageal resection is performed for benign lesions requiring resection or confirmed short segment Barrett esophagus with HGD that is recalcitrant to efforts at endoscopic ablation. Pedicled jejunal flaps with proximal microvascular augmentation will allow for total esophageal replacement with the small bowel.

Finally, musculocutaneous flaps are also frequently used for segmental cervical reconstruction and can be harvested from any of multiple areas with minimal physiological or aesthetic effect.

Few prospective studies have been performed to evaluate the use of different replacement conduits, but evidence from several nonrandomized and small randomized trials supports that overall survival is unchanged regardless of the technique used. A review performed by Urschel (2001) was unable to reach definitive results that would cause one technique to be favored over another. The basic principles are that the stomach has the most reliable blood supply, is a hearty conduit, and is associated with the lowest immediate postoperative morbidity. Cervical leaks from a colon interposition tend to be well tolerated and stricture rarely occurs. If strictures do occur, they are more easily dilated than those in esophagogastric anastomoses. Graft loss can occur with any conduit in any position. Pyloroplasty or pyloromyotomy may be required to avoid gastric stasis secondary to the division of the vagus nerves during esophagectomy; however this remains somewhat controversial and several centers are omitting this step without significant change in outcomes.

Results of Surgical Therapy

Mortality rates for transhiatal or transthoracic esophagectomies are now less than 5%, and realistic morbidity rates range from 35% to 65%. Overall survival rates after surgical resection correspond to the stage of the disease and vary drastically. The 5-year survival rates have been reported to be 60% to 95% for stage I, 30% to 60% for stage II, 5% to 30% for stage III, and 0% to 20% for stage IV (Fig. 8.1). Unfortunately, the vast majority (70%) of patients present with advanced stage III or IV disease at diagnosis.

When examining the pattern of failure after surgical resection, one finds that most patients experience either distant metastasis or both locoregional and distant

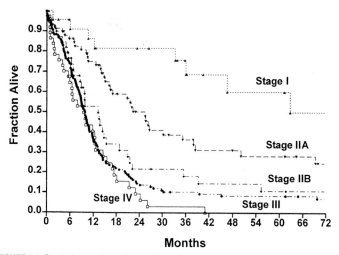

FIGURE 8.1 Survival curves for patients with esophageal cancer.

recurrence, and a small percentage experience solely a recurrence of localized disease. Novel treatment modalities focusing on the patterns of failure need to be explored to improve on the relatively poor prognosis afforded by surgery alone in most patients with esophageal carcinoma.

Adjuvant Therapy

Results of several randomized prospective trials on the use of adjuvant radiation therapy (45–56 Gy) after resection have been published. Traditionally clinicians would consider radiation therapy in patients with unexpected locally advanced disease, positive margins, or an R2 resection although there is no scientific proof of benefit. Treatment-related toxicity can be severe. Overall, although reductions in local recurrences have been noted and specific subsets may benefit, no significant survival advantage has been found using adjuvant radiotherapy for esophageal carcinoma.

According to the results of prospective randomized trials, postoperative combination chemotherapy with various agents, including 5-fluorouracil (5-FU), cisplatin, mitomycin C, vindesine, and paclitaxel, also has no proven role in the treatment of completely resected lesions. Furthermore, adjuvant chemotherapy is generally poorly tolerated, and many patients fail to complete their treatment regimen. This treatment modality, therefore, is not recommended outside clinical trial settings.

Adjuvant chemoradiotherapy may benefit patients with esophageal carcinoma. This modality has the advantage of better patient selection because the pathological stage will guide the decision to proceed to therapy. Patients with a high risk of recurrence (stage IIb and above) would be considered to selectively undergo treatment. In theory, chemoradiotherapy may increase survival by decreasing both distant and local disease. To date, there is some phase III evidence that has shown favorable results in a select group of patients with gastroesophageal junction adenocarcinomas treated with adjuvant chemoradiation, but compliance with treatment was not ideal. Patients with squamous cancers, on the other hand, have not been shown to benefit from adjuvant chemoradiation after complete resection.

Neoadjuvant Therapy

Largely because of the difficulty administering adjuvant therapy to postesophagec-tomy patients and the disappointing results of trials with adjuvant chemotherapy or radiation monotherapy, researchers have turned their attention toward the use of preoperative or neoadjuvant therapy. Preoperative radiation therapy has been investigated in several prospective randomized trials, and the results have been subjected to meta-analysis. Despite some initial response, the results of these trials have shown marginal overall benefit in terms of survival rate. Preoperative radia-tion therapy alone is therefore not generally recommended, even in the face of clinical trials.

Although results of phase II studies of induction chemotherapy had been promising, most of the subsequent prospective randomized trials using multiple different agents and combinations have failed to show any advantage in recurrence or survival. Evidence that neoadjuvant chemotherapy was capable of significant tumor response and even complete responses was reported by multiple authors. Complete responders were also found to have better survival rates than partial or nonresponders, and the R0 resection rate seemed to improve overall. However, the net gain in survival was not significantly different from controls (surgery alone). Conjecture on the reasons for this are that nonresponders frequently fare worse than controls; the overall resection rate was lower in patients undergoing neoadju-vant therapy, thereby abolishing any overall benefit; or there was a study design flaw, possibly representing a β-error. Unfortunately, the benefits seen in phase II trials were mainly believed to be secondary to selection bias. In contrast, the largest trial on induction chemotherapy involving more than 800 patients with esophageal carcinoma (squamous and adeno) performed in Europe (MRC Trial, 2002) did show a significant survival advantage over surgery alone. The fact that the largest U.S. intergroup trial, however, failed to find any advantage in survival rate with the same agents in more than 400 patients was disappointing. Furthermore, although the long-term follow-up of the MRC trial continued to show a survival advantage in the treatment arm, the advantage was very small. At this point, interest in chemo-therapy as a neoadjuvant monotherapy has been mostly diverted to combined chemoradiotherapy.

Neoadjuvant chemoradiation therapy for esophageal carcinoma has been shown to be feasible and effective. Radiation to 50.4 Gy is given concurrently with a doublet of chemotherapy (fluorouracil and a platinum combination is the most common at this time) which is well tolerated without significantly increasing peri-operative mortality (in experienced centers). Phase II trials reported excellent over-all response rates (complete responses in 25% to 35%) and relatively decent compliance with therapy. Survival and local control compare favorable to historical controls. However, despite that there have been many prospective randomized studies published, only the Walsh (University of Dublin) and the CALGB trials have shown a benefit to this therapy over surgery alone. The Walsh trial has been widely criticized, and the results have not been repeated in any other randomized trial. This trial, conducted at the University of Dublin with 113 patients with adenocar-cinoma, evaluated neoadjuvant cisplatin plus 5-FU and 40 Gy of radiation with surgery alone. The investigators reported a 25% complete pathological response, as well as a significant increase in median survival (16 vs. 11 months) and 3-year survival rate (32% vs. 6%) for the patients receiving the neoadjuvant treatment. Much of the debate over this study has focused on the poor survival in the surgery-only arm of 6% at 3 years, erratic preoperative clinical staging, and questions of miscalculations within the statistics. Two trials published thus far only in abstract form (CROSS and POET trials) are expected to confirm a survival advantage with preoperative chemoradiation therapy. Finally, three separate meta-analyses have been published comparing neoadjuvant therapy to a surgery-alone arm. All favored the treatment arm, although squamous cancers and the Walsh trial may be adding a significant amount of weight to the calculated hazard ratios.

Definitive Chemoradiation Therapy

Although surgical resection remains the preferred therapy for esophageal cancer, definitive radiation therapy and chemoradiation therapy have been used in patients who opt out of or who are not candidates for surgical resection. Local control rates ranged between 40% and 75%, and median and 2-year survival rates ranged from 9 to 24 months and from 18% to 38%, respectively. Several prospective randomized trials have shown that definitive chemoradiation therapy is superior to radiation therapy alone in the treatment of esophageal cancer. A trial published by Stahl et al. (2005) from Germany sought to evaluate the additional benefit of surgery in patients with SCCA after neoadjuvant chemoradiotherapy. The trial showed significantly improved locoregional control in the surgery arm compared with chemoradiotherapy alone and greater freedom from the use of palliative procedures after surgery. However, despite a local-regional recurrence rate approaching 60% in both the German and the French (FFCD, Bedenne et al., 2007) definitive chemoradiation trials, neither trial was able to demonstrate a statistically significant difference in overall survival after surgery, largely due to the fact that these multicenter trials had an initially poor survival after surgery, and both modalities failed to prevent death from distant disease.

Other Therapeutic Modalities

In certain parts of the world, particularly in areas where esophageal cancer is endemic, mass screening and advances in diagnostic techniques have led to the detection of increased numbers of superficial esophageal cancers. Studies from Japan and the United States have suggested that for lesions confined to the epithelium and lamina propria, lymphatic spread is rare. In some of these patients, EMR is a feasible option, although experience with this technique is still limited. Endoscopic ablative therapy using radio-frequency ablation, cryotherapy, and photodynamic therapy can be used for palliating large otherwise untreatable tumors, but in patients with superficial cancers and carcinoma in situ, these methods can also be curative. Although experience with these techniques is limited, investigators have reported tumor-free survival for several months after therapy, although recurrence rates after about 1 year can be significant. Similarly, photodynamic therapy has been used in nonsurgical candidates, and results of preliminary studies in patients with early-stage tumors have suggested that tumor-free survival can last several months and that complete remission is possible in some patients (at 2-year follow-up). However, long-term studies are still needed.

Palliation for Unresectable Tumors

Common indications for palliation in patients with advanced disease include dysphagia, presence of esophagorespiratory fistula, recurrent bleeding, and prolongation of survival. Tumor debulking surgery has been performed, and although survival duration seems somewhat improved relative to that in patients who did not undergo resection, few randomized trials have been performed, and morbidity can be significant. Other options for palliation include (a) dilation, which is a safe and effective method to relieve dysphagia, although it usually requires multiple procedures; (b) stents, both rigid and expandable, which have become very popular in recent years for relieving dysphagia and for treating fistulas and bleeding; (c) laser therapy, which has been effective in relieving dysphagia from shorter strictures and those with intraluminal rather than infiltrative growth; (d) photodynamic therapy, which results in fewer perforations than do dilations or laser therapy and is tolerated better but requires more frequent sessions; (e) bipolar electrocautery and coagulation with tumor probes that use heat to destroy tumor cells and cause circumferential injury; and (f) brachytherapy, which delivers radioactive seeds intraluminally.

All of these techniques have advantages and disadvantages, and short-term success rates of 80% to 100% have been reported. If these treatment options fail, an endoscopic prosthesis can often be placed with good results. These techniques are not without complications, however, and ulceration, obstruction, dislocation, and aspiration have all been reported. Recently, improvements in definitive radiation therapy and chemotherapy have also provided excellent means for short-term palliation. With nonoperative treatment, however, long-term local control is still poor (40% locoregional failure). Which method to use therefore depends on the experience of the physician and the particular needs and condition of the patient.

Surveillance

A barium swallow study should be obtained in the first postoperative month as a baseline study. Asymptomatic patients can be assessed with yearly physical examinations and chest radiography. Any symptoms (e.g., pain, dysphagia, and weight loss) should be evaluated aggressively with CT scanning, barium studies, or endoscopy. Benign strictures at the anastomosis should be treated with dilation. Unfortunately, treatment options are limited for locoregional or distant recurrences. If radiation therapy was not given preoperatively or postoperatively, it can be used along with the previously mentioned nonoperative methods of palliation (i.e., dilation, stenting, laser, photodynamic, or thermal resection).

Recommended Readings

Ajani JA. Current status of new drugs and multidisciplinary approaches in patients with carcinoma of the esophagus. *Chest.* 1998;113(suppl 1):112S.

Akiyama H, Tsurumaru M, Udagawa H, et al. Esophageal cancer. *Curr Probl Surg.* 1997; 34:767.

Bedenne L, Michel P, Bouche O, et al. Randomized phase III trial in locally advanced esophageal cancer: radiochemotherapy followed by surgery versus radiochemotherapy alone (FFCD 9102) [abstract 519]. *Proc Am Soc Clin Oncol.* 2002;21:130a.

Bedenne L, Michel P, Bouché O, et al. Chemoradiation followed by surgery compared with chemoradiation alone in squamous cancer of the esophagus: FFCD 9102. *J Clin Oncol.* 2007;25(10):1160–1168.

Bosset JF, Gignoux M, Triboulet JP, et al. Chemoradiotherapy followed by surgery compared with surgery alone in squamous-cell cancer of the esophagus. *N Engl J Med.* 1997;337:161.

Goldminc M, Maddern G, LePrise E, et al. Oesophagectomy by transhiatal approach or thoracotomy: a prospective randomized controlled trial. *Br J Surg.* 1993;80: 367.

Gore RM. Esophageal cancer: clinical and pathologic features. *Radiol Clin North Am.* 1997;35:243.

Herskovic A, Martz K, Al-Sarraf M, et al. Combined chemotherapy and radiotherapy compared with radiotherapy alone in patients with cancer of the esophagus. *N Engl J Med.* 1992;326:1593.

Kelsen DP, Ginsberg R, Pajak TF, et al. Chemotherapy followed by surgery compared with surgery alone for localized esophageal cancer. *N Engl J Med.* 1998; 339:1979.

Knyrim K, Wagner HJ, Bethge N, et al. A controlled trial of an expansile metal stent for palliation of esophageal obstruction due to inoperable cancer. *N Engl J Med.* 1993;329:1302.

Kolh P, Honore P, Degauque C, et al. Early stage results after oesophageal resection for malignancy-colon interposition versus gastric pull-up. *Eur J Cardiothorac Surg.* 2000;18:293–300.

Medical Research Council Oesophageal Cancer Working Party. Surgical resection with or without preoperative chemotherapy in oesophageal cancer: a randomised controlled trial. *Lancet.* 2002; 359:1727–1733.

Omloo JM, Lagarde SM, Hulscher JB, et al. Extended transthoracic resection compared with limited transhiatal resection for adenocarcinoma of the mid/distal esophagus: five-year survival of a randomized clinical trial. *Ann Surg.* 2007; 246(6):992–1000.

Orringer MB, Marshall B, Iannettoni MD. Transhiatal esophagectomy: clinical experience and refinements. *Ann Surg.* 1999;230:392.

Pech O, Behrens A, May A, et al. Long-term results and risk factor analysis for recurrence after curative endoscopic therapy in 349 patients with high-grade intraepithelial neoplasia and mucosal adenocarcinoma in Barrett's oesophagus. *Gut.* 2008;57(9):1200–1206.

Rizk NP, Ishwaran H, Rice TW, et al. Optimum lymphadenectomy for esophageal cancer. *Ann Surg.* 2010;251(1):46–50.

Roth JA, Pass HI, Flanagan MM, et al. Randomized clinical trial of preoperative and postoperative adjuvant chemotherapy with cisplatin, vindesine and bleomycin for carcinoma of the esophagus. *J Thorac Cardiovasc Surg.* 1988;96:242.

Stahl M, Stuschke M, Lehmann N, et al. Chemoradiation with and without surgery in patients with locally advanced squamous cell carcinoma of the esophagus. *J Clin Oncol.* 2005;23(10):2310–2317. Erratum in *J Clin Oncol.* 2006; 24(3):531.

Tepper J, Krasna MJ, Niedzwiecki D, et al. Phase III trial of trimodality therapy with cisplatin, fluorouracil, radiotherapy, and surgery compared with surgery alone for esophageal cancer: CALGB 9781. *J Clin Oncol.* 2008;26(7):1086–1092.

Urba SG, Orringer MB, Turrisi A, et al. Randomized trial of preoperative chemoradiation versus surgery alone in patients with locoregional esophageal carcinoma. *J Clin Oncol.* 2001;19:305.

Urschel JD. Does the interponat affect outcome after esophagectomy for cancer? *Dis Esophagus.* 2001;14(2):124–130.

Walsh TN, Noonan N, Hollywood D, et al. A comparison of multimodal therapy and surgery for esophageal adenocarcinoma. *N Engl J Med.* 1996;335:462.

9 Primary Gastric Malignancies

Maria C. Russell, Cary Hsu, and Paul F. Mansfield

Because 95% of gastric cancers are adenocarcinomas, they are the primary focus of this chapter. Advances in the evaluation and treatment of gastric adenocarcinoma since the mid-1990s has led to a shift in the management of this disease. Currently, laparoscopy is an essential component of pretreatment staging for resectable gastric adenocarcinoma. The American Joint Committee on Cancer (AJCC) staging system was previously altered to consider the number rather than the location of nodes involved by metastatic tumor, based on data which showed this to yield a more accurate prognosis. This has been further refined in the 2010 edition; however, this is not without some controversy. Finally, evidence that the combination of chemotherapy or chemoradiation therapy and potentially curative surgical resection increases disease-free and overall survival has led many investigators to recommend multimodality treatment in patients with advanced resectable gastric adenocarcinomas. This chapter covers the epidemiology, preoperative evaluation, and surgical and adjuvant treatment of gastric cancer, as well as management of advanced disease. Less common tumors such as gastric lymphoma, gastric neuroendocrine tumors (NETs), and gastrointestinal stromal tumors (GISTs) of the stomach are also briefly discussed.

EPIDEMIOLOGY

The American Cancer Society estimates that approximately 21,000 new cases of adenocarcinoma of the stomach will be diagnosed in 2010 and that 10,570 patients will die from the disease in the United States (Jemal et al., 2009). Despite a sharp worldwide decline in incidence and mortality during the second half of the 20th century, gastric cancer remains the world's second leading cause of cancer-related deaths. Stomach cancer incidence rates show substantial variation internationally, with highest rates in Japan and eastern Asia followed by South America, whereas it is less common in Europe and North America.

Gastric tumors are classified according to their site in the proximal (cardia) and distal (noncardia) stomach. Proximal tumors are now staged as esophageal tumors in the latest edition of the *AJCC Staging Manual*. Although the incidence of distal gastric cancer is decreasing in the United States, the incidence of proximal gastric tumors continues to increase. Cancers of the gastric cardia currently account for nearly 50% of all cases of gastric adenocarcinoma. Gastric cardia tumors are five times more common in men than women, whereas noncardia gastric tumors are twice as common in men as in women. While an increased trend for gastroesophageal junction (GEJ) adenocarcinoma is suggested in the United States, there is conflicting data on the trends in Asia, although the rates appear to be stable or increasing at a slow rate (Dean et al., 2011). These tumors are associated with poorer outcomes than more distal cancers.

Stomach cancer incidence is twice as high in African American and Asian American/Pacific Islanders when compared with Caucasians (16.7 and 17.5, respectively, vs. 8.9 per 100,000), perhaps reflecting an increased prevalence of chronic infection with *Helicobacter pylori* in this population. Additionally, African American males have a higher death rate due to gastric cancer than Caucasian men (11.0 vs. 4.8 per 100,000). Data originating from both endemic and nonendemic areas indicate a male predominance in elderly gastric cancer patients, but in young patients

(<40 years old), a significant number of studies have reported either no gender difference or a female predominance.

RISK FACTORS

There are wide variations in the incidence of gastric cancer between Asian and Western countries suggesting ethnic origin as a possible risk factor. The National Cancer Institute, in an examination of ethnicity as a risk factor for gastric tumors, identified three groups: those with high (Koreans, Vietnamese, Japanese, Native American, and Hawaiian), intermediate (Latino, Chinese, and African American), and low (Filipino and Caucasian) age-adjusted incidence of gastric cancer. Follow up of first-generation migrants from high-incidence to low-incidence countries demonstrated the same risk rate of their native country. Subsequent generations acquired the risk rate of their new environment, indicating that the risk might not be influenced by the ethnicity but rather by the environment.

Atrophic gastritis, intestinal metaplasia, dysplasia, and infection with *H. pylori* have been identified as important steps in the pathogenesis of gastric cancer (Correa, 1996). Epidemiological evidence has indicated that the bacterium *H. pylori* plays a critical role in the development of gastric cancer. *H. pylori* is common in patients with distal (noncardia) cancer but not in patients with proximal cancer. A falling incidence of *H. pylori* infection and noncardia gastric cancer in developed countries coincides with increasing incidence rates of cardia and GEJ tumors (Sharma & Vakil, 2003). *H. pylori* infection is more prevalent in the populations of developing nations than in industrialized nations. Similarly, *H. pylori* is essential for the development of mucosa-associated lymphoid tissue (MALT) and gastric lymphoma. Almost 90% of patients with intestinal-type gastric cancer have *H. pylori* detected in adjacent, histologically normal mucosa, while only 32% of patients with diffuse-type gastric cancer have this finding. The risk of adenocarcinoma appears to be increased in patients with serologic evidence of immunoglobulin G antibody to *H. pylori* bacterial proteins and with infection of greater than 10 years duration. Furthermore, *H. pylori* is capable of adhering to the Lewis blood group antigen and may be an important factor facilitating chronic infection. An association between blood group A and gastric carcinoma was first described in 1953; however, the relative risk is only 1.2.

Diet is believed to play a major role in the development of gastric carcinoma. Diets rich in salt, smoked or poorly preserved foods, nitrates, nitrites, and secondary amines have been associated with an increase in gastric cancer. The prolonged exposure to this type of diet is believed to result in alteration in the gastric environment with the generation of carcinogenic N-nitroso compounds. Indeed, animal studies have shown that polycyclic hydrocarbons and dimethylnitrosamines, substances produced after prolonged smoking of fish and meat, can induce malignant gastric tumors. Conversely, diets high in raw vegetables, fresh fruits, vitamin C, vitamin A, calcium, and antioxidants are associated with a decreased risk of cancer.

In the United States, male gender, African American race, and low socioeconomic class are associated with a higher risk of gastric carcinoma. Obesity is associated with proximal gastric cancers. A specific occupational hazard may exist for metal workers, miners, and rubber workers, as well as for workers exposed to wood or asbestos dust. Cigarette smokers have a two to three times increased risk of proximal gastric cancer, most likely due to the associated decreased vitamin C levels. Alcohol consumption has not been correlated with the development of gastric carcinoma.

Most gastric carcinomas occur sporadically; however, 8 to 10% of gastric carcinomas have an inherited familial component. Gastric carcinoma occasionally develops in families with germline mutations in p53 (Li–Fraumeni syndrome) and BRCA2. Germline mutations in the gene *CDH1* encoding the cell adhesion protein E-cadherin results in an autosomal-dominant predisposition to gastric carcinoma, referred to as hereditary diffuse gastric cancer. This mutation is seen in 1% to 3% of gastric cancers and has a penetrance of about 70% in women and 80% in men. Prophylactic gastrectomy is offered to carriers of this mutation. Virtually all carriers of this mutation have been found to harbor an early malignancy in the resected specimen, despite negative endoscopic findings, pointing to the advisability of gastrectomy. Gastric cancer can also develop as part of the hereditary nonpolyposis colon cancer syndrome, as well as part of the gastrointestinal polyposis syndromes, including familial adenomatous polyposis and Peutz–Jeghers syndrome.

Gastric polyps are unusual and rarely precursors of gastric cancer. Hyperplastic polyps, the polyps most commonly found in the stomach, are benign lesions. The finding of villous adenomas does, however, indicate an increased risk of malignancy, not only within the polyp itself, but also elsewhere in the stomach. However, villous adenomas represent only 2% of all gastric polyps. There are rare patients who have extensive polyps present in the stomach precluding meaningful surveillance. In these patients, resection can be considered.

Pernicious anemia is associated with a 10% incidence of gastric cancer, higher than in the normal population. Even though the risk of carcinoma developing in a chronic gastric ulcer is small, of concern is the fact that up to 10% of patients with gastric carcinoma are misdiagnosed as having a benign gastric ulcer when evaluated by only a double-contrast study of the upper gastrointestinal tract, though these are rarely performed anymore with the widespread availability of upper endoscopy. Also, initial endoscopic biopsies may miss the cancer, thus requiring the endoscopy to be repeated to ensure that the ulcer has resolved. Operations for benign peptic ulcers also appear to be associated with an increased risk of stomach cancer. Gastric stump cancer typically appears 25 or more years after gastrectomy for the treatment of gastric ulcers and has been reported to occur from zero to five times more often in patients who have had gastrectomy than in individuals without previous gastric resection. Chronic atrophic gastritis and the intestinal metaplasia that often result from these procedures are also risk factors for gastric carcinoma but may not be direct precursor conditions. To date, no association has been demonstrated between long-term H_2 blockade and gastric cancer incidence, though there is suggestion of association with carcinoid tumors.

Finally, other reported risk factors include prior radiation therapy and Epstein–Barr virus infection. Interestingly, a meta-analysis evaluating the clinicopathological and molecular characteristics of Epstein–Barr virus -associated gastric carcinoma demonstrated that it is more prevalent in Caucasian and Hispanic patients, most often developed in the proximal stomach and as diffuse histological type.

PATHOLOGY

Ninety-five percent of gastric cancers are adenocarcinomas that arise almost exclusively from the mucous-producing rather than the acid-producing cells of the gastric mucosa. Lymphoma, carcinoid, leiomyosarcoma, GISTs of the stomach, and adenosquamous and squamous cell carcinoma comprise the remaining 5% of gastric cancers. Adenocarcinoma of the stomach is an aggressive tumor, often metastasizing early by both lymphatic and hematogenous routes and can extend directly into adjacent structures. Extension through the serosal surface is associated with an increased risk of peritoneal tumor spread.

According to the Lauren classification, there are two histologic types of gastric adenocarcinoma: intestinal and diffuse. Each type has distinct clinical and pathological features (Crew & Neugut, 2004; Kelley & Duggan, 2003; Lauren, 1965; Munoz et al., 1968). The intestinal type is found in geographic regions where there is a high incidence of gastric cancer and is characterized pathologically by the tendency of malignant cells to form glands. These tumors are usually well to moderately differentiated and associated with metaplasia or chronic gastritis. They occur more commonly in males and older patients. These tumors tend to spread through the lymphatics and hematologically to distant organs, often the liver. The diffuse type typically lacks organized gland formation, is usually poorly differentiated, and has many signet ring cells. If more than 50% of the tumor contains intracytoplasmic mucin, then it is designated signet ring type. Diffuse-type tumors are more common in younger patients with no history of gastritis and spread transmurally and by lymphatic invasion. Diffuse-type tumors appear to be associated with obesity. Although the incidence of these tumors varies little from country to country, their overall incidence appears to be increasing worldwide. Although Lauren classification separates gastric tumors into two types, the World Health Organization classifies them according to their histomorphologic appearance, which includes tubular, mucinous, papillary, and signet ring cell types.

In the past, most gastric carcinomas (60% to 70%) were found in the antrum. However, the proportion of gastric carcinomas arising in the antrum have decreased, and the proportion arising in the cardia have increased. Nine percent of patients have tumor that involves the entire stomach; this is known as linitis plastica or "leather bottle" stomach, and the prognosis for these patients is dismal. In general, gastric tumors are more common on the lesser curve of the stomach than on the greater curve. In the United States, the incidence of synchronous gastric lesions is 2.2%, compared with an incidence of up to 10% in Japanese patients with pernicious anemia.

CLINICAL PRESENTATION

Gastric adenocarcinoma is usually not associated with specific symptoms early in the course of the disease. Patients often ignore the vague epigastric discomfort and indigestion that portend the cancer and may be treated presumptively for benign disease for 6 to 12 months or longer before diagnostic studies are performed. Rapid weight loss, anorexia, and vomiting are usually a sign of advanced disease. These presenting features are simply due to the presence of a partially obstructing (either mechanical or physiological) lesion. The most frequent presenting symptoms of 1,121 patients at Memorial Sloan-Kettering Cancer Center were weight loss, pain, vomiting, and anorexia. The epigastric pain is usually similar to the pain caused by benign ulcers and is often relieved by eating food; however, it can mimic angina. Dysphagia is usually associated with tumors of the cardia or GEJ. Antral tumors may cause symptoms of gastric outlet obstruction. Although rare, large tumors that directly invade the transverse colon may present with colonic obstruction. Physical examination will reveal a palpable mass in up to 30% of patients.

Approximately 10% of patients present with one or more signs of metastatic disease. The most common indications of distant metastasis are a palpable supraclavicular lymph node (Virchow node), a mass palpable on rectal examination (Blumer shelf), a palpable periumbilical mass (Sister Mary Joseph node), ascites, jaundice, or a liver mass. The most common site of hematogenous spread is the liver (intestinal type); tumor also often spreads to the lining of the peritoneal cavity (diffuse type).

Gastric tumors may be associated with chronic blood loss, though massive upper gastrointestinal bleeding is rare. In Japan, the high incidence of gastric cancer has led to routine endoscopic screening; as a result, in that country, more than 50% of gastric cancers are diagnosed at an early stage.

PREOPERATIVE EVALUATION

National Comprehensive Cancer Network Guidelines for Initial Evaluation

The National Comprehensive Cancer Network has developed consensus guidelines for the clinical evaluation and staging of patients suspected of having gastric adenocarcinoma. The recommended initial evaluation includes complete history and physical examination, laboratory studies (e.g., complete blood cell, chemistry and liver function tests), and computed tomography (CT) of the chest, abdomen, and pelvis. Esophagogastroduodenoscopy is necessary and provides both tissue for a pathological diagnosis and anatomically localizes the primary tumor in more than 90% of patients. Four to six biopsy specimens and cytologic brushings are usually sufficient for establishing an accurate diagnosis. Endoscopic ultrasound (EUS) should be considered if there is no evidence of M1 disease. This initial workup enables the stratification of patients into two clinical stage groups: those with locoregional disease (AJCC stages I–III) and those with systemic disease (AJCC stage IV) (Table 9.1). Palliative therapy is considered in patients with systemic disease, depending on their symptoms and functional status, because several randomized studies have shown a quality of life benefit from treatment in patients with stage IV disease. Patients with locoregional disease are divided into early gastric cancer (EGC) and advanced gastric cancer (AGC) with primary consideration as to the feasibility of more limited resections such as endoscopic mucosal resection (EMR). Patients are further stratified on the basis of their functional status and comorbid conditions. Patients with locoregional disease who are considered candidates for surgery receive definitive (frequently multimodality) therapy, including laparoscopy followed by laparotomy and resection. Patients with M1 disease are considered for palliative therapy.

Upper Gastrointestinal Endoscopy and Endoscopic Ultrasonography

Upper gastrointestinal endoscopy with biopsy is essential for the diagnosis of gastric tumors and enables anatomic assessment of the proximal extent of the tumor, tumor size, and, provided that luminal obstruction does not prevent passage of the gastroscope beyond the tumor, the distal extent of the tumor. Tumor location can guide surgical or palliative treatment planning. In selected patients with advanced disease, esophagogastroduodenoscopy enables palliative treatment consisting of laser ablation, dilatation, or tumor stenting to be performed.

Depth of tumor invasion is a major determinant of stage and directly correlates with prognosis. Gastric mural EUS can achieve spatial resolution of 0.1 mm, which allows for a reasonably accurate assessment of the degree of tumor penetration through the layers of the gastric wall. However, because EUS cannot reliably distinguish between tumor and fibrosis (either treatment related or secondary to ulceration and scarring), EUS is used primarily for initial staging rather than for assessing response to neoadjuvant therapy.

Pathological confirmation of preoperative EUS findings has shown the overall staging accuracy of EUS to be 75%. However, EUS correctly identifies T2 lesions only 38.5% of the time; it is better at identifying T1 (80%) and T3 (90%) lesions. Technical improvements and experience have improved the accuracy of EUS in the nodal evaluation of N1 disease to approximately 65%. The information yielded by EUS-guided fine-needle aspiration may further improve the accuracy of nodal staging, but this technique is technically more challenging. Given the operator dependence of EUS, it is largely performed at regional referral centers.

Computed Tomography

Chest, abdominal, and pelvic CT are performed early in the overall staging of patients with newly diagnosed gastric cancer. This allows unnecessary laparotomy

TABLE 9.1 TNM Classification of Carcinoma of the Stomach

Category	Criteria
Primary Tumor (T)	
Tx	Primary tumor cannot be assessed
T0	No evidence of primary tumor
Tis	Carcinoma in situ
T1	Tumor invades lamina propria, muscularis mucosae or submucosa
T1a	Tumor invades lamina propria or muscularis mucosae
T1b	Tumor invades submucosa
T2	Tumor invades muscularis propria[a]
T3	Tumor penetrates subserosal connective tissue without invasion of visceral peritoneum or adjacent structures[b,c]
T4	Tumor invades serosa (visceral peritoneum) or adjacent structures[b,c]
T4a	Tumor invades serosa (visceral peritoneum)
T4b	Tumor invades adjacent structures

[a]*Note:* A tumor may penetrate the muscularis propria with extension into the gastrocolic or gastrohepatic ligaments, or into the greater or lesser omentum, without perforation of the visceral peritoneum covering these structures. In this case, the tumor is classified T3. If there is perforation of the visceral peritoneum covering the gastric ligaments or the omentum, the tumor should be classified as T4.

[b]The adjacent structures of the stomach include the spleen, transverse colon, liver, diaphragm, pancreas, abdominal wall, adrenal gland, kidney, small intestine, and retroperitoneum.

[c]Intramural extension to the duodenum or esophagus is classified by the depth of the greatest invasion in any of these sites, including the stomach.

Regional Lymph Nodes (N)

Nx	Regional lymph nodes cannot be assessed
N0	No regional lymph node metastasis[a]
N1	Metastasis in 1–2 lymph nodes
N2	Metastasis in 3–6 lymph nodes
N3	Metastasis in seven or more regional lymph nodes
N3a	Metastasis in 7–15 regional lymph nodes
N3b	Metastasis in 16 or more regional lymph nodes

[a]A designation of pN0 should be used if all examined lymph nodes are negative, regardless of the total number removed and examined.

Distant Metastasis (M)

M0	No distant metastasis
M1	Distant metastasis

Stage Grouping

Stage 0	Tis	N0	M0
Stage IA	T1	N0	M0
Stage IB	T2	N0	M0
	T1	N1	M0
Stage IIA	T3	N0	M0
	T2	N1	M0
	T1	N2	M0

(*continued*)

TABLE 9.1	TNM Classification of Carcinoma of the Stomach (*continued*)		
Stage IIB	T4a	N0	M0
	T3	N1	M0
	T2	N2	M0
	T1	N3	M0
Stage IIIA	T4a	N0	M0
	T3	N2	M0
	T2	N3	M0
Stage IIIB	T4b	N0	M0
	T4b	N1	M0
	T4a	N2	M0
	T3	N3	M0
Stage IIIC	T4b	N2	M0
	T4b	N3	M0
	T4a	N3	M0
Stage IV	Any T	Any N	M1

Adapted from Stomach. In: Edge SB, Byrd DR, Compton CC, eds. *AJCC Cancer Staging Manual.* 7th ed. New York, NY: Springer; 2010.
Used with permission of the American Joint Committee on Cancer (AJCC), Chicago, Illinois. The original source for this material is the AJCC Cancer Staging Manual, Seventh Edition (2010) published by Springer Science and Business Media LLC, www.springer.com.

to be avoided in many patients with visceral metastatic disease or malignant ascites. The major limitations of CT as a staging tool are in the evaluation of early gastric tumors and small (<5 mm) metastases on peritoneal surfaces or in the liver.
Even with the use of helical CT scan, the overall accuracy in determining tumor
stage is approximately 66% to 77%. CT is accurate in determining nodal stage in
25% to 86% of patients.

Laparoscopy and Laparoscopic Ultrasonography
The value of further staging with laparoscopy is apparent on recognition of the low
sensitivity of CT for the detection of small (<5 mm) metastases on the peritoneal
surface. Laparoscopy can be done either separately or immediately before surgical
resection. In brief, a laparoscopic inspection is usually performed in a systematic
manner and includes a search for metastases on the peritoneal surfaces and the
liver. Biopsy of perigastric or other nodal basins for staging purposes is not routinely
performed. The identification of advanced disease afforded by laparoscopy allows
many patients to be spared an ultimately nontherapeutic laparotomy. Patients with
small-volume metastatic disease at laparoscopy have a life expectancy of only 3 to
9 months; thus, despite some reports that palliative gastrectomy may confer a survival advantage, such patients rarely benefit from expectant palliative resection.
There is an ongoing joint study between Japan and Korea, examining the role of
gastrectomy in this patient population. An argument for performing a second-look
laparoscopy can be made in the case of patients who receive neoadjuvant chemotherapy for unresectable disease and appear to have a good clinical response, but
more importantly in patients with only stable disease or a minor response.

Researchers at Memorial Sloan-Kettering Cancer Center and M. D. Anderson
Cancer Center have evaluated the feasibility, yield, and clinical benefit of laparoscopic staging after high-quality abdominal CT staging and found that laparoscopy

identified CT-occult metastatic disease in 23% to 37% of patients. Moreover, less than 2% of the patients in whom CT-occult metastases were identified by laparoscopy required subsequent laparotomy for palliation. On the basis of the available data, the National Comprehensive Cancer Network has integrated laparoscopy into the recommended routine staging algorithm for patients with locoregional gastric cancers and select patients with AGC.

Laparoscopic ultrasonography (LUS) has been proposed as a means to overcome some of the limitations of laparoscopy and to improve the diagnostic yield. However, the majority of studies of LUS in the staging of gastric cancer are difficult to interpret because the use of state-of-the-art prelaparoscopy staging (particularly CT) has varied, and results have been reported in a manner that makes it difficult to determine the specific added benefit of LUS over high-quality CT plus laparoscopy alone. Given the limitations of the available data, the high cost of LUS equipment, and the operator-dependent nature of the technique, it is best to regard LUS as requiring further investigation to define its role.

Peritoneal Cytology

Cytologic analysis of peritoneal fluid or fluid obtained by peritoneal lavage may identify occult carcinomatosis. The fluid is usually obtained by percutaneous or laparoscopic aspiration (with or without peritoneal lavage) performed at the time of staging laparoscopy. Peritoneal cytologic analysis can be relatively simple and fast and is therefore also feasible intraoperatively, although one must be on the watch for false-positive readings.

In most series, patients with positive peritoneal cytology findings have a prognosis similar to that of patients with macroscopic visceral or peritoneal disease (3- to 9-month median survival). Some researchers have investigated the impact of peritoneal cytology findings on outcome and noted that the median survival in those with positive cytology findings was 122 days; others have used it as an indication for neoadjuvant treatment rather than an absolute contraindication to resection. Regardless, the AJCC has found the data for positive peritoneal cytology convincing enough to include it as M1 disease in the most recent TNM classification.

The primary concerns regarding the use of peritoneal cytology are the possibility of false-positive results and the fact that some reports do not confirm the uniformly poor prognosis in patients with positive findings. Given that cytologic analysis is very much an operator-dependent visual interpretation, efforts are ongoing to develop more sensitive and specific techniques for identifying peritoneal dissemination, including immunostaining and reverse transcriptase–polymerase chain reaction testing for carcinoembryonic antigen (CEA) mRNA. Although some success has been seen using these techniques, because they take more time than peritoneal cytology, they may not be practical for use in the operating room.

Lymphatic Mapping

Given the essential role of nodal status in gastric cancer staging and the controversy that surrounds the extent of lymphadenectomy, there has been interest in evaluating the feasibility of sentinel lymph node mapping in gastric cancer. Lymphatic drainage of the stomach is more complex and variable than what has seen for breast cancer and melanoma, and thus there is a risk of a "skip" metastasis in up to 15% of cases. Although lymphatic mapping of stomach tumors has been most commonly performed via an open laparotomy, it has also been done using a laparoscopic approach. Mapping agents such as radiocolloid with or without vital dye and activated carbon particles have been used. The identification rate varies from 90% to 100%, and the sensitivity of the findings ranges from 61% to 100%. However, lymphatic mapping has several drawbacks. First, the number of patients with gastric cancer in which it has been studied is small in comparison with melanoma or breast cancer. Second, it is associated with a false-negative rate as high as 39%. Third, the number of sentinel lymph nodes per patient is quite varied (two to seven sentinel nodes per patient). Fourth, the findings are significantly different in the typically obese Western patients from those in Asian patients, in whom most of the studies of lymphatic mapping have been done. Finally, if accurate mapping requires a separate operation, the implications of a repeat laparotomy are vastly different than they are for an axillary or inguinal lymph node dissection. For these reasons, sentinel lymph node mapping for stomach cancer remains investigational.

Other Studies

Positron emission tomography (PET), which estimates tumor metabolism on the basis of the uptake of a radiotracer—most commonly, fluorodeoxyglucose (FDG)—is currently being evaluated as a staging tool for gastric cancer. This technique may reveal CT-occult metastases (particularly extra-abdominal disease) and may be used to assess response to neoadjuvant therapy. Current drawbacks to PET are its high cost and its limited availability. While intestinal-type tumors may have some benefit from PET imaging, most diffuse-type tumors are not FDG avid and thus PET is useless. The additional benefit of PET over standard staging studies in the evaluation of gastric cancer has thus far not been shown.

Increased levels of CEA are seen in about 30% of patients with gastric carcinoma. Because the CEA level is usually normal in EGC, CEA is not a useful screening marker. Serial determinations of the CEA level may be helpful, however, in detecting tumor recurrence or in monitoring response to treatment in patients who present with an increased CEA level.

STAGING SYSTEMS

Many staging systems for gastric adenocarcinoma have been proposed. The pathological staging system currently in use worldwide is the Union Internationale Contre le Cancer/AJCC TNM staging system. In 2009, the AJCC published the 7th edition *TNM Classification Of Malignant Tumors for Gastric Cancer.* Gastric cancer is one of the solid tumors most reassessed in this latest edition (Sobin et al., 2009). Several other largely abandoned systems have been developed in an attempt to describe both the extent of *disease* and the resultant extent of *resection* or *lymphadenectomy* necessary in a given patient. The various staging systems in use are explained below.

American Joint Committee on Cancer Staging System

The staging of gastric adenocarcinoma has changed significantly since the mid-1990s. The validity of the newer TNM staging system is now well established. Because it is a pathological rather than a clinical staging system, a patient's TNM status is only fully known following resection. Three important clinicopathological factors have been shown to reliably stratify patients into distinct groups with different risks of tumor-related death: the depth of penetration of the primary tumor through the gastric wall (T), the absence or presence and extent of lymph node involvement (N), and the absence or presence of distant metastases (M). In 2009, the TNM staging system for gastric cancer underwent significant revision in the tumor, node, and metastasis categories.

One area of contention in gastric cancer has always revolved around the esophagogastric junction (EGJ) and the proximal stomach, which some argue should be treated as a separate entity from distal cancers. These have been staged variably as gastric or esophageal cancers and left up to some personal interpretation. The 7th edition of AJCC addresses this controversy by assigning tumors with mid-point in the lower thoracic esophagus, EGJ, or within the proximal 5 cm of stomach that extend into the EGJ or esophagus to be staged as esophageal adenocarcinoma. This has lead to significant further discussion. Additional changes in the T staging of gastric cancer include defining tumors that invade the lamina propria or muscularis mucosa as T1a and those that invade the submucosa as T1b. Finally, T3 tumors now are classified as those penetrating the subserosal connective tissue without invasion of visceral peritoneum, whereas tumors that invade the serosa (visceral peritoneum) and adjacent structures now are classified as T4a and T4b, respectively.

The nodal classification of tumors has also changed substantially with fewer nodes necessary for higher nodal status. Metastases in 1–2 nodes is now N1, whereas formerly this included 1–6 regional lymph nodes. N2 disease is now defined as 3–6 nodes positive, a decrease from the 7–14 in 6th edition of *AJCC*. N3 is split into N3a for 7–15 positive nodes and N3b for metastases in 16 or more regional lymph nodes. Some sources suggest that the decrease in numbers of lymph nodes required for higher N status attempts to compensate for the "unhomogene-ity" of surgical lymphadenectomy between Europe and the United States and Asia (Rausei et al., 2010). Since there is still marked variability in the extent of dissection between the Japanese operations and those performed in much of Europe and the United States, the intention is to obtain some prognostic information regardless of the extent of dissection. Additionally, the "requirement" of 15 lymph nodes no longer exists and has been replaced by the suggestion that at least 16 regional lymph nodes should be assessed or else the designation of pN0 is assigned. These changes are the focus of a significant multinational review by a work group from the International Gastric Cancer Association.

For distant metastases, there have been two changes. First, the Mx category no longer exists. Not being able to evaluate distant metastases is no longer considered appropriate as it prevents accurate staging of patients, as well as the inability to assess the response to neoadjuvant and adjuvant treatment. In addition, to reflect the poor prognosis of patients with positive peritoneal cytology, this is now considered M1 disease.

Residual Disease: R Status

The *R status*, which was first formally described by Hermanek and Wittekind in 1994, is commonly used to describe the tumor status in a patient following resection and is designated following pathological evaluation of the resection margins (Table 9.2). R0 indicates that microscopic margins are free of tumor and that no gross or microscopic disease remains. R1 indicates that all gross disease has been extirpated but that microscopic margins are positive for tumor. R2 indicates that gross residual disease remains. Long-term survival can be expected only in patients who undergo an R0 resection for gastric adenocarcinoma and significant effort is therefore made to avoid R1 or R2 resections.

Japanese Classification: Extent of Resection

The extent of pathological lymph node involvement relative to the scope of the lymphadenectomy performed is the distinguishing characteristic of the Japanese

TABLE 9.2	Current Description of Completeness of Resection Based on Presence or Absence of Residual Disease Following Resection and Pathological Evaluation of Resection Margins
Description	**Gross or Pathological Extent of Residual Disease**
R0	No residual gross disease and negative microscopic margins
R1	Microscopic residual disease only
R2	Gross residual disease

TABLE 9.3	"D" Nomenclature: Extent of Surgical Resection and Lymphadenectomy
Description	**Regions Included in Resection**
D1	Removal of all nodal tissue within 3 cm of the primary tumor
D2	D1 plus clearance of hepatic, splenic, celiac, and left gastric lymph nodes
D3	D2 plus omentectomy, splenectomy, distal pancreatomy, and clearance of porta hepatis lymph nodes and paraaortic lymph nodes

classification scheme, which is based on the assumption that extended lymph node clearance beyond the level of pathological involvement may prolong survival. In yet another Japanese system (Table 9.3), the completeness of nodal dissection is designated D1 (removal of all nodal tissue within 3 cm of the primary tumor), D2 (D1 plus clearance of hepatic, splenic, celiac, and left gastric nodes), or D3 (total gastrectomy, omentectomy, with or without splenectomy and distal pancreatectomy, and celiac and portal and paraaortic lymphadenectomy). Although these classifications are not part of the AJCC staging system, the D terminology is important in comparing the results of surgical therapy, as is discussed later in the chapter.

SURGICAL TREATMENT

Surgical resection offers the only significant potential for cure of gastric cancer. Preoperative staging should demonstrate the extent of disease, define the patient's prognosis, and permit treatment planning. The type of surgery is then dependent upon tumor depth, growth pattern, and tumor localization (Ott, 2011). EGC confined to the mucosa can be treated endoscopically. All other surgical resections are based on the location of the tumor and potential lymph node metastases. We recommend a wide macroscopically negative margin of 5 to 6 cm, along with the en bloc resection of adjacent lymph nodes. D2 lymphadenectomy, sparing the spleen and distal pancreas, is employed if it can be done with low morbidity and mortality. The appropriate surgical procedure for a given patient must take into account the location of the lesion and the known pattern of spread.

Endoscopic Mucosal Resection

The risk of lymph node metastases is highly associated with the depth of tumor in EGC. Those confined to the mucosa have a 0.36% to 5% chance of involving lymph nodes (Ott, 2011; Yamao, 1996); therefore, the Japanese Gastric Cancer Association has set forth guidelines for EMR of EGCs. According to these guidelines, endoscopic therapy is appropriate with (1) well-differentiated adenocarcinoma, (2) tumor 20 mm or less in size for elevated types, (3) tumor 10 mm or less in size for depressed types, (4) tumor not associated with peptic ulcer, and (5) invasion limited to mucosa (Tada et al., 2000). It is critical that the specimen be carefully evaluated, particularly the deep margin, to determine whether a more formal resection is required. In appropriately selected patients, EMR holds many potential benefits including better quality of life, low incidence of postoperative complications, and decreased cost, with outstanding survival rates similar to conventional surgery (Kojima et al., 1998; Suzuki et al., 1999; Tada et al., 2000; Takeshita et al., 1997). Using these standard criteria for EMR leads to a local cure rate of 98%. However, reports have described the use of expanded criteria such as resection of larger tumors, tumors with submucosal invasion, and for patients whose comorbidities preclude standard treatment with gastrectomy (Amano et al., 1998; Hiki et al., 1995; Kojima et al., 1998). This leads to a drop in local cure rate to 67%. Overall mortality due to EMR is low, with the two main complications being bleeding and perforation, which range from 1.2 to 20.5% and 0.4 to 5.2%, respectively (Kondo et al., 2001; Ono et al., 2001; Tanabe et al., 1999). The results from the published Japanese studies are attractive; however, it should be stressed that the vast majority of Western institutions have limited experience or expertise with EMR. The Cochrane Collaboration published a review in 2009 evaluating EMR for EGC and found that there were no randomized controlled trials comparing the safety and effectiveness of EMR with gastrectomy (Bennett et al., 2009). While they call for a randomized trial, it is not likely that such a trial will ever be done. Those utilizing this technique should proceed with caution.

Proximal Tumors

In the new *AJCC*, seventh edition, proximal gastric cancers, those arising at the GEJ or in the stomach less than 5 cm from the GEJ are now staged as esophageal cancers. It has been shown by multivariate analysis that an R0 resection is independent of other strong predictors of survival like TNM status. The primary goal of therapy for any proximal gastric cancer, therefore, should be complete resection. The manner in which to achieve this resection is debatable. Surgical strategies have included en bloc esophagogastrectomy, subtotal esophagectomy with resection of the proximal stomach, total gastrectomy with resection of the distal esophagus, and limited resection of the EGJ. Approaches include abdominal, abdominothoracic, transhiatal, and transthoracic. To delineate the appropriate treatments based on pathophysiology and location, tumors of the EGJ have been further divided according to the Siewert classification, also referred to as "adenocarcinoma of the esophageal junction": type I tumors are associated with Barrett esophagus or true esophageal cancer growing into the GEJ; type II cancers are true junctional tumors that lie within 2 cm of the squamocolumnar junction at the level of the cardia; and type III cancers are present within the subcardial region of the stomach. The treatment of adenocarcinoma of the esophageal junction I tumors is usually esophagectomy via either a transthoracic or a transhiatal approach. The surgeon must balance the benefit of a mediastinal lymph node dissection in a transthoracic approach with the perceived decreased morbidity of a transhiatal approach. The optimal surgical management of type II and III cancers is controversial. The incidence of lower mediastinal lymph node metastasis is 10% to 40% (Dresner et al., 2001; Husemann, 1989; Kawaura et al., 1988; Kodama et al., 1998; Maruyama et al., 1996; Wang et al., 1993; Yonemura et al., 1995). It is debatable whether a thoracotomy is necessary for lymph node dissection and adequate margin since these patients have such a poor prognosis even with a more extensive procedure. Sasako et al. started a multicenter, prospective randomized phase III trial which was prematurely closed after there were no proven significant benefits to a left thoracoabdominal approach compared to a transabdominal approach, with substantially increased morbidity from the thoracoabdominal approach. Some authors argue that one should perform a proximal subtotal gastrectomy, noting that total gastrectomy does not improve prognosis for patients with stage III and IV disease. However, some studies have shown a poorer quality of life (primarily due to reflux) in patients who undergo a proximal subtotal gastrectomy than in patients who undergo a total gastrectomy.

For GEJ tumors, we often approach them with a multidisciplinary and multiteam approach. For these tumors, after neoadjuvant therapy, we often make the final decision for the surgical approach at the time of surgery with input from both thoracic surgery and surgical oncology. At M. D. Anderson, we usually perform a total gastrectomy with a Roux-en-Y reconstruction and regional lymphadenectomy for proximal gastric lesions. This procedure has the advantage of avoiding the alkaline reflux esophagitis often associated with proximal subtotal gastrectomy. Furthermore, lymph nodes along the lesser curvature, a common site of spread, are easily removed during a total gastrectomy. There is also no greater mortality or morbidity in patients who undergo total gastrectomy compared with those who undergo a proximal subtotal gastrectomy.

Midbody Tumors

Midstomach tumors account for 15% to 30% of all gastric cancers. While there are numerous publications debating the role of partial gastrectomy versus total gastrectomy for proximal and distal gastric cancer, there is much less literature on midbody gastric cancers. Jang et al. retrospectively reviewed over 400 patients with midbody tumors who either received total gastrectomy or distal gastrectomy and found that the extent of gastric resection and the length of proximal resection margin did not affect the long-term outcome for patients as long as a curative resection was achieved. While those patients undergoing a distal gastrectomy had a significantly higher overall survival rate, this was explained by the more favorable stage gastric cancer in those patients that were able to undergo distal gastrectomy instead of total gastrectomy. Other authors recommend total gastrectomy for all tumors localized in the middle third of the stomach (Ott, 2010). For these tumors, our surgical approach is to perform either subtotal or total gastrectomy based on the adequacy of the proximal margin as noted above, as well as on the amount of gastric remnant that remains for reconstruction.

Distal Tumors

Distal tumors account for approximately 35% of all gastric cancers. The standard operation for these lesions is a distal subtotal gastrectomy with appropriate lymphadenectomy. In a multicenter randomized trial of 618 patients, Bozzetti in 1997 reported that tumors of the mid- and distal stomach treated with subtotal or total gastrectomy had the same 5-year survival. They further concluded that based on the association with better nutritional status and quality of life, subtotal gastrectomy should be the procedure of choice, as long as the proximal resection margin included healthy tissue. Other studies have reported similar findings of increased morbidity with no increase in survival following a total gastrectomy for distal gastric cancers.

Because studies have shown that microscopic invasion beyond 6 cm from the gross tumor is rare, we recommend a 5- to 6-cm luminal resection margin when possible. Even if this distance is achieved, the surgical margins should be evaluated by frozen section.

Splenectomy

Multiple trials have demonstrated that routine splenectomy for gastric cancer does not increase survival and is associated with increased morbidity or mortality (Bozzetti et al., 1997; Csendes et al., 2002; Wu et al., 2006). In 2006, Yu et al. published a randomized clinical trial of patients with proximal gastric adenocarcinoma who underwent total gastrectomy with or without splenectomy. They reported no significant difference in 5-year survival or in morbidity or mortality. The conclusion was that prophylactic splenectomy to remove macroscopically negative splenic lymph nodes was not supported. A large randomized trial addressing this question has been conducted in Japan; the results of which are not currently available.

At M. D. Anderson Cancer Center, splenectomy is not performed unless the tumor adheres to or invades the spleen or its vascular supply. If a splenectomy is anticipated preoperatively, pneumococcal polysaccharide, meningococcal, and *Haemophilus* influenza vaccines are administered prior to surgery.

Lymphadenectomy

Despite prospective randomized trials, controversy still exists regarding the role of extended lymphadenectomy in the treatment of gastric cancer. Radical lymphadenectomy was adopted based on an initial report published in 1981 by Kodama et al. that described a survival benefit for patients with serosal or regional lymph node involvement who underwent a D2 or D3 lymphadenectomy (R2 or R3 in the old Japanese nomenclature). Specifically, the 5-year survival rate in patients who underwent radical lymphadenectomy was 39% as opposed to only 18% in patients who underwent D1 lymphadenectomy. Many other nonrandomized studies from Japan have shown a similarly significant survival benefit in patients undergoing radical lymphadenectomy. Unfortunately, Western studies evaluating extended lymphadenectomy have not demonstrated any improvement in survival.

There may be multiple explanations for the divergent outcomes seen in comparing Japanese and Western studies. One potential reason is that most Japanese patients present with early-stage disease, which makes overall survival appears better. However, stage for stage, the differences are not quite so dramatic. Furthermore, the Japanese approach to nodal dissection and pathological analysis is much more meticulous than the approach used in the West, and there is likely to be an element of stage migration. Also, proximal tumors, which behave more aggressively, are less common in Japan than in the West. Finally, there are significant differences in both surgeon experience and patient characteristics (including comorbidities) between the Japanese and the Western patient populations.

Multiple randomized trials evaluating the extent of lymphadenectomy for gastric cancer have been conducted. There are trials which have compared D1 versus D2 lymphadenectomy, as well as additional trials comparing the more extensive D3 versus D2 or D1 lymphadenectomy.

The first randomized trial of D1 and D2 lymphadenectomy performed by Dent et al., from South Africa, included only 43 patients. Those who underwent D2 dissection had a higher blood transfusion requirement (D1, 4 units; D2, 25 units; $P <$ 0.005), longer hospital stay (D1, 9.3 days; D2, 13.9 days; $0.05 > P > 0.025$), and longer operative time (D1, 1.7 hours; D2, 2.3 hours; $P < 0.005$). However, there was no difference in survival and the procedure was advised not to be performed outside a clinical trial.

In 1999, Bonenkamp et al. reported on a study conducted by the Dutch Gastric Cancer Group in which 711 patients were prospectively randomized to undergo D1 or D2 lymphadenectomy. Patients undergoing the more extended lymphadenectomy (D2) had a significantly higher operative morbidity rate (D2, 43%; D1, 25%; $P < 0.001$), significantly higher mortality rate (D2, 10%; D1, 4%; $P = 0.004$), and a higher reoperation rate (D2, 18%; D1 8%; $P = 0.00016$). The 5-year relapse rates (D1, 43%; D2, 37%) and 5-year survival rates (D1, 45%; D2, 47%) were similar. The longer term results published in 2004 indicate that of all subgroups analyzed, only those with N2 disease may have benefited from extended lymphadenectomy (Hartgrink et al., 2004). They found increased morbidity and mortality for D2 dissections, splenectomy, pancreatectomy, and age older than 70 years. The 15-year follow-up from this study was recently published (Songun et al., 2010). This chapter demonstrates that after a median follow-up of 15 years, D2 lymphadenectomy provides lower locoregional recurrence (22% in D1 vs. 12% in D2) and lower gastric-cancer-associated deaths (48% in D1 vs. 37% in D2, $P = 0.01$). The increased morbidity and mortality associated with D2 dissection in this study, likely obscured any potential advantage from the more aggressive surgery.

The results obtained in the Medical Research Council trial reported by Cuschieri et al. (1999) proved to be similar. In this study, 400 patients with gastric adenocarcinoma were prospectively randomized to undergo D1 or D2 lymphadenectomy. There was no difference in the overall 5-year survival rate between the two groups (D1, 35%; D2, 33%). Morbidity for this trial was 25% for D1 and 43% for D2 ($P < 0.001$), while mortality was 4% and 10%, respectively ($P = 0.004$). In this study, pancreaticosplenectomy performed as part of the D2 resection accounted for much of the postoperative morbidity (D1 28%; D2 46%; $P < 0.001$) and mortality (D1 6.5%; D2 13%; $P = 0.04$). Approximately one-third of patients in the D1 group had a splenectomy. The authors cautiously suggested that a D2 resection without pancreaticosplenectomy may be better than the standard D1 resection.

In comparison, the Italian Gastric Cancer Study Group recently published their randomized clinical trial comparing D1 and D2 gastrectomy in 267 patients treated at specialized hospitals (Deguili et al., 2010). The caveats of this study included staging laparotomy with washings, elimination of splenopancreatectomy as a routine part of D2 dissection, and the surgeons were trained and then proctored for their first three operations to ensure the surgeons were experienced with the D2 technique. The overall morbidity rates after D2 and D1 dissections were 17.9% and 12%, respectively ($P = 0.178$). Postoperative 30-day mortality was 2.2% after D2 and 3% after D1 dissection ($P = 0.722$). The conclusion from this trial is that specialized centers may have much lower rates of complications with a D2 dissection and therefore make it a safe option for management of gastric cancer patients even in Western countries.

In 2006, Wu et al. published a randomized controlled trial of 221 patients undergoing a D1 and D3 lymphadenectomy with curative intent (D3 in this trial is equivalent to D2 in the Japanese classification of surgery). The surgeons in this trial were required to have done at least 25 independent D3 resections. There was no pre- or postoperative chemotherapy or radiotherapy. The overall survival for the D3 group was 59.5% and for the D1 group was 53.6% (log rank $P = 0.041$). Disease-specific survival was significantly higher in the D3 group who did not require a splenectomy or pancreatectomy. The reported morbidity for the D2 versus D1 dissection was 17.1% versus 7.3%, respectively, significantly higher in the D2 group, predominantly secondary to abdominal abscesses. The conclusion from this study was that extended lymphadenectomy was associated with more complications but also offered a survival benefit to gastric cancer patients.

In 2004, the Japanese Cooperative Oncology Group (JCOG 9501) reported the findings from a prospective multicenter randomized trial evaluating R0 gastrectomy with D2 lymphadenectomy versus D2 plus paraaortic lymphadenectomy in 523 patients. There were two deaths in each arm, accounting for a remarkably low hospital mortality rate of 0.8% though the morbidity rate in patients who underwent the D2 plus paraaortic lymphadenectomy (28.1%) was higher than that in the patients who underwent the D2 lymphadenectomy (20.9%) ($P = 0.07$). Patients who underwent the D2 plus paraaortic lymphadenectomy had longer operations ($P < 0.001$) with increased blood loss ($P < 0.001$) and hence higher blood transfusion requirements ($P < 0.001$) than did those who had only a D2 lymphadenectomy. Long-term survival results were published in 2008 (Sasako, 2008). Five-year survival was 69.2% after D2 and 70.3% after D2 plus paraaortic node dissection ($P = 0.85$). There were no significant differences in recurrence-free survival. The conclusion was that D2 plus paraaortic lymph node dissection does not improve survival.

Current standard recommendations include a D1 dissection (perigastric lymphadenectomy), although major centers employ more extended nodal dissections in the setting of low operative mortality. At M. D. Anderson, spleen-sparing D2 lymphadenectomy is our standard approach. Analysis of patients who underwent curative resection after neoadjuvant therapy at M. D. Anderson between 1991 and 1998 showed a perioperative mortality rate of 2%.

Laparoscopic Resection

When considering a laparoscopic resection for any cancer operation, there are two points of paramount importance: safety and oncologic integrity. A recent publication in the *Journal of the American College of Surgeons* provides a review of laparoscopic surgery for gastric cancer (Kodera et al., 2010). The first laparoscopic-assisted operation for gastric cancer dates to 1994; however, in the 2010 revised version of the Japanese *Gastric Cancer Treatment Guidelines*, a laparoscopic-assisted gastrectomy, remains classified as an investigational procedure for stage IA and IB cancers. There have been many studies of laparoscopic gastrectomy, mainly in the Asian literature and focusing primarily on distal gastrectomy for EGC. The majority of these trials seem to conclude that a laparoscopic gastrectomy is associated with a longer operating time and less blood loss. Extent of lymphadenectomy based on number of lymph nodes retrieved is variable and the effects of this in terms of survival are unknown at this time. The largest of these trials is the KLASS trial which reported its interim analysis on a phase III multicenter, prospective randomized trial in preoperative stage I gastric cancer patients (Kim et al., 2010). In a total of 342 patients, the postoperative complication rates were similar for laparoscopic-assisted distal gastrectomy (10.5%) and open distal gastrectomy (14.7%, $P = 0.137$). Postoperative mortality was 1.1% and 0% ($P = 0.497$) in the laparoscopic and open groups, respectively. They concluded that the approach was safe and were continuing to evaluate the oncologic safety of laparoscopic distal gastrectomy. A series of retrospective analyses for long-term outcomes similarly show no difference in the 5-year survival between the groups.

While these trials address EGC, there are fewer reports in the literature of the laparoscopic approach for AGCs. A recent meta-analysis published in 2011 by Martinez-Ramos et al. compared seven trials (one prospective randomized, one comparative prospective, and five comparative retrospective) on laparoscopic versus open surgery for advanced resectable gastric cancer. Interestingly, the majority of these trials were in Europe or the United States and all contained small sample sizes (<120 patients). They concluded that laparoscopic total and partial gastrectomy for advanced disease is associated with a longer operative time, but there may be decreased blood loss and shorter postoperative stay without detrimental effect on lymph node dissection. Strong et al. published a review of the Western literature for laparoscopic resections and concluded that this approach should be limited to high volume centers and EGCs until more definitive studies are performed evaluating advanced cancers.

Overall, there are still controversies that must be addressed in determining the applicability of laparoscopic gastrectomy. First, since proximal gastric cancers are less common in the East, there is much less laparoscopic experience with total gastrectomy than distal gastrectomy. While circular stapling and flexible stapling devices may make this operation technically feasible, there is some controversy over the safety of the esophagojejunostomy. The preponderance of early stage gastric cancers in the East compared to that in the West makes much of this literature less relevant when discussing safety and efficacy of the operation in the United States.

SURGICAL TECHNIQUE

Total Gastrectomy

Our approach for a total gastrectomy begins with separating the omentum from the mesocolon. The right gastroepiploic vessels are ligated at their origin, and the subpyloric nodes are resected with the specimen. The first portion of the duodenum is mobilized and divided 2 cm distal to the pylorus. The gastrohepatic ligament is opened, and the left gastric artery is ligated at its origin. It is important to remember that a replaced or accessory left hepatic artery may originate from the left gastric artery and reside in the gastrohepatic ligament. If an extended lymphadenectomy is done, the celiac, hepatic artery, and splenic artery nodes are cleared of nodal tissue and removed along with the specimen. The short gastric vessels are ligated sequentially. Dissection around the GEJ can free up 7 to 8 cm of distal esophagus, which facilitates transection of the esophagus with an adequate proximal margin. Stay sutures of 2–0 silk are placed, and after the esophagus is divided, the resection margins are evaluated by frozen-section examination. If the tumor adheres to the spleen, pancreas, liver, diaphragm, colon, or mesocolon, the involved organ or organs are removed en bloc.

There are many types of reconstructions, but the one most frequently used is a Roux-en-Y anastomosis. If a significant portion of the distal esophagus is resected, a left thoracoabdominal or right thoracotomy incision (Ivor–Lewis approach) may be necessary, with the former being rarely employed. Although several studies have shown that reconstruction with pouches and loops to act as reservoirs appear to be beneficial, there are results to the contrary and the technique is not widely accepted. Jejunal interposition, utilizing a 45-cm long segment of the small bowel between the esophagus and duodenum is rarely employed. While this reconstruction makes physiologic sense and may be associated with a lower incidence of cholelithiasis and less weight loss, it is also more complex, requires an additional anastomosis (esophagojejunostomy, duodenojejunostomy, and jejunojejunostomy), and results of studies are not supportive. A feeding jejunostomy tube is placed for postoperative nutritional support.

Subtotal Gastrectomy

The mobilization for subtotal gastrectomy is identical to that for total gastrectomy described in the preceding section, except that the short gastrics are preserved and only approximately 75% to 80% of the distal stomach is resected. The dissection of the distal one or two short gastric vessels is performed early to ensure splenic preservation. The small remnant of stomach that is left is supplied by the remaining short gastric vessels and the posterior gastric artery arising from the splenic artery. We often use Roux-en-Y reconstruction after subtotal gastrectomy, although a loop gastrojejunostomy (Billroth II) or less frequently a gastroduodenostomy (Billroth I) are also employed.

Figure 9.1 shows the M. D. Anderson treatment algorithm for potentially resectable gastric carcinoma.

COMPLICATIONS OF SURGERY

Complications of gastric resection and their relative frequencies are given in Table 9.4. One of the most potentially devastating complications is an anastomotic leak, which occurs in 3% to 21% of patients. Because leaks can occur late, an intact anastomosis early in the postoperative period is not a guarantee of an uncomplicated course. Oral feeding is typically started 4 to 7 days postoperatively, often after return of bowel function. Upper gastrointestinal tract contrast studies are performed on the basis of clinical indications only (e.g., fever, tachycardia, and tachypnea). Because the food reservoir is gone, most patients must initially change their eating habits such that they consume several small meals per day. A significant proportion of patients will eventually eat regular meals plus snacks. Supplemental jejunostomy feedings are started the day after surgery and continued until oral intake is adequate. Within several months, most patients are able to increase their oral intake capacity and eat larger meals less frequently (three or four meals per day).

About 10% of patients will develop clinically significant dumping syndrome. Early dumping typically occurs 15 to 30 minutes after a meal: signs and symptoms

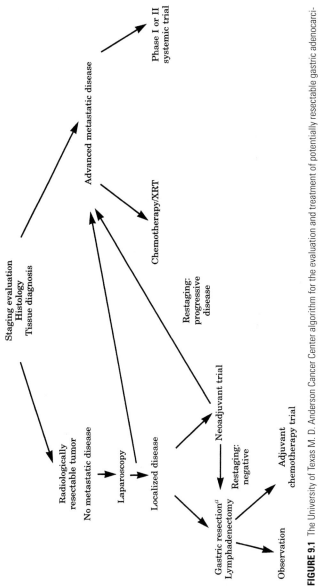

FIGURE 9.1 The University of Texas M. D. Anderson Cancer Center algorithm for the evaluation and treatment of potentially resectable gastric adenocarcinoma. [a]Occasionally, metastatic disease is found at the time of open surgical exploration for tumors believed to be resectable on the basis of radiologic and laparoscopic staging. In this situation, the decision to perform palliative resection is made on an individualized basis. Patients with metastatic disease have a dismal prognosis (see text).

TABLE 9.4	Complications of Gastric Resection

Complication	Percentage of Patients Affected
Pulmonary	3–55
Infectious	3–22
Anastomotic	3–21
Cardiac	1–10
Renal	1–8
Bleeding	0.3–5
Pulmonary embolus	1–4

include diaphoresis, abdominal cramps, palpitations, and watery diarrhea. Late dumping is usually associated with hypoglycemia and hyperinsulinemia. The medical management for dumping symptoms should include dietary modification (increased fiber diet, avoidance of concentrated sweets, and avoidance of hyperosmolar liquids) and, if refractory, a somatostatin analog.

OUTCOMES OF SURGERY

The overall 5-year survival rate of patients with gastric cancer in most Western series is 10% to 21%, which is a consequence of the high proportion of patients who present at an advanced stage. A retrospective study by Hundahl et al. (2000), involving 50,169 gastric carcinoma cases in the United States, demonstrated that 65% of patients present at an advanced stage (T3/T4), with approximately 85% of tumors containing lymph node metastasis at diagnosis. There is a median survival of 24 months (20% to 30% 5-year survival) in patients who undergo surgery with curative intent, a median survival of 8.1 months after palliative procedures, and a median survival of 5.4 months for advanced disease if no interventions are performed. Patients who undergo potentially curative resection (R0) have a slightly better prognosis (5-year survival rate of 24% to 57%), heavily influenced by stage of disease. The 5-year survival rate in patients who undergo curative resection in Japan is reported to be at least 50% and as high as 70% in some series. Overall 5-year survival rates in Japan and the United States by TNM stage are listed in Table 9.5.

To evaluate differences in disease-specific survival after an R0 resection between the East and the West, Strong et al. published a comparison using a previously validated nomogram by Kattan et al. looking at two independent, single-institution prospective databases from the United States (711 patients and Korea, 1,646 patients) (Kattan et al., 2003; Strong et al., 2010). They found significant differences in age, BMI, site of tumor (more proximal in United States), early-stage tumors (more common in Korea), and higher number of lymph nodes identified in Korean patients. After multivariate analysis, the disease-specific survival was still significantly better in Korean patients. The authors noted that it was likely that lower node positivity and early-stage tumors accounted for the differences in disease-specific survival.

Disease recurrence has been analyzed in autopsy, reoperative, and clinical series. In 1982, Gunderson and Sosin analyzed patterns of recurrence in a prospective study of 109 patients who underwent gastric resection and subsequent reoperation at the University of Minnesota. Of the 107 evaluable patients, 86 (80%) had recurrent disease. Locoregional recurrence alone was found in 53.7% of these patients, but if peritoneal seeding was included as a component of recurrence, then

Five-Year Survival Rates After Gastrectomy with Complete Resection and >15 Lymph Nodes Examined

	5-Year Survival Rate (%)			
	United States[a]			
AJCC Stage	**All** **($n = 32,532$)**	**Japanese Americans** **($n = 697$)**	**Japan**[b] **($n = 587$)**	**Germany**[c] **($n = 1,017$)**
IA	78	95	95	86
IB	58	75	86	72
II	34	46	71	47
IIIA	20	48	59	34
IIIB	8	18	35	25
IV	7	5	17	16
Overall	28	42	NR	NR

AJCC, American Joint Committee on Cancer; n, number of patients; NR, not reported.
[a]Data from Hundahl SA, Phillips JL, Menck HR. The National Cancer Data Base Report on poor survival of U.S. gastric carcinoma patients treated with gastrectomy: fifth edition American Joint Committee on Cancer staging, proximal disease, and the "different disease" hypothesis. *Cancer.* 2000;88:921–932.
[b]Data from Ichikura T, Tomimatsu S, Uefuji K, et al. Evaluation of the New American Joint Committee on Cancer/International Union against cancer classification of lymph node metastasis from gastric carcinoma in comparison with the Japanese classification. *Cancer.* 1999;86:553–558.
[c]Data from Roder JO, Bottcher K, Busch R, et al. Classification of regional lymph node metastasis from gastric carcinoma. German Gastric Cancer Study Group. *Cancer.* 1998;82:621–631.

87.8% of the recurrent disease patients (67.3% of total 107) were included. Isolated distant metastases were uncommon but occurred as some component of recurrence in 25.6% of the failure patients.

In 1990, Landry et al. from Massachusetts General Hospital analyzed disease recurrence in 130 patients treated by resection with curative intent. The overall locoregional recurrence rate was 38% (49/130); 21 patients (16%) had locoregional recurrence alone; 28 patients (22%) had locoregional recurrence and distant metastasis; and 39 patients (30%) had distant metastasis alone. However, when viewed only in terms of the 88 (68%) patients in whom treatment failed, locoregional recurrence developed in 57% (49/88). The risk of locoregional recurrence increased with the degree of tumor penetration through the gastric wall. The most frequent sites of locoregional recurrence were the gastric remnant at the anastomosis, the gastric bed, and the regional nodes. The overall incidence of distant metastasis was 52% (67 patients), and the incidence of distant metastasis increased with advancing stage of disease.

In 2004, D'Angelica reported the patterns of recurrence in 1,172 patients who underwent R0 resection at Memorial Sloan-Kettering Cancer Center. At a median follow-up of 22 months, tumor recurrence had developed in 42.3% of the 1,172 patients. In the patients in whom disease recurred, 79% did so within the first 2 years of treatment. Locoregional recurrence was the most frequent (54%), followed by distant (51%) and peritoneal (29%) recurrence. On multivariate analysis, factors predictive of locoregional recurrence were male gender and proximal lesions. The median time to death from the time of recurrence was 6 months. Interestingly, the nodal status and the extent of lymphadenectomy were not associated with locoregional recurrence. Although this analysis identified the recurrence pattern and predictors of recurrence, this retrospective study had some limitations. First, 26% of patients with recurrence did not have a recurrence pattern documented. Second, postoperative follow-up and adjuvant treatments were not consistent. The effect of adjuvant therapy on recurrence was also not evaluated.

Reported factors influencing patterns of recurrence may differ significantly. Youn et al. from Samsung Medical Center in Seoul retrospectively reviewed over 3,800 patients with EGC undergoing curative gastrectomy and found an overall recurrence rate of 2.2% (85 patients). Of these 85 patients with recurrence, 43.5%, 67.1%, and 85.6% were noted after 2, 3, and 5 years of follow-up, respectively. Age, tumor size (but not depth of penetration), number of tumors, N category, and N2 station metastases were predictive factors, and in this study, lymph node metastases was the most significant factor. Another study from Japan looking at more advanced disease demonstrated that early recurrence (within 1 year) was associated with a high level of lymph node metastases (or N2), stage IIIB, and the presence of vascular invasion. On multiple logistic regression analysis, the depth of wall invasion (T3 and above), level of lymph node metastases (N2), and degree of vascular invasion were significantly correlated with early recurrence.

EARLY GASTRIC CANCER

In the early 1960s, the Japanese defined EGC as carcinoma limited to the mucosa and submucosa, regardless of whether there were lymph node metastasis. This pathological classification was based on the high cure rate in this group of patients. In the United States, the proportion of patients with EGC at diagnosis has increased since the mid-1980s to approximately 10% to 15%. In Japan, aggressive screening has resulted in EGC being diagnosed in greater than 50% of Japanese patients. The mean age of patients at diagnosis is 63 years in Western studies, whereas it is 55 years in Japanese studies. Most patients with EGC present with gastrointestinal symptoms similar to those of peptic ulcer disease, including epigastric pain and dyspepsia or even no symptoms.

Endoscopy is critical for the diagnosis of EGC. For example, in collected Western series, although only 22% of EGCs were diagnosed with an upper gastrointestinal tract barium study, 80% were diagnosed with endoscopy. The Japanese have classified EGC pathologically on the basis of gross endoscopic appearance into three basic morphologic types: type I, protruded or polypoid; type II, superficial (IIA, elevated; Iib, flat; and IIc, depressed); and type III, excavated or ulcerated. EGCs include all TNM T1 tumors.

Despite a high potential cure rate, up to 10% to 15% of early gastric tumors may be associated with positive lymph nodes. Therefore, although gastrectomy with D1 or D2 lymphadenectomy generally remains the treatment of choice in Japan, specific criteria have been developed for identifying patients who can be managed safely by EMR. Recognition that tumor size (mucosal area), differentiation, lymphovascular invasion, and submucosal invasion are significant predictors of nodal metastases in patients with T1 tumors has also provided the means of identifying select patients with early tumors who require less aggressive treatment. In 1994, Takekoshi reported the findings from an analysis of cases of EGC from 104 centers in Japan. In particular, analysis of the endoscopic appearance (previously described) of early tumors in patients who underwent mucosal resection enabled the formulation of specific criteria for the mucosal resection of EGCs without submucosal invasion. Subsequent analyses have led to refinements in the criteria that must be met to ensure the safe EMR of AJCC T1 gastric cancers. These are described in the EMR section. Importantly, conventional gastrectomy with at least a D1 lymphadenectomy is mandated if submucosal invasion is found on permanent serial sectioning in a patient after an EMR.

ADJUVANT THERAPY

Patients with localized node-negative gastric cancer have 5-year survival rates approaching 75% when treated with surgery alone (Middleton & Cunningham, 1995). Lymph node involvement, unfortunately, drops this survival to 10% to 30% (Msika et al., 2000). Some form of recurrence develops in most patients who undergo a potentially curative resection for gastric cancer. However, until recently, the studies on both adjuvant and neoadjuvant chemotherapy have produced variable results.

Postoperative Chemotherapy

Randomized trials investigating the effects of adjuvant chemotherapy alone on survival after complete resection of gastric adenocarcinoma have produced inconsistent results. Meta-analyses performed to resolve this issue have also yielded inconsistent findings regarding the impact of postoperative chemotherapy in gastric cancer. There are several meta-analyses suggesting a small advantage to postoperative chemotherapy in the treatment of resected gastric cancer. Earle et al. studied 13 randomized controlled trials of adjuvant chemotherapy versus observation following curative resection of stomach cancer in non-Asian countries and cautiously concluded that adjuvant chemotherapy may produce a small survival benefit of borderline significance in patients with gastric carcinoma resected for cure. Likewise, Mari et al. noted in their 2000 meta-analysis of 20 randomized trials that adjuvant chemotherapy was associated with a survival benefit (hazard ratio [HR] = 0.82, 95% confidence interval [CI] = 0.75–0.89, $P < 0.001$). However, these authors were reluctant to recommend adjuvant chemotherapy in patients with gastric cancer because of the inconsistencies in the findings from meta-analyses. Hu et al. also refused to support their own conclusion that intravenous chemotherapy may have a positive treatment effect on gastric cancer based on the poor quality of the randomized trials in their meta-analysis. In 2002, Janunger conducted a meta-analysis of 21 randomized studies of adjuvant systemic chemotherapy from around the world and found survival duration was significantly better in those who received postoperative chemotherapy than in controls (odds ratio [OR] = 0.84, 95% CI = 0.74–0.96). However, when the data from Asian and Western studies were analyzed separately, no survival benefits were seen for the Western patients treated with chemotherapy (OR = 0.96; 95% CI = 0.83–1.12). Given the flaws in the conduct of some of the randomized trials, the authors noted that the results of their meta-analysis should be interpreted with caution when it came to recommending postoperative chemotherapy in patients with gastric cancer. More recently, a meta-analysis retrieved 31 eligible trials of purely adjuvant chemotherapy for resectable gastric cancer. They examined the 17 randomized controlled trials in which individual patient data were available and accrual was completed before 2004 and found that postoperative adjuvant chemotherapy was associated with a statistically significant reduced risk compared to surgery alone (HR = 0.82; 95% CI = 0.76–0.90; $P < 0.001$) (GASTRIC Group, 2010). With no evidence of statistical difference based on specific regimen grouping, the authors recommended fluorouracil (FU)-based regimens. In one of the largest studies, Japanese investigators randomized stage II and III gastric cancer in patients who underwent gastrectomy plus D2 dissection to adjuvant S-1 for 1 year versus observation and did show a statistically significant higher rate of survival than those receiving surgery alone (Sakuramoto et al., 2007). Overall, given the frequent smaller size of studies, varied regimens used, and concerns with the design and conduct of many studies, there has been a reluctance to recommend any specific adjuvant chemotherapy in Western patients. The conclusions of the meta-analyses are somewhat contradictory and are often subject to the usual criticisms of meta-analyses such as publication bias, differences in patient characteristics, and differences in inclusion and exclusion criteria. More trials may be required before any final recommendations on postoperative chemotherapy for resectable gastric cancer can be made, particularly in Western patients.

Postoperative Radiation Therapy

Gastric cancer is considered by some to be a relatively radioresistant cancer and radiation alone is usually reserved for palliation of advanced disease. One trial randomized patients to surgery alone versus adjuvant external beam radiation therapy versus adjuvant chemotherapy and found no benefit to adjuvant radiation therapy or adjuvant chemotherapy over surgery alone (Hallissey et al., 1994). The consequences of postoperative external beam radiation without chemotherapy at this time are unproven.

Postoperative Chemoradiation Therapy

Most studies of radiation therapy for gastric cancer have examined radiation therapy as an adjuvant to surgery or combined with sensitizing chemotherapy (usually 5-FU). Studies from the Mayo Clinic in the 1960s of low-dose bolus 5-FU with 40 Gy external-beam radiation therapy versus radiation therapy alone showed that combination therapy improved survival. The improvement in survival was attributed to a radiation-sensitizing effect of chemotherapy because the 5-FU dose was relatively low.

Two randomized studies have examined patients assigned to receive no additional therapy or radiation therapy with 5-FU only during radiation, after complete tumor resection. In their 1979 study of 142 patients, Dent et al. found no benefit from this combined regimen, although the findings may have been influenced by the fact that some patients may have had an incomplete resection and the radiation therapy dose was only 20 Gy. In a second study in 1984, Moertel et al. found a benefit to chemotherapy plus radiation therapy, but the study results may have been skewed because 10 patients who were randomized to the experimental arm refused treatment. Nonetheless, interest was generated by this study because the 5-year survival rate was slightly higher and the local recurrence rate was lower in the adjuvant therapy group than in the surgery-only group.

Many investigators believe that the standard of care for patients with resectable gastric cancer has changed in the past 10 years based on the national intergroup trial (INT-0116) initiated by the Southwest Oncology Group that evaluated two cycles of 5-FU and leucovorin followed by radiation therapy with concurrent chemotherapy following R0 resection of gastric adenocarcinoma (MacDonald et al., 2001). More than 600 patients were randomized after confirmation of an R0 resection; of these, 556 were evaluable and were randomly assigned to observation ($n = 275$ patients) or observation with chemoradiation therapy ($n = 281$ patients) consisting of 45 Gy external-beam radiation therapy delivered concurrently with 5-FU and leucovorin. The first cycle used the Mayo Clinic regimen (425 mg/m^2 5-FU and 20 mg/m^2 leucovorin) for four consecutive days, followed by concurrent chemoradiation therapy, with chemotherapy doses decreased at this point and near the end of radiation therapy. One month after the completion of radiation therapy, two additional cycles of 5-FU and leucovorin were given. Three deaths were attributed to the adjuvant therapy (1%), and morbidity was acceptable; however, only 65% of the patients were able to complete the full adjuvant treatment. Nonetheless, adjuvant therapy produced a significant improvement in the disease-free and overall 3-year survival rates. The median survival in the surgery-only group was 27 months, compared with 36 months in the chemoradiation therapy group; the 3-year survival rates were 41% and 52%, respectively. Concerns have been voiced regarding the surgery performed and the high percentage of what are described as D0 lymphadenectomies, with some investigators arguing that the principal benefit of this regimen is that it makes up for suboptimal surgery. Although 54% of patients had what was described as less than a D1 lymphadenectomy, this trial did not demonstrate any difference in overall or relapse-free survival among the three node dissection groups, D0, D1, or D2 ($P = 0.80$).

Since the MacDonald trial, there have been several meta-analyses that looked at various combinations of radiotherapy, chemoradiotherapy, and surgery in reduction of mortality in patients with resectable gastric cancer. Fiorica et al. (2007) found a significant reduction in the 5-year mortality rate when surgery was followed by chemoradiation when compared to surgery alone, but they were cautious to point out that the magnitude of this result was relatively small. Valentini et al. (2009) in their study evaluated radiotherapy (pre-, post-, or intraoperative) compared to surgery alone or surgery with chemotherapy. The authors concluded that radiotherapy treatment had a significant 5-year survival benefit and that subsequent trials should include new conformational radiotherapy technology.

Based on the results of the MacDonald trial, adjuvant chemoradiotherapy has become the standard of care *following* curative resection in North America and serves as the control arm for the current intergroup postoperative therapy study.

NEOADJUVANT THERAPY

The use of neoadjuvant chemotherapy in the treatment of gastric cancer evolved from preoperative treatment strategies used for esophageal and rectal cancers. While several investigators were evaluating preoperative approaches, it was the 1980s report by Wilke et al. that really sparked interest in this treatment. They found impressive results in patients with locally AGC (who were deemed unresectable either clinically or intraoperatively) who underwent R0 resection after receiving systemic preoperative chemotherapy.

There are several potential advantages of neoadjuvant therapy for gastric cancer. These include theoretical biological advantages (decreased tumor seeding at surgery) and the potential opportunity to assess in vivo tumor sensitivity to a chemotherapeutic regimen. If the tumor responds to the neoadjuvant therapy, the same treatment can be continued postoperatively. Another theoretical advantage is an improved R0 resection rate. Patients are generally better able to tolerate intensive chemotherapy preoperatively. As patients do not typically die of their primary tumor, the micrometastases from which they would eventually die are treated early. Finally, the interval required for neoadjuvant therapy provides a time in which to evaluate for progression of disease in those patients with extremely aggressive disease, thus improving patient selection for resection. Additionally an advantage to preoperative radiation therapy is smaller treatment volume and displacement of contiguous structures by the intact tumor leading to reduced radiation therapy toxicity.

A potential disadvantage of neoadjuvant treatment is that patients with initially resectable cancers may progress during therapy rendering them unresectable. Whether this is simply a reflection of extremely aggressive disease as most believe or an actual loss of window of opportunity may not be possible to discern. It is also possible that the toxicity from preoperative treatment may delay operative interventions or increase surgical morbidity. Finally, there is a risk of overtreating patients with early-stage disease although improved pretreatment staging with EUS minimizes this risk.

CHEMOTHERAPY

Various combinations of etoposide, cisplatin, 5-FU (ECF), and doxorubicin as neoadjuvant treatment have been evaluated in several trials. Clinical response rates have ranged from 21% to 31%, and complete pathological response rates have ranged from 0% to 15%. Multivariate analysis of three phase II trials of neoadjuvant therapy at M. D. Anderson (Lowy et al., 1999) revealed that the response to neoadjuvant chemotherapy was the single most important predictor of overall survival after such treatment for gastric cancer.

Survival results of the UK Medical Research Council Adjuvant Gastric Infusion Chemotherapy (MAGIC) trial were reported in 2006 (Cunningham et al., 2006). In this multi-institutional, prospective randomized trial, 503 patients with stage II or higher gastric cancer were randomized to receive perioperative chemotherapy (preoperative chemotherapy followed by surgery followed by additional postoperative chemotherapy) or to undergo surgery alone. Those randomized to the perioperative treatment arm received three cycles of ECF, followed by surgery and then three cycles of ECF. While completion of the preoperative therapy was 88%, only 42% of patients completed the postoperative portion of treatment even though they had up to 12 weeks after surgery to begin. Both progression-free survival and overall survival were improved in the treatment arm ($P < 0.001$ and $P = 0.009$, respectively). The 5-year survival rate was 36% in the treatment plus surgery group and 23% in the surgery-only group. Despite these promising results, the MAGIC trial is not without some criticism. First, the trial included patients with distal esophageal cancers, which may affect the results of the trial. Second, the staging in this trial may have been suboptimal due to lack of EUS or staging laparoscopy. Finally, only 40% of patients had a D2 resection. Nevertheless, the positive impact in survival was very similar to that seen in the intergroup trial discussed above and these results were reproduced in a French trial which confirmed that preoperative FU and cisplatin improved disease-free and 5-year overall survival (Boige et al., 2007).

RADIATION

There are several older studies that looked at preoperative radiation in resectable gastric cancer. Skoropad et al. (2002) published a 20-year follow-up on their randomized trial of surgery alone or with 20 Gy of radiotherapy. There was no significant change in survival. Zhang et al. (1998) published on a prospective randomized trial on preoperative radiotherapy versus surgery alone in 370 patients with advanced gastric cardia adenocarcinoma. They found significant improvements in resection rate, pathologic stage after resection, and lymph node metastases; however, inclusion of only gastric cardia patients makes this difficult to extrapolate to distal tumors. It is unlikely that future studies will evaluate radiation alone as the current focus seems to incorporate chemotherapy with radiation.

CHEMORADIATION

The approach to gastric adenocarcinoma at M. D. Anderson has been largely to deliver chemotherapy and chemoradiation therapy preoperatively, except in selected patients with very early-stage cancers. Multimodality neoadjuvant therapy combining chemotherapy with external-beam radiation therapy is continuing to be studied.

In 2004, Ajani et al. demonstrated that a pathological complete response (30%) can be achieved through a three-step approach in patients with localized gastric adenocarcinoma. In this trial, 28 of 34 patients received induction chemotherapy (5-FU [200 mg/m^2/day], leucovorin [20 mg/m^2], and cisplatin [20 mg/m^2/day]), followed by chemoradiation therapy (45 Gy plus concurrent 5-FU) and gastrectomy. R0 resection was achieved in 70% of patients, and a complete pathological response was noted in 30%. At a median follow-up of 50 months, the median survival was 33.7 months, and 2-year survival rate was 54%. There were two treatment-related deaths. This trial also demonstrated that a pathological response to treatment is associated with a significant survival benefit.

In an attempt to discern whether it is the pathological response to preoperative chemotherapy, and not pretreatment parameters, that determine a patient's outcome, Ajani et al. (2005) reported a prospective nonrandomized study of preoperative paclitaxel-based chemoradiation therapy. In this analysis, 43 patients received two cycles of 5-FU, cisplatin, and paclitaxel for 28 days, followed by chemoradiation therapy. The radiation regimen included 25 fractions of 1.8 Gy up to a total dose of 45 Gy. Then, patients underwent gastrectomy with spleen-preserving D2 lymphadenectomy after radiographic and endoscopic restaging. At the time of analysis, 78% of patients had undergone an R0 resection, 20% had had a complete pathological response, and 15% had had a partial pathological response. In this study, R0 resection ($P < 0.001$), pathological complete response ($P = 0.02$), pathological partial response ($P = 0.006$), and postsurgical T and N status ($P = 0.01$ and $P < 0.001$, respectively) were factors associated with overall survival. This was followed by a multi-institutional study, in 2006, evaluating two cycles of FU, leucovorin, and cisplatin followed by concurrent radiation and chemotherapy (infusional FU and weekly paclitaxel). The pathologic complete response rate was 26% with a R0 resection rate of 77%. Although the authors acknowledged the importance of pretreatment parameters in the staging of gastric cancer, pathological response was a major determinant of outcome. Attempts to compare preoperative and postoperative therapies, while attractive, have met with resistance.

In summary, current trials of neoadjuvant chemotherapy and chemoradiation therapy are yielding promising results; however, these results need to be validated in the setting of large, prospective randomized trials. The current existing trials are insufficient to draw definitive conclusions. There are a number of ongoing trials including the MAGIC-B examining the addition of bevacizumab to perioperative chemotherapy; the CALGB 80101 evaluating a postoperative regimen of ECF followed by chemoradiation, followed by additional ECF; the Dutch Gastric Cancer Group CRITICS is studying the addition of postoperative chemo-radiation to ECX; and the SAKK trial in which patients with resectable gastric cancer were randomly assigned to docetaxel, cisplatin, and 5-FU either before or after operative intervention. These trials will yield important information regarding the multimodal treatment of gastric cancer.

Intraoperative Radiation Therapy

Most of the data available on intraoperative radiation therapy (IORT) for gastric cancer comes from the 1981 report of Abe and Takahashi from Japan. In a prospective nonrandomized trial, these authors compared 110 patients treated with surgery alone with 84 patients treated with surgery plus IORT. The 5-year survival rates were similar in patients with stage I disease; however, a suggestion of a survival benefit from IORT was seen in patients with stage II, III, or IV disease. In contrast, a small (<40 patients) randomized study of IORT done at the National Cancer Institute showed neither a disease-free nor an overall survival benefit from IORT, despite a marked decrease in the frequency of locoregional recurrence. In 2001, Lowy et al. described a pilot study of preoperative chemoradiation therapy combined with IORT for resectable gastric cancer done at M. D. Anderson in which 24 patients were treated with 45 Gy external-beam radiation therapy and concurrent infusional 5-FU (300 mg/m^2). Patients were restaged 4 to 6 weeks after completing treatment and, if free of disease, underwent resection and IORT (10 Gy). Several findings were of significant interest. Twenty-three (96%) of the 24 patients completed their chemoradiation therapy, a rate significantly higher than that seen in trials of postoperative adjuvant therapy. Four patients had progression of disease and did not undergo resection; the remaining 19 patients underwent resection with D2 lymphadenectomy and IORT. The morbidity and mortality rates were acceptable (32% and one death, respectively). Of the patients who underwent resection, two (11%) had complete pathological responses and 12 (63%) had significant pathological evidence of a treatment effect. Other studies of IORT have generally examined it in combination with other therapies (see Management of Advanced Disease).

MANAGEMENT OF ADVANCED DISEASE

Many patients (20% to 30%) present with obvious stage IV disease, and an additional 28% to 37% initially believed to have localized disease are found to have metastatic disease after complete staging. The 5-year survival rate for patients with stage IV disease approaches zero—hence, a large percentage of newly diagnosed gastric cancer patients are incurable. Because of this advanced disease stage at presentation and the overall low cure rate for gastric cancer, in many patients, palliation is an essential component of gastric cancer management. An appropriate understanding and use of palliative techniques is therefore essential. It is critical in any consideration of palliative therapy to separate true palliation from what can best be defined as expectant palliation or relieving symptoms that the patient may or may not eventually develop. Many investigators and clinicians often blur the distinction.

Optimal palliation relieves or abates symptoms, while causing minimal morbidity and improving the patient's quality of life. Prolonged survival is generally not a goal of palliative treatment, but palliation may relieve debilitating and potentially life-threatening problems, such as gastrointestinal bleeding or gastric outlet obstruction, which may acutely impact survival.

Palliative Surgery

Surgical palliation of AGC may include resection or bypass alone or in combination with other interventions. Complete staging is required for determination of the best palliative approach.

Palliation by endoscopic means may be appropriate for patients with peritoneal disease, hepatic metastases, extensive nodal metastases, or ascites and for patients with problems that include bleeding or proximal or distal gastric obstruction. Both morbidity and mortality are relatively high in these patients with a short life expectancy. Laser recanalization or simple dilatation with or without stent placement can be used to treat obstruction. Repeat endoscopy may be required at periodic intervals. Patients who undergo stent placement for gastric outlet obstruction are frequently able to eat solid or semisolid food for a short period of time and may not require any further intervention before death. Though stents carry their own complications, their use should be considered carefully.

The selection of patients for palliative resection is complex. In patients with an excellent performance status, experienced surgeons can perform palliative distal gastrectomy with minimal morbidity and acceptable mortality rates. Palliative total gastrectomy and esophagogastrectomy, however, should be approached with great caution because the morbidity from these procedures is higher. One also needs to be aware that surgery may not achieve good palliation. In 2004, Miner et al. retrospectively reviewed patients who underwent R1 or R2 resections and divided them into palliative (R1/R2) resections and nonpalliative resections (R1/R2). They reported a perioperative mortality rate of 7% associated with palliative resections versus 4% associated with nonpalliative resections; the median survival was 8.3 and 13.5 months, respectively ($P < 0.001$).

Specific indications for palliative resection, surgical bypass (open or laparoscopic), and endoscopic palliation remain undefined. However, assessment of morbidity, mortality, and quality of life has revealed that carefully selected patients may benefit from palliative resection. While palliative bypass may work in some patients, an equal or larger percent will fail to benefit. Advanced endoscopic techniques, including laser or argon-beam tumor ablation and endoscopic placement of coated metallic stents, provide better palliation of dysphagia than surgical bypass with lower morbidity. Multimodality therapy consisting of radiotherapy, surgery, and endoscopy is likely to lead to improvements in quality of life and lower morbidity with palliative therapy. Additionally, the employment of surgical approaches in these patients should be considered against the backdrop that many patients with some symptoms, particularly dysphagia, will have them improve with systemic therapy. However, earlier diagnosis and advances in curative therapy are ultimately the only way in which the high incidence of morbidity associated with advanced disease in patients with gastric adenocarcinoma will definitively be reduced.

Palliative Chemotherapy

Historically, investigators have debated the role of chemotherapy versus that of best supportive care. As a result, four randomized trials have been conducted to assess the impact of combination chemotherapy on survival and quality of life. The combination regimens included FAMTX (5-FU, doxorubicin, and high-dose methotrexate), FEMTX (5-FU, epirubicin, and high-dose methotrexate), and ELF (etoposide, leucovorin, and 5-FU). Patients who received combination chemotherapy had both better survival (3 to 9 months) and quality of life than did patients given best supportive care. Despite these benefits, the outcome from AGC remains poor.

Palliative Radiation Therapy

There are several isolated case reports describing the benefit of radiation therapy for the palliative treatment of advanced gastric carcinoma. However, no large prospective trial has demonstrated a long-term benefit from radiation therapy alone in patients with advanced disease. This modality is most likely best used in combination with chemotherapy, as described previously in this chapter.

Intraperitoneal Hyperthermic Perfusion

Intraperitoneal hyperthermic perfusion has been examined in several trials as a treatment for AGC. In 1988, Koga et al. reviewed their experience with a combination of hyperthermia and mitomycin C as treatment for patients with peritoneal recurrence of gastric cancer. These researchers reported that this procedure was technically feasible and safe. In 1990, Fujimoto et al. evaluated 59 patients with AGC who underwent gastrectomy and were then randomly assigned to receive either no further therapy or intraperitoneal hyperthermic perfusion. The patients treated with perfusion survived longer than did the controls (1-year survival rate of 80% vs. 34%). A significant survival benefit was also seen in patients with peritoneal seeding who underwent perfusion with hyperthermic mitomycin C. Similarly, Yonemura et al. (1996) reported that adjuvant hyperthermic intraperitoneal chemotherapy with mitomycin C, etoposide, and cisplatin after gastric resection in patients with peritoneal seeding resulted in complete response in 8 (19%) of 43 patients and partial responses in 9 (21%) of 43 patients. A randomized trial conducted by Yu in patients who were treated at the time of complete resection of tumors that penetrated the gastric serosa but had no evidence of peritoneal metastases showed that hyperthermic intraperitoneal chemotherapy with mitomycin C led to a reduced incidence of peritoneal recurrence and a small survival advantage at 3 years. In 2005, Yonemura et al. prospectively reviewed 107 patients with peritoneal dissemination from gastric adenocarcinoma. Over a 10-year period, 65 patients underwent cytoreductive surgery in combination with intraperitoneal hyperthermic perfusion before 1995, and 42 patients underwent cytoreductive surgery in combination with intraperitoneal hyperthermic perfusion with peritonectomy after 1995. The perfusion regimen included mitomycin C, cisplatin, and etoposide. Complete cytoreductive surgery was achieved in 43% of 107 patients. There was a 21% postoperative complication rate, and there were three postoperative deaths (all in the peritonectomy group), accounting for 7% of the patients in this group. At a median follow-up of 46 months, the 5-year survival rates in those who had complete and incomplete cytoreductive surgery were 13% and 2%, respectively ($P < 0.001$), with a median survival of 19 and 7.8 months, respectively. Furthermore, the 5-year survival rate for patients who underwent cytoreductive surgery by peritonectomy was 27% ($P < 0.001$). Multivariate analysis showed that complete cytoreductive surgery ($P = 0.010$) and peritonectomy ($P = 0.012$) were associated with a more favorable outcome. However, peritonectomy was also associated with higher postoperative morbidity (43%) and mortality (7%) rates.

More recently, Yang et al. conducted a randomized phase III study to evaluate the efficacy and safety of cytoreductive surgery plus hyperthermic intraperitoneal chemotherapy with cisplatin and mitomycin C for peritoneal carcinomatosis from gastric cancer (Yang, 2010). They reported a small but significant survival advantage with acceptable mortality when compared with cytoreduction alone. A French collaborative effort by Glehen et al. (2010) was the largest cohort of peritoneal carcinomatosis patients. With a median follow-up of 20.4 months overall median survival was 9.2 months, not that dissimilar from survival of low-volume patients with chemotherapy. They did note a 5-year survival of 13%. For those patients with complete macroscopic resection 5-year actuarial survival was 23% and median survival was 15 months. Interestingly, in the manuscript the survival curves do not actually go all the way to 5 years. Unfortunately, the study does not report the actual number of patients alive or evaluable at the various time points, thereby precluding meaningful evaluation. Furthermore, even among the patients with a complete cytoreduction it appears that only a handful of patients who had low-volume disease even survived past 2 years. This coupled with the fact that it took 15 centers over 18 years to accrue 159 patients suggests an enormous selection bias. It should be noted that this survival does not appear to be much better than similar patients receiving systemic therapy and it comes at a high price. Operative mortality was 6.5%, with 14% of patients having to be taken back to the OR and 16% of patients developing a fistula. Median hospitalization was 3.5 weeks, not an insignificant amount of time for the vast majority of patients with this disease who have a limited survival time. Other centers have not found such encouraging results. This technique is currently under investigation in a few centers around the world.

In summary, there is no standard treatment for patients with peritoneal carcinomatosis stemming from gastric adenocarcinoma other than systemic chemotherapy. Cytoreductive surgery and intraperitoneal chemotherapy may be of benefit in selected patients; however, the overall survival in these patients remains dismal and such procedures are associated with significant morbidity and mortality. Further investigation will be required to clarify the role of cytoreductive surgery and intraperitoneal therapy in this setting. We believe that this technique should not be considered outside of a formal clinical trial and that while a very small handful of patients might benefit from this approach, it may harm more patients than it helps.

SURVEILLANCE

We typically see patients every 3 months for the first 2 years following curative resection of gastric adenocarcinoma. At each follow-up, a careful history and physical examination are performed, along with laboratory studies (complete blood cell count liver function tests, chemistry, prealbumin, and vitamin B12 and vitamin D levels) Chest radiographs are obtained every 6 months, and abdominal and pelvic CT is performed every 6 months after surgery for 2 years and then yearly thereafter. It is important to balance patients' needs for nutritional evaluation and the radiographic and laboratory testing done with the likely ability to benefit a patient who does have a recurrence. In patients who have undergone a subtotal gastrectomy, endoscopy should be considered at the end of the first postsurgical year, once more the following year, and then will likely need not be repeated until the patient is

5 years out. Patients who receive protocol-based therapy often have more frequent staging studies, but this has never been proven to impact patient survival. Perhaps the most important reasons to follow patients closely are to enable any postgastrectomy sequelae to be dealt with and to acquire accurate recurrence and survival data on patients in clinical trials.

GASTRIC LYMPHOMA

Two-thirds of gastrointestinal lymphomas occur in the stomach and the worldwide incidence of gastric lymphoma is steadily increasing. Approximately 3,000 new cases are diagnosed annually each year in the United States. The median age of diagnosis is 60 years and the disease affects an equal number of men and women. Lymphomas of the stomach are generally non-Hodgkin lymphomas and represent an estimated 5% of primary gastric malignancies. The two primary histologic types are low-grade marginal zone B-cell lymphomas of the MALT-type and high-grade diffuse large B-cell lymphoma (DLBCL); the latter contains a low-grade MALT component in approximately one-third of cases. Whether high-grade lymphomas derive from MALT lymphomas remains unresolved; however, pathogenesis for both is frequently attributed to chronic gastritis and infection with *H. pylori*. The initial symptomatology of gastric lymphoma is often nonspecific and delay in diagnosis is common. The most frequent symptoms at the time of presentation are pain (68%), weight loss (28%), bleeding (28%), and fatigue (16%). Obstruction, perforation, and massive bleeding, while they can occur, are uncommon.

Diagnosis is established with upper endoscopic evaluation and biopsy. Multiple biopsies should be taken in each region of the stomach, duodenum, GEJ, and all suspicious lesions should be sampled. Endoscopic ultrasound is of modest utility in determining the depth of invasion and the presence of involved perigastric lymph nodes but likely has no impact on treatment decisions. The presence of *H. pylori* must be determined through histopathology, urease enzyme levels (breath test), and serology. Laboratory evaluation includes lactate dehydrogenase and beta-2-microglobulin levels as well as bone marrow aspiration and biopsy. The extent of disease is assessed with axial imaging of the chest, abdomen, and pelvis.

Initial therapy for early-stage, low-grade MALT lymphoma consists of regimens of antibiotics and proton pump inhibitors for the eradication of *H. pylori* and results in long-term remission in 60% to 100% of patients. Diligent endoscopic surveillance is required to monitor for treatment response and recurrence. Disappearance of the lymphoma takes several months. There is evidence that patients with limited residual disease may be safely observed, illustrating the indolent course of this disease. For patients with stage I and stage II MALT lymphomas persistent after *H. pylori* therapy or those without evidence of *H. pylori* infection, external beam radiation therapy (30 Gy) has a 90% to 100% rate of complete response and results in durable remission in a majority of patients. Alternatively, single-agent chemotherapy or rituximab (anti-CD20 monoclonal antibody) may be administered if radiation is contraindicated or may be preferential to receiving radiotherapy since that may impact future treatment options should a patient subsequently develop a gastric or GEJ adenocarcinoma (which we have seen on several occasions). Combination chemotherapy, often combined with rituximab, is reserved for patients with GI bleeding, bulky local disease, or progressive systemic disease.

The treatment of high-grade gastric DLBCL varies among institutions and typically consists of aggressive anthracycline-based combination chemotherapy: epirubicin, Adriamycin, or mitoxantrone combined with cyclophosphamide, vincristine, and prednisone (CHOP, CEOP, or CNOP). Rituximab has not been extensively studied in gastric lymphoma but is typically included because of its proven efficacy in nodal DLBCL. In patients with gastric DLBCL containing a low-grade MALT component, *H. Pylori* eradication can result in complete response and sustained remission. The role of consolidation radiotherapy remains unclear. Retrospective studies suggest that patients with localized disease (stages I and II) may have lower local relapse rates with the addition of consolidation radiotherapy. The development of these regimens has resulted in a significant improvement in overall survival rates. Patients who relapse are treated with high-dose chemotherapy followed by autologous stem-cell transplantation. Gastrectomy may be suitable for patients with limited relapse and contraindications to salvage chemotherapy.

In a previous era, surgery played a central role in the acquisition of diagnostic information and was believed to be an important component of therapy for gastric lymphoma. With the refinements in axial imaging and recognition that for most patients systemic therapy is indicated, surgical staging is now obsolete. Several retrospective and prospective trials over the last two decades have compared surgical and nonsurgical management of early-stage gastric lymphoma and collectively demonstrated no compromise in survival with nonsurgical treatment. Furthermore, these studies addressed several theoretical concerns regarding nonsurgical therapy, revealing that perforation and GI bleeding rarely occur. Primary surgical resection for gastric lymphomas has a proven record of excellent oncologic outcomes but has been abandoned because conservative therapies result in superior quality of life and fewer treatment-related complications with comparable oncologic outcomes. Currently, the most common indications for surgical intervention in gastric lymphoma include bleeding, perforation, obstruction, and the rare finding of localized residual disease after primary therapy.

GASTRIC NEUROENDOCRINE TUMORS

When Oberndorfer coined the term "carcinoid" in 1907, the designation reflected the belief that these tumors had a uniformly indolent behavior. After a century of investigation, it is clear that neuroendocrine cells throughout the body give rise to neoplasms of varying morphology and clinical behavior. As such, the World Health Organization classification of 2000 utilizes the term NET and presented a classification scheme to better categorize and define these fascinating, heterogeneous neoplasms.

Gastric NETs constitute approximately 6% of all NETs. Population-based studies indicate that the incidence of gastric NETs increased 10-fold over the last 35 years and is currently 3.0/1,000,000 persons/year in the United States. This is partially attributed to the increasing use of endoscopy. Incidental NETs are being detected more frequently while the proportion of patients with advanced tumor stages at diagnosis has decreased. The current 5-year survival of patients with gastric NETs has increased to 71% from 51% in the 1970s. Four distinct clinicopathologic categories of gastric NETs have been described.

Type 1 gastric NETs are the most frequent, accounting for 70% to 80% of all cases. Typically these are asymptomatic, small (usually <1 cm), well-differentiated, multifocal tumors. The majority of patients are women (70% to 80%) and the condition develops in the setting of chronic atrophic gastritis and enterochromaffin-like (ECL) cell hyperplasia. These patients have elevated plasma gastrin levels and low gastric acid production. Regional lymph node metastases occur rarely and usually only in larger tumors that penetrate the muscularis propria. Endoscopic resection is the treatment of choice for small tumors (<2 cm). Surgical excision or resection is considered for larger or more invasive tumors. Type 1 tumors have a tendency to recur and require endoscopic surveillance. Nevertheless, these patients have an excellent prognosis with 5- and 10-year survivals that are comparable to the general population.

Type 2 gastric NETs account for 5% to 6% of gastric endocrine tumors and occur in the association with multiple endocrine neoplasia type 1 (MEN-1)-associated Zollinger–Ellison syndrome (ZES). These tumors rarely develop in sporadic ZES patients (<0.1%); in contrast, 15% to 30% of MEN-1/ZES patients develop type 2 gastric NETs. The disease tends to develop late in the course (15 to 20 years) of MEN-1/ZES disease. The tumors are typically well-differentiated, multifocal, small (<1.5 cm), and limited to the mucosa/submucosa. ECL hyperplasia is common. These patients have elevated plasma gastrin levels and high gastric acid production. In tumors larger than 2 cm and/or invading the muscularis propria, regional lymph node spread or metastatic disease may be present in up to 30% of patients. Therapy is directed toward localizing and removing the source of hypergastrinemia; most commonly this requires local excision of a duodenal gastrinoma(s) or pancreaticoduodenectomy. Somatostatin analogs are used to inhibit tumor growth, particularly in patients in whom hypergastrinemia cannot be surgically corrected. Resection of type 2 NETS is reserved for tumors with suspicious or proven signs of malignancy. Type 2 gastric NET patients have 5-year survival rates of 60% to 75%.

Between 14% and 25% of gastric NETs are type 3. These are more aggressive sporadic neoplasms that are not associated with ECL hyperplasia, hypergastrinemia, or any other disease of the stomach. There is a predilection for the male sex. The tumors tend to be solitary, historically large (3 to 5 cm), and are well-differentiated. Plasma gastrin levels and gastric acid production are usually within normal limits (though the use of PPIs may impact this and should be accounted for during evaluation). Penetration of the muscularis propria is common and invasion of all layers of the gastric wall is seen in approximately 50% of patients. Metastases are present in greater than 50% of patients with larger lesions. Treatment has been similar to gastric adenocarcinoma and consists of extirpative surgery and possible chemotherapy. Recently more patients with small type 3 lesions are being seen and a reconsideration of the extent of required surgery is being discussed. Because of the generally favorable biology, aggressive surgical or ablative therapies should be considered even in patients with metastatic disease. The 5-year survival is no better than 50%.

Type 4 gastric NET is the newest classification and accounts for 6% to 8% of gastric NETs. These tumors occur more frequently in men and consist of highly malignant, poorly differentiated (small cell) neuroendocrine carcinoma. Patients commonly present at an advanced stage with large (>5 cm), often ulcerated primary masses exhibiting local invasion and frequently disseminated metastases. As such, surgical intervention is rarely appropriate but may be considered in the rare event of localized disease. Median survival is less than 1 year.

Recently, everolimus has been demonstrated to have significant impact on the survival of patients with pancreatic NETs. While it has not been approved for the indication of gastric NET and there is no conclusive data to support it, this may be a potential treatment option for some patients with gastric NET (Yao et al., 2011).

The range of clinicopathologic behavior of gastric NETs is diverse. Accordingly, the management recommendations vary. Several general points are worth noting. For type 1 and 2 gastric NETs, surgical resection is recommended for NETs greater than 2 to 3 cm in diameter because of the heightened risk of invasion and metastasis. Because of the indolent nature of type 1 and type 2 gastric NETs, nonsurgical management may be preferable in the elderly or infirm. Somatostatin analogs can mediate the regression of small (<1 cm) gastric NETs and may also prevent recurrence after resection. When complete cytoreduction is feasible, aggressive surgical and/or ablative therapy may be considered in carefully selected type 1, 2, and 3 patients with metastatic disease.

GASTROINTESTINAL STROMAL TUMORS OF THE STOMACH

Approximately 4,000 to 6,000 new cases of GISTs are diagnosed annually in the United States each year. These rare neoplasms arise from the interstitial cells of Cajal and are the most common mesenchymal tumors of the gastrointestinal tract. GISTs occur most frequently in the stomach (60 to 70%). The most common presenting symptoms include bleeding (53%), abdominal pain or fullness (32%), and palpable mass (13%). Greater than 50% of patients undergoing surgical resection alone of a primary GIST will recur within 5 years. The Miettinen–Lasota/AFIP risk stratification system summarizes the known prognostic factors for relapse including large tumor size, high mitotic index, and primary tumor site. Gastric GISTs have favorable outcomes compared to GISTs of the small bowel or rectum.

Microscopic GISTs of the stomach (0.2 to 10 mm) are a newly recognized entity. These lesions have been identified incidentally in up to a third of resected stomach specimens removed for carcinoma and autopsy series of patients greater than 50 years of age. While all GISTs are considered to have malignant potential, the majority of microscopic GISTs will not progress to clinically relevant malignancy. Consensus guidelines recommend annual endoscopic surveillance for gastric GISTs less than 2 cm in size in the absence of symptoms or worrisome features.

Surgical resection remains the primary therapy for GISTs at any location. Principles of surgery for primary gastric GISTs have been defined and simple wedge resection is favored. For tumors located near the lesser curvature, segmental gastric resection is occasionally required to prevent luminal narrowing. A resection margin of 1 to 2 cm is generally deemed sufficient. Routine lymphadenectomy is not recommended because lymphatic metastases are extremely rare. Although long-term survival data remains limited, laparoscopic resection of gastric GISTs is considered technically feasible and is associated with shorter hospital stays. Laparoscopic resection of tumors >8 cm remains very controversial.

Therapy for GISTs has been revolutionized by the development of tyrosine kinase inhibitors (TKI) such as imatinib (IM) and sunitinib. As such, the optimal surgical management of GISTs has become increasingly complex and should be approached in a multidisciplinary setting. Neoadjuvant therapy with a TKI is recommended if the need for multivisceral resection is anticipated; a significant response may decrease the extent of resection required, diminish the vascularity of the tumor, and facilitate the achievement of an R0 resection. Total gastrectomy is rarely required as it was in the past and should not be undertaken without a trial of TKI therapy. Less than 5% of patients develop progressive disease during neoadjuvant therapy and objective responses may be seen in up to 60% of patients. Patients are typically treated until maximal response is achieved and may continue treatment up to the date of surgery without any apparent increase in surgical morbidity or mortality. In the ACOSOG Z9001 trial, adjuvant IM improved 1-year recurrence-free survival from 83% to 98% in patients with intermediate to high-risk GISTs. Ongoing studies of adjuvant IM will clarify issues of patient selection and optimal duration of therapy. Prior to the development of TKIs, it had been reported that the occasional patient undergoing complete (R0) metastasectomy could achieve long-term survival. Patients with metastatic disease are now treated with TKIs as first-line therapy and, remarkably, have an approximately 50% 5-year survival. It is suspected that surgical resection in selected patients may further enhance disease control in this setting. Retrospective studies have demonstrated that patients with metastatic GISTs with responding or stable disease after TKI have favorable outcomes after metastasectomy and should be evaluated for surgical resection. TKI therapy should be continued indefinitely after metastasectomy; prompt recurrence is almost a certainty in the absence of TKI, even after resection of all visible disease.

CONCLUSION

Strides are being made in the treatment of gastric cancer. Although several diagnostic modalities are available for staging gastric cancer and ongoing trials of neoadjuvant treatment are yielding promising results, better systemic agents and better-designed trials are still needed. Despite the current progress, the outcome in most patients with all but EGC generally remains poor. As we enter the era of targeted therapy, it is imperative that such therapy also be developed for gastric cancer and that molecular predictors are identified to help in selecting appropriate treatment for patients. However, for the foreseeable future surgery will continue to play an essential role in the diagnosis, staging, and treatment of gastric cancer.

Recommended Readings

Abe M, Takahashi M. Intraoperative radiotherapy: the Japanese experience. *Int J Radiat Oncol Biol Phys.* 1981;7(7):863–868.

Ajani JA, Mansfield PF, Crane CH. Paclitaxel-based chemoradiotherapy in localized gastric carcinoma: degree of pathologic response and not clinical parameters dictated patient outcome. *J Clin Oncol.* 2005;23:1237–1244.

Ajani JA, Mansfield PF, Janjan J, et al. Multi-institutional trials of preoperative chemoradiotherapy in patients with potentially resectable gastric carcinoma. *J Clin Oncol.* 2004;22:2274–2280.

Ajani JA, Mansfield PF, Lynch PM, et al. Enhanced staging and all chemotherapy preoperatively in patients with potentially resectable gastric carcinoma. *J Clin Oncol.* 1999;17:2403–2411.

Ajani JA, Ota DM, Jessup JM, et al. Resectable gastric carcinoma. An evaluation of preoperative and postoperative chemotherapy. *Cancer.* 1991;68:1501–1506.

Amano Y, Ishihara S, Amano K, et al. An assessment of local curability of endoscopic surgery in early gastric cancer without satisfaction of current therapeutic indications. *Endoscopy.* 1998;30(6):548–552.

Bennett C, Wang Y, Pan T. Endoscopic mucosal resection for early gastric cancer. *Cochrane Database Sys Rev.* 2009;4:CD004276.

Boige V, Pignon J, Saint-Aubert B, et al. Final results of a randomized trial comparing preoperative 5-fluorouracil/cisplatin to surgery alone in adenocarcinoma of the stomach and lower esophagus (ASLE):FNLCC ACCORD01-FFCD 0703 trial. *J Clin Oncol.* 2007; ASCO Annual Meeting Proceedings Par I:25(suppl 18):4510.

Bonenkamp JJ, Hermans J, Sasako M, et al. Extended lymph-node dissection for gastric cancer. Dutch Gastric Cancer Group. *N Engl J Med.* 1999;340:908–914.

Bonenkamp JJ, Songun I, Hermans J, et al. Randomised comparison of morbidity after D1 and D2 dissection for gastric cancer in 996 Dutch patients. *Lancet.* 1995;345:745–748.

Bozzetti F, Bonfanti G, Bufalino R, et al. Adequacy of margins of resection in gastrectomy for cancer. *Ann Surg.* 1982;196:685–690.

Bozzetti F, Marubini E, Bonfanti G, et al. Total versus subtotal gastrectomy: surgical morbidity and mortality rates in multicenter Italian randomized trial. The Italian Gastrointestinal Tumor Study Group. *Ann Surg.* 1997;226:613.

Burke EC, Karpeh MS, Conlon KC, et al. Laparoscopy in the management of gastric adenocarcinoma. *Ann Surg.* 1997;225:262–267.

Burke EC, Karpeh MS, Conlon KC, et al. Peritoneal lavage cytology in gastric cancer: an independent predictor of outcome. *Ann Surg Oncol.* 1998;5:411–415.

Cady B, Rossi RL, Silverman ML, et al. Gastric adenocarcinoma. A disease in transition. *Arch Surg.* 1989;124:303–308.

Conlon KC, Karpeh MS. Laparoscopy and laparoscopic ultrasound in the staging of gastric cancer. *Semin Oncol.* 1996;23:347–351.

Correa P. *Helicobacter pylori* and gastric cancer: state of the art. *Cancer Epidemiol Biomarkers Prev.* 1996;5(6):477–481.

Correa P, Shiao YH. Phenotypic and genotypic events in gastric carcinogenesis. *Cancer Res.* 1994;54:1941s–1943s.

Crew KD, Neugut AI. Epidemiology of upper gastrointestinal malignancies. *Semin Oncol.* 2004;31:450–464.

Csendes A, Burdiles P, Rojas J, et al. A prospective randomized study comparing D2 total gastrectomy versus D2 total gastrectomy plus splenectomy in 187 patients with gastric carcinoma. *Surgery.* 2002;131:401–407.

Cunningham D, Allum WH, Stenning SP, et al. Perioperative chemotherapy versus surgery alone for resectable gastroesophageal cancer. *N Engl J Med.* 2006;355(1): 11–20.

Cuschieri A, Weeden S, Fielding J, et al. Patient survival after D1 and D2 resections for gastric cancer: long-term results of the MRC randomized surgical trial. Surgical Cooperative Group. *Br J Cancer.* 1999;79:1522–1530.

D'Angelica M, Gonen M, Brennan M, et al. Pattern of initial recurrence in completely resected gastric adenocarcinoma. *Ann Surg.* 2004;240:808–816.

D'Ugo DM, Pende V, Persiani R, et al. Laparoscopic staging of gastric cancer: an overview. *J Am Coll Surg.* 2003;196(6):965–974.

Dean C, Yeo MS, Soe MY, et al. Cancer of the gastric cardia is rising in incidence in an Asian population and is associated with adverse outcome. *World J Surg.* 2011; 35(3):617–624.

Deguili M, Sasako M, Ponti A, et al. Morbidity and mortality in the Italian Gastric Cancer Study Group randomized clinical trial of D1 versus D2 resection for gastric cancer. *Br J Surg.* 2010;97:643–649.

Dematteo RP, Ballman KV, Antonescu CR, et al. Adjuvant imatinib mesylate after resection of localized, primary gastrointestinal stromal tumour: a randomized, double-blind, placebo-controlled trial. *Lancet.* 2009;373(9669):1097–1104.

Dent DM, Madden MV, Price SK. Randomized comparison of R1 and R2 gastrectomy for gastric carcinoma. *Br J Surg.* 1988;75(2):110–112.

Dent DM, Werner ID, Novis B, et al. Prospective randomized trial of combined oncological therapy for gastric carcinoma. *Cancer.* 1979;44:385–391.

Dresner SM, Lamb PJ, Bennett MK, et al. The pattern of metastatic lymph node dissemination from adenocarcinoma of the esophagogastric junction. *Surgery.* 2001;129:103–109.

Earle CC, Maroun JA. Adjuvant chemotherapy after curative resection for gastric cancer in non-Asian patients: revisiting a meta-analysis of randomised trials. *Eur J Cancer.* 1999;35:1059–1064.

Eguchi T, Gotoda T, Oda I, et al. Is endoscopic one-piece mucosal resection essential for early gastric cancer? *Digestive Endoscopy.* 2003;15:113–116.

Ell C, May A. Self-expanding metal stents for palliation of stenosing tumors of the esophagus and cardia: a critical review. *Endoscopy.* 1997;29:392–398.

Estape J, Grau JJ, Alcobendas F, et al. Mitomycin C as an adjuvant treatment to resected gastric cancer. A 10-year follow-up. *Ann Surg.* 1991;213:219–221.

Fiorica F, Cartei F, Enea M, et al. The impact of radiotherapy on survival in resectable gastric carcinoma: a meta-analysis of literature data. *Cancer Treat Rev.* 2007; 33(8):729–740.

Fujii K, Isozaki H, Okajima K, et al. Clinical evaluation of lymph node metastasis in gastric cancer defined by the fifth edition of the TNM classification in comparison with the Japanese system. *Br J Surg.* 1999; 86:685–689.

Fujimoto S, Shrestha RD, Kokubun M, et al. Positive results of combined therapy of surgery and intraperitoneal hyperthermic perfusion for far-advanced gastric cancer. *Ann Surg.* 1990;212:592–596.

GASTRIC (Global Advanced/Adjuvant Stomach Tumor Research International Collaboration). Benefit of adjuvant chemotherapy for resectable gastric cancer: a meta-analysis. *JAMA* 2010;303(1): 1729–1737.

Gastrointestinal Tumor Study Group. A comparison of combination chemotherapy and combined modality therapy for locally advanced gastric carcinoma. *Cancer.* 1982;49:1771–1777.

Glehen O, Gilly FN, Arvieux C, et al. Peritoneal carcinomatosis from gastric cancer: a multi-institutional study of 159 patients treated by cytoreductive surgery combined with perioperative intraperitoneal chemotherapy. *Ann Surg Oncol.* 2010:17(9):2370–2377.

Goh PM, So JB. Role of laparoscopy in the management of stomach cancer. *Semin Surg Oncol.* 1999;16:321–326.

Greenlee RT, Murray T, Bolden S, et al. Cancer statistics, 2000. *CA Cancer J Clin.* 2000;50:7–33.

Gunderson LL, Sosin H. Adenocarcinoma of the stomach: areas of failure in a re-operation series (second or symptomatic look): clinicopathologic correlation and implications for adjuvant therapy. *Int J Radiat Oncol Biol Phys.* 1982;8:1–11.

Hallissey MT, Dunn JA, Ward LC, et al. The second British Stomach Cancer Group trial of adjuvant radiotherapy or chemotherapy in resectable gastric cancer: five-year follow up. *Lancet.* 1994; 343:1309–1312.

Hamazoe R, Maeta M, Kaibara N. Intraperitoneal thermochemotherapy for prevention of peritoneal recurrence of gastric cancer. Final results of a randomized controlled study. *Cancer.* 1994;73:2048–2052.

Hartgrink HH, van de Velde CJ, Putter H, et al. Extended lymph node dissection for gastric cancer: who may benefit? Final results of the randomized Dutch gastric cancer group trial. *J Clin Oncol.* 2004; 22:2069–2077.

Hermanek P, Wittekind C. Residual tumor (R) classification and prognosis. *Semin Surg Oncol.* 1994;10:12–20.

Hiki Y, Shimao H, Mieno H, et al. Modified treatment of early gastric cancer: evaluation of endoscopic treatment of early gastric cancers with respect to treatment indication groups. *World J Surg.* 1995; 19(4):517–522.

Hohenberger P, Eisenberg B. Role of surgery combined with kinase inhibition in the management of gastrointestinal stromal tumor (GIST). *Ann Surg Oncol.* 2010; 17:2585–2600.

Hu JK, Chen ZX, Zhou ZG, et al. Intravenous chemotherapy for resected gastric cancer: meta-analysis of randomized controlled trials. *World J Gastroenterol.* 2002; 8:1023–1028.

Hundahl SA, Phillips JL, Menck HR. The National Cancer Data Base Report on poor survival of U.S. gastric carcinoma patients treated with gastrectomy: fifth edition American Joint Committee on Cancer staging, proximal disease, and the "different disease" hypothesis. *Cancer.* 2000;88:921–932.

Husemann B. Cardia carcinoma considered a distinct entity. *Br J Surg.* 1989;76: 136–139.

Ichikura T, Tomimatsu S, Uefuji K, et al. Evaluation of the New American Joint Committee on Cancer/International Union against Cancer classification of lymph node metastasis from gastric carcinoma in comparison with the Japanese classification. *Cancer.* 1999;86:553–558.

Jang YJ, Park MS, Kim JH, et al. Advanced gastric cancer in the middle one-third of the stomach: should surgeons perform total gastrectomy? *J Surg Oncol.* 2010;101:451–456.

Janunger KG, Hafstrom L, Glimerlius B. Chemotherapy in gastric cancer: a review and updated meta-analysis. *Eur J Surg.* 2002;168(11):597–608.

Jatzko GR, Lisborg PH, Dent H, et al. A 10-year experience with Japanese-type radical lymph node dissection for gastric cancer outside of Japan. *Cancer.* 1995; 76: 1302–1312.

Jemal A, Seigel R, Ward E, et al. Cancer statistics 2009. *CA Cancer J Clin.* 2009;59(4): 225–249.

Jentschura D, Winkler M, Strohmeier N, et al. Quality-of-life after curative surgery for gastric cancer: a comparison between total gastrectomy and subtotal gastric resection. *Hepatogastroenterology.* 1997;44: 1137–1142.

Kattan MW, Karpeh MS, Mazumdar M, et al. Postoperative nomogram for disease-specific survival after an R0 resection for gastric carcinoma. *J Clin Oncol.* 2003; 19:3647–3650.

Karpeh MS, Kelsen DP, Tepper JE. Cancer of the stomach. In: DeVita VT, Hellman S, Rosenberg SA, eds. *Cancer: Principles and Practice of Oncology,* 6th ed. Philadelphia, PA: Lippincott Williams & Wilkins; 2001:1092–1126.

Kawaura Y, Mori Y, Nakajima H, et al. Total gastrectomy with left oblique abdominothoracic approach for gastric cancer involving the esophagus. *Arch Surg.* 1988;123:514–601.

Kelley JR, Duggan JM. Gastric cancer epidemiology and risk factors. *J Clin Epidemiol.* 2003;56(1):1–9.

Kim H, Hyung W, Cho G, et al. Morbidity and mortality of laparoscopic gastrectomy versus open gastrectomy for gastric cancer: an interim report—a phase III multicenter, prospective, randomized trial (KLASS Trial). *Ann Surg Oncol.* 2010;251:417–420.

Kitano S, Iso Y, Moriyama M, et al. Laparoscopy-assisted Billroth I gastrectomy. *Surg Laparosc Endosc.* 1994;4:146–148.

Kloppel G, Perren A, Heitz PU. The gastroenteropancreatic neuroendocrine cell system and its tumors: The WHO classification. *Ann NY Acad Sci.* 2004; 1014:13–27.

Kodama I, Kofuji K, Yano S, et al. Lymph node metastasis and lymphadenectomy for carcinoma in the gastric cardia: clinical experience. *Int Surg.* 1998;83:205–209.

Kodama Y, Sugimachi K, Soejima K, et al. Evaluation of extensive lymph node dissection for carcinoma of the stomach. *World J Surg.* 1981;5:241–248.

Kodera Y, Fujiwara M, Ohashi N, et al. Laparoscopic surgery for gastric cancer: a collective review with meta analysis of randomized trials. *J Amer Coll Surg.* 2010; 11(5):677–686.

Koga S, Hamazoe R, Maeta M, et al. Prophylactic therapy for peritoneal recurrence of gastric cancer by continuous hyperthermic peritoneal perfusion with mitomycin C. *Cancer.* 1988;61:232–237.

Kojima T, Parra-Blanco A, Takahaski H, et al. Outcome of endoscopic resection for early gastric cancer: review of the Japanese literature. *Gastrointest Endosc.* 1998; 48(5):550–555.

Kondo H, Gotoda T, Ono H, et al. Early gastric cancer: endoscopic mucosal resection. *Ann Ital Chir.* 2001;72(1):27–31.

Landry J, Tepper JE, Wood WC, et al. Patterns of failure following curative resection of gastric carcinoma. *Int J Radiat Oncol Biol Phys.* 1990;19:1357–1362.

Lauren P. The two histological main types of gastric carcinoma: diffuse and so-called intestinal-type carcinoma. An attempt at histo-clinical classification. *Acta Pathol Microbiol Scand.* 1965;64:31–49.

Lightdale CJ. Endoscopic ultrasonography in the diagnosis, staging and follow-up of esophageal and gastric cancer. *Endoscopy.* 1992;24(suppl 1):297–303.

Lordick F, Stein HJ, Peschel C, et al. Neoadjuvant therapy for esophagogastric cancer. *Br J Surg.* 2004;91:540–551.

Lowy AM, Feig BW, Janjan N, et al. A pilot study of preoperative chemoradiotherapy for resectable gastric cancer. *Ann Surg Oncol.* 2001;8:519–524.

Lowy AM, Mansfield PF, Leach SD, et al. Laparoscopic staging for gastric cancer. *Surgery.* 1996;119:611–614.

Lowy AM, Mansfield PF, Leach SD, et al. Response to neoadjuvant chemotherapy best predicts survival after curative resection of gastric cancer. *Ann Surg.* 1999;229:303–308.

MacDonald JS. Gastric cancer: chemotherapy of advanced disease. *Hematol Oncol.* 1992;10:3–42.

MacDonald JS, Smalley S, Benedetti J, et al. Chemoradiotherapy after surgery compared with surgery alone for adenocarcinoma of the stomach or gastroesophageal junction. *N Engl J Med.* 2001;345:725–730.

Makuuchi H, Kise Y, Shimada H, et al. Endoscopic mucosal resection for early gastric cancer. *Semin Surg Oncol.* 1999;17:108–116.

Mansfield PF. Lymphadenectomy for gastric cancer. *J Clin Oncol.* 2004;22:2759–2760.

Mari E, Floriani I, Tinazzi A, et al. Efficacy of adjuvant chemotherapy after curative resection for gastric cancer: a meta-analysis of published randomized trials. A study of the GISCAD (Gruppo Italiano per lo Studio dei Carcinomi dell' Apparato Digerente). *Ann Oncol.* 2000;11(7):837–843.

Martinez-Ramos D, Miralles-Tena JM, Cuesta MA, et al. Laparoscopy versus open surgery for advanced and resectable gastric cancer: a meta-analysis. *Rev Esp Enferm Dig.* 2011;103(3):133–141.

Maruyama K, Sasako M, Kinoshita T, et al. Surgical treatment for gastric cancer: the Japanese approach. *Semin Oncol.* 1996; 23:360–368.

Middleton G, Cunningham D. Current options in the management of gastrointestinal cancer. *Ann Oncol.* 1995;6(suppl 1):17–25.

Miettinen M, Lasota J. Gastrointestinal stromal tumors: pathology and prognosis at different sites. *Semin Diagn Pathol.* 2006;23:70–83.

Miner TJ, Jaques DP, Karpeh MS, et al. Defining palliative surgery in patients receiving noncurative resections for gastric cancer. *J Am Coll Surg.* 2004;198(6):1013–1021.

Minsky BD. The role of radiation therapy in gastric cancer. *Semin Oncol.* 1996;23: 390–396.

Moertel CG, Childs DS, O'Fallon JR, et al. Combined 5-fluorouracil and radiation therapy as a surgical adjuvant for poor prognosis gastric carcinoma. *J Clin Oncol.* 1984;2:1249–1254.

Monson JR, Donohue JH, McIlrath DC, et al. Total gastrectomy for advanced cancer. A worthwhile palliative procedure. *Cancer.* 1991;68:1863–1868.

Msika S, Benhamiche A, Jouve J-L, et al. Prognostic factors after curative resection of gastric cancer. A population-based study. *Eur J Cancer.* 2000;36:390–396.

Munoz N, Correa P, Cuello C, et al. Histologic types of gastric carcinoma in high- and low-risk areas. *Int J Cancer.* 1968;3(6):809–818.

National Comprehensive Cancer Network. NCCN practice guidelines for upper gastrointestinal carcinomas. *Oncology (Hunting).* 1998;12:179–223.

Nomura A, Stemmermann GN, Chyou PH, et al. *Helicobacter pylori* infection and gastric carcinoma among Japanese Americans in Hawaii. *N Engl J Med.* 1991;325: 1132–1136.

Ogata K, Mochiki E, Yanai M, et al. Factors correlated with early and late recurrence after curative gastrectomy for gastric cancer. *Hepatogastroenterology.* 2009;56(96):1760–1764.

Oiwa H, Maehara Y, Ohno S, et al. Growth pattern and $p53$ overexpression in patients with early gastric cancer. *Cancer.* 1995;75(suppl):1454–1459.

Ono H, Kondo H, Gotoda T, et al. Endoscopic mucosal resection for treatment of early gastric cancer. *Gut.* 2001;48:225–229.

Ott K, Lordick F, Blank S, et al. Gastric cancer: surgery in 2011 [published online ahead of print January 14, 2011]. *Langenbecks Arch Surg.*

Parsonnet J, Vandersteen D, Goates J, et al. *Helicobacter pylori* infection in intestinal- and diffuse-type gastric adenocarcinomas. *J Natl Cancer Inst.* 1991;83: 640–643.

Psyrri A, Papageorgiou S, Economopoulos T. Primary extranodal lymphomas of the stomach: clinical presentation, diagnostic pitfalls and management. *Ann Oncol.* 2008;12:1992–1999.

Rausei S, Dionigi G, Boni L, et al. How does the 7th TNM Edition fit in gastric cancer management? *Ann Surg Oncol.* 2010; 18(5):1219–1221.

Rugge M, Cassaro M, Leandro G, et al. *Helicobacter pylori* in promotion of gastric carcinogenesis. *Dig Dis Sci.* 1996;41:950–955.

Sakuramoto S, Sasako M, Yamaguchi T, et al. Adjuvant chemotherapy for gastric cancer with S-1, an oral fluoropyrimidine. *N Engl J Med.* 2007;357(18):1810–1820.

Sano T, Sasako M, Yamamoto S. Gastric cancer surgery: results of mortality and morbidity of prospective randomized controlled trials (JCOG 9501) comparing D2 and extended para-aortic lymphadenectomy. *J Clin Oncol.* 2004a;22:2767–2773.

Sano T, Sasako M, Yamamoto S, et al. Gastric cancer surgery: morbidity and mortality results from a prospective randomized controlled trial comparing D2 and extended para-aortic lymphadenectomy – Japan Clinical Oncology Group study 9501. *J Clin Oncol.* 2004b;22:2767–2773.

Sarbia M, Becker KF, Hofler H. Pathology of upper gastrointestinal malignancies. *Semin Oncol.* 2004;31:465–475.

Sasako M, Sano T, Yamamoto S, et al. (Left thoracoabdominal approach versus abdominal-transhiatal approach for gastric cancer of the cardia or subcardia: a randomised controlled trial. *Lancet Oncol.* 2006;7(8):644–651.

Sasako M, Sano T, Yamamoto S, et al. D2 lymphadenectomy alone or with para-aortic nodal dissection for gastric cancer. *N Engl J Med.* 2008;359(5):453–462.

Sawyers JL. Gastric carcinoma. *Curr Probl Surg.* 1995;32:101–178.

Sepe PS, Brugge WR. A guide for the diagnosis and management of gastrointestinal stromal cell tumors. *Nat Rev Gastroenterol Hepatol.* 2009;6:363–371.

Sharma P, Vakil N. Review article: *Helicobacter pylori* and reflux disease. *Aliment Pharmacol Ther.* 2003;17(3):297–305.

Skoropad VY, Berdov BA, Mardynski YS, et al. A prospective, randomized trial of preoperative and intraoperative radiotherapy versus surgery alone in resectable gastric cancer. *Eur J Surg Oncol.* 2000;26:773–779.

Skoropad V, Berdov B, Zagrebin V. Concentrated preoperative radiotherapy for resectable gastric cancer: 20-years follow-up of a randomized trial. *J Surg Oncol.* 2002;80:72–78.

Smith JW, Brennan MF. Surgical treatment of gastric cancer. Proximal, mid, and distal stomach. *Surg Clin North Am.* 1992; 72:381–399.

Smith JW, Shiu MH, Kelsey L, et al. Morbidity of radical lymphadenectomy in the curative resection of gastric carcinoma. *Arch Surg.* 1991;126:1469–1473.

Sobin L, Gospodarowicz M, Wittekind C. *TNM Classification of Malignant Tumours.* 7th ed. New York, NY: Wiley; 2009.

Songun I, Keizer HJ, Hermans J, et al. Chemotherapy for operable gastric cancer: results of the Dutch randomised FAMTX trial. The Dutch Gastric Cancer Group (DGCG). *Eur J Cancer.* 1999;35:558–562.

Songun I, Putter H, Kranenbarg EM, et al. Surgical treatment of gastric cancer: 15-year follow-up results of the randomised nationwide Dutch D1D2 trial. *Lancet Oncol.* 2010;11:439–449.

Greene FL, Page DL, Fleming ID, et al. Exocrine pancreas In: Greene FL, Page DL, Fleming ID, et al, eds. *AJCC Cancer Staging Manual.* 6th ed. New York, NY: Springer; 2002:157–164.

Strong VE, Devaud N, Allen PJ, Gonen M, et al. Laparoscopic versus open subtotal gastrectomy for adenocarcinoma: as case-control study. *Ann Surg Oncol.* 2009;16(6):1507–1513.

Strong VE, Song KY, Park CH, et al. Comparison of gastric cancer survival following R0 resection in the United States and Korea using an internationally validated nomogram. *Ann Surg.* 2010;251(4):640–646.

Sugarbaker PH, Yonemura Y. Clinical pathway for the management of resectable gastric cancer with peritoneal seeding: best palliation with a ray of hope for cure. *Oncology.* 2000;58:96–107.

Suzuki Y, Hiraishi H, Kanke K, et al. Treatment of gastric tumors by endoscopic mucosal resection with ligating device. *Gastrointest Endosc.* 1999;49(2):192–198.

Svedlund J, Sullivan M, Liedman B, et al. Quality of life after gastrectomy for gastric carcinoma: controlled study of reconstructive procedures. *World J Surg.* 1997;21:422–433.

Tada M, Tanaka Y, Matsuo N, et al. Mucosectomy for gastric cancer: current status in Japan. *J Gastroenterol Hepatol.* 2000; 15(suppl):D98–D102.

Tada M, Tokiyama H, Nakamura H, et al. Endoscopic resection for early gastric cancer. *Acta Endoscopica.* 1998;28:87–95.

Takekoshi T. General view of gastric cancer with depth invasion into muscle layer (M cancer) from a survey of reports of the Japanese Research Society for Gastric Cancer. *J Gastroenterol Mass Survey.* 1994;32:93–132.

Takeshita K, Tani M, Inoue H, et al. Endoscopic treatment for early oesophageal or gastric cancer. *Gut.* 1997;40(1):123–127.

Talamonti MS, Dawes LG, Joehl RJ, et al. Gastrointestinal lymphoma. A case for primary surgical resection. *Arch Surg.* 1990;125:972–976.

Tanabe S, Koizumi W, Kokutou M, et al. Usefulness of endoscopic aspiration mucosectomy as compared with strip biopsy for treatment of gastric mucosal cancer. *Gastrointest Endosc.* 1999;50(6):819–822.

Valentini V, Cellini F, Minsky BD, et al. *Radiother Oncol.* 2009;92(2):176–183.

Wanebo HJ, Kennedy BJ, Chmiel J, et al. Cancer of the stomach. A patient care study by the American College of Surgeons. *Ann Surg.* 1993;218:583–592.

Wanebo HJ, Kennedy BJ, Winchester DP, et al. Gastric carcinoma: does lymph node dissection alter survival? *J Am Coll Surg.* 1996;183:616–624.

Wang LS, Wu CW, Hseih MJ, et al. Lymph node metastasis in patients with adenocarcinoma of gastric cardia. *Cancer.* 1993;71:1948–1953.

Weese JL, Harbison SP, Stiller GD, et al. Neoadjuvant chemotherapy, radical resection with intraoperative radiation therapy (IORT): improved treatment for gastric adenocarcinoma. *Surgery.* 2000;128:564–571.

Wilke H, Shahl M, Fink U, et al. Preoperative chemotherapy for unresectable gastric cancer. *World J Surg.* 1995;19(2):210–215.

Wu CW, Chang IS, Lo SS, et al. Complications following D3 gastrectomy post hoc analysis of a randomized trial. *World J Surg.* 2006;30(1):12–16.

Yamao T, Shirao K, Ono H, et al. Risk factors for lymph node metastasis from intramucosal gastric carcinoma. *Cancer.* 1996;77(4):602–606.

Yang XJ, Huang CQ, Suo T, et al. Cytoreductive surgery and hyperthermic intraperitoneal chemotherapy improves survival of patients with peritoneal carcinomatosis from gastric cancer: final results. *Ann Surg Oncol.* 2011;18(6):1575–1581.

Yao JC, Shah MH, Ito T, et al. Everolimus for advanced pancreatic neuroendocrine tumors. *N Engl J Med.* 2011;364(6):514–523.

Yim HB, Jacobson BC, Saltzman JR, et al. Clinical outcome of the use of enteral stents for palliation of patients with malignant upper GI obstruction. *Gastrointest Endosc.* 2001;53:329–332.

Yonemura Y, Fujimura T, Nishimura G, et al. Effects of intraoperative chemohyperthermia in patients with gastric cancer with peritoneal dissemination. *Surgery.* 1996;199(4):437–444.

Yonemura Y, Kawamura T, Bandou E, et al. Treatment of peritoneal dissemination from gastric cancer by peritonectomy and chemohyperthermic peritoneal perfusion. *Br J Surg.* 2005;92:370–375.

Yonemura Y, Tsugawa K, Fushida S, et al. Lymph node metastasis and surgical management of gastric cancer invading the esophagus. *Hepatogastroenterology.* 1995;42:37–42.

Yonemura Y, Wu CC, Fukushima N, et al. Randomized clinical trial of D2 and extended paraaortic lymphadenectomy in patients with gastric cancer. *Int J Clin Oncol.* 2008;13:132–137.

Yoon SS, Coit DG, Portlock CS, et al. The diminishing role of surgery in the treatment of gastric lymphoma. *Ann Surg.* 2004;240:28–37.

Youn HG, An JY, Choi MG, et al. Recurrence after curative resection of early gastric cancer. *Ann Surg Oncol.* 2010;17(2):448–454.

Yu W, Choi GS, Chung HY. Randomized clinical trial of splenectomy versus splenic preservation in patients with proximal gastric cancer. *Br J Surg.* 2006;93:559–563.

Zhang ZX, Gu XZ, Yin WB, et al. Randomized clinical trial of the combination of preoperative radiation and surgery in the treatment of adenocarcinoma of the gastric cardia—report on 370 patients. *Int J Radiat Oncol Biol Phys.* 1998;42:929–934.

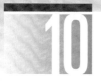

Small Bowel Malignancies and Carcinoid Tumors

Tawnya L. Bowles, Keith D. Amos, Rosa F. Hwang, and Jason B. Fleming

Malignancies of the small intestine are rare, with an estimated 6,230 new cases diagnosed in the United States in 2009. Small intestine malignancies account for only 1% of all gastrointestinal (GI) neoplasms. Adenocarcinoma, carcinoid, lymphoma, and sarcoma account for the majority of primary small bowel malignancies. Metastases to the small bowel from melanoma, colon, lung, and ovarian primaries are also observed. The diagnosis of small bowel malignancies is often delayed due to nonspecific clinical presentation of vague abdominal pain and the inherent technical difficulties in imaging the entire small bowel. Treatment varies with the type of tumor but most often includes surgical resection.

EPIDEMIOLOGY

The annual age-adjusted incidence of small bowel malignancies has increased from 11.8 per 1 million persons in 1973 to 22.7 per 1 million persons in 2004. This increase is mostly due to the increased incidence of carcinoid tumors. Historically, adenocarcinomas were the most common small bowel malignancy, but in a recent analysis by Bilimoria et al. (2009) using the Surveillance, Epidemiology, and End Results (SEER) program and National Cancer Data Base (NCDB) registry, carcinoid was the most common histology (37.4%), followed by adenocarcinoma (36.9%), stromal tumors (8.4%), and lymphoma (7.3%). Adenocarcinoma is the most common malignancy in the proximal small intestine, whereas carcinoid is the most common malignancy in the ileum. Sarcoma and lymphoma may develop throughout the small intestine but are more prevalent in the distal small bowel. The median age at presentation across all histologic subtypes was 67 years.

Small bowel malignancies may be found in association with familial polyposis, Gardner syndrome, Peutz–Jeghers syndrome, adult (nontropical) celiac sprue, von Recklinghausen neurofibromatosis, and Crohn's disease. In addition, immunosuppressed patients such as those with immunoglobulin A (IgA) deficiency are believed to be at increased risk of small bowel malignancies. As many as 25% of affected patients have synchronous malignancies, including neoplasms of the colon, endometrium, breast, and prostate gland.

Mutations of the Ki-*ras* gene are found in 14% to 53% of small intestine adenocarcinomas and are more prevalent in duodenal, rather than jejunal or ileal, adenocarcinomas. In contrast, mutations of the *APC* gene are uncommon in small bowel carcinomas, suggesting that these tumors arise through a different genetic pathway than colorectal carcinomas.

RISK FACTORS

While the small intestine represents 75% of the length and 90% of the surface area of the alimentary tract, small bowel malignancies account for only 1% of all GI neoplasms. The secretion of protective substances in the small bowel and the lack of pro-carcinogenic factors may explain its relative sparing from malignancy.

Benzopyrene hydroxylase, an enzyme that converts benzopyrene to a less carcinogenic compound, and secretory IgA, which may protect against oncogenic viruses, are found in large amounts in the mucosa of the small intestine. The small intestine is not exposed to the acidic environment of the stomach or to the potentially carcinogenic effect of solid GI contents found in the colon. Anaerobic bacteria, which convert bile salts into potential carcinogens, are generally lacking in the small intestine. The rapid transit of liquid succus entericus through the small bowel is also believed to reduce its tumorigenicity by minimizing the contact time between potential enteric carcinogens and the mucosa.

GI dysfunction may disrupt the normal physiology of the small intestine and predispose to tumorigenesis. Stasis secondary to partial obstruction or blind loop syndrome leads to bacterial overgrowth and has been implicated in the development of small intestine malignancies.

CLINICAL PRESENTATION

GI symptoms develop in 75% of patients with malignant lesions of the small bowel, compared with only 50% of patients with benign tumors. Sixty-five percent of patients will present with dull, colicky abdominal pain that radiates to the back, 50% with anorexia and weight loss, and 25% with signs and symptoms of bowel obstruction. Only 10% of the patients with small bowel malignancies will develop bowel perforation, most commonly those with lymphomas or sarcomas. A palpable abdominal mass is present in 25% of the patients. Jaundice may be present in patients with common bile duct obstruction from ampullary cancer. Episodic jaundice associated with guaiac-positive stool suggests the presence of an ampullary malignancy.

The nonspecific nature of symptoms frequently results in a 6- to 8-month delay in diagnosis. The correct diagnosis is established preoperatively in only 50% of cases. Delayed detection and inaccurate diagnoses contribute to the advanced stage of the disease at presentation and surgery which translates into an overall poor prognosis for these patients.

DIAGNOSTIC WORKUP

A high index of suspicion is essential to the early diagnosis and treatment of small intestine malignancies. The patient presenting with nonspecific abdominal symptoms should undergo a complete history, physical examination, and screening for occult fecal blood. Laboratory workup should include a complete blood cell count, measurement of serum electrolyte levels, and liver function tests. Further laboratory testing, including measurement of urinary 5-hydroxyindoleacetic acid (5-HIAA) to detect functioning carcinoid tumors, should be directed by clinical suspicion.

Retrospective reviews report that 50% to 60% of small intestine neoplasms are detected using conventional radiographic techniques, including upper GI series with small bowel follow-through (UGI/SBFT) and enteroclysis. Hypotonic duodenography, using anticholinergic agents or glucagon to reduce duodenal peristalsis, may enhance diagnostic yield to as high as 86% for more proximally located duodenal malignancies. Traditionally, computed tomography (CT) was not believed to be helpful in diagnosing small bowel neoplasms. However, several recent reviews have shown that CT is able to detect abnormalities in 97% of patients with small bowel tumors. Angiography demonstrates a tumor blush in specific subtypes of small bowel malignancies, most notably carcinoid and leiomyosarcoma, but is rarely indicated in the initial diagnostic workup.

Upper endoscopy is efficient in diagnosing tumors of the duodenum. However, endoscopy of the small bowel distal to the duodenal papilla has been limited by the practical difficulties of negotiating an endoscope through the tortuous length of the small bowel. Current options for an endoluminal investigation of the small bowel include push enteroscopy, push-and-pull (double-balloon) enteroscopy, video capsule endoscopy (VCE), and intraoperative endoscopy. Push enteroscopy utilizes a pediatric colonoscope that is passed orally and then pushed distally through the small intestine, facilitating intubation of the jejunum 40 to 60 cm distal to the ligament of Treitz. To evaluate the remainder of the small bowel, the newer technique of push-and-pull enteroscopy has been utilized. In push-and-pull enteroscopy, a high resolution 200 cm video endoscope with latex balloons attached at the tip of the enteroscope and on an overtube can be alternately inflated and deflated to permit the threading of the small bowel over the scope. The completion rate of push-and-pull enteroscopy is 80% and the diagnostic yield is ~60% in most studies. VCE was introduced in 2001 as a novel, noninvasive method of examining the entire small bowel mucosa. The system consists of an ingestible capsule equipped with a camera that transmits pictures from the capsule to sensing pads that are placed on the patient's abdomen. The data is then transmitted to a data recorder the patient wears on a belt. The completion rate for VCE is similar to push-and-pull enteroscopy (80%) but is decreased for patients with prior abdominal surgery, poor bowel preparation, or delayed gastric emptying. The diagnostic yield of VCE is approximately 50% to 60% for small bowel tumors. VCE and push-and-pull enteroscopy can be used as complementary diagnostic techniques in difficult cases. The capsule retention rate requiring repeat endoscopy or surgery was 1% in one large series.

Despite the advances in small bowel endoscopy, most retrospective studies report only moderate success in diagnosing small bowel neoplasms preoperatively. Many large series report a correct preoperative diagnosis in only 50% of cases. Exploratory laparotomy remains the most sensitive diagnostic modality in evaluating a patient in whom small bowel neoplasm is suspected and should be considered in patients with occult GI bleeding, unexplained weight loss, or vague abdominal pain. At exploration, intraoperative enteroscopy can be utilized to help localize small bowel tumors. The gastroenterologist can pass the enteroscope transorally, allowing the surgeon to guide the scope through the length of the small bowel.

Distally located small bowel adenocarcinoma at or near the ileum is diagnosed with laparotomy in 57% of patients, with UGI in 21% of patients, and CT scan in only 7% of patients. Because most tumors present as large, bulky lesions with lymph node metastasis, laparoscopy is potentially useful for establishing the diagnosis of malignancy when the workup is otherwise negative and for obtaining adequate tissue samples if a diagnosis of lymphoma is suspected.

In summary, early detection and treatment remain the most significant variables in improving outcome from small bowel malignancy, necessitating thoughtful and expedient diagnostic workup of patients presenting with vague abdominal symptoms.

SPECIFIC TYPES OF SMALL BOWEL MALIGNANCIES

Adenocarcinoma

Pathology

Adenocarcinoma of the small intestine occurs most commonly in the duodenum, with 65% of the neoplasms clustered in the periampullary region. These tumors infiltrate into the muscularis propria and may extend through the serosa and into adjacent tissues. Ulceration is commonly observed and can cause occult GI bleeding and chronic anemia. Obstruction may develop from progressive growth of apple core lesions or large intraluminal polypoid masses. Obstructing duodenal lesions can manifest clinically as gastric outlet obstruction, while more distally located lesions can result in severe cramping abdominal pain. Approximately 60%

of tumors are well- or moderately differentiated tumors, and 37% are signet ring and poorly differentiated tumors.

Staging

The American Joint Committee on Cancer (AJCC) staging system for small bowel adenocarcinoma is shown in Table 10.1.

Clinical Course

Adenocarcinoma of the small bowel follows a pattern of tumor progression similar to that of colon cancer, with similar survival rates when compared stage for stage. Most small bowel adenocarcinomas (70% to 80%) are resectable at the time of diagnosis, with a 5-year survival rate of 20% to 30% reported for patients undergoing resection. Approximately 35% of patients will have metastasis to regional lymph

---

TABLE 10.1 AJCC (7th ed) Staging of Small Intestine Malignancies (Excluding Lymphomas, Carcinoid Tumors, and Visceral Sarcomas)

Primary Tumor (T)

T0	No evidence of primary tumor
Tis	Carcinoma in situ
T1a	Tumor invades lamina propria
T1b	Tumor invades submucosa
T2	Tumor invades muscularis propria
T3	Tumor invades through the muscularis propria into the subserosa or into the nonperitonealized perimuscular tissue (mesentery or retroperitoneum) with extension ≤2 cm
T4	Tumor perforates the visceral peritoneum or directly invades other organs or structures (includes other loops of the small intestine, mesentery, or retroperitoneum >2 cm, and abdominal wall by way of serosa; for duodenum only, invasion of pancreas or bile duct)

Regional Lymph Nodes (N)

N0	No regional lymph node metastasis
N1	Metastasis in 1–3 regional lymph nodes
N2	Metastasis in four or more regional lymph nodes

Distant Metastasis (M)

M0	No distant metastasis
M1	Distant metastasis

Staging

Stage 0	Tis	N0	M0
Stage I	T1-T2	N0	M0
Stage IIA	T3	N0	M0
Stage IIB	T4	N0	M0
Stage IIIA	Any T	N1	M0
Stage IIIB	Any T	N2	M0
Stage IV	Any T	Any N	M1

AJCC, American Joint Committee on Cancer staging.
Adapted from Edge SB, Byrd DR, Compton CC, et al., eds. AJCC Cancer Staging Handbook. 7th ed. Philadelphia, PA: Springer-Verlag; 2010.

nodes at the time of diagnosis, and an additional 20% will have distant metastasis. The liver is the most common site of distant metastasis. Mural penetration, nodal involvement, distant metastasis, and perineural invasion correlate with a poor prognosis. In a single institution series from the University of California, Los Angeles, large tumor size and poor histologic grade were also associated with decreased survival, but this association has not been confirmed by other investigators.

Adenocarcinoma of the small bowel is also associated with Crohn's disease, usually occurring in the distal ileum. Risk factors associated with the development of a small bowel cancer in Crohn's disease include duration of disease, male gender, associated fistulous disease, and the presence of surgically excluded bowel loops.

Surgical Treatment

Surgical resection of the primary tumor with resection of the associated lymph node basin is the primary treatment of small bowel adenocarcinomas for patients without evidence of distant disease. A retrospective review of 217 patients diagnosed with small bowel adenocarcinoma treated at The University of Texas M. D. Anderson Cancer Center found that surgery was the primary definitive treatment modality in 67% of patients. For tumors localized in the jejunum and ileum, a standard small bowel resection with resection of the mesentery to ensure resection of the draining lymph nodes is performed.

Duodenal adenocarcinomas have been managed with a variety of surgical strategies ranging from wide local excision to pancreaticoduodenectomy. Pancreaticoduodenectomy has been touted as a superior operation for duodenal adenocarcinoma because of its more radical clearance of the tumor bed and regional lymph nodes. In a 1994 comparison of pancreaticoduodenectomy to segmental resection for management of duodenal adenocarcinoma at M. D. Anderson Cancer Center, Barnes et al. found no significant difference in survival rates, but did find a difference in 5-year local control rates—76% for pancreaticoduodenectomy and 49% for segmental resection. Several other reviews, including those of Lowell et al. (1992), Joestling et al. (1981), van Ooijen and Kalsbeek (1988), and Bakaeen et al. (2000), which compared survival following pancreaticoduodenectomy to segmental resection for lesions in the third and fourth portions of the duodenum, have demonstrated no significant difference in 5-year survival. In these studies, a more limited resection, with a lower rate of associated morbidity and mortality, provided a survival benefit equal to that of a more extensive resection. In a multivariate analysis of 101 patients by Bakaeen et al., nodal metastases, advanced tumor stage, and positive resection margins had a negative impact on survival.

At M. D. Anderson, a pancreaticoduodenectomy is performed for lesions involving the proximal duodenum to the right of the superior mesenteric artery (SMA). A segmental resection is performed for duodenal lesions to the left of the SMA. Local excision is considered for small lesions on the antimesenteric wall of the second portion of the duodenum. Two studies have found a higher rate of postoperative complications from pancreaticoduodenectomy in patients with periampullary malignancies than in those with pancreatic adenocarcinoma, although this did not result in a higher rate of perioperative mortality in either study. An increased pancreatic anastomotic leak rate was present in the group with duodenal carcinoma, presumably due to a normal, soft pancreas which increased the technical difficulty of the pancreatic anastomosis.

Chemoradiation Therapy

5-Fluorouracil (5-FU) based chemotherapy has been recommended both in the adjuvant setting and in cases of unresectable disease, although the benefit has not been clearly shown. Adjuvant 5-FU in patients treated with margin-negative resection at M. D. Anderson Cancer Center resulted in an improved disease-free survival but not overall survival. For patients with metastatic disease, the addition of a platinum compound to 5-FU chemotherapy resulted in a higher response rate and improved progression-free survival compared to other chemotherapeutic treatments. Because most centers have only limited experience treating adenocarcinoma of the small intestine, the efficacy of chemotherapy needs further study, and patients should continue to be enrolled in prospective randomized clinical trials.

Electron-beam intraoperative radiation therapy and external-beam radiation therapy have been administered at M. D. Anderson in a limited number of cases with microscopic involvement of resection margins or unresectable disease. However, adenocarcinoma of the small intestine is generally considered to be radiation resistant.

Carcinoid Tumors

Epidemiology

The peak incidence of carcinoid tumors is in the sixth and seventh decades of life, although these tumors have been reported in patients as young as 10 years. While carcinoid tumors are considered rare tumors, a recent population-based review of more than 35,600 patients by Yao et al. (2008) showed that their incidence is increasing. The estimated 29-year limited-duration prevalence of carcinoid tumors (defined as the number of people alive in 2004 who were diagnosed with a carcinoid in the preceding 29 years) was 103,312 cases, making carcinoid significantly more common than esophageal (28,664), gastric (65,836), and pancreatic cancer (32,353).

The sites of origin of carcinoid tumors are shown in Table 10.2. Approximately 85% of carcinoid tumors are found in the GI tract, with the appendix being the most common site. Nonintestinal sites include the lungs, pancreas, biliary tract, thymus, and ovary. Ileal carcinoids are the most likely to metastasize, even when small, in contrast to appendiceal carcinoids, which rarely metastasize.

Pathology

Carcinoids are characterized by their ability to produce peptides, such as serotonin, that can result in characteristic hormonal syndromes. Carcinoids arise from

TABLE 10.2 | Sites of Origin of Carcinoid Tumors

Tumor Site	% of Cases
GI tract	54.5
Small intestine	44.7
Rectum	19.6
Appendix	16.7
Colon	10.6
Stomach	7.2
Lung/Bronchus	30.1
Pancreas	2.3
Gynecologic/Ovarian	1.2
Biliary	1.0
Head and neck	0.4
Other (soft tissue, etc.)	9.7

Modified from Maggard MA, O'Connell JB, Ko CY. Updated population-based review of carcinoid tumors. *Ann Surg.* 2004;240(1):117–122.

enterochromaffin cells, which are located predominantly in the GI tract and mainstem bronchi. In addition to serotonin, these tumors can secrete a number of biologically active substances, including amines, tachykinins, and prostaglandins. Small bowel carcinoids occur most commonly in the terminal 60 cm of the ileum as tan, yellow, or gray-brown intramural or submucosal nodules. The presence of multiple synchronous nodules in 30% of patients mandates careful inspection of the entire small intestine in these patients.

Staging
The AJCC staging system for small bowel carcinoids is shown in Table 10.3.

Clinical Presentation
The presentation of carcinoids varies depending on physical characteristics, site of origin, and production of hormonally active substances such as serotonin. In general, most carcinoids are small, indolent tumors that can be categorized either by microscopic pathologic features or by embryologic site of origin. The embryologic classification divides carcinoids into tumors of the foregut (stomach, pancreas, lungs), midgut (small bowel and appendix), and hindgut (colon and rectum) (Table 10.4).

T A B L E 10.3	AJCC (7th ed) Staging of Small Intestine Carcinoids

Primary Tumor (T)

T0	No evidence of primary tumor
T1	Tumor invades lamina propria or submucosa and size ≤1 cm (small intestinal tumors); tumor ≤1 cm (ampullary tumors)
T2	Tumor invades muscularis propria or size >1 cm (small intestinal tumors); tumor >1 cm (ampullary tumors)
T3	Tumor invades through the muscularis propria into subserosal tissue without penetration of overlying serosa (jejuna or ileal tumors) or invades pancreas or retroperitoneum (ampullary/duodenal tumors) or into nonperitonealized tissues
T4	Tumor invades visceral peritoneum (serosa) or invades other organs

Regional Lymph Nodes (N)

N0	No regional lymph node metastasis
N1	Regional lymph node metastases

Distant Metastasis (M)

M0	No distant metastasis
M1	Distant metastasis

Staging

Stage I	T1	N0	M0
Stage IIA	T2	N0	M0
Stage IIB	T3	N0	M0
Stage IIIA	T4	N0	M0
Stage IIIB	Any T	N1	M0
Stage IV	Any T	Any N	M1

AJCC, American Joint Committee on Cancer.
Adapted from Edge SB, Byrd DR, Compton CC, et al., eds. *AJCC Cancer Staging Handbook.* 7th ed. Philadelphia, PA: Springer-Verlag; 2010.

TABLE 10.4	Characteristics of Carcinoid Tumors by Embryologic Site of Origin		
Characteristics	**Foregut**	**Midgut**	**Hindgut**
Location	Bronchus	Jejunum	Colon
	Stomach	Ileum	Rectum
	Pancreas	Appendix	
Histology	Trabecular	Nodular, solid nest of cells	Trabecular
Secretion			
Tumor 5-HT	Low	High	None
Urinary 5-HIAA	High	High	Normal
Carcinoid syndrome	Yes	Yes	No
Other endocrine secretions	Frequent	Frequent	No

5-HIAA, 5-hydroxyindoleacetic acid; 5-HT, 5-hydroxytryptamine or serotonin.

Foregut carcinoids are more commonly associated with an atypical presentation due to secretion of peptide hormone products other than serotonin, such as gastrin, adrenocorticotropic hormone, or growth hormone. Pulmonary carcinoids are usually perihilar, and patients present with recurrent pneumonia, cough, hemoptysis, or chest pain. Ectopic secretion of corticotropin or growth hormone-releasing factor from these tumors can produce Cushing syndrome or acromegaly, respectively. Gastric carcinoids are associated with chronic atrophic gastritis type A (CAG-A) in 75% of cases, predominantly occurring in women, roughly half of whom are also diagnosed with pernicious anemia. These tumors are usually identified on endoscopic evaluation for anemia or abdominal pain and are located in the body or fundus of the stomach. Another 5% to 10% of gastric carcinoids are associated with Zollinger-Ellison syndrome in patients with multiple endocrine neoplasia type I. The remaining 15% to 25% of gastric carcinoids are sporadic and more frequently appear in men. Sporadic foregut carcinoids are associated with an atypical carcinoid syndrome, which is believed to be histamine mediated and exhibited mainly as intense erythematous flushing, itching, conjunctival suffusion, facial edema, and occasional urticaria.

Midgut carcinoids produce symptoms of hormone excess only when they are bulky or metastatic. Most midgut carcinoids are located in the distal one-third of the small bowel and less than 10% cause symptoms. The vast majority of appendiceal carcinoids are found incidentally. When symptomatic, these patients usually present with symptoms similar to those described for other small bowel tumors (nonspecific, colicky abdominal pain). Sometimes, as a small bowel carcinoid progresses, it induces fibrosis of the mesentery, which may contribute to intestinal obstruction and lead to varying degrees of mesenteric ischemia. Most patients with small bowel carcinoids present with metastases to lymph nodes or to the liver.

Hindgut carcinoids tend to be clinically silent tumors until they are advanced. Two-thirds are found in the right colon with the average tumor diameter at presentation being 5 cm. They rarely produce serotonin, even in the presence of metastatic disease. Patients with hindgut tumors most commonly present with bleeding and occasionally experience abdominal pain.

The hormonal manifestations of carcinoid tumors (carcinoid syndrome) are seen in only 10% of patients and occur when the secretory products of these tumors gain direct access to the systemic circulation and avoid metabolism in the liver. This clinical

TABLE 10.5	Clinical Symptoms of Carcinoid Syndrome
Symptom	**Causative Tumor Product**
Flushing	Bradykinin
	Hydroxytryptophan
	Prostaglandins
Telangiectasia	Vasoactive intestinal polypeptide
	Serotonin
	Prostaglandins
	Bradykinin
Bronchospasm	Bradykinin
	Histamine
	Prostaglandins
Endocardial fibrosis	Serotonin
Glucose intolerance	Serotonin
Arthropathy	Serotonin
Hypotension	Serotonin

syndrome occurs in the following situations: (a) when hepatic metastases are present; (b) when retroperitoneal disease is extensive, with venous drainage directly into the paravertebral veins; and (c) when the primary carcinoid tumor is outside the GI tract, as with bronchial, ovarian, or testicular tumors. Ninety percent of cases of carcinoid syndrome are seen in patients with midgut tumors.

The main symptoms of carcinoid syndrome are watery diarrhea, flushing, sweating, wheezing, dyspnea, abdominal pain, hypotension, right heart failure due to tricuspid regurgitation, or pulmonic stenosis caused by endocardial fibrosis (Table 10.5). The flushing of carcinoid syndrome is often dramatic and is an intense purple color on the upper body and arms. Facial edema is often present. Repeated attacks can lead to the development of telangiectasias and permanent skin discoloration. The flush can be precipitated by consuming alcohol, blue cheese, chocolate, or red wine, and by exercise.

A life-threatening form of carcinoid syndrome called *carcinoid crisis* is usually precipitated by anesthesia, surgery, or chemotherapy. The manifestations include an intense flush, diarrhea, tachycardia, hypertension or hypotension, bronchospasm, and altered mental status. The symptoms are usually refractory to fluid resuscitation and administration of vasopressors. The somatostatin analog octreotide should be given preoperatively to all patients with metastatic carcinoid to prevent carcinoid crisis intraoperatively.

Diagnosis
The diagnosis of carcinoid tumor is made using a combination of biochemical tests and imaging studies. Overall, approximately 50% of patients with carcinoids have elevated urinary levels of 5-HIAA, irrespective of whether they have symptoms of carcinoid syndrome. One study reported 100% specificity and 70% sensitivity of urinary 5-HIAA for the presence of carcinoid syndrome. 5-HIAA levels may also correlate with tumor burden. Urinary 5-HIAA levels can be altered by medications and certain foods (e.g., bananas, walnuts, pineapples). When urinary 5-HIAA levels are nondiagnostic, a more extensive workup should be undertaken, consisting of the measurement of urinary 5-hydroxytryptamine (5-HT, serotonin) and

5-hydroxytryptophan (5-HPT), plasma 5-HPT, platelet 5-HT, and serum levels of other secretory products such as chromogranin A, neuron-specific enolase (NSE), substance P, and neuropeptide K. In well-differentiated tumors, the sensitivity of serum chromogranin A is between 80% and 100% and also reflects tumor load. Chromogranin A can be used in the detection of functional and nonfunctional tumors.

Localization of the tumor may also help confirm the diagnosis. Bronchial carcinoids are best visualized with a chest radiograph or CT scan. Gastric, duodenal, colonic, and rectal carcinoids are usually seen on endoscopy and barium studies. Small intestine carcinoids are initially evaluated as described for other small bowel malignancies. Abdominal CT scan is useful for assessing the involvement of the retroperitoneum and the presence of liver metastasis. In addition, small bowel carcinoids have a spoke-wheel appearance on CT due to extensive mesenteric fibrosis, and 70% of the cases demonstrate calcifications.

Nuclear medicine scans have also been used in localization. Scans using Indium 111 (^{111}In-penetreotide) or metaiodobenzylguanidine (MIBG) radiolabeled with iodine 131 (^{131}I) can identify primary or metastatic carcinoid tumors approximately 70% of the time, when MIBG is taken up by the tumor and stored in its neurosecretory granules. The combination of these two imaging modalities increases sensitivity to 95%. However, the sensitivity of detecting bone metastases is only 20% to 50%.

On occasion, a patient may benefit from angiography or selective venous sampling if other diagnostic maneuvers prove unsuccessful.

Clinical Course

Primary carcinoid tumors are indolent, slow-growing lesions that become symptomatic late in the course of the disease. Carcinoid tumors can infiltrate the muscularis propria and extend through the serosa to involve the mesentery or retroperitoneum, producing a characteristically intense desmoplastic reaction. Mesenteric lymph nodes are also frequently involved. Distant sites of metastases include the liver and, to a lesser degree, the lungs and bone. Metastatic disease correlates with primary tumor size, depth of invasion, and site.

There is no widely accepted histologic classification of carcinoids that accurately predicts metastatic behavior. Morphologic criteria such as mitotic activity, cytologic atypia, and tumor necrosis have been evaluated; however, these features can be affected by ischemia secondary to mesenteric sclerosis in GI carcinoids. An analysis by Moyana et al. in 2000 revealed that positive immunohistochemical staining for MIB-1 (a marker of proliferation) and p53 was associated with metastatic behavior. In addition, high levels of the nuclear antigen Ki-67 appears to correlate with decreased survival in patients with carcinoid tumors.

Treatment of Localized Disease

Surgical extirpation is the definitive treatment for localized primary carcinoid tumors. The extent of resection is determined by the size of the primary lesion and is based on the likelihood of mesenteric lymph node involvement.

Appendiceal carcinoids smaller than 1 cm rarely metastasize and are adequately treated by appendectomy alone unless the base of the appendix is involved, in which case a partial cecectomy may be necessary. Because the incidence of metastasis increases with primary tumor size, treatment of appendiceal carcinoids between 1 and 2 cm is more controversial. In general, most authors recommend appendectomy alone for lesions smaller than 1.5 cm and right hemicolectomy for lesions larger than 1.5 cm or for any lesion with invasion of the mesoappendix, blood vessels, or regional lymph nodes.

In contrast to appendiceal carcinoids, carcinoids of the small bowel are more likely to metastasize even when smaller than 1 cm. As a result, most surgeons recommend a wide en bloc resection that includes the adjacent mesentery and lymph nodes.

Mesenteric resection may be more difficult due to fibrosis and foreshortening, secondary to the desmoplastic reaction often incited by carcinoid tumors. Although some surgeons advocate local excision for small midgut carcinoids, up to 70% of these tumors metastasize to the lymph nodes. Therefore, a wide resection may not only cure some of these patients, but should also provide better local disease control than local excision. Furthermore, a careful and thorough examination of the entire length of bowel is important because 20% to 40% of small bowel carcinoids are multicentric. Because of the slow-growing nature of these tumors, wide excision is advocated even when distant metastases are present. In addition, approximately 40% of patients with midgut carcinoids have a second GI malignancy. Therefore, the entire bowel and colon should be evaluated before any planned surgical intervention.

Surgical management of rectal carcinoids is dependent on the size of the tumor and depth of invasion. Like all GI carcinoids, rectal carcinoids can metastasize to regional lymph nodes and distant sites. The risk of lymph node metastases increases with tumor size; rectal carcinoids <1 cm have a 3.4% incidence of lymph node metastases while tumors >2 cm have a 74% incidence. The majority of rectal carcinoids are small (<1 cm) when detected. Tumors <1 cm that lack lymphovascular invasion and have no lymph node metastases are adequately treated by local excision (transanal or endoscopic, if possible). Transanal endoscopic microsurgery is an emerging technique for small benign and malignant tumors of the rectum that may have utility in small rectal carcinoids. The management of tumors between 1 and 2 cm is more controversial. Wide local excision may be appropriate for tumors 1 to 2 cm that have no lymphovascular invasion or lymph node metastases and do not invade the muscularis propria. However, if the tumor invades the muscularis propria, total mesorectal excision (TME) is recommended. For patients with rectal carcinoids >2 cm, TME is also typically the procedure of choice. If more extensive surgery is indicated, every attempt should be made for sphincter preservation.

Long-term prognosis after surgical treatment of patients with GI carcinoids was evaluated in a study from the Mayo Clinic. With a median follow-up of 18 years, survival was significantly associated with the embryologic origin of the tumor and the patient's age. Increased survival was found in those patients with midgut carcinoids, compared to those with foregut tumors, as well as in patients younger than 62 years. Overall survival rates at 5- and 10 years were 69% and 53%, respectively.

Treatment of Advanced Disease

The role for surgery in patients with unresectable and metastatic disease is not clearly defined, but it appears that surgery may benefit some patients. When metastatic disease is present, it is necessary to establish whether the patient has symptoms of carcinoid syndrome and whether curative resection is possible. If the patient has no contraindications to surgery and the metastatic disease is resectable, then an attempt at complete extirpation should be made because it may lead to prolonged disease-free survival and symptomatic relief. All patients with metastatic carcinoid should receive octreotide therapy preoperatively to prevent a carcinoid crisis. Prophylactic cholecystectomy should be considered in patients who may require octreotide therapy in the future due to the increased risk of gallstones.

Surgical resection of liver metastases has resulted in long-term relief of symptoms. Eighty-two percent of patients with midgut carcinoids metastatic to the liver who underwent resection demonstrated partial or complete relief of symptoms with a mean duration of 5.3 years. Patients in whom liver metastases from carcinoid tumor are suspected should undergo an abdominal CT scan. The study should be done before and after the administration of the intravenous (IV) contrast material to better visualize carcinoid liver metastases, which are usually hypervascular and can be difficult to distinguish from normal liver after the injection of the IV contrast material.

Patients with mildly symptomatic carcinoid syndrome can be treated medically. Diarrhea can usually be controlled with loperamide, diphenoxylate, or serotonin receptor antagonist cyproheptadine. Flushing can frequently be controlled with either adrenergic blocking agents (e.g., clonidine or phenoxybenzamine) or a combination of type 1 and 2 histamine receptor antagonists. Albuterol (a beta-adrenergic blocking agent) and aminophylline are effective in relieving bronchospasm and wheezing.

For patients whose symptoms cannot be controlled with these conservative measures or in whom a carcinoid crisis develops, the somatostatin analog octreotide has shown tremendous promise. A trial from the Mayo Clinic found that flushing and diarrhea could be controlled in the vast majority of patients with as little as 150 µg of octreotide administered subcutaneously three times per day. The duration of the responses was, on the average, more than 1 year. Interestingly, a number of studies have now shown that octreotide is also able to significantly slow down tumor growth in more than 50% of patients and to cause tumor regression for variable periods in another 10% to 20% of patients. The long-acting release (LAR) formulation of octreotide, given as a 20 to 30 mg intramuscular injection every 4 weeks, is also effective at suppressing tumor growth in functionally active and inactive tumors. In a double-blind, randomized controlled trial of LAR in unresectable metastatic carcinoid, the median time to tumor progression was 6 months in the placebo group and 14.3 months in LAR-treated patients.

Asymptomatic patients with unresectable metastatic disease should be monitored. Local complications related to the tumor can be addressed if and when they develop. Our current indications for surgical intervention in unresectable and widely metastatic disease include complications of bulky carcinoid tumors such as obstruction and perforation. In addition, surgical debulking is considered for severe intractable symptoms unresponsive to medical treatment, if a dominant mass or liver metastasis can be identified. For patients who have undergone liver resection for metastatic carcinoid tumors, R2 (vs. R0) resection and pancreatic location of the carcinoid have been associated with poorer prognosis.

Despite the advanced stage of disease at presentation and the limited effectiveness of currently available therapies, the natural history of carcinoids affords affected patients a better prognosis than other malignancies of the small bowel. The 5-year survival rate for localized disease approaches 100% after complete resection. Resection of metastatic disease is associated with a 68% 5-year survival rate, whereas unresectable disease has a 38% 5-year survival rate.

Experimental Therapy

A number of chemotherapeutic agents have been studied in patients with carcinoid tumors. Results of chemotherapy trials with such agents as doxorubicin, dacarbazine, and streptozotocin, either alone or in combination, have been disappointing. Most chemotherapy trials show response rates of less than 30%, with responses lasting only a few months. The role of chemotherapy is still investigational, but for patients with advanced disease that cannot be controlled with standard measures, monitored clinical trials should be recommended.

One biologic agent, interferon, in both alfa-2a and alfa-2b forms, has demonstrated promising results in diminishing urinary levels of 5-HIAA and symptoms of carcinoid syndrome. Most patients in various studies experienced either partial regression or stabilization of their disease for a prolonged period. Unfortunately, objective responses with reduction of tumor size occurred in only approximately 15% of patients.

In some centers, hepatic artery occlusion or embolization has been used with some success to diminish the size of liver metastases and decrease levels of biologically active mediators of carcinoid syndrome. However, the duration of response is usually short, with median duration ranging from 7 months for hepatic artery occlusion alone to 20 months in a study using hepatic artery occlusion followed by systemic chemotherapy. Furthermore, side effects may be substantial. Liver embolization with Gelfoam performed in patients with neuroendocrine tumors resulted in serious complications in 10%, including renal failure, liver necrosis, and bowel ischemia. Another option for management of carcinoid hepatic metastases is radiofrequency ablation (RFA). In one small series, RFA was used as a salvage therapy in patients with hepatic metastases who were not amenable to surgical resection and unresponsive to embolization. Although only three patients were treated, all three demonstrated decreases in both the size of the lesions and the severity of symptoms. Because RFA can be performed percutaneously or laparoscopically, this may be a useful treatment alternative for patients with disseminated carcinoid tumors.

Targeted therapies, alone or in combination with octreotide, are under investigation. Vascular endothelial growth factor (VEGF) pathway inhibitors (bevacizumab, sunitinib, sorafenib) are being evaluated in phase II and III trials. Everolimus, a novel oral inhibitor of mammalian target of rapamycin (mTOR), in combination with long-acting octreotide slowed tumor growth in a Phase II trial of carcinoid tumors performed at M. D. Anderson Cancer Center and is currently being evaluated in a Phase III trial.

Although external-beam radiation has not proven effective in treating carcinoid tumors, targeted radiation in the form of radioactive iodine coupled to either MIBG or octreotide is a therapeutic strategy that may hold some promise for the future.

Sarcoma

Pathology

Sarcomas of the small intestine occur most frequently in the jejunum and the ileum and are typically slow-growing lesions. Small intestine sarcomas can invade adjacent tissues and metastasize hematogenously to the liver, lungs, and bones. Leiomyosarcoma and gastrointestinal stromal tumor (GIST) account for 75% of small intestine sarcomas; fibrosarcoma, liposarcoma, and angiosarcoma are seen less frequently. The various subtypes of small intestine sarcoma encompass a broad range of biologic behavior, the scope of which exceeds this review.

Clinical Presentation

The most common clinical presentations of small intestine sarcomas are pain (65%), abdominal mass (50%), and bleeding. More than 75% of tumors exceed 5 cm in diameter at diagnosis, but because most of the tumor extension is extramural, as opposed to intramural or intraluminal, obstruction is rarely seen. CT scan of these lesions typically demonstrates a heterogeneous mass with focal areas of necrosis where the tumor has outgrown its nutrient blood supply creating the potential to form localized abscesses.

Treatment

Surgical resection is the primary treatment modality for sarcoma of the small bowel. Because sarcoma rarely metastasizes to regional mesenteric lymph nodes, unlike adenocarcinoma and carcinoid, an extensive mesenteric lymphadenectomy is unnecessary and will not prolong survival. En bloc resection of the lesion with tumor-free margins is recommended for a potentially curative resection; however, at the time of diagnosis, 50% of lesions are unresectable and most of them exceed 5 cm in diameter. In the presence of widely metastatic disease, local resection should be considered if necessary to control bleeding or to relieve obstruction.

Chemoradiation therapy plays a limited role in the treatment of small bowel sarcomas.

Leiomyosarcomas are relatively resistant to chemoradiation therapy. Combined chemotherapy and radiation therapy should be offered to patients with leiomyosarcomas only as part of an experimental protocol in an attempt to downstage the disease or render an unresectable lesion resectable. Chemotherapy may be used in the treatment of recurrent or metastatic disease as part of an experimental protocol. Sarcomas of other histologic subtypes, most importantly, the GISTs, are discussed in Chapter 5.

Lymphoma

Pathology

Lymphoma may arise as a primary GI neoplasm or as a component of systemic disease with GI involvement. The small intestine is the second most common site of primary GI lymphoma (the stomach is the most common site). The distribution of lymphoma in the small intestine parallels the distribution of lymphoid follicles in the small intestine, with the lymphoid-rich ileum representing the most common location of small bowel lymphoma. When lymphoma arises from the lymphoid aggregates in the submucosa, infiltration of the mucosa can result in ulceration and bleeding. The tumor may also extend to the serosa and adjacent tissues, producing a large obstructing mass associated with cramping abdominal pain. Perforation occurs in as many as 25% of the patients. As with sarcoma, bulky disease is a characteristic of lymphoma, with approximately 70% of the tumors larger than 5 cm in diameter.

The most common histologic type of primary small bowel lymphoma is diffuse large B-cell. Other less common histologies include mucosa-associated lymphoid tissue [MALT] lymphoma, Burkitt/atypical Burkitt lymphoma, mantle cell, and follicular lymphoma. There are several staging systems for GI lymphomas, including the Ann Arbor Staging System which is detailed in Chapter 17 (Hematologic Malignancies and Splenic Tumors). Prognostic factors for small bowel lymphoma include tumor grade, extent of tumor penetration, nodal involvement, peritoneal disease, and distant metastasis. The 5-year survival rates range from 20% to 33%.

Treatment

The initial treatment for primary lymphoma of the small bowel is chemotherapy. The first-line chemotherapy regimen currently used at the M. D. Anderson Cancer Center is anthracycline-based combination chemotherapy, such as cyclophosphamide, doxorubicin, vincristine, and prednisone (CHOP).

Unfortunately, intra-abdominal complications of the tumor, most notably obstruction and perforation, can preempt or prohibit the use of cytotoxic chemotherapy. After initiating chemotherapy, perforation of the bowel may result due to tumor involvement of the inherent thin wall of the small intestine. In these clinical situations, surgical resection of the primary tumor extending to grossly normal bowel may be a safer treatment than chemotherapy. There is no role for frozen-section evaluation of margins because potential microscopic disease will be adequately treated by adjuvant chemotherapy. Lymph node metastases are frequent, but en bloc resection of the adjoining mesentery is only indicated if necessary to achieve complete gross resection of the primary tumor mass. Otherwise, the tumor burden in the lymph nodes is better treated with adjuvant chemotherapy.

Experimental Therapy

Chemoradiation has been used at some institutions for nodal metastasis, positive resection margins, and unresectable disease. However, a survival benefit from such treatment regimens has not been demonstrated. The use of radiation therapy alone has been associated with significant tumor necrosis, bleeding, and bowel perforation, but may be considered in elderly patients unable to tolerate the toxicity of chemotherapy.

Metastatic Malignancies

Pathology

Metastases are the most common form of malignancy in the small intestine and develop as a result of hematogenous or lymphatic spread from a primary tumor to the mucosa or submucosal lymphatics of the small intestine. The primary tumors that most commonly metastasize to the small bowel include ovarian, colon, lung, and melanoma. Metastatic melanoma is unique in that once localized in the small bowel, the metastatic focus may further disseminate to the small bowel mesentery and draining lymph nodes. In general, however, small bowel metastases remain localized to the bowel wall, and they may produce small bowel obstruction (frequently due to intussusception with melanoma metastases) or perforation.

Although the typical presentation of metastatic lesions is obstruction or perforation, recurrence of the primary tumor or adhesions resulting from the initial exploration are more common causes of obstruction and perforation in patients with a history of surgical resection of a GI primary tumor. In general, a segmental bowel resection without regional lymphadenectomy is the primary treatment for small bowel metastases. An exception is melanoma metastases, where a regional lymphadenectomy is recommended to remove adjacent lymph nodes at risk of harboring metastatic foci.

Palliation

At the time of diagnosis, primary or metastatic malignancies involving the small bowel are often locally advanced, with significant bulky disease or metastases. When the advanced stage of disease precludes surgical resection, enteric bypass should be performed for palliation. In the event of bleeding from an unresectable small bowel malignancy, superselective arterial embolization of small bowel mesenteric arteries can be considered. The patient should be closely monitored for postembolectomy bowel ischemia and perforation, although the risk of complications has decreased with improvement in superselective angiography techniques.

Chemotherapy or chemoradiation may offer effective control of locally advanced unresectable disease, particularly in the case of lymphoma, and should be considered as a palliative treatment option.

SURVEILLANCE

Routine follow-up for patients should include a complete history and physical examination, complete blood cell count, serum electrolyte determination, and liver function tests performed at regular intervals. A chest radiograph should be obtained every 6 months for the first 3 years after resection, followed by subsequent yearly examinations. Assessment of locoregional recurrence in patients who have undergone segmental resection for duodenal malignancy should include endoscopy at 6-month intervals. Assessment for recurrence at other sites may include CT scan, UGI/SBFT, angiography, or enteroscopy and must be directed by clinical suspicion based on patient history and physical and laboratory findings.

Recommended Readings

Ajani JA, Carrasco H, Samaan NA, et al. Therapeutic options in patients with advanced islet cell and carcinoid tumors. *Reg Cancer Treat.* 1990;3:235.

Arai M, Shimizu S, Imai Y, et al. Mutations of the Ki-*ras*, *p53* and *APC* genes in adenocarcinomas of the human small intestine. *Int J Cancer.* 1997;70:390.

Bakaeen FG, Murr MM, Sarr MG, et al. What prognostic factors are important in duodenal adenocarcinoma? *Arch Surg.* 2000;135:635–642.

Barnes G, Romero L, Hess KR, et al. Primary adenocarcinoma of the duodenum: management and survival in 67 patients. *Ann Surg Oncol.* 1994;1:73.

Bilimoria KY, Bentrem DJ, Wayne JD, et al. Small bowel cancer in the United States. Changes in epidemiology, treatment, and survival over the last 20 years. *Ann Surg.* 2009;249(1):63–71.

Bomanji J, Mather S, Moyes J, et al. A scintigraphic comparison of iodine-123 metaiodobenzylguanidine and iodine-labeled somatostatin analog (tyr-3-octreotide) in metastatic carcinoid tumors. *J Nucl Med.* 1992;33:1121.

Cancer Facts and Figures 2009, American Cancer Society, www.cancer.org

Carrasco CH, Charnsangavej C, Ajani J, et al. The carcinoid syndrome palliation by hepatic artery embolization. *AJR Am J Roentgenol.* 1986;147:149.

Cattell RB, Braasch JW. A technique for the exposure of the third and fourth portions of the duodenum. *Surg Gynecol Obstet.* 1960;11:379.

Cheek RC, Wilson H. Carcinoid tumors. *Curr Probl Surg.* 1970;11:4–31.

Crist DW, Sitzman JV, Cameron JL. Improved hospital morbidity, mortality, and survival after the Whipple procedure. *Ann Surg.* 1987;206:358.

Dabaja BS, Suki D, Pro B, et al. Adenocarcinoma of the small bowel. *Cancer.* 2004; 101:518.

Dematteo RP, Lewis JJ, Leung D, et al. Two hundred gastrointestinal stromal tumors: recurrence patterns and prognostic factors for survival. *Ann Surg.* 2000; 231:51.

Eriksson BK, Larsson EG, Skogseid BM, et al. Liver embolizations of patients with malignant neuroendocrine gastrointestinal tumors. *Cancer.* 1998;81:2293.

Farouk M, Niotis M, Branum GD, et al. Indications for and the techniques of local resection of tumors of the papilla of Vater. *Arch Surg.* 1991;126:650.

Feldman JM. Carcinoid tumors and syndrome. *Semin Oncol.* 1987;14:237.

Gill SS, Heuman DH, Mihas AA. Small intestinal neoplasms. *J Clin Gastroenterol.* 2001;33(4):267–282.

Graadt van Roggen JF, van Velthuysen MLF, Hogendoorn PCW. The histopathological differential diagnosis of gastrointestinal stromal tumours. *J Clin Pathol.* 2001; 54:96.

Hanson MW, Feldman JE, Blinder RA, et al. Carcinoid tumors: iodine-131 MIBG scintigraphy. *Radiology.* 1989;172:699.

Howe JR, Karnell LH, Menck HR, et al. The American College of Surgeons Commission on Cancer and the American Cancer Society. Adenocarcinoma of the small bowel: review of the National Cancer Data Base, 1985–1995. *Cancer.* 1999;86: 2693–2706.

Howe JR, Karnell LH, Scott-Conner C. Small bowel sarcoma: analysis of survival from the National Cancer Data Base. *Ann Surg Oncol.* 2001;8(6):496–508.

Joensuu H, Roberts PJ, Sarlomo-Rikala M, et al. Effect of the tyrosine kinase inhibitor STI571 in a patient with a metastatic gastrointestinal stromal tumor. *N Engl J Med.* 2001;344:1052.

Joestling DR, Beart RW, van Heerden JA, et al. Improving survival in adenocarcinoma of the duodenum. *Am J Surg.* 1981;141:228.

Kim CY, Suhocki PV, Miller MJ Jr, et al. Provocative mesenteric angiography for lower gastrointestinal hemorrhage: results from a single institution study. *J Vasc Interv Radiol.* 2010;21(4):477–483.

Kulke MH, Mayer RJ. Medical progress: carcinoid tumors. *N Engl J Med.* 1999;340:858.

Kvols LK, Moertel CG, O'Connell MJ, et al. Treatment of the malignant carcinoid syndrome: evaluation of a long acting somatostatin analogue. *N Engl J Med.* 1986;315:663.

Kwaan MR, Goldberg JE, Bleday R. Rectal carcinoid tumors: review of results after endoscopic and surgical therapy. *Arch Surg.* 2008;143(5):471–475.

Ladas SD, Triantafyllou K, Spada C, et al. European Society of Gastrointestinal Endoscopy (ESGE): Recommendations (2009) on clinical use of video capsule endoscopy to investigate small-bowel, esophageal, and colonic disease. *Endoscopy.* 2010;42(3):220–227.

Lamberts SW, Bakker WH, Reubi JC, et al. Somatostatin-receptor imaging in the localization of endocrine tumors. *N Engl J Med.* 1990;323:1246.

Landry CS, Brock G, Scoggins CR, et al. A proposed staging system for rectal carcinoid tumors based on an analysis of 4701 tumors. *Surgery.* 2008;144(3):460–466.

Lewis BS, Kornbluth A, Waye JD. Small bowel tumors: yield of enteroscopy. *Gut.* 1991; 32:763.

Lowell JA, Rossi RL, Munson L, et al. Primary adenocarcinoma of third and fourth portions of duodenum. *Arch Surg.* 1992;127: 557.

Maggard MA, O'Connell JB, Ko CY. Updated population-based review of carcinoid tumors. *Ann Surg.* 2004;240(1):117–122.

Maglinte DT, O'Connor K, Bessette J, et al. The role of the physician in the late diagnosis of primary malignant tumors of the small intestine. *J Gastroenterol.* 1991; 86:304.

Makridis C, Rastad J, Oberg K, et al. Progression of metastases and symptom improvement from laparotomy in midgut carcinoid tumors. *World J Surg.* 1996; 20:900.

Moertel CG, Weiland LH, Nagorney DM, et al. Carcinoid tumor of the appendix: treatment and prognosis. *N Engl J Med.* 1987;317:1699.

Motojima K, Tsukasa T, Kanematsu T, et al. Distinguishing pancreatic cancer from other periampullary carcinomas by analysis of mutations in the Kirsten-ras oncogene. *Ann Surg.* 1991;214:657.

Moyana TN, Xiang J, Senthilselvan A, et al. The spectrum of neuroendocrine differentiation among gastrointestinal carcinoids. *Arch Pathol Lab Med.* 2000; 124:570.

Naunheim KS, Zeitels J, Kaplan EL, et al. Rectal carcinoid tumors—treatment and prognosis. *Surgery.* 1983;94(4):67–76.

Nave H, Mossinger E, Feist H, et al. Surgery as primary treatment in patients with liver metastases from carcinoid tumors: a retrospective, unicentric study over 13 years. *Surgery.* 2001;129:170.

Ng EH, Pollock RE, Munsell MF, et al. Prognostic factors influencing survival in gastrointestinal leiomyosarcomas. Implications for surgical management and staging. *Ann Surg.* 1992;215(1):68–77.

North JH, Pack MS. Malignant tumors of the small intestine: a review of 144 cases. *Am Surg.* 2000;66:46.

O'Rourke MG, Lancashire RP, Vattoune JR. Lymphoma of the small intestine. *Aust N Z J Surg.* 1986;56:351.

Oberg K. Carcinoid tumors: current concepts in diagnosis and treatment. *Oncologist.* 1998;3:339.

Oberg K, Eriksson B. The role of interferons in the management of carcinoid tumors. *Br J Haematol.* 1991;79:74.

Ouriel K, Adams JT. Adenocarcinoma of the small intestine. *Am J Surg.* 1984;147:66.

Overman MJ, Kopetz S, Lin E, et al. Is there a role for adjuvant therapy in resected adenocarcinoma of the small intestine. *Acta Oncologica.* 2010;49:474–479.

Overman MJ, Kopetz S, Wen S, et al. Chemotherapy with 5-fluorouracil and a platinum compound improves outcomes in metastatic small bowel adenocarcinoma. *Cancer.* 2008;113:2038–2045.

Patel SR, Benjamin RS. Management of peritoneal and hepatic metastases from gastrointestinal stromal tumors. *Surg Oncol.* 2000;9:67.

Pidhorecky I, Cheney RT, Kraybill WG, et al. Gastrointestinal stromal tumors: current diagnosis, biologic behavior, and management. *Ann Surg Oncol.* 2000;7:705.

Rinke A, Muller HH, Schade-Brittinger C, et al. Placebo-controlled, double-blind, prospective, randomized study on the effect of octreotide LAR in the control of tumor growth in patients with metastatic neuroendocrine midgut tumors: a report from the PROMID Study Group. *J Clin Oncol.* 2009;27(28):4656–4663.

Rothmund M, Kisker O. Surgical treatment of carcinoid tumors of the small bowel, appendix, colon and rectum. *Digestion.* 1994;55(suppl 3):86.

Ryder NM, Ko CY, Hines OJ, et al. Primary duodenal adenocarcinoma. *Arch Surg.* 2000;135:1070.

Sohn TA, Lillemoe KD, Cameron JL, et al. Adenocarcinoma of the duodenum: factors influencing long-term survival. *J Gastrointest Surg.* 1998;2:79.

Stinner B, Kisker L, Zielke A, et al. Surgical management for carcinoid tumors of small bowel, appendix, colon and rectum. *World J Surg.* 1996;20:183.

Strodel WE, Talpos G, Eckhauser F, et al. Surgical therapy for small bowel carcinoid tumors. *Arch Surg.* 1983;118:391.

Talamini MA, Moesinger RC, Pitt HA, et al. Adenocarcinoma of the ampulla of Vater. A 28-year experience. *Ann Surg.* 1997;225:590.

Thompson GB, van Heerden JA, Martin JK Jr, et al. Carcinoid tumors of the gastrointestinal tract: presentation, management, and prognosis. *Surgery.* 1985;98:1054.

Tsai BM, Finne CO, Nordenstam JF, et al. Transanal endoscopic microsurgery resection of rectal tumors: outcomes and recommendations. *Dis Colon Rectum.* 2010;53(1):16–23.

Van Ooijen B, Kalsbeek HL. Carcinoma of the duodenum. *Surg Gynecol Obstet.* 1988; 166:343.

Verman D, Stroehlein JR. Adenocarcinoma of the small bowel: a 60-yr perspective derived from M. D. Anderson Cancer Center tumor registry. *Am J Gastroenterol.* 2006;101:1657–1654.

Vinik AI, Thompson N, Eckhauser F, et al. Clinical features of carcinoid syndrome and the use of somatostatin analogue in its management. *Acta Oncol.* 1989;28:389.

Wallace S, Ajani JA, Charnsangavej C, et al. Carcinoid tumors: imaging procedures and interventional radiology. *World J Surg.* 1996;20:147.

Welch JP, Malt RA. Management of carcinoid tumors of the gastrointestinal tract. *Surg Gynecol Obstet.* 1977;145:223.

Wessels FJ, Schell SR. Radiofrequency ablation treatment of refractory carcinoid hepatic metastases. *J Surg Res.* 2001;95:8.

Willett CG, Warshaw AL, Connery K, et al. Patterns of failure after pancreaticoduodenectomy for ampullary carcinoma. *Surg Gynecol Obstet.* 1993;176:33.

Yao JC. Neuroendocrine tumors. Molecular targeted therapy for carcinoid and islet-cell carcinoma. *Best Pract Res Clin Endocrinol Metab.* 2007;21(1):163–172.

Yao JC, Hassan M, Phan A, et al. One hundred years after "carcinoid": epidemiology of and prognostic factors for neuroendocrine tumors in 35,825 cases in the United States. *J Clin Onc.* 2008;26(18): 3063–3072.

Yao JC, Phan AT, Chang DZ, et al. Efficacy of RAD001 (everolimus) and octreotide LAR in advanced low-to intermediate grade neuroendocrine tumors: results of a phase II study. *J Clin Onc.* 2008;26(26): 4311–4318.

Yeo CJ, Cameron JL, Sohn TA, et al. Six hundred fifty consecutive pancreaticoduodenectomies in the 1990s: pathology, complications, and outcomes. *Ann Surg.* 1997;226:248.

Younes N, Fulton N, Tanaka R, et al. The presence of K-12 *ras* mutations in duodenal adenocarcinomas and the absence of *ras* mutations in other small bowel adenocarcinomas and carcinoid tumors. *Cancer.* 1997;79:1804.

Zuetenhorst JM, Taal BG. Metastatic carcinoid tumors: a clinical review. *Oncologist.* 2005;10:123.

Cancer of the Colon, Rectum, and Anus

Eric J. Silberfein, George J. Chang,
Yi-Qian Nancy You, and Barry W. Feig

EPIDEMIOLOGY

Colorectal cancer is the third most commonly diagnosed cancer and the third leading cause of cancer deaths in both men and women in the United States. In 2009, there were an estimated 146,970 cases diagnosed in the United States, including 106,102 cases of colon cancer and 40,870 cases of rectal cancer. Colorectal cancer incidence rates have continued to decline since 1985, a decline partly believed to be due to improved screening and treatment of polyps before their progression to invasive cancers. However, colorectal cancer still accounts for approximately 9% of cancer deaths. Estimates for the year 2009 show 49,920 deaths from colon and rectal cancer.

In the United States, the cumulative lifetime risk of developing colorectal cancer is about 6%. The median age at onset is 72 years for colon cancer and 68 years for rectal cancer. The risk of colorectal cancer clearly increases with age. Except in the setting of hereditary forms of colorectal cancer, this disease rarely occurs before age 40. After age 50, there is a rapid increase in the rate of disease as the incidence is more than 14 times higher in adults 50 years and older than in those younger than 50. This is represented by 91% of new cases and 94% of deaths occurring in patients older than 50. These facts are responsible for the recommendations to begin screening at age 50. Based on data between 1996 and 2004, the 5-year relative survival for colon cancer is 65% and for rectal cancer is 67% overall.

When diagnosed, 40% of patients have localized disease, 37% have regional disease, 20% have distant metastasis, and 5% are unstaged. The survival rates for local, regional, and distant disease at 5 years are 90%, 68%, and 11%, respectively, and at 10 years are 85%, 58%, and 6.6%, respectively.

Approximately 75% of colorectal cancer cases are sporadic, with the remainder of cases occurring in patients who are at increased risk. The patients with increased risk include those with inflammatory bowel disease, familial adenomatous polyposis (FAP), and hereditary nonpolyposis colorectal cancer (HNPCC), as well as patients with a strong family history of colorectal cancer. Men are at slightly increased risk as the age-adjusted incidence is 58.5 per 100,000 in men and 44.2 per 100,000 in women.

RISK FACTORS

Diet

Many dietary factors have been studied regarding their effect on colorectal cancer. Consumption of red meat, processed meat, and animal fat, as well as the presence of high fecal levels of cholesterol, correlate with and may be causally related to an increased risk of colorectal carcinoma. Smoking increases the development of adenomatous polyps, particularly more aggressive adenomas, and some studies have shown that long-term smoking increases the risk of developing colorectal cancer, particularly rectal cancer. Furthermore, colorectal cancer has been linked to moderate alcohol consumption (30 g or approximately two drinks/day). Folate supplements have been shown to be protective against colorectal cancer. Calcium supplements have been shown to decrease the formation of new adenomas in patients with a history of adenomas. Vitamins with antioxidant properties including beta-carotene, vitamin C, vitamin D, and vitamin E have been studied, and at present there are no prospective data that demonstrate a protective effect from colorectal cancer with their use. Dietary fiber has also been studied and is epidemiologically associated with a decreased colorectal cancer risk; however, no prospective data support its use for protection from the development of colorectal cancer. Increasing garlic consumption may be associated with a decreased risk.

Medications
Several medications have demonstrated protective effects for colorectal cancer. Hormone replacement therapy has been shown to significantly decrease mortality from colorectal cancer in women. Aspirin and other nonsteroidal anti-inflammatory drugs have also demonstrated protective effects. Recent studies with sulindac and the selective cyclooxygenase-2 inhibitor celecoxib demonstrated the ability of these agents to cause regression of colon polyps in patients with FAP. However, the cyclooxygenase-2 inhibitors have been associated with an increased risk for cardiovascular complications; therefore, their role in chemoprevention remains unclear.

Polyps
Most colorectal cancers arise from polyps. Colorectal polyps are classified histologically as either neoplastic (adenomatous including serrated adenomatous) polyps (which may be benign or malignant) or non-neoplastic (including hyperplastic, mucosal, inflammatory, and hamartomatous) polyps. Adenomatous polyps are found in approximately 33% of the general population by age 50 and in approximately 50% of the general population by age 70. Most lesions are less than 1 cm in size, with 60% of people having a single adenoma and 40% having multiple lesions. Sixty percent of lesions will be located distal to the splenic flexure.

A genetic model for colon carcinogenesis has been developed from the genetic analysis of colorectal adenomas and carcinomas. This model demonstrates a sequence of genetic alterations responsible for the development of colorectal adenomas and their progression to invasive carcinoma and involves separate pathways. The traditional pathway begins with a mutation in the adenomatous polyposis coli (APC) gene leading to a small tubular adenoma which, through a series of genetic mutations including *p53*, progresses to a large adenoma with severe dysplasia and eventual carcinoma. The serrated pathway begins with a *BRAF* mutation leading to a hyperplastic polyp which may or may not be predisposed to high levels of methylation leading to the development of a sessile serrated adenoma. The National Polyp Study showed that colonoscopic removal of adenomatous polyps significantly reduced the risk of developing colorectal cancer.

Polyps coexist with colorectal cancer in 60% of patients and are associated with an increased incidence of synchronous and metachronous colonic neoplasms. Patients with a primary cancer and a solitary associated polyp have a lower incidence of synchronous and metachronous lesions when compared to patients with multiple polyps. The natural history of polyps supports an aggressive approach to their treatment: invasive cancer will develop in 24% of patients with untreated polyps at the site of that polyp within 20 years.

There are three main histologic variants of adenomatous polyps. *Tubular adenomas* represent 75% to 87% of polyps and are found with equal frequency throughout all segments of the bowel. Less than 5% of tubular adenomas are malignant. *Tubulovillous adenomas* constitute 8% to 15% of polyps. They are also equally distributed throughout the bowel, and 20% to 25% are malignant. The remaining 5% to 10% of polyps are *villous adenomas*, which are most commonly found in the rectum; 35% to 40% of these polyps are malignant. Polyps may be pedunculated (usually tubular or tubulovillous), sessile (usually tubulovillous or villous), or non-polypoid (flat or depressed). Nonpolypoid neoplasms are more difficult to detect because of subtle similarities to normal mucosa. Depressed nonpolypoid lesions have been shown to carry a high risk of cancer at the time of diagnosis. Besides histologic characteristics, the size of a polyp and the degree of dysplasia has been associated with malignant potential. Malignancy was found in 1.3% of adenomas less than 1 cm, 9.5% between 1 and 2 cm, and 46% greater than 2 cm. Similarly, 5.7% of mild, 18% of moderate, and 34.5% of adenomatous polyps with severe dysplasia were found to have malignant cells on complete excision of the polyp. Therefore, although only 2% to 5% of adenomatous polyps harbor malignancy at the time of diagnosis, the histologic characteristics, size, and degree of dysplasia can help predict which polyps will be malignant.

The terms *carcinoma in situ, intramucosal carcinoma,* and *high-grade dysplasia* are used to describe severely dysplastic adenomas where the cancerous cells have not invaded through the muscularis mucosae and therefore do not have a risk of lymph node metastases. Some degree of dysplasia exists in all adenomas. In an effort to avoid confusion, standardized use of the term *high-grade dysplasia* is advocated. Approximately 5% to 7% of adenomatous polyps contain high-grade dysplasia and 3% to 5% have invasive carcinoma at the time of diagnosis. Increasing dysplasia and malignant potential correlate with increasing size, villous component, and patient age. If a polyp containing high-grade dysplasia is completely excised endoscopically, the patient may be considered cured.

Overall, 8.5% to 25% of polyps harboring invasive carcinoma will metastasize to regional lymph nodes. Unfavorable pathological features of malignant colorectal polyps increase the probability that regional lymph nodes will be involved with tumor and include (a) poor differentiation, (b) vascular and/or lymphatic invasion, (c) invasion below the submucosa, and (d) positive resection margin as defined by the presence of tumor within 1 to 2 mm from the transected margin and the presence of tumor cells within the diathermy of the transected margin. Poorly differentiated lesions (grade 3) are associated with a higher incidence of lymphovascular involvement and recurrent disease when compared with well- and moderately differentiated lesions (grades 1 and 2, respectively). Approximately 4% to 8% of malignant polyps will be poorly differentiated. The presence of one or more of these adverse features should prompt evaluation for surgical resection. Depth of invasion is an important prognostic factor for mesenteric lymph node involvement with invasive cancer arising in a polyp. In 1985, Haggitt et al. classified the level of invasion from the head of the polyp to the submucosa of the underlying colonic wall (Table 11.1). In a multivariate analysis, only invasion into the submucosa of the underlying bowel wall (level 4) was a significant prognostic factor. This is in keeping with previous pathological studies that have shown that the lymphatic channels do

T A B L E 11.1	Haggitt Classification for Colorectal Carcinomas Arising in Adenomas
Classification	**Depth of Invasion**
0	Carcinoma confined to the mucosa
1	Head of polyp
2	Neck of polyp
3	Stalk of polyp
4	Submucosa of the underlying colonic wall

not penetrate above the muscularis mucosa. Although these findings have been confirmed by other studies, there are frequently multiple adverse prognostic factors seen in patients with higher levels of invasion (i.e., levels 3 and 4), which makes it difficult to assign depth as the most important factor. A negative resection margin has consistently been shown to be associated with a decreased risk for adverse outcome (recurrence, residual carcinoma, lymph node metastases, decreased survival). Twenty-seven percent of patients with positive or indeterminate tumor margins will have adverse outcomes, compared with 18% with negative margins and poor prognostic features and 0.8% with negative margins and no other poor prognostic features. Therefore, a negative margin is only one component in risk factor assessment.

An additional classification system for malignant colorectal polyps may be applicable to malignant sessile polyps and was described by Kikuchi in 1995. It classifies invasive cancer as Sm1 (slight carcinoma invasion of the muscularis mucosa, 200 to 300 μm), Sm2 (intermediate invasion), or Sm3 (deep submucosal invasion extending to the inner surface of the muscularis propria). Sm1 depth of invasion is associated with a low risk for local recurrence or lymph node metastasis. In a Mayo Clinic series, Sm3 depth of invasion was associated with a 23% risk for lymph node metastasis.

Although clinical factors such as age, location, number of polyps, and gender are collectively known to be prognostic factors, only age greater than 60 years has been identified as an independent risk factor for invasion.

Treatment

When adenomatous polyps are found by sigmoidoscopy, we recommend complete colonoscopy with colonoscopic removal of the polyp and colonoscopic surveillance every 1 to 3 years until the examination result is normal. Colonoscopic polypectomy is a safe, effective treatment for nearly all pedunculated polyps. For those polyps not amenable to safe colonoscopic removal, endoscopic mucosal resection (EMR) provides a way of treating small flat and depressed (not >1 cm) lesions that may have a high risk of deep invasion into the submucosa. Furthermore, EMR is a curative procedure for early cancers without lymphovascular invasion or lesions capable of harboring a focal cancer. By resecting in the deep submucosal layer, EMR provides an en-bloc resection for pathologic analysis. A surgical resection is recommended for large sessile villous lesions. Fungating, ulcerated, or distorted lesions destroying the surrounding bowel wall indicate the presence of invasive cancer and are contraindications to polypectomy.

Colectomy is indicated for patients with residual invasive carcinoma and for those at high risk for lymph node metastases despite complete endoscopic polypectomy. The high-risk pathological features previously described (margin <3 mm, poor differentiation, Haggitt level 4, and vascular or lymphatic invasion) and the resultant increased risk of lymph node metastasis should be weighed against the risk of surgical resection.

In a review of 17 studies to evaluate the frequency of lymph node metastases or residual carcinoma in low-risk patients with pedunculated polyps, only a 1% incidence was found. In sessile polyps with low-risk features, the incidence was increased to 4.1%. Because the incidence of nodal metastases is higher in sessile polyps with invasive cancer, those patients at low operative risk should be considered for resection even if no high-risk pathological features are observed. Stalk invasion in pedunculated polyps is not considered an adverse histologic feature, and treatment of polyps with stalk invasion is the same as that of polyps without stalk invasion (based on risk stratification). Polypoid cancers (almost all the polyp is invaded with carcinoma) are treated no differently from other malignant polypoid lesions. Large villous adenomas of the rectum may be amenable to transanal local excision. This provides a complete diagnostic evaluation for malignancy, and if excised with negative margins (with other favorable prognostic features), it may be the only therapeutic procedure needed.

Hereditary Colorectal Cancer Syndromes

The majority of colorectal cancers are sporadic cancers that occur in patients without a significant family history of colorectal cancer. Approximately 5% to 10% of all colorectal cancers are associated with a familial colorectal cancer syndrome in which highly penetrant inherited mutations are associated with well-characterized clinical presentations. An additional 15% to 20% are associated with a familial predisposition. The hereditary colorectal cancer syndromes expressing adenomatous polyps include HNPCC (Lynch syndrome), FAP, attenuated FAP, and MUTYH-associated polyposis (MAP). Hamartomatous polyps are expressed in Peutz–Jeghers syndrome (PJS) and juvenile polyposis syndrome (JPS). All of these conditions are inherited in an autosomal dominant fashion except MAP which is inherited in an autosomal recessive fashion.

HNPCC (Lynch syndrome) is the most common inherited colorectal cancer syndrome and accounts for 2% to 4% of all colorectal cancers. Individuals with HNPCC are predisposed to a number of other cancers including tumors of the endometrium, ovary, stomach, small bowel, hepatobiliary tract, pancreas, ureter, and renal pelvis. Penetrance is between 30% and 70%. There is an estimated 50% to 85% lifetime risk of developing colorectal cancer. Compared with patients with sporadic colon cancer, patients with HNPCC have cancers that are more right sided (60% to 70% occur proximal to the splenic flexure), occur earlier (at about 45 years of age), have a lower stage, have better survival, and have an increased rate of metachronous and synchronous tumors (20%).

The genetic mutations causing HNPCC are DNA mismatch repair (MMR) genes that cause a microsatellite repeat replication error to go unfixed, thereby inactivating tumor suppressor genes; hence the term genetic instability. The cancers that develop are said to be characterized by a high level of microsatellite instability (MSI-H) and afford a better overall prognosis compared to those without MSI. Four of the DNA MMR genes have been linked to HNPCC and include hMLH1, hMSH2, hMSH6, and hPMS2. Mutations in hMLH1 and hMLH2 account for up to 90% of Lynch syndrome cases; mutations in hMSH6 account for approximately 10%, and mutations in hPMS2 are detected on rare occasions. One of the main difficulties in the management of patients with HNPCC is the identification of those individuals who should be tested. A detailed family history should be obtained in all patients with colorectal cancer and may identify high-risk conditions for which genetic counseling should be obtained. Potentially affected individuals may also be identified by screening using Amsterdam criteria or Bethesda guidelines (Table 11.2). Although lacking in specificity, the use of these criteria and guidelines is associated with 60% to 94% sensitivity for identifying individuals with HNPCC. Furthermore, histopathological evaluation of the surgical specimen may reveal the presence of features associated with HNPCC, including a "Crohn-like" inflammatory cell infiltrate and signet ring cells. At M. D. Anderson Cancer Center (MDACC), immunohistochemistry for MMR gene protein expression is performed in the colorectal tumors of suspected individuals. If loss of one of the repair proteins is noted, genetic testing is performed.

The treatment of HNPCC begins with early surveillance. Screening colonoscopy in affected individuals should begin by 20 to 25 years of age and should be repeated every 1 to 2 years. Surgical treatment in those with confirmation of cancer includes subtotal colectomy with ileorectal anastomosis (IRA). Annual rectal surveillance is indicated thereafter. Segmental resection may be considered if annual colonoscopy can be performed. Prophylactic hysterectomy and bilateral salpingo-oophorectomy should be discussed as an option in women after the completion of childbearing.

T A B L E **11.2**	Amsterdam Criteria and Bethesda Guidelines

Amsterdam I

At least three relatives must have histologically verified colorectal cancer

1. One must be a first-degree relative of the other two
2. At least two successive generations must be affected
3. At least one of the relatives must have received the diagnosis before age 50

Amsterdam II

Similar to Amsterdam I, but may include any combination of cancers associated with HNPCC (e.g., colorectal, endometrial, gastric, ovarian, ureter or renal pelvis, brain, small bowel, hepatobiliary tract, sebaceous gland adenomas, keratoacanthomas)

Bethesda Guidelines

1. Amsterdam criteria are met
2. Two colorectal or HNPCC-related cancers, including synchronous and metachronous presentation
3. Colorectal cancer and a first-degree relative with colorectal and/or an HNPCC-related cancer and/or a colonic adenoma; one of the cancers must be diagnosed before age 45 and the adenoma diagnosed before age 40
4. Colorectal or endometrial cancer diagnosed before age 45
5. Right-sided colorectal cancer with an undifferentiated pattern (solid/cribriform) on histopathology, diagnosed before age 45
6. Signet ring cell-type colorectal cancer diagnosed before age 45 (>50% signet ring cells)
7. Colorectal adenomas diagnosed before age 40

Revised Bethesda Guidelines

1. Early onset colorectal cancer (before age 50)
2. Synchronous, metachronous, or other HNPCC-associated tumors, regardless of age
3. Colorectal cancer with high microsatellite instability diagnosed before age 60
4. Colorectal cancer diagnosed in one or more first-degree relatives with an HNPCC-related tumor, with one of the cancers being diagnosed before age 50
5. Colorectal cancer diagnosed in two or more first- or second-degree relatives with HNPCC-related tumors, regardless of age

HNPCC, hereditary nonpolyposis colorectal cancer.

FAP is the second most common inherited colorectal cancer syndrome; 1% to 2% of patients diagnosed with colon carcinoma will have FAP. Germ-line mutations in the APC gene on chromosome 5q are characteristic of FAP. The majority of the mutations result in a truncated APC protein; however, some mutations can only be identified with gene sequencing. The pattern of inheritance is autosomal dominant, with 90% penetrance. The incidence of new mutations in FAP patients is high; approximately 25% of all FAP cases are the result of a de novo germ-line mutation. In patients with FAP, thousands of polyps develop throughout the gastrointestinal (GI) tract but are most common in the colon. The median age of adenoma diagnosis is 15 years. Without prophylactic colectomy, colorectal cancer will develop in virtually all affected individuals by the end of the third decade of life. A milder phenotype known as *attenuated* FAP is associated with fewer polyps (average 30) with the typical age of onset for colorectal cancer by the early fifties. Attenuated FAP is a less severe form of the disease with an average 69% lifetime risk of colorectal cancer. Patients with FAP may also develop extracolonic manifestations including gastric polyps, duodenal adenomas and carcinomas, desmoid tumors, thyroid carcinoma, mandibular osteomas, congenital hypertrophy of the retinal pigmented epithelium, sebaceous and epidermoid cysts and fibromas (previously Gardner syndrome), or central nervous system tumors (Turcot syndrome). Commercial genetic testing can now identify the APC gene mutation by sequencing. Since the complete sequencing of the APC gene, studies have correlated the specific genetic mutations identified with the differing phenotypes of extraintestinal manifestations of FAP. Genetic testing and counseling should be offered to all patients in whom FAP is suspected. Surveillance for FAP should begin at the age of 10 to 12 with annual endoscopic evaluations. Once a mutation is identified within a family, unaffected individuals can be spared such an intensive surveillance regimen.

The primary treatment for FAP is prophylactic colectomy. Surgical options include abdominal colectomy with IRA, restorative proctocolectomy with ileal-pouch anal anastomosis (IPAA), and less commonly proctocolectomy with end ileostomy. Patients who have polyp burdens within the rectum that cannot be endoscopically controlled should not undergo IRA. It should be emphasized that after prophylactic colectomy or proctocolectomy, these patients must continue life-long surveillance because there remains a risk for cancer in the remaining rectum after IRA or at the anastomosis or within the ileal pouch itself after IPAA.

MAP has recently been identified from subgroups of patients in FAP registries who have tested negative for APC gene mutations. The pattern of inheritance is autosomal recessive, and the phenotype demonstrates multiple colorectal polyps (>10) but typically fewer than in individuals with classic FAP. The age of onset of colorectal cancer in patients younger than 50 years has been reported in those with biallelic MYH mutations. Colorectal cancers in MYH polyposis syndrome are associated with G : C to T : A transversions resulting from defects in base excision repair. Sub-total colectomy is advised for patients who develop colon cancer and should be considered when endoscopic management becomes problematic or when polyps become large or exhibit high-grade dysplasia. This colorectal cancer-associated polyposis syndrome continues to be defined.

Other less common hereditary colorectal cancer syndromes may be associated with hamartomatous polyposis such as PJS, JPS, Cowden syndrome, and Bannayan–Ruvalcaba–Riley syndrome. Germ-line mutations in STK11 (LKB1) are associated with PJS, mutations in SMAD4 and BMPR1-A are associated with JPS, and PTEN mutations are associated with Cowden syndrome and Bannayan–Ruvalcaba–Riley syndrome. The hamartomatous polyposis syndromes are associated with a significantly increased risk for colorectal cancer and are present in <1% of patients with colorectal cancer in North America (Table 11.3).

People with a first-degree relative with colorectal cancer have a 1.8- to 8-fold higher risk of colorectal cancer than the general population. The risk is higher if more than one relative is affected and higher if the cancer developed in the relative at a young age (<45). The role of inheritable genetic defects in predisposition to colorectal cancer in such patients is not well understood.

Inflammatory Bowel Disease
Chronic ulcerative colitis (CUC) carries a risk of colorectal carcinoma that is 30 times greater than that of the general population. The risk of cancer increases 0.5% to 1% per year after 10 years and is 18% to 35% at 30 years. The severity, extent, and duration of inflammation, as well as family history of colorectal cancer and history of primary sclerosing cholangitis, are risk factors for the development of cancer. In contrast to sporadic colorectal cancers, CUC-related cancers are more often multiple, broadly infiltrating, and poorly differentiated. It can be extremely difficult to

| TABLE 11.3 | Indications for Evaluation of High-Risk Colorectal Cancer Conditions |

Earlier age of cancer onset than the general population
   Colorectal or endometrial cancer before age 50 years
   Colorectal cancer with MSI-H histology
Multiple close family members with colorectal cancer or other Lynch syndrome cancers
Individual with multiple primary colorectal cancers or other Lynch syndrome cancers
Multiple cumulative gastrointestinal polyps

- Ten colorectal adenomatous polyps
- Twenty colonic serrated polyps
- Five serrated polyps in the proximal colon, two of which are >1 cm
- Five hamartomatous gastrointestinal polyps or any histologically distinct Peutz-Jeghers gastrointestinal polyp

Individual from a family with confirmed hereditary colorectal cancer syndrome

identify small tumors in a CUC colon due to the chronic changes resulting from the inflammatory process. Therefore, random surveillance biopsies should be routinely performed in patients with CUC, and prophylactic colectomy or proctocolectomy should be recommended for high-grade dysplasia and considered for low-grade dysplasia. Crohn disease is also associated with an increased risk for colorectal cancer that is related to the duration and severity of disease. Its risk is similar to that with CUC. The risk associated with inflammatory bowel disease underscores the importance of surveillance in this patient population.

Previous Colon Carcinoma
A second primary colon carcinoma is three times more likely to develop in patients with a history of colon cancer than in the general population; metachronous lesions develop in 5% to 8% of these patients.

SCREENING
The value of routine screening of asymptomatic populations who lack high-risk factors for development of colorectal cancer has been established. Screening should be initiated at age 50. As many as 19% of the general population are at risk of developing adenomatous polyps, and 5% of sporadic polyps may progress to colorectal carcinoma. The goals of screening are detection of early cancers and prevention of cancer by finding and removing adenomas. Five randomized trials have shown that fecal occult blood screening followed by colonoscopy has been shown to detect cancers at an earlier stage. One of these trials, the Minnesota Colon Cancer Control Study, has demonstrated a significantly improved cancer-related survival, and a meta-analysis of the randomized trials indicates that Hemoccult testing is associated with a 15% to 43% reduction in the mortality rate from colorectal carcinoma. However, the sensitivity of fecal occult blood tests (FOBTs) has been reported to be 30% to 90%. Therefore, alternative methods have been investigated, including immunochemical FOBTs and fecal tests for DNA mutations. If FOBT is positive, total colonoscopy should be performed.

Four case-control studies have demonstrated that sigmoidoscopy is associated with a reduced mortality for colorectal cancer. The utility of flexible sigmoidoscopy as a screening test for colorectal neoplasia is limited by the amount of colon visualized with a 60-cm sigmoidoscope. Therefore, flexible sigmoidoscopy should be used in conjunction with radiographic evaluation of the more proximal colon or annual fecal occult blood testing. As a screening test, flexible sigmoidoscopy, when normal, should be repeated every 5 years. If adenomatous disease is found, a full colonoscopy is warranted.

The value of colonoscopy in screening can be appreciated if one considers that approximately 40% of colon cancers arise proximal to the splenic flexure and that 75% of proximal colon cancers do not have an index lesion within reach of the flexible sigmoidoscope. All roads eventually lead to colonoscopy for diagnosis or therapy (as in the case of a lesion on barium enema). Most studies using screening colonoscopy in average-risk patients report an average of 30% of neoplastic lesions detected. Cost is an important issue, however, if colonoscopy is considered the ultimate screening tool. Currently, screening colonoscopy is cost-effective if a 10-year interval is used once the colon is cleared of polyps.

Double-contrast barium enema (DCBE) is used less frequently than colonoscopy for screening and can detect colorectal carcinoma and polyps greater than 1 cm with accuracy equal to that of colonoscopy. It has been used in patients who refuse or cannot have full colonoscopy to the cecum as an adjunct to flexible sigmoidoscopy to evaluate the remainder of the colon and for difficult-to-visualize turns in the colon. The difficulty with this method is that lesions detected by DCBE require further evaluation, decreasing the cost-effectiveness of the method. Current American Cancer Society screening recommendations are for DCBE every 5 years with subsequent colonoscopy if test results are positive.

Computed tomography (CT) colonography (virtual colonoscopy) has emerged as a technique for the diagnosis of colonic polyps in the screening population that uses three-dimensional reconstruction of the air-distended colon. At the National Naval Medical Center, in 1,223 average-risk adults who subsequently underwent conventional (optical) colonoscopy, virtual colonoscopy was as good or better at detecting relevant lesions. A more recent multi-institutional study looking at 2,600 asymptomatic patients 50 years of age or older found that CT colonography identified 90% of patients with adenomas or cancers measuring 10 mm or more in diameter and further strengthened published data on the role of CT colonography in screening patients with an average risk of colorectal cancer. However, some of the major limitations included the need for full bowel preparation and follow-up colonoscopy for tissue diagnosis of radiographic abnormalities. Because virtual colonoscopy is considerably time and labor intensive from the standpoint of the radiologist, active investigations into methods of automating the evaluation process are ongoing. Current American Cancer Society screening recommendations are for virtual colonoscopy every 5 years with subsequent colonoscopy if a lesion is found.

Carcinoembryonic antigen (CEA) is a glycoprotein found in the cell membranes of many tissues, including colorectal cancer. Some of the antigen enters the circulation and is detected by radioimmunoassay of serum; CEA is also detectable in various other body fluids, urine, and feces. Elevated serum CEA is not specifically associated with colorectal cancer; abnormally high levels are also found in sera of patients with malignancies of the pancreas, breast, ovary, prostate gland, head and neck, bladder, and kidney. CEA levels are high in approximately 30% to 80% of patients with cancer of the colon, but less than half of patients with localized disease are CEA positive. Therefore, CEA has no role in screening for primary lesions. False-positive results occur in benign disease (lung, liver, and bowel). The CEA level is also increased in smokers. Overall, 60% of tumors will be missed by CEA screening alone.

Screening Recommendations

In 2008, the U.S. Multisociety Task Force on Colorectal cancer met to update the 2002 consensus guidelines for colorectal cancer screening and surveillance and made recommendations regarding screening (Table 11.4).

T A B L E **11.4**	Colorectal Cancer Screening Recommendations

Risk Category	Screening Recommendations
Average risk, asymptomatic (age ≥50, consider ≥45 years for African American)	FOBT each year (full colonoscopy or CT colonography if +) Flexible sigmoidoscopy every 5 years (consider full colonoscopy if +) Colonoscopy every 5–10 years CT colonography every 5–10 years
First-degree relative with CRC or adenomatous polyps at age ≤60 years, or two second-degree relatives affected with CRC	Same as for average risk but starting at age 40 years Colonoscopy every 5 years beginning at age 40 or 10 years younger than the earliest diagnosis in the family
Gene carrier or at risk for FAP	Annual flexible sigmoidoscopy beginning at 10–12 years
Gene carrier or at risk for HNPCC	Colonoscopy every 1–2 years beginning at age 20–25 years or 10 years younger than the earliest case in the family

FOBT, fecal occult blood test; DCBE, double-contrast barium enema; CRC, colorectal cancer; FAP, familial adenomatous polyposis; HNPCC, hereditary nonpolyposis colorectal cancer.

PATHOLOGY

Histologically, more than 90% of colon cancers are adenocarcinomas. On gross appearance, there are four morphologic variants of adenocarcinoma. Ulcerative adenocarcinoma is the most common configuration seen and is most characteristic of tumors in the descending and sigmoid colon. Exophytic (also known as polypoid or fungating) tumors are most commonly found in the ascending colon, particularly in the cecum. These tumors tend to project into the bowel lumen, and patients often present with a right-sided abdominal mass and anemia. Annular (scirrhous) adenocarcinoma tends to grow circumferentially into the wall of the colon, resulting in the classic apple core lesion seen on barium enema radiologic study. Rarely, a submucosal infiltrative pattern can be observed that is similar to linitis plastica seen with gastric adenocarcinoma.

Other epithelial histologic variants of colon cancer that are occasionally seen include mucinous (colloid) carcinoma, signet-ring cell carcinoma, adenosquamous and squamous cell carcinoma (SCC), and undifferentiated carcinoma. Other rare tumors include carcinoids and leiomyosarcomas.

A commonly used grading system is based on the degree of formation of glandular structures, nuclear pleomorphism, and number of mitoses. Grade 1 tumors have the most developed glandular structures with the fewest mitoses, grade 3 is the least differentiated with a high incidence of mitoses, and grade 2 is intermediate between grades 1 and 3.

STAGING

The Dukes and TNM staging systems for colorectal carcinoma are presented in Tables 11.5 and 11.6. Although most clinicians are familiar with both staging systems, clinical trial and treatment planning should be based on the TNM staging system. The Dukes staging system is important for historical perspective.

TABLE 11.5	Modified Astler–Coller Classification of the Dukes Staging System for Colorectal Cancer

Stage	Description
A	Lesion not penetrating submucosa
B1	Lesion invades but not through the muscularis propria
B2	Lesion through intestinal wall, no adjacent organ involvement
B3	Lesion involves adjacent organs
C1	Lesion B1 invasion depth; regional lymph node metastasis
C2	Lesion B2 invasion depth; regional lymph node metastasis
C3	Lesion B3 invasion depth; regional lymph node metastasis
D	Distant metastatic disease

CLINICAL PRESENTATION

Patients with colorectal cancer present with bleeding, anemia, abdominal pain, change in bowel habits, anorexia, weight loss, nausea, vomiting, fatigue, and anemia. Pelvic pain or tenesmus in rectal cancer may be associated with an advanced stage of disease indicating involvement of the pelvic floor muscles or nerves. Metastatic disease is suspected in patients with right upper quadrant pain, fevers and sweats, hepatomegaly, ascites, effusions, and supraclavicular adenopathy. Central nervous system and bone metastases are seen in less than 10% of autopsy cases and are very rare in the absence of advanced liver or lung disease. The incidence of complete obstruction in newly diagnosed colorectal cancer is 5% to 15%. In a large study from the United Kingdom, 49% of obstructions occurred at the splenic flexure, 23% occurred in the left colon, 23% occurred in the right colon, and 7% occurred in the rectum. Obstruction increases the risk of death from colorectal cancer 1.4-fold and is an independent covariate in multivariate analyses. Perforation occurs in 6% to 8% of colorectal carcinoma cases. Perforation increases the risk of death from cancer 3.4-fold. Using TMN staging and surveillance, epidemiology, and end results (SEER) program data, 15% of patients present with stage I disease, 30% with stage II, 20% with stage III, and 25% with stage IV. The remainder have unknown staging.

DIAGNOSIS

Colon Cancer

Clinical evaluation of carcinoma of the colon should include colonoscopy and biopsy (CT colonography should be considered if the entire colon could not be visualized by colonoscopy), chest radiograph, complete blood cell count, CEA determination, urinalysis, and liver function tests (LFTs).

The use of CT in the preoperative evaluation of patients with colon cancer is controversial. We evaluate the abdomen and pelvis with CT to detect involvement of contiguous organs, para-aortic lymph nodes, and the liver. Abnormal LFTs are present in only approximately 15% of patients with liver metastases and may be elevated without liver metastases in up to 40%; therefore, LFTs are not a useful screen for determining the need for obtaining a CT scan.

The preoperative CEA level can also reflect the extent of the disease and prognosis: CEA levels surpassing 10 to 20 ng/mL are associated with increased chances of disease failure for both node-negative and node-positive patients. About 15% to 20% of liver metastases will be nonpalpable at the time of surgery. However, up to 15% of lesions can be missed by combined preoperative and operative evaluation. Intraoperative ultrasonography has been shown to be the most accurate method of detecting liver metastasis. Approximately 20% of patients will have synchronous

TABLE 11.6   TNM Staging Classification of Colorectal Cancer

Primary Tumor (T)

TX	Primary tumor cannot be assessed
T0	No evidence of primary tumor
Tis	Carcinoma in situ: intraepithelial or invasion of the lamina propria without invasion through the muscularis mucosae into the submucosa
T1	Tumor invades submucosa
T2	Tumor invades muscularis propria
T3	Tumor invades through the muscularis propria into the subserosa or into nonperitonealized pericolic or perirectal tissues
T4a	Tumor penetrates to the surface of the visceral peritoneum
T4b	Tumor directly invades or is adherent to other organs or structures

Regional Lymph Nodes (N)

NX	Regional lymph nodes cannot be assessed
N0	No regional lymph node metastasis
N1	Metastasis in one to three regional lymph nodes
N1a	Metastasis in one regional lymph node
N1b	Metastasis in two to three regional lymph nodes
N1c	Tumor deposit(s) in the subserosa, mesentery, or nonperitonealized pericolic or perirectal tissues without regional nodal metastases
N2	Metastasis in four or more regional lymph nodes
N2a	Metastasis in four to six regional lymph nodes
N2b	Metastasis in seven or more regional lymph nodes

Distant Metastases (M)

MX	Distant metastasis cannot be assessed
M0	No distant metastasis
M1	Distant metastases present
M1a	Metastasis confined to one organ or site (e.g., liver, lung, ovary, nonregional node)
M1b	Metastases in more than one organ/site or the peritoneum

Stage Grouping

0	Tis	N0	M0
I	T1	N0	M0
	T2	N0	M0
IIA	T3	N0	M0
IIB	T4a	N0	M0
IIC	T4b	N0	M0
IIIA	T1–T2	N1/N1c	M0
	T1	N2a	M0
IIIB	T3–T4a	N1/N1c	M0
	T2–T3	N2a	M0
	T1–T2	N2b	M0
IIIC	T4a	N2a	M0
	T3–T4a	N2b	M0
	T4b	N1-N2	M0
IVA	Any T	Any N	M1a
IVB	Any T	Any N	M1b

liver metastasis at the time of diagnosis; therefore, the preoperative identification of liver metastasis is necessary for the surgical planning of combined resections of the primary tumor and the liver metastasis or for the treatment of tumors involving contiguous organs. Magnetic resonance imaging (MRI) may be helpful in circumstances when intravenous contrast-enhanced CT scanning is contraindicated. Patients who are symptomatic or have large, bulky lesions should have a preoperative intravenous pyelogram, CT scan, or cystoscopy to evaluate the urinary tract. At MDACC, CT scan is our initial test of choice in this scenario.

Positron emission tomography (PET), and now PET–CT, is a potentially important imaging modality for colorectal cancer. The technique uses the glucose analog fluorodeoxyglucose, which accumulates in metabolically active tissues. The standardized uptake value can provide a semi-quantitative determination to help discriminate benign from malignant disease. Although potentially useful in recurrent cancer, it has not been helpful in the primary evaluation of patients with colon cancer due to poor sensitivity, false positives, and high costs.

Rectal Cancer

In addition to the history and physical examination, chest radiograph, complete blood cell count, CEA, proctoscopic examination, endorectal ultrasound (ERUS), or dedicated rectal MRI, full colonoscopy and CT scan of the abdomen and pelvis should be performed to accurately stage and evaluate patients with rectal cancer. Symptomatic patients undergo evaluation of their urinary tract as described earlier for colon cancer.

Accurate preoperative staging tools are critical in rectal cancer because disease stage may influence treatment decisions such as local excision or preoperative multimodality therapy. ERUS is an accurate tool in determining tumor (T) stage. Performed using rigid or flexible probes, the layers of the rectal wall can be identified with 67% to 93% accuracy. The ERUS characteristics of T1 and T3 tumors make them relatively easy to differentiate. However, the distinction between T2 and T3 tumors is more difficult. ERUS is highly operator-dependent, and it can be difficult to differentiate lymph nodes from blood vessels and other structures or peritumoral edema from tumor. Furthermore, ERUS is limited in its ability to evaluate tumors that are large or bulky or associated with large villous tumors. As a result of these factors, overstaging occurs in approximately 20% of cases and understaging in approximately 10% to 20%. Stenotic lesions may make ERUS impossible secondary to the inability to pass the probe. ERUS evaluation of T stage is superior to that of CT scanning (52% to 83% accuracy) and compares to rectal MRI (59% to 95% accuracy). The relative accuracy of ERUS or MRI for rectal cancer staging is institution-dependent, and ERUS is preferred at MDACC. CT and MRI can delineate the relationship of the tumor to surrounding viscera and pelvic structures as well as predict risk for involvement of circumferential margins. The MERCURY Study Group (2006) found that MRI accurately predicted whether surgical margins would be clear or affected by tumor.

Lymph node staging in rectal cancer has proven more difficult than primary tumor staging, with ERUS accuracies of 62% to 83%, CT accuracies of 35% to 73%, and MRI accuracies of 39% to 84% reported. Despite descriptions of methods to radiologically predict metastases in lymph nodes, only nodal enlargements can be detected with most current technologies. About 50% to 75% of positive lymph nodes in rectal cancer may be normal in size, thereby limiting accurate evaluation. Similarly, lymph nodes may be enlarged from inflammation, giving false-positive results. Combining size and ultrasonographic characteristics can increase accuracy. Lymph nodes that are greater than 3 mm and hypoechoic are more likely to contain metastatic deposits. In addition, it is possible to perform fine-needle aspiration of suspicious lymph nodes under ERUS guidance. ERUS is invaluable when evaluating patients for preoperative adjuvant therapy, but it cannot accurately assess response to preoperative adjuvant therapy due to the obliteration of tissue planes by edema and fibrosis secondary to the treatment.

Abdominopelvic CT scanning is important in assessing the presence of distant spread of disease and involvement of adjacent organs. In the management of rectal cancer, it is extremely important to accurately assess the local spread of disease, including the potential involvement of the levator muscles and other pelvic structures. Although ERUS is superior to CT in detecting depth of penetration, CT provides a better assessment of contiguous organ involvement. MRI is a useful adjunct in the evaluation of locally advanced rectal cancer by providing multiple views of the relationships of the tumor to adjacent pelvic structures.

The staging of recurrent rectal cancer is complicated by radiation and post-treatment changes that are often difficult to distinguish from tumor. There is poor correlation of postradiation therapy ERUS in preoperative regimens to final pathological findings (postresection), indicating the limited value of ERUS in assessing tumor in an irradiated milieu. The use of ERUS for postoperative surveillance is limited due to difficulty in distinguishing scar from tumor. CT is useful to assess the extent of the disease and adjacent organ involvement if recurrent tumor is obvious. MRI may yield added information by providing sagittal images that give additional information on resectability. In cases where recurrence is unknown but suspected, CT is more useful if a baseline study is available for comparison. PET may be helpful in identifying recurrent tumor and in a selected series has been shown to be up to 95% sensitive, 98% specific, and 96% accurate in the detection of cancer recurrence. When used appropriately, it can help distinguish patients who would benefit from surgery for recurrent cancer from those who have unresectable disease, particularly when the other imaging modalities fail to localize the disease. However, further studies are required before this test can be recommended for use on a routine basis. Currently at MDACC, we obtain both a CT scan and an MRI of the pelvis in cases of isolated recurrent rectal carcinoma because we believe these studies are complementary in their provision of critical staging and resectability information.

MANAGEMENT OF COLON CANCER

The goal of primary surgical treatment of colon carcinoma is to eradicate disease in the colon, the draining nodal basins, and contiguous organs. Careful surgical planning is essential. The stage of disease, presence of synchronous colonic tumors, and the presence of underlying colorectal cancer syndromes are significant factors in determining the optimal surgical approach. The patient's general medical condition is also important because most perioperative deaths result from cardiovascular or pulmonary complications.

Anatomy

Thorough knowledge of the arterial, venous and lymphatic anatomy of the colon and rectum is essential for appropriate surgical management (Fig. 11.1). The ascending and proximal transverse colons are embryologically derived from the midgut and receive their arterial blood supply from the superior mesenteric artery via the ileocolic, right, and middle colic arteries. The distal transverse, descending, and sigmoid colon are hindgut derivatives whose arterial blood supply arises from the inferior mesenteric artery (IMA) through the left colic and sigmoid arteries. The rectum, also a hindgut derivative, receives its blood supply to the upper third from the IMA via the superior hemorrhoidal artery. The middle and lower thirds of the rectum are supplied by the middle and inferior hemorrhoidal arteries, which are branches of the hypogastric artery. Collateral blood supply for the colon is provided through the marginal artery of Drummond and the arc of Riolan. The venous drainage of the colon and rectum parallels the arterial supply, with the majority draining directly into the portal

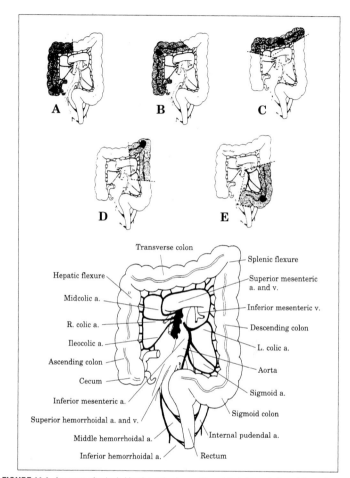

FIGURE 11.1 Anatomy of colonic blood supply along with a pictorial description of the various anatomical resections used for colon carcinoma. **A:** Right hemicolectomy. **B:** Extended right hemicolectomy. **C:** Transverse colectomy. **D:** Left hemicolectomy. **E:** Low anterior resection. (From Sugarbaker PH, MacDonald J, Gunderson L. Colorectal cancer. In: DeVita VT, Hellman S, Rosenberg SA, eds. *Cancer: Principles and Practice of Oncology*. 3rd ed. Philadelphia, PA: Lippincott; 1984, with permission.)

venous system. This provides a direct route for metastatic spread of tumor to the liver. The only minor anatomical variation in the venous drainage compared with the arterial supply is that the inferior mesenteric vein (IMV) joins the splenic vein before emptying into the portal system. The rectum has dual venous drainage; the upper rectum drains into the portal system, and the distal one-third of the rectum drains into the inferior vena cava via the middle and inferior hemorrhoidal veins, providing a direct route for hematogenous spread outside the abdomen.

The lymphatic drainage of the bowel is more complex than the vascular supply. Lymphatics begin in the bowel wall as a plexus beneath the lamina propria and drain into the submucosal and intramuscular lymphatics. The epicolic lymph nodes drain the subserosa and are located in the colon wall. This nodal group runs along the inner bowel margin between the intestinal wall and the arterial arcades. These nodes in turn drain into the paracolic nodes, which follow the routes of the marginal arteries. The epicolic and paracolic nodes represent the majority of the colonic lymph nodes and are the most likely sites of regional metastatic disease. The paracolic nodes drain into the intermediate nodes, which follow the main colic vessels. Finally, the intermediate nodes drain into the principal nodes, which begin at the origins of the superior and inferior mesenteric arteries and are contiguous with the para-aortic chain.

The route of lymphatic flow parallels the arterial and venous distribution of the colon. The right colon will drain to the superior mesenteric nodes through the intermediate nodes or to the portal system via the lymphatics of the superior mesenteric vein. The left colon's lymphatic drainage follows the marginal artery to the left colic intermediate nodes and finally to the inferior mesenteric nodes. The lymphatic drainage of the upper third of the rectum follows the IMV, whereas the lower two-thirds drain into the hypogastric nodes, which, in turn, drain into the para-aortic nodes. The lower third of the rectum can also drain along the pudendal vessels to the inguinal nodes.

Surgical Options

At resection, the primary tumor and its lymphatic, venous, and arterial supply are extirpated, as well as any contiguously involved organs. Our current use of intraoperative ultrasound is limited to the evaluation of nonpalpable hepatic abnormalities identified on preoperative CT scan. We do not believe that the "no touch" isolation technique is necessary; we support high ligation of appropriate vessels in colon cancer resections.

The various surgical options, as well as their indications and major morbidities, are briefly discussed next.

Right Hemicolectomy

This operation involves removal of the distal 5 to 8 cm of the ileum, right colon, hepatic flexure, and transverse colon just proximal to the middle colic artery. This procedure is indicated for cecal and ascending colonic lesions. Major morbidities include ureteral injury, duodenal injury, and rarely bile acid deficiency. Anastomotic dehiscence is a risk with all bowel resections that include reconstruction.

Extended Right Hemicolectomy

This procedure includes resection of the transverse colon (including resection of the middle colic artery at its origin) in addition to the structures removed in the right hemicolectomy. It generally requires mobilization of the splenic flexure to allow a tension-free anastomosis. Indications for the procedure are hepatic flexure or transverse colon lesions. Morbidities include splenic injury in addition to the complications associated with right hemicolectomy. Ninety percent of the fecal water is absorbed in the proximal colon; therefore, extended resections are associated with the potential for diarrhea.

Transverse Colectomy

This procedure involves the segmental resection of the transverse colon and is indicated for middle transverse colon lesions. This operation is infrequently performed because the mid-transverse colon is one of the least common locations for primary colon cancers. To prevent anastomotic dehiscence, a well-vascularized and tension-free anastomosis is mandated. This requires mobilization of both the right and the left colons, along with both flexures with an ascending-to-descending colon anastomosis.

Left Hemicolectomy

This resection involves the removal of the transverse colon distal to the right branch of the middle colic artery and the descending colon up to, but not including, the rectum and proximal ligation and division of the left colic vessels or IMA. This operation may be tailored to the location of the lesion. Indications for the procedure are left colon and splenic flexure lesions. Morbidities include splenic and ureteral injury.

Low Anterior Resection

When performed for lesions within the sigmoid colon or proximal rectum, this procedure includes removal of the sigmoid colon and the involved rectum, and ligation of the superior rectal vessels at their origin. The splenic flexure is routinely mobilized and the reconstruction is performed using the descending colon. The use of the sigmoid colon is discouraged, especially for distal reconstruction as the thickened and hypertrophic muscle of the sigmoid is less compliant and well vascularized than the descending colon. To achieve a tension-free anastomosis, the IMA may need to be divided at its origin, along with the IMV at the inferior border of the pancreas. For lesions involving the rectum, the mesorectum should be divided at least 5 cm distal to the distal aspect of the tumor. Morbidities include anastomotic dehiscence, which is higher with more distal reconstruction and has been reported to be less than 10%, and bowel ischemia (secondary to inadequate flow through the marginal artery of Drummond). For routine low anterior resections (LARs) for sigmoid or upper rectal lesions without radiation, a defunctioning ileostomy is not typically necessary.

Subtotal Colectomy

This resection involves the removal of the entire colon to the rectum with an IRA. This procedure is indicated for multiple synchronous colonic tumors that are not confined to a single anatomical distribution, for selected patients with FAP with minimal rectal involvement, or for selected patients with HNPCC and colon cancer. Although an excellent quality of life can be achieved after ileorectostomy, frequent loose bowel movements are the norm. Patients should be counseled regarding a bowel regimen and perianal care. The risk for anastomotic leak after IRA is approximately 5% or less.

The surgical treatment of the familial polyposis syndromes depends on the age of the patient and the polyp density in the rectum. Surgical options include proctocolectomy with Brooke ileostomy, total abdominal colectomy with IRA, or restorative proctocolectomy with IPAA. Proctocolectomy with continent ileostomy is rarely performed today. Total abdominal colectomy with IRA has a low complication rate, provides good functional results, and is a viable option for patients with fewer than 20 adenomas in the rectum. These patients must be observed with 6-month proctoscopic examinations to remove polyps and detect signs of cancer. If rectal polyps become too numerous, completion proctectomy with Brooke ileostomy or IPAA, when technically possible, is warranted. The Cleveland Clinic Foundation recently evaluated their registry of patients with FAP who were treated with IRA or IPAA. Prior to the use of IPAA for patients with high rectal polyp burdens, the risk of cancer in the retained rectum was 12.9% at a median follow-up of 212 months. Because of the use of IPAA for patients with large rectal polyp burdens and the selected use of IRA for those with small rectal polyp burdens, no patient has developed rectal cancer in the remaining rectum at a median follow-up of 60 months. Restorative proctocolectomy with IPAA has the advantage of removing all or nearly all large intestine mucosa at risk for cancer while preserving transanal defecation. Complication rates are low when this procedure is done in large centers. Morbidity from the procedure includes incontinence, multiple loose stools, impotence, retrograde ejaculation, dyspareunia, and pouchitis. Approximately 7% of patients have to be converted to permanent ileostomy due to complications after the procedure.

Obstructing Colorectal Cancers

Obstructing left-sided colorectal cancers are usually treated in two stages: resection and Hartmann procedure, followed by colostomy takedown and anastomosis. An alternative is a one-stage procedure with either subtotal colectomy and primary anastomosis or a segmental resection and intraoperative colonic lavage for carefully selected patients. (Contraindications include multiple primary cancers, advanced peritonitis, hemodynamic instability, poor general health, steroid therapy, or immunosuppressed state.) In the SCOTIA prospective randomized trial using these two treatment modalities in 91 patients with malignant left-sided colonic obstruction, the morbidity and mortality rates were similar. Laser fulguration and endoscopic stenting of obstructive lesions can be used for palliation and to allow for bowel preparation and subsequent single-step resection. Obstructing right-sided cancers can be effectively treated with resection and anastomosis in one stage.

Survival

Five-year survival rates for all stages is 64%. Nodal involvement is the primary determinant of 5-year survival. In node-negative disease, the 5-year survival rate is 90% for patients with T1 and T2 lesions and 80% for those with T3 lesions. For node-positive cancers, the 5-year survival ranges from 74% with N1 disease to 51% with N2 disease. These figures also vary depending on the number of lymph nodes evaluated in the surgical specimen, with improved survival associated with a higher number of lymph nodes evaluated. Other factors that are proven prognostic indicators include grade, bowel perforation, and obstruction. Patients who present with unresectable metastatic disease have historically had an 11% 5-year survival rate.

Adjuvant Therapy for Stage III Disease

Most patients with colon cancer present with disease that appears localized and can be completely resected with surgery. However, almost 33% of patients undergoing curative resection will relapse with recurrent disease secondary to unresected occult microscopic metastasis. Adjuvant therapy is administered to treat and hopefully eradicate this residual micrometastatic disease. Historically, 5-fluorouracil (5-FU) was the only effective agent for colon carcinoma, with response rates of 15% to 30% in patients with advanced disease. Several new agents have shown excellent activity in colorectal cancer, including irinotecan, oxaliplatin, and biological agents.

5-Fluorouracil/Levamisole

With the identification of the anticancer activity of 5-FU in patients with colorectal cancers, there have been numerous studies of 5-FU in combination therapies. The first major success of adjuvant therapy for colon cancer was demonstrated in trials of 5-FU in combination with levamisole, an antihelmintic agent with immunostimulatory properties. A pilot prospective randomized study comparing 5-FU/levamisole, levamisole, and surgery alone conducted by the North Central Cancer Treatment Group (NCCTG) demonstrated improved 5-year disease-free survival with levamisole and 5-FU/levamisole given for 1 year as compared with surgery alone. The improvement in the levamisole-only arm was less significant than that of the 5-FU/levamisole arm when examining the overall 5-year survival. These results were confirmed by the National Cancer Institute Intergroup Trial protocol 035, a larger study comparing the same treatment arms. In this study, patients with stage III disease were shown to have a 41% reduction in the risk of recurrence when treated with 5-FU/levamisole. These patients also demonstrated a 33% improvement in overall 5-year survival. Based on these results, the National Institutes of Health Consensus Conference in 1990 recommended that all patients with stage III colon carcinoma receive adjuvant chemotherapy with 5-FU and levamisole. Adjuvant chemotherapy for patients with stage II colon carcinoma remained of unproven benefit.

5-Fluorouracil/Leucovorin

The addition of leucovorin (LV) to 5-FU has been shown to increase antitumor activity in both in vitro and in vivo models. LV works by stabilizing the 5-FU thymidylate synthase complex, thus prolonging the inhibition of thymidylate synthase and increasing tumor cytotoxicity. In the United States, the two most commonly used regimens are the Mayo Clinic regimen of bolus 5-FU 425 mg/m^2/day and LV 20 mg/m^2/day days 1 to 5 every 28 days and the Roswell Park regimen using bolus 5-FU 500 mg/m^2 and LV 500 mg/m^2 weekly for 6 weeks on an every 8-week cycle. These regimens have shown efficacy in the metastatic cancer setting and quickly led to studies of this combination in the adjuvant setting. Initial efficacy of this combination was demonstrated in the National Cancer Institute Intergroup Trial protocol 089, which demonstrated a 30% improvement in 5-year survival when compared with surgery alone. The NSABP C-03 trial compared 5-FU/LV to MOF (MeCCNU, Vincristine, and 5-FU) chemotherapy (MOF was used in NSABP C-01). This study was reported early because 5-FU/LV was significantly superior to MOF in terms of overall survival, and it was much less toxic than MOF. NSABP C-04 compared 5-FU/LV with 5-FU/levamisole and 5-FU/LV/levamisole and showed that the 5-FU/LV combination was superior to 5-FU/levamisole, with disease-free survival of 64% versus 60% and overall survival of 74% versus 69%, respectively ($P = 0.05$). The 5-FU/LV/levamisole combination did not improve outcome but had marked increased toxicity. Finally, NSABP C-05 compared 5-FU/LV with 5-FU/LV and interferon. No difference in disease-free and overall survival was demonstrated with the addition of interferon.

Oral Fluoropyrimidines

Two new oral agents, UFT and capecitabine, have been tested in large, well-designed trials. UFT, a combination of oral uracil and the 5-FU prodrug Tegafur, has been studied in the NSABP C-06 trial comparing 6 months of UFT with LV to 5-FU and LV using the Roswell Park regimen. No differences were seen in 5-year survival with these regimens.

Capecitabine is a drug with rapid GI absorption that undergoes a three-step enzymatic conversion to 5-FU in tumor tissue. When used in first-line treatment of metastatic colorectal cancer, it was associated with a better toxicity profile than 5-FU. The phase III "X-ACT" trial investigated the use of capecitabine in the adjuvant setting for resected stage III colon cancer and also noted an improved safety profile when compared with 5-FU and LV using the Mayo Clinic regimen, with significantly less diarrhea, nausea/vomiting, stomatitis, and neutropenia. Capecitabine was associated with an increased risk for severe hand and foot syndrome.

Irinotecan

Irinotecan has shown significant activity in metastatic colorectal cancer and its use in the adjuvant setting has been studied in several trials. The most important are the Cancer and Leukemia Group B (CALGB) C89803 trial and European PETACC-3 trial. In the CALGB study, 1,260 patients with resected stage III colon cancer were randomized to Roswell Park regimen 5-FU and LV with or without irinotecan (IFL). The IFL arm noted an increased 60-day mortality of 2.5% versus 0.8% in the control group, primarily due to GI and thromboembolic toxicities. The PETACC-3 and Accord02/FFCD9802 trials used two different schedules of 5-FU infusion alone or with irinotecan for 6 months in the adjuvant setting for stages II and III colon cancer and found increased toxicities in the experimental arm with no improvement in disease-free survival in patients with stage III cancer. Based on these trials, irinotecan-based regimens cannot be recommended in the adjuvant setting.

Oxaliplatin
Oxaliplatin, a new platinum derivative with activity against colorectal cancer, has shown impressive antitumor activity against advanced colorectal cancer. The Multicenter International Study of Oxaliplatin, 5-FU, and LV in the adjuvant treatment of colon cancer (MOSAIC) trial enrolled 2,246 patients with completely resected stage II/III colorectal cancer to receive either the infusional LV5-FU2 regimen or FOLFOX-4, which is LV5-FU2 plus oxaliplatin (85 mg/m^2) given every 2 weeks for 12 cycles. The primary endpoint of 3-year disease-free survival was significantly better for the FOLFOX-4 arm (78.2% vs. 72.9%, $P = 0.002$). These results were more significant in stage III patients than in stage II patients. The NSABP C-07 trial studied the Roswell Park regimen of bolus 5-FU and LV with or without oxaliplatin and also showed significant improvement in disease-free survival in the oxaliplatin arm in patients with stage II and III colon cancer.

Adjuvant Therapy for Stage II Disease
Although adjuvant therapy has been proven to benefit patients with stage III disease, the issue of benefit for patients with stage II disease remains controversial. Although many of the adjuvant trials included patients with stage II disease, subgroup analysis shows trends toward benefit without reaching statistical significance as these trials were not powered to see a difference in this subgroup. This issue has been addressed in three meta-analyses from NSABP, NCCTG, and International Multi-Center Pooled Analysis of Colon cancer Trials. All have suggested marginal improvements in disease-free and overall survival with 5-FU and LV in stage II colon cancer patients. Adjuvant chemotherapy in stage II patients provides a relative improvement in overall 5-year survival that was comparable to that of stage III patients (approximately 30% relative improvement). However, the absolute improvement in overall survival is only 2% to 7%. Therefore, the routine use of adjuvant chemotherapy for stage II patients is still not common practice. Generally, patients with stage II disease are offered FOLFOX or 5-FU if adverse prognostic features such as lymphovascular invasion, perforation, T4 status, obstruction, or poor differentiation are present. For stage II patients with no high-risk features, observation or enrollment in a clinical trial is recommended. The determination of molecular and genetic prognostic markers that will be useful in selecting those stage II patients who would benefit most from routine use of adjuvant therapy is an area of active investigation.

Treatment of Metastatic Disease
One of the most important recent advances in the treatment of metastatic colorectal cancer has been the availability of biological agents directed against tumor-specific targets. The epidermal growth factor receptor (EGFR)-mediated pathways are important for tumor proliferation and metastases. Monoclonal antibodies directed against EGFR include cetuximab and panitumumab. Cetuximab is a chimeric antibody with activity against colorectal cancer that has been demonstrated by the European randomized phase II "BOND" trial, which randomized irinotecan failure patients to receive cetuximab and irinotecan or cetuximab monotherapy. The response rate was 10.8% with cetuximab alone and 22.9% with combination therapy.

Currently, cetuximab and panitumumab are approved for second- and third-line treatment for metastatic colon cancer alone or in combination with other chemotherapy. Until recently the role of cetuximab in the adjuvant setting of stage III disease was unknown. The results of the Intergroup/NCCTG NO147 trial comparing adjuvant cetuximab in combination with FOLFOX versus FOLFOX alone for stage III colon cancer have recently been reported and showed no benefit of the addition of cetuximab in this setting. PETACC-8 is a similar ongoing trial comparing the disease-free survival rates in patients with completely resected stage III colon cancer treated with adjuvant oxaliplatin, LV, and FU with and without cetuximab and has yet to report.

It was previously thought that there must be overexpression of EGFR in colorectal tumors in order for these agents to be effective. It is now known that this is not true. The EGFR leads to a downstream activation of a k-ras/MAPK pathway involved in regulation of tumor growth and survival. Therefore, a mutation in k-ras may be associated with resistance to cetuximab and panitumumab. A k-ras mutation in codon 12 and 13 is seen in approximately 30% to 40% of colorectal tumors. The results of the CRYSTAL trial for patients with metastatic colorectal cancer showed improved progression-free survival for patients with wild-type (nonmutated) k-ras tumors who were randomly assigned to receive cetuximab and FOLFIRI (irinotecan + 5-FU) compared to those treated with FOLFIRI. Furthermore, the interpretation of the presence of the serine-threonine kinase B-RAF V600 mutation (a direct downstream effector of k-ras) may further impact the benefit of anti-EGFR therapy. B-RAF tumor mutation status has been shown to be a poor prognostic factor in patients with metastatic colorectal cancer but has not shown to serve a role as a predictive biomarker.

Currently, patients who are being considered for treatment with either cetuximab or panitumumab should undergo k-ras testing and only those with wild-type k-ras tumors should be offered these agents. Although B-RAF appears to denote a poorer prognosis, further analysis is needed to justify the routine use of its determination for patients who are potential candidates for anti-EGFR therapy.

The vascular endothelial growth factor family of glycoproteins is also important for tumor growth. Bevacizumab is a humanized monoclonal antibody that targets circulating vascular endothelial growth factor. In previously untreated metastatic colorectal cancer, the addition of bevacizumab to IFL improved the response rate from 35% to 45% ($P = 0.0029$) and the overall survival from 15.6 to 20.3 months ($P = 0.00003$). The ECOG 3200 trial compared FOLFOX with single-agent bevacizumab or FOLFOX and bevacizumab as second line for metastatic colorectal cancer. Addition of bevacizumab prolonged median survival from 10.7 months for FOLFOX to 12.5 months for the combination regimen. In contrast to these studies, results of the NSABP C08 trial indicated that adding bevacizumab to standard adjuvant chemotherapy of FOLFOX did not improve disease-free survival in patients with stage II or stage III colon cancer. Currently, bevacizumab is indicated in combination with 5-FU-based chemotherapy for first- and second-line treatment of metastatic colorectal cancer.

Treatment of Locally Advanced Colon Cancer

Colon cancers that are adherent to adjacent structures have a 36% to 53% chance of local failure after complete resection. Approximately 10% of carcinomas present in this fashion. Strategies designed to reduce local recurrence would benefit these patients.

Surgical Strategy

Resection of colorectal cancer that has invaded adjacent structures involves en bloc resection of all involved structures; failure to do so results in significantly increased local recurrence and decreased survival. Importantly, all adhesions between the carcinoma and adjacent structures should be assumed to be malignant and not taken down because 33% to 84% are malignant when examined histologically. The affected organ should have resection limited to the involved area with a rim of normal tissue. A patient who has a margin-negative multivisceral resection has the same survival as a patient with no adjacent organ involvement on a stage-matched basis.

Adjuvant Radiation Therapy

Retrospective series have shown subsets of patients who have benefited from postoperative radiation therapy with or without 5-FU-based chemotherapy. Unfortunately, there are no consistent criteria to use in assessing increased risk of local failure. The value of adjuvant radiation therapy after complete resection of high-risk colon cancer is currently being evaluated in a randomized prospective fashion (NCCTG 91–46-52). In this trial, patients with B3 or C3 (modified Astler-Coller) tumors are randomized to receive postoperative 5-FU/levamisole or 5-FU/levamisole and radiation therapy. Patients with subtotally resected cancers fare worse than those with positive microscopic disease, as one would expect. It has been found that radiation therapy is more effective in microscopic than in macroscopic disease and that it is more effective when combined with 5-FU. In a recent retrospective Mayo Clinic study of 103 mostly stage B3 and C3 (modified Astler-Coller) patients, in which 49% had no residual disease, 17% had microscopic residual disease, and 34% had gross residual disease; the local failure rate was 10% for patients with no residual disease, 54% for those with microscopic residual disease, and 79% for those with gross residual disease. More recently, improved local control with adjuvant radiation has been demonstrated in a small set of patients with T4 cancers with perforation or fistula. Although a margin-negative resection should be performed whenever possible, if circumstances prohibit it, surgical clips should be used to outline the area of the tumor bed. If the margin is positive on final pathological studies, radiation should be administered with concomitant 5-FU-based chemotherapy.

MANAGEMENT OF RECTAL CANCER

The primary principle in the management of localized rectal cancer is similar to that for colon cancer (i.e., complete oncologic resection). In line with this principle are the goals of cancer control (negative margin resection of tumor and resection of all draining lymph nodes), restoration of intestinal continuity, and preservation of anorectal sphincter, sexual, and urinary function. Achieving these goals can be difficult due to the anatomical constraints of the bony pelvis. Local control is clearly related to the adequacy of the surgical procedure. Although local control is critical for increasing the chances of cure, many patient- and tumor-related factors are associated with overall outcome. Data suggest that there is a significant surgeon- and center-related variation in patient outcome after treatment for rectal cancer. The Stockholm Rectal Cancer Study Group found that specialists and high volume centers had lower local failure rates and improved survival rates. It was previously not unusual to see local recurrence rates ranging from 3.7% to 43% in various series for curative surgical resection, with or without adjuvant therapy. This is due to multiple other factors being involved, such as methods of adjuvant therapy, patient selection, and disease factors. These factors have hindered an accurate assessment of the vital components of adequate oncologic treatment and prevented an accurate assessment of the value of adjuvant chemoradiation in rectal cancer. There may be instances where adjuvant chemoradiation treatment may be avoided for favorable risk lesions when the oncologic resection has been performed by an experienced surgeon. Nevertheless, surgical technique is clearly critical to the success of the treatment of rectal cancer.

When planning surgical treatment of rectal cancer, the rectum can be generally divided into three regions: lower, middle, and upper thirds. The upper rectum is generally defined as extending 11 to 15 cm from the anal verge. The length of the rectum varies significantly depending on the size of the individual, and therefore these distinctions should be individualized. Tumors of the proximal rectum, at the level of the sacral promontory, behave similarly to colonic cancers and are therefore generally considered to be "rectosigmoid" cancers. Tumors 6 to 10 cm from the anal verge are defined as middle rectal cancers, and tumors from 0 to 5 cm are defined as low rectal cancers. Note that low rectal cancers can be associated with the internal and external sphincters, anal canal, or levator muscles, or can be above the pelvic floor.

Surgical Aspects

In addition to understanding the anatomical site of the tumor, it is important to understand the principles influencing the extent of radical extirpative surgery, regardless of the type of resection planned.

Resection Margin

Optimal treatment of all malignancies requires an adequate margin of resection. Histologic examination of the bowel wall distal to the gross rectal tumor reveals that only 2.5% of patients will have submucosal spread of disease greater than 2.5 cm. However, the most important margin is the radial margin. For many, particularly distal, rectal cancers, this is the most difficult margin to achieve. In 1986, Quirke et al. were the first to characterize the critical importance of the negative radial margin in preventing rectal cancer recurrence. In their series, the rate of local recurrence was 86% in the setting of a positive radial resection margin. At MDACC, we try to obtain a distal resection margin of at least 2 cm. The oncologic impact of irrigation of the rectum remains controversial.

Lymphadenectomy

Adequate lymphadenectomy should be performed for accurate staging and local control and should include proximal vascular ligation at the origin of the superior rectal vessels from the IMA just distal to the origin of the left colic. Spread from the primary tumor occurs along the mesorectum. Therefore, although a 2-cm bowel margin is considered adequate for rectal cancer, the mesorectal margin should be at least 5 cm distal to the inferior aspect of the tumor or to the end of the mesorectum at the pelvic floor. The technique of total mesorectal excision (TME) provides adequate lymphadenectomy for most rectal cancers. It involves sharp excision and extirpation of the mesorectum by dissecting outside the investing fascia of the mesorectum. TME optimizes the oncologic operation by not only removing draining lymph nodes but also maximizing lateral resection margins around the tumor. Although no randomized trials have compared TME with conventional mesorectal excision, there is overwhelmingly comparative observational evidence that demonstrates a significant decrease in the local recurrence rate (in the range of 6.3% to 7.3%) compared with conventional surgery (15% to 30%). The major morbidity associated with TME may be the increased rate of anastomotic leak believed to be due to devascularization of the rectal stump. Leak rates of 11% to 16% have been reported for TME as compared with 8% for non-TME.

The TME dissection can be facilitated by ligation of the IMA (and IMV) at or near its origin ("high ligation"). This allows for maximal mobilization of the proximal bowel to facilitate a tension-free low pelvic or coloanal anastomosis (CAA). The data on whether high ligation results in a decreased local recurrence remain equivocal. It has been well documented that negative lateral (radial) margins are major determinants of local recurrence and survival and may be more important than longitudinal resection margins. Lateral margin clearance can be maximized by sharp dissection between the fascia propria of the mesorectum and the endopelvic fascia. The bony pelvis, which inherently limits the maximal extent of lateral dissection, may serve as the best explanation of why distal rectal cancers have a higher local recurrence rate than their more proximal counterparts when comparing patients with tumors of similar stage. At MDACC, we perform a *tumor-specific* mesorectal excision. The mesorectum is transected 5 cm distal to the distal aspect of the tumor. This would include the entire mesorectum for the lower and lower-middle rectal cancers, while preserving a portion of the mesorectum for the upper and upper-middle rectal cancers. This *tumor-specific* mesorectal excision does not compromise an adequate oncologic operation and may decrease the risk for anastomotic dehiscence from devascularization of the rectum. No benefit in survival or local disease control has been attainable with the use of more extended lymphadenectomy (iliac/periaortic nodes, obturator), and the complication rates are higher with these more extensive surgical procedures.

Surgical Approaches to Rectal Cancer

Surgical approaches to the rectum include transabdominal procedures (abdomino-perineal resection [APR], LAR, CAA), transanal approaches, and trans-sacral approaches (York-Mason, Kraske). The latter two approaches will be discussed in detail in the section Local Approaches to Rectal Cancer. Historically, APR, an operation devised by Ernest Miles in the 1930s, was the treatment for all rectal cancers. With the advent of better preoperative staging, neoadjuvant therapy, and improved surgical techniques and stapler technology, the use of APR has decreased significantly. APR is now reserved for patients with primary sphincter dysfunction and incontinence, patients with direct tumor invasion into the sphincter complex, and patients with large or poorly differentiated lesions in the lower third of the rectum that do not have adequate tumor clearance for sphincter preservation.

Sphincter Preservation Procedures

Besides local excision, sphincter preservation procedures include LAR and proctectomy/CAA either alone or combined with neoadjuvant radiation and chemoradiation. Another option includes the addition of a colonic reservoir for improved short-term function. These procedures can only be performed if the oncologic result is not compromised and the functional results are acceptable. It was demonstrated more than 20 years ago that there is no difference in local recurrence rate or survival in patients with midrectal cancers who undergo LAR rather than APR. The technical feasibility of LAR in this setting was increased with the advent of circular stapling devices and the knowledge that distal mucosal margins of resection of 2 cm were adequate in the setting of TME. Survival was found to depend on the distance of the tumor from the anal verge, the presence of positive lymph nodes, and the lateral extent of dissection. An alternative to LAR is proctectomy with CAA. It is used in low rectal cancers, with the stapled or hand-sewn anastomosis just above or at the dentate line. Temporary fecal diversion is routinely performed. The use of proctectomy and CAA for low rectal cancers is usually in the context of preoperative radiation or chemoradiation. Using either LAR or proctectomy with CAA (and adjuvant therapy), local recurrence rates of 5.3% to 7.9% have been reported by MDACC and others. Functional results have been good, with 60% to 86% of patients attaining continence by 1 year, 10% to 15% requiring laxative use, and some with mild soiling at night. Preoperative chemoradiation does not seem to have a negative impact on these functional results. Obviously, the lower the anastomosis (i.e., coloanal), the greater the potential for bowel dysfunction. Many patient factors are related to the decision to avoid a colostomy; however, there have been no randomized comparative studies of quality of life after CAA versus APR.

Colonic J Pouch

Although continence can be maintained in patients with CAA, there is a degree of incontinence in some patients, and others require antidiarrheal agents. This is partly due to lack of compliance in the neorectum. This led to the introduction of the colonic J pouch for low rectal cancers that showed better results in terms of stool frequency, urgency, nocturnal movements, and continence than straight colo-anal anastomoses. These advantages are principally during the first 12 to 24 months after which time functional improvements after straight anastomosis improves. One potential problem, especially when the pouch is longer than 5 or 6 cm, is dif-ficulty in pouch evacuation (approximately 20% of patients). As in anterior resec-tion, the functional outcome of patients with CAA (with or without a J pouch) may take 1 to 3 years to stabilize and is related to the level of the anastomosis (lower anastomoses tend to have poorer function). Unfortunately, many, particularly male, patients with low rectal cancers do not have enough room within the pelvis to accommodate a colonic J pouch. An alternative approach of a transverse coloplasty pouch has been proposed but it has not been shown to demonstrate significant benefit over a straight anastomosis. Postoperative radiation therapy has not been shown to have a significant adverse effect on pouch function.

Proximal Diversion

Proximal diversion after sphincter preservation is indicated in the following circum-stances: (a) anastomosis less than 5 cm above the anal verge, (b) patients who have received preoperative radiation therapy, (c) patients on corticosteroids, (d) when the integrity of the anastomosis is in question, and (e) any case of intraoperative hemo-dynamic instability.

Local Approaches to Rectal Cancer

Local treatment alone as definitive therapy of rectal cancer was first applied to patients with severe coexisting medical conditions unable to tolerate radical sur-gery. Currently, conservative, sphincter-saving local approaches are being more widely considered and have the benefits of potentially avoiding a colostomy sparing major perioperative risks and obtaining favorable functional results. Local excision has been associated with up to 97% local control rate and 92% disease-specific sur-vival for properly selected individuals with early cancers. Local treatment is best applied to rectal cancers within 10 cm of the anal verge, less than 3 cm in diameter involving less than one-fourth of the circumference of the rectal wall, tumors staged less than T2 by EUS, highly mobile and of low histologic grade. The decision to use local excision alone or to employ adjuvant therapy after local excision is based on the pathological characteristics of the primary cancer (with negative margins) and the potential for micrometastases in the draining lymph nodes. T1 lesions have been associated with positive lymph nodes in up to 18% of cases, whereas the rate for T2 and T3 lesions is up to 38% and 70%, respectively. T2 tumors treated with local resection alone have local recurrence rates of 25% to 62%. T1 lesions with poor prognostic features and all T2 tumors should be resected with radical surgery; how-ever, when local excision is performed, adjuvant chemoradiation and close surveil-lance should also be performed. Two phase II cooperative group studies evaluated local excision for T1 lesions and local excision with adjuvant chemoradiation using a 5-FU-based regimen for T2 lesions. The CALGB 8984 trial evaluated 177 patients who underwent transanal excision for T1 or T2 lesions. T2 patients were given adju-vant chemoradiation and T1 patients were followed for recurrence and survival. At a median follow-up of 7.1 years, 4 of 59 patients with T1 lesions (2 local, 1 local and distant, and 1 distant) and 10 of 51 patients with T2 lesions (5 local, 2 local and distant, and 3 distant) had recurrences. Overall survival rates were 84% and 66% and disease-free survival 75% and 64%, respectively. Local recurrence rates for patients with T1 and T2 lesions were 8% and 18%, respectively. The Radiation Therapy Oncology Group (RTOG) protocol 89–02 used a similar strategy with a median follow-up of 6.1 years in 52 patients with T1/T2 rectal cancers and demonstrated a 4% local failure rate for T1 lesions and 16% local failure rate for T2 lesions. An additional 3 of 13 (23%) patients with T3 disease treated with local excision and chemoradiation were noted to have local failure. These data should be considered in the background of data from other studies demonstrating a recurrence rate of 18% and 37% in patients undergoing local excision alone for T1 and T2 tumors, respectively. The ACOSOG Z6041 trial is a phase II study looking at neoadjuvant chemoradiation followed by local excision for uT2N0 rectal cancers with primary endpoints being disease-free survival at 3 years. Results should be available in the upcoming year.

Local therapy of distal rectal cancers can be accomplished by transanal excision, posterior proctectomy, fulguration, or endocavitary irradiation.

Transanal excision is the most straightforward approach to removing distal rectal cancers. The deep plane of dissection is the perirectal fat. Tumors should be excised with a 1 cm mucosal margin and an adequate circumferential margin.

Posterior proctotomy involves a posterior incision just above the anus (Kraske procedure) or including the anus (York-Mason procedure), the coccyx is removed, and the fascia is divided. The rectum can then be mobilized for a sleeve resection, or a proctotomy is performed for excision of the tumor. This procedure presently has limited application for rectal tumors.

Fulguration uses either standard electrocautery or laser to ablate the tumor. *Endocavitary radiation* is a high-dose, low-voltage irradiation technique that applies contact radiation to a small rectal cancer through a special proctoscope. Fulguration and endocavitary radiation are used for palliation and do not have a role in treatments with curative intent.

Transanal endoscopic microsurgery (TEM) provides accessibility to tumors of the middle and upper rectum, which would otherwise require a laparotomy or transsacral approach, through improved visibility and instrumentation. This approach can be used for selected lesions up to 15 cm from the anal verge. Caution must be taken with higher lesions because full-thickness excision can result in perforation into the abdomen that will result in leakage of gas into the abdominal cavity and potential for injury to intraperitoneal organs. The procedure is technically demanding and requires special equipment and is not recommended for tumors within 5 cm of the anal verge. These tumors are optimally treated with a standard transanal approach. Patient selection is important, and it is recommended that patients have preoperative EUS to select superficial lesions. Patients with deeper lesions and metastatic disease or comorbid conditions that would preclude laparotomy are also potential candidates. Although local procedures have become more commonly used, few randomized prospective trials have evaluated oncologic and functional outcomes compared with anterior resection or APR. In 1996, Winde et al. prospectively randomized 50 patients with T1 adenocarcinoma of the rectum to either anterior resection or TEM. Similar local recurrence and survival rates, as well as decreased morbidity rates for local excision, were found in the two study arms, confirming the advantages of local excision.

At MDACC, transanal excision is used for select low rectal cancers, whereas a radical resection is used for higher rectal lesions. Optimal local excision includes at least a 1-cm mucosal resection margin circumferentially, a full-thickness excision, and an excision that is not fragmented or piecemeal. An inadequate local excision mandates an alternate resection strategy, not merely the addition of adjuvant therapy. If preoperative T stage is increased after pathological evaluation following local excision, the appropriate standard resection is recommended. T1 tumors are treated with local therapy alone unless any of the following poor prognostic features are identified: tumor greater than 4 cm, poorly differentiated histologic type, lymphatic or vascular invasion, or clinical or radiologic evidence of enlarged lymph nodes. Those T1 tumors with poor prognostic features are treated with radical surgery. Patients with T2 tumors are offered local excision with chemoradiotherapy in the neoadjuvant setting or adjuvant setting but are generally treated with radical resection unless contraindicated. T3 lesions are treated with local excision alone only if radical resection is contraindicated. However, MDACC recently reported a series of selected T3 rectal cancer patients who demonstrated an excellent response to preoperative chemoradiation therapy and underwent full-thickness local excision with resulting comparable local control, disease-free survival, and overall survival to that achieved with proctectomy.

Treatment for Locally Advanced Rectal Cancer

Occasionally, patients will present with involvement of adjacent structures (bladder, vagina, ureters, seminal vesicles, and sacrum). These patients benefit from multimodality therapy, including preoperative or postoperative chemoradiation treatment. Intraoperative radiation therapy (IORT) or brachytherapy has been shown to provide additional potential benefit. The goal of surgical therapy is resection of the primary tumor, with en bloc resection of adjacent involved structures to obtain negative margins. The confines of the pelvis and the proximity to nerves and blood vessels that cannot be resected decrease the resectability of rectal tumors compared with locally advanced colon cancer. Improved resectability and decreased locoregional recurrence have been demonstrated for locally advanced rectal cancers after preoperative chemoradiation treatment. As reported by the Mayo Clinic, the addition of IORT to standard external-beam radiation therapy with 5-FU in patients with locally advanced rectal cancer has been associated with improved local disease control and possibly some improvement in survival. Preoperative chemoradiation has also been shown to improve rates of sphincter preservation in patients who were initially believed to need APR for curative resection by as much as twofold when compared with postoperative chemoradiation regimens. The best chance of cure in patients with locally advanced disease appears to involve preoperative chemoradiation treatment, maximal surgical resection, and IORT in selected cases.

At MDACC preoperative chemoradiation is standard treatment for locally advanced rectal cancer. An evaluation of 40 patients (29 with locally advanced disease; 11 with recurrence) requiring pelvic exenteration for local disease control with negative margins demonstrated that chemoradiation may significantly improve survival and that chemoradiation response and S-phase fraction were important determinants of survival. Patients with low-risk factors had a 65% 5-year survival, whereas high-risk patients had only a 20% survival. Table 11.7 summarizes the treatment strategy for patients with rectal cancer at MDACC.

Laparoscopic and Robotic Approaches to Colorectal Cancer

Studies have confirmed that laparoscopy for colorectal carcinoma resection is technically feasible and safe, yielding an equivalent number of resected lymph nodes and length of resected bowel when compared with open colectomy. Early concerns regarding port-site metastases have now been laid to rest. A number of landmark-randomized trials have demonstrated oncologic noninferiority of laparoscopic versus open surgery for colon cancer.

The National Cancer Institute-sponsored multicenter clinical outcomes of surgical therapy (COST) trial enrolled nearly 800 patients and validated the oncologic safety and efficacy of laparoscopy for colon cancer. Laparoscopic-assisted colectomy for cancer was associated with equivalent recurrence-free and overall survival when compared with open surgery with no increase in wound recurrences. Statistically significant patient-related benefits included reduced length of hospital stay (one day shorter in the laparoscopic group, 5 vs. 6 days, $P < 0.001$) and

TABLE 117. Recommended Surgical Treatment Strategy for Rectal Cancer

Location	T Stage	N Stage	Resection	Mesorectal Excision to
Upper rectum	T1	N0	TEM	—
	≥T2	N0	LAR	5 cm distal to tumor
	T1–T2	N1–N2	± CXRT followed by LAR	5 cm distal to tumor
	≥T3	N0–N2	± CXRT followed by LAR	5 cm distal to tumor
Middle rectum	T1	N0	TAE, Kraske	—
	T2	N0	LAR[a]	5 cm distal to resection margin or entire
	T1–T2	N1–N2	CXRT followed by LAR[a]	5 cm distal to resection margin or entire
	≥T3	N0–N2	CXRT followed by LAR[a]	5 cm distal to resection margin or entire
Low rectum	T1	N0	TAE or proctectomy with CAA	—
	T2	N0	Proctectomy/CAA,[b] (± J pouch), APR	Entire
	T1–T2	N1–N2	CXRT followed by proctectomy/CAA,[b] (± J pouch), APR	Entire
	≥T3	N0–N2	CXRT followed by proctectomy/CAA,[b] (± J pouch), APR	Entire

[a]LAR distal bowel resection margin >2 cm.
[b]CAA ± protective ileostomy.
TEM, transanal endoscopic microsurgery; LAR, low anterior resection; CXRT, preoperative chemoradiation; TAE, transanal excision; CAA, coloanal anastomosis; APR, abdominoperineal resection.

decreased pain (one day less each of parenteral narcotics [3 vs. 4 days, $P < 0.001$] and oral analgesics [1 vs. 2 days, $P = 0.02$]). There was only a small improvement in short-term quality of life which was able to be shown in the trial. Even in a recent long-term follow-up study of the quality of life analysis from the COST trial, only a small benefit was able to be documented for the patients treated with laparoscopic resection.

The Medical Research Council-sponsored conventional versus laparoscopic-assisted surgery in patients with colorectal cancer multicentered trial in the United Kingdom has shown no differences in local recurrence or disease-free survival at 3 years in patients undergoing laparoscopic versus open colectomy for cancer. In a subset analysis, bladder dysfunction was worse with laparoscopic rectal resection and male sexual function trended to be worse with laparoscopic resection. Similar patient-related benefits as in the COST trial were observed. The European multi-centered colon carcinoma laparoscopic or open resection trial compared 3-year disease-free survival and overall survival after laparoscopic and open resection of solitary colon cancer and could not rule out a difference in disease-free survival at 3 years in favor of open colectomy. An additional trial from Hong Kong demonstrated oncologic equivalency with laparoscopy for sigmoid and rectosigmoid tumors. The colon carcinoma laparoscopic or open resection II trial is an ongoing international randomized clinical trial comparing laparoscopic and open surgery for rectal cancer with primary endpoints being locoregional recurrence rates at 3 years and secondary endpoints including overall and disease-free survival. ACOSOG Z6051 opened in 2008 and is a phase III randomized controlled trial with a noninferiority design and 1:1 randomization of laparoscopic versus open rectal resection. Primary endpoints include circumferential resection margin, distal margins, number of lymph nodes recovered, and integrity of the mesorectum. Secondary endpoints include disease-free survival and local recurrence at 2 years. Finally, the Japanese Clinical Oncology Group 0404 study is an ongoing trial comparing laparoscopic versus open resection for colorectal cancer with overall survival and relapse-free survival as clinical endpoints. The laparoscopic-assisted approach has consistently been associated with reductions in hospital stay, postoperative pain, and duration of postoperative ileus when compared with open surgery. However, the magnitude of these effects in randomized trials have been modest, approximately 20% to 35%, and remains the subject of further investigation. Unproven additional benefits of laparoscopy include potentially decreased morbidity, decreased convalescence, improved quality of life, and decreased costs.

With respect to clinical trials of laparoscopy for colorectal cancer, it should be noted that experienced surgeons who have demonstrated proficiency in laparoscopic colectomy for cancer obtained these results. Furthermore, although laparoscopic-assisted techniques have been validated for colon carcinoma, its use for rectal cancer has not yet been definitively established. Additional indications for laparoscopy include resection of polyps, creation of intestinal stomas, and diagnostic procedures.

The appeal of laparoscopic colon surgery is a simple one: minimally invasive techniques result in faster recovery and therefore may result in improved quality of life and lower health care costs when compared with open laparotomy. These benefits have been dramatically realized with surgery for other sites such as for benign gallbladder disease. When considering colectomy, reduction in postoperative pain and narcotic use, faster resolution of ileus, and shorter duration of hospitalization are unifying observations of the laparoscopic approach. Added benefits may include the potential for improved short- and long-term complications and a reduction in costs. However, owing to the relatively increased complexity of laparoscopic colectomy and the ongoing evolution of the techniques, the magnitude of these benefits is still being determined. Further investigation will be required to determine whether the small statistical benefits which have been seen in the randomized clinical trials are clinically significant as well.

Furthermore, the importance of these effects may in part depend on the underlying diagnosis. Most patients with colon cancer are candidates for laparoscopic-assisted techniques. Transverse colon tumors require extensive bilateral colonic mobilization and therefore are technically more difficult. Factors associated with an increased need for conversion include tumor-related factors such as proximal left-sided lesions and large bulky tumors, as well as patient obesity, adhesions, and the presence of an associated abscess that was not preoperatively identified. Cancers with perforation, obstruction, or invasion of the retroperitoneum or abdominal wall are not approached laparoscopically.

A special mention should be made regarding the use of robotics in rectal surgery. This approach has been suggested to address many of the inherent drawbacks of conventional laparoscopy including assistant-dependent unstable camera, two-dimensional views, limited dexterity, and fixed instrument tips. Other benefits include excellent ergonomics, tremor elimination, ambidextrous capability, motion scaling, and instruments with seven degrees of freedom. Robotic surgery fundamentally represents an extension of laparoscopy but some of the drawbacks include cost, longer operating times, lack of haptic feedback, and need for significant training and supervision. Currently there is a paucity of long-term data and there is a need for critical evaluation of its application.

Survival After Surgical Therapy

About 75% to 90% of node-negative rectal cancers are cured by radical surgical resection. Five-year disease-free survival in stage III patients remains approximately 60% or less. Local failure still remains a significant problem, although its risk has decreased in the era of TME.

The survival rate after local therapy varies from 70% to 86%, with recurrence rates of 10% to 50%. The overall local recurrence rate is 30% and increasing recurrence rates are seen with increasing stage of disease and decreasing distance from the anal verge. Many of these patients can be salvaged with radical surgery after a local recurrence; however, survival after salvage surgery may not be as good as after initial curative radical surgery. When considering local therapy for rectal cancer, patient selection is of paramount importance.

Complications of Surgical and Adjuvant Therapy for Rectal Cancer

Complications of surgical and adjuvant therapy for rectal cancer include all complications associated with major abdominal surgery (e.g., bleeding, infection, adjacent organ injury, ureteral injury, and bowel obstruction), with the addition of some complications that are unique to pelvic surgery. Specifically, anastomotic leak occurs in 5% to 10% of cases overall, with increasing rates seen in lower anastomoses, those associated with immunocompromised states, and those associated with preoperative radiation therapy. A defunctioning stoma will decrease the consequences of such a leak and may decrease leak incidence. At MDACC, a defunctioning loop ileostomy is used in all anastomoses below the peritoneal reflection in patients who have received preoperative radiotherapy and in most patients after CAA. Autonomic nerve preservation is always performed during pelvic dissections, unless tumor involvement necessitates the sacrifice of these structures. With careful dissection during TME, 75% to 85% of patients have a return to preoperative sexual and urinary function. Other complications include urinary dysfunction, stoma dysfunction, perineal wound complications, hemorrhage from presacral vessels, and anastomotic stricture. The mortality rate from surgical resection varies from less than 2% to 6%.

The complications associated with chemoradiation treatment include radiation enteritis and dermatitis, autonomic neuropathy, hematologic toxicity, stomatitis (mostly with continuous 5-FU infusions), and venous access infections. The frequency and intensity of these complications depend on multiple factors, including radiation therapy total dosing, fractionation, field technique, and whether the radiation therapy is given preoperatively or postoperatively. There are no good predictors of which patients will have these complications and to what degree they will have them.

Adjuvant Therapy of Rectal Cancer

There is limited data for chemotherapy in the adjuvant setting for rectal cancer and most treatment strategies borrow treatment recommendations from the colon data. Regardless, the two main components of adjuvant therapy for rectal cancer are radiation therapy to the pelvis and 5-FU-based chemotherapy. The goal of chemotherapy is to increase tumor radiation sensitivity and to decrease the chance of distant failure. The goal of radiation therapy is to increase local control and in the preoperative setting to increase margin-negative resection rates and sphincter preservation. It must be emphasized that successful multimodality treatment of rectal cancer requires close collaboration between radiation therapists, medical oncologists, and surgeons.

Postoperative Radiation

A number of trials in the United States have examined the role of postoperative radiotherapy for improved local control for stage II and stage III cancers. Only the NSABP R-01 study demonstrated a benefit with 46–47 Gy following conventional rectal resection. Local recurrence was decreased from 25% in the surgical arm to 16% in the postoperative radiation therapy arm ($P = 0.06$). Several nonrandomized trials have shown a decrease in local recurrence rates to the 6% to 8% level; the differences between these trials may reflect radiotherapy dosing and patient selection. These trials showed that postoperative radiation therapy could reduce local recurrence, but total radiation therapy dose and technique were important to achieve this effect.

Postoperative Radiation Therapy and Chemotherapy

The addition of chemotherapy to radiation therapy has been used to enhance the radiation responsiveness of tumors and impact distant failure. Several landmark studies have shown both improved local control and survival. The Gastrointestinal Tumor Study Group (1985) 7175 trial compared the following treatment arms: (a) surgery alone, (b) surgery followed by postoperative radiotherapy (40–48 Gy), (c) surgery followed by postoperative chemotherapy (bolus 5-FU and semustine), and (d) surgery followed by concurrent chemotherapy and radiotherapy. It demonstrated a decrease in pelvic failure for the group treated by surgery and postoperative chemoradiation therapy (11% vs. 24% for surgery alone). In addition, a significant survival advantage was found at 7 years using the combination of resection, radiation, and chemotherapy. The NCCTG subsequently conducted a trial randomizing 204 patients to radiotherapy (45–50.4 Gy in 25–28 fractions) with or without concurrent chemotherapy (bolus 5-FU). There was a significant decrease in pelvic recurrence (14% vs. 25%) and a significant decrease in cancer-related deaths for the group treated by resection, radiation, and chemotherapy compared with the group treated with resection and radiation therapy alone.

The findings from these studies prompted the publication of a clinical advisory by the National Cancer Institute Consensus Conference in 1990 recommending adjuvant treatment for patients with Dukes B2 and C rectal carcinoma (T3–T4, N0; T3–T4, N1–N3, now stage II–III) consisting of six cycles of FU-based chemotherapy and concurrent radiation therapy to the pelvis. This regimen has remained the standard by which all current adjuvant rectal cancer protocols are compared. In the United States, postoperative chemoradiation is by far the most common mode of delivering adjuvant therapy. This is usually given as a continuous infusion of 5-FU and approximately 50.4 Gy of irradiation delivered to the pelvis in 1.8 to 2.0 Gy fractions (6-week treatment). Although the trend in Europe has been treatment with radiation therapy and no chemotherapy, the addition of chemotherapy in the United States has been shown to decrease the rate of distant metastases, something not attainable with radiation therapy alone. In addition, there has consistently been a 10% to 15% survival advantage when radiotherapy with chemotherapy is compared to radiotherapy alone. The Intergroup 0114 trial was designed to study the effects of biochemical modulation of 5-FU during radiotherapy. It demonstrated no significant survival advantage to the addition of levamisole and/or LV to adjuvant bolus 5-FU and pelvic radiation in the postoperative period. Protracted infusion 5-FU has been compared to bolus 5-FU by the NCCTG and has been demonstrated to result in improved disease-free and overall survival. This finding has been confirmed in subsequent studies.

Preoperative Radiation Therapy (±Chemotherapy)
Several advantages to the use of preoperative compared with postoperative radiation therapy have been identified, including the following:

1. A reduction in tumor size increases rates of sphincter preservation in those patients initially deemed to require APR and improves overall resectability.
2. There is a decreased risk of local failure due to improved compliance with the chemoradiation regimen and improved tumor response in the preoperative setting.
3. There is a decreased risk of toxicity because the small bowel can more readily be excluded from the radiation field in a preoperative setting.
4. There is less bowel dysfunction because the colon used for reconstruction is not in the radiation field.
5. There is no delay of therapy as in some cases of postoperative therapy due to operative morbidity.

Until now, there have been several randomized trials evaluating the role of preoperative radiation therapy in resectable rectal cancer. Although most report significant decreases in local recurrence, only the 1997 Swedish Rectal Cancer Trial has shown a significant survival advantage for the total patient group. This trial gave short-course radiotherapy (25 Gy in five fractions, 1 week), followed by curative resection to the experimental group, and curative surgery alone to the control group. The local recurrence rate and 9-year disease-specific survival were 11% and 74%, respectively, versus 27% and 65% for the control group. One limitation of this study compared to more recent trials is the lack of surgical quality control, which is believed to be the reason for the high local recurrence rate in the control group. This was addressed in the Dutch Colorectal Cancer Group trial in which more than 1,800 patients with rectal cancer located within 15 cm from the anal verge were randomized to receive preoperative short-course radiotherapy followed by TME versus TME alone. The local recurrence rate in the surgery alone group was 8.2%. Preoperative radiotherapy improved this to 2.4%. However, there was no difference in overall survival. Also, subgroup analysis of data from this trial showed no significant benefit for irradiation of lesions located in the upper rectum greater than 10 cm from the anal verge ($P = 0.17$).

In the United States, preoperative radiation therapy trials have usually included chemotherapy in a more protracted course rather than using short-course radiotherapy alone. This practice has been based on data demonstrating the importance of the addition of chemotherapy to radiation in the adjuvant setting.

Generally a 6-week interval is given after the completion of chemoradiation before surgery. Longer intervals after radiotherapy have been associated with improved pathological complete response rates. The most definitive randomized data demonstrating the superiority of preoperative versus postoperative chemoradiation comes from the German Rectal Cancer Study Group. Four-hundred and twenty-one patients with tumors located within 16 cm from the anal verge were randomly assigned to preoperative long-course radiation (50.4 Gy in 28 fractions) with concurrent infusional 5-FU (1,000 mg/m^2/day) during weeks 1 and 5 followed by TME or to TME followed by postoperative radiation (45 Gy in 25 fractions) and concurrent infusional 5-FU. All patients in the preoperative group and those patients with stage II or greater disease in the postoperative group also received four cycles of bolus 5-FU in the adjuvant setting. Patients assigned to the preoperative arm had a lower 5-year cumulative risk of local failure (6% vs. 13%, $P = 0.006$) and decreased toxicity, both severe acute (27% vs. 40%, $P = 0.001$) and late (14% vs. 24%, $P = 0.01$). Moreover, improved sphincter preservation rates were noted in those patients who were initially deemed to require APR (39% vs. 19%, $P = 0.004$), preoperative versus postoperative, respectively. However, there was no difference in survival between the two arms.

Two multicentered randomized trials have attempted to address the question of preoperative versus postoperative chemoradiation for rectal cancer, RTOG 94-01, which closed early due to poor accrual, and NSABP R-03, which failed to accrue its intended sample size, but did report in 2009 an improved disease-free survival and trend toward improved overall survival when preoperative chemoradiotherapy was compared to postoperative chemoradiotherapy with no difference in local recurrence.

The main disadvantage of the preoperative regimens is that approximately 20% of patients with rectal cancer will be preoperatively overstaged and therefore may undergo potentially unnecessary radiation and chemotherapy with their associated toxicities. In the German study, 20% of the patients randomized to the postoperative arm were noted to actually have stage I disease once the specimen was available for evaluation. These patients do not need adjuvant therapy and would have been overtreated if they were treated preoperatively. Recently, a number of groups have demonstrated efficacy of the oral fluoropyrimidine, capecitabine, as the chemotherapeutic radiation sensitizer in neoadjuvant regimens. Capecitabine has the advantages of convenient oral administration and reduced toxicity when compared to intravenous 5-FU. The NSABP R-04 study hopes to address this issue in a multi-institutional trial comparing conventional 5-FU with or without oxaliplatin versus capecitabine with or without oxaliplatin in the neoadjuvant setting.

Intraoperative Radiation Therapy

IORT can be used for both recurrent and locally advanced rectal cancer. Its advantages include increased local control in high-risk cancers, accurate treatment of focal areas at risk, and the ability to shield sensitive structures. Even preoperative chemoradiation in high-risk tumors can result in high local recurrence rates. IORT allows treatment of areas with close or microscopically positive margins in this situation. IORT dosing depends on the clinical situation and the total preoperative radiotherapy dose: 12–13 Gy is given for close margins (<3 mm), 15 Gy is given for microscopically positive margins, and 17–20 Gy is used for areas of gross residual disease. An alternative approach is intraoperative brachytherapy. This allows radiation access in areas where the IORT beam cannot be focused due to anatomical constraints of the pelvis. At MDACC, intraoperative brachytherapy (10–20 Gy) is used selectively in patients with locally advanced or recurrent disease where there is a close or positive margin as demonstrated by frozen section.

M. D. Anderson Experience

Our preferred management of locally advanced rectal cancer (T3–T4, N0, or any T, N1–N2) includes preoperative radiation therapy with a protracted intravenous infusion of 5-FU or capecitabine. We deliver 45 Gy of preoperative radiation therapy in 25 fractions with a boost to the tumor bed of 5.4 Gy in three fractions for a total of 50.4 Gy in 28 fractions. A continuous infusion of 5-FU at a dose of 300 mg/m^2/day or capecitabine 850 mg/m^2/day is given 5 days/week. Surgery is performed 6 to 8 weeks after completion of therapy. With this regimen, more than 60% of patients experience a T-stage decrease and 17% achieve a pathological complete response. In patients with T3 disease, 44% of patients with rectal cancers located within 3 cm of the anal verge are now able to undergo sphincter-preserving procedures, with a local control rate in excess of 90% and a 3-year survival rate of 88% in node-negative patients. In patients with fixed T3 and T4 tumors, the same regimen was used with the addition of an IORT boost for positive or close margins. The local control rate was 97% with 82% 5-year survival.

Although some institutions will advocate TME alone for most rectal cancers, surgeons globally are now looking to identify those patients who will benefit most from adjuvant therapy and what therapy should be used (chemotherapy and radiation therapy and dosing). Ongoing studies are investigating combinations of different agents and the timing of surgery following multimodal therapy in an effort to improve the pathological response rate. The role of local excision with multimodality therapy is still controversial, particularly in the era of newer biologically active chemotherapeutic agents. Some centers are exploring the use of IORT and brachytherapy as adjuncts to neoadjuvant chemoradiation treatments to increase the local disease control in select patients who are at high risk for local recurrence. Various molecular markers are being evaluated in fresh or archival specimens to aid in identifying patients who will benefit from treatment.

SURVEILLANCE

Patients with a history of colorectal carcinoma require close surveillance. The data to support this, however, are lacking. In a Danish prospective randomized study in 597 colorectal cancer patients, patients had either close follow-up (every 6 months for the first 3 years) or yearly for 3 years (including examination/stool heme test, colonoscopy, laboratory testing [except CEA], and chest radiograph). The frequency of recurrent cancer was the same in both groups, but it was diagnosed earlier in the close follow-up group. The close follow-up group had more resections for curative intent (local and distant), but cancer-specific survival differences have been more difficult to demonstrate. Multiple surveillance regimens have been advocated by several national societies. In general, close follow-up including regularly scheduled CEA level determination during the first 2 years followed by less intensive follow-up during years 3 to 5 are advocated.

History and physical examination and laboratory tests including CEA are performed at MDACC every 3 to 4 months for the first 2 years after surgery, every 6 months during years 3 through 5, and yearly thereafter. Colonoscopy should be performed after 1 year and then at 3 years if normal. A baseline CT scan of the abdomen and pelvis is obtained preoperatively followed by annual intervals unless otherwise indicated by disease biology. A chest radiograph is obtained every 6 months for the first 2 years and yearly thereafter. It has traditionally been proposed that patients should be monitored closely for local recurrence during the first 2 years postoperatively (the time at which most local recurrences appear). Recent data show that the addition of adjuvant radiation therapy may extend this period of vulnerability such that 50% of local recurrences may occur more than 2 years from surgery. Finally, it should be noted that these are *general* guidelines that may need to be tailored to individual patients.

RECURRENT AND METASTATIC DISEASE

More than 50% of patients who undergo curative surgery for colorectal cancer have tumor recurrences. Of the patients who have recurrences, 85% do so during the first 2.5 years after surgery. The remaining 15% experience recurrence during the subsequent 2.5 years. Recurrence develops in less than 5% of patients who are disease-free at 5 years. The risk of recurrence is higher with stage II or III disease. Other recurrence risk modifiers include race, presentation, grade of tumor, aneuploidy, and adjacent organ invasion. Many molecular markers are currently being evaluated for their usefulness in predicting recurrence risk. Recurrences may be local, regional, or distant. Distant disease recurrence, the most common presentation, occurs either alone or concomitantly with locoregional recurrence. Local recurrence develops in 20% to 30% of patients who undergo initial curative resections for rectal cancer, and in 50% to 80% of these patients, the local recurrence is the only site of disease. For all recurrence sites, complete resection results in a 25% to 30% cure rate. Recurrence isolated to the anastomosis (intramural) is rare and can indicate inadequate surgical resection. Liver involvement occurs in approximately 50% of patients with colon cancer, whereas lung, bone, and brain involvement occurs in 10%, 5%, and less than 5%, respectively. Symptomatic recurrences present with a constellation of symptoms ranging from the vague and nonspecific to the clinically overt.

CEA is invaluable for postoperative monitoring. It is most useful in patients in whom levels are increased preoperatively and return to normal following surgery. Levels should be determined preoperatively, 6 weeks postoperatively, and then according to the schedule described in the surveillance section. The absolute level and rate of increase in CEA and the patient's clinical status are important in determining prognosis and treatment. Postoperative CEA levels that do not normalize within 4 to 6 weeks suggest incomplete resection or recurrent disease, although false-positive results do occur. CEA levels that normalize postoperatively and then start to increase are indicative of recurrence. This may represent occult or clinically obvious disease. A rapidly increasing CEA level suggests liver or lung involvement, whereas a slow, gradual rise is more likely to be associated with locoregional disease. Despite the reliability of an increased CEA level in predicting tumor recurrence, 20% to 30% of patients with locoregionally recurrent tumors have a normal CEA level. Poorly differentiated tumors may not make CEA, which is one explanation for such false-negative results. In contrast, CEA is increased in 80% to 90% of patients with hepatic recurrences. A prospective randomized trial of the value of CEA in follow-up in 311 patients followed asymptomatic patients with increased CEA levels until symptoms developed; then a full workup was initiated. The sensitivity, specificity, and positive predictive values of an increased CEA level were 58%, 93%, and 79%, respectively. The median lead-time of the increased CEA to detection by other means was 6 months. Seven percent of patients who had an increased CEA failed to have identifiable recurrent disease on workup. Two meta-analyses have been performed pooling results from five randomized studies and a survival advantage in patients allocated to intensive follow-up, including CEA has been shown. The German Colorectal Cancer Study Group evaluated follow-up CEA levels in 1,321 patients after curative resection and determined that CEA monitoring was beneficial in 47% of patients with recurrence and 11% of patients overall; however, only 2.3% underwent a curative R0 resection of recurrent disease. Results from a UK multicenter randomized prospective trial of protracted infusion 5-FU versus bolus 5-FU in the adjuvant setting demonstrated that both CT and CEA were valuable components for postoperative follow-up and resulted in improved survival. Despite significant interest, the use of radiolabeled monoclonal antibodies (mAb) directed against tumor-specific antigens and CEA have not been shown to be useful for imaging the extent and location of metastases.

PET with 2-(^{18}F)fluorodeoxy-D-glucose (FDG) has been reported to have 89% positive predictive value and 100% negative predictive value in patients who had a rising CEA and normal conventional radiography. FDG–PET imaging relies on the increased metabolic uptake of glucose (fluorine-labeled analog of 2-deoxyglucose or FDG) in tumors compared with normal tissues and sometimes may help to distinguish postsurgical and postradiation changes from recurrent tumor. Treatment of the asymptomatic patient with an increased CEA level can be challenging. An increased level should be confirmed by a repeat CEA determination. A thorough clinical investigation should include LFTs, CT scan of the chest, abdomen, pelvis, and brain (when indicated), and colonoscopy. At MDACC, we routinely monitor CEA values because of the potential to detect resectable metastases, especially within the liver. This allows for the potential identification of a subgroup of patients who may benefit from early recurrence intervention. PET scans are performed to evaluate patients with rising CEA values where conventional radiography is not able to identify the site of recurrence.

If the metastatic evaluation is negative in the face of increased CEA level, a second-look laparotomy may be indicated. In studies conducted prior to modern imaging technology, approximately 60% to 90% of patients with asymptomatically increased CEA levels will have recurrent disease at laparotomy; 12% to 60% of whom will have resectable disease. Early detection of asymptomatic disease results in a higher resectability rate than when resection is attempted for symptomatic disease (60% vs. 27%). The liver is the most common site of recurrence, followed by adjacent organs, the anastomotic site, and the mesentery. Resectability rates correspond to the level of CEA elevation, with CEA levels less than 11 ng/mL being associated with higher resectability rates.

Treatment

The appropriate treatment of resectable recurrent disease depends on the location of the disease. If two disease sites are detected that are completely resectable, the procedure is undertaken in select patients. Otherwise, individual treatment modalities are used as needed for palliation of symptoms. As in locally advanced disease, potentially resectable recurrent disease is treated in a multimodality fashion using preoperative chemotherapy (with or without radiation), surgery, IORT (if available), and brachytherapy. For recurrence involving the sacrum, en bloc sacral resection can sometimes result in 4-year survival rates of 30%. Contraindications to sacral resection include pelvic sidewall involvement, sciatic notch involvement, bilateral S2 involvement, encasement of common or external iliac vessels, and extrapelvic disease. Symptoms of recurrent disease could be adequately palliated with surgery. At MDACC, potentially resectable pelvic recurrences are treated with preoperative chemoradiation, followed by surgery and the use of intraoperative brachytherapy as needed. Using this approach in 171 patients with locally recurrent and re-recurrent rectal cancer, multimodality salvage therapy resulted in a 5-year overall and recurrence-free survival of 42% and 30%, respectively. Although the usual surgical procedure for resectable recurrent rectal cancer is APR, select cases can be treated with sphincter preservation.

Median survival for metastatic colorectal cancer without systemic chemotherapy ranges from 6 to 9 months in early series. The addition of 5-FU-based regimens improves survival to 10 to 12 months. The addition of irinotecan or oxaliplatin to 5-FU further improves survival to 14 to 17 months. As described previously, the addition of the monoclonal antibodies have improved median survival to greater than 20 months.

Liver

The liver is the most common site of visceral metastases, and it is the only site affected in up to 20% of patients. Recent data from MDACC demonstrates that surgical resection of hepatic metastases now offers the potential for 5-year survival up to 58%. Colorectal hepatic metastases are discussed in detail in Chapter 12.

Lung

Pulmonary metastases occur in 10% to 20% of patients with colorectal cancer. They are most commonly seen in the setting of a large hepatic tumor burden or extensive metastatic disease. Isolated pulmonary metastases occur most commonly with distal rectal lesions because the venous drainage of the distal rectum bypasses the portal system and allows metastasis to travel directly to the lungs.

The finding of a solitary lesion on a chest radiograph should prompt evaluation with thoracic CT scanning and, for a centrally located lesion, bronchoscopy with biopsy. Peripheral lesions may be amenable to CT-guided needle biopsy or video-assisted thoracoscopic surgery. Fifty percent of patients with solitary pulmonary nodules will have primary lung tumors rather than colorectal metastases.

Patients with locally controlled primary tumors, no evidence of metastases elsewhere, good pulmonary reserve, and good medical condition are candidates for resection. Patients with solitary metastases experience the best survival, but patients with as many as three lesions (unilateral or bilateral) can experience up to a 40% 5-year survival. As in liver resection for metastatic disease, the optimum surgery includes achievement of negative margins at resection without the routine use of pneumonectomy.

The overall 5-year survival rate following resection of pulmonary metastases can approach 40%. Age, gender, location of the primary disease, disease-free interval, or involvement of hilar or mediastinal lymph nodes does not seem to influence survival. The number of metastases in most series is inversely correlated with 5-year survival. Recurrence confined to the lung after resection is an indication by some for repeat resection.

Bone and Brain

Metastatic disease to the brain is uncommon and usually occurs after established lung involvement. Symptomatic solitary lesions can be treated by palliative craniotomy and resection. In a very small subpopulation of patients, cranial disease may be the only site of involvement, and excision in this setting may increase survival. Bone metastases are quite uncommon and are best managed with radiation therapy.

Ovary

Because 1% to 8% of women who undergo potentially curative resections subsequently develop ovarian metastases, prophylactic oophorectomy at the time of colectomy has been considered for postmenopausal patients. However, prophylactic oophorectomy has not been shown to improve survival and therefore is not routinely performed, but grossly abnormal ovaries should be removed. When isolated metastatic disease to the one ovary is identified, a bilateral oophorectomy is performed because of high risk of bilateral involvement.

UNCOMMON COLORECTAL TUMORS

Lymphoma

Lymphoma is an uncommon tumor that occurs in 0.4% of patients with intestinal lymphoma presenting anywhere between the second and eighth decades of life. Almost all are non-Hodgkin lymphomas. Twenty-five percent of patients may present with fever, occult blood loss, anemia, a palpable mass, or an acute abdomen. The diagnosis is often made intraoperatively. A history of abdominal pain, fever, and weight loss in a patient who is younger than the expected age for a colorectal tumor should raise the suspicion of intestinal lymphoma.

Abdominal CT and endoscopy with biopsy are the most useful diagnostic tests because lesions are often missed on barium enema examination. A thickened bowel, adjacent organ extension, or nodal enlargement may be seen. If the lesion is intraluminal, endoscopic biopsy will facilitate the diagnosis. Most of these lesions are intermediate- to high-grade B-cell lymphomas. If a diagnosis is made preoperatively in an otherwise asymptomatic patient, bone marrow biopsy should be performed. A primary lesion is defined as a lesion with no associated organ or lymphatic involvement, negative chest CT, and a negative peripheral blood smear and bone marrow.

Surgery is performed in the clinical setting of obstruction, bleeding, perforation, or an uncertain diagnosis. In rare cases, surgery may be performed for complete resection of a primary lesion. A thorough exploration is performed, and all suspicious nodes or organs are biopsied to assess the stage of disease. The primary intestinal lesion should be resected with negative margins whenever possible. The bowel mesentery should be resected with the tumor so regional nodes can be assessed pathologically. Intestinal continuity should be restored whenever possible. If a large tumor is found to be unresectable and is not obstructing the bowel, a bypass can be performed. Surgical clips should be placed to facilitate identification of the tumor by the radiation oncologist.

Intestinal lymphoma requires a combined-modality approach using surgery and chemotherapy with or without radiation. For rectal lymphoma, complete resection is followed by radiation treatments to the pelvis. Chemoradiation is used if the resection was incomplete. The overall survival for stage I and II disease is approximately 80%. This decreases to 35% with advanced disease.

Gastrointestinal Stromal Tumors

Gastrointestinal stromal tumors (GISTs) account for most mesenchymal tumors arising in the wall of the colon or rectum. Primary colorectal GISTs are rare and comprise less than 1% of colonic tumors. GISTs have recently been characterized, but historically classified, as leiomyomas, leiomyosarcomas, neurofibromas, and schwannomas and are further discussed in detail elsewhere in this text. In a review of 1,458 cases of malignant GISTs from 1992 to 2000 in the SEER database, 7% were located in the colon and 5% in the rectum. These tumors can present as small submucosal or as large intramural masses. Patients can present with pain, bleeding, obstruction, nausea, vomiting, anemia, tenesmus, or hematuria. Ulceration may be present in 30% to 50% of patients. A thorough clinical evaluation should be conducted to exclude metastatic disease. Excision with negative surgical margins is the treatment of choice. Colonic tumors are excised with adjacent mesentery. Wide nodal excision is not indicated in the absence of clinically evident disease. Small tumors of the rectum and anal canal can be removed transrectally or endoscopically. Criteria similar to GISTs elsewhere in the GI tract are used for determining the need for adjuvant therapy with imatinib mesylate (STI-571, Gleevec), a monoclonal antibody to the tyrosine kinase receptor. Further details regarding GISTS are discussed in Chapter 5.

Neuroendocrine Tumors

Neuroendocrine tumors classified as low grade (carcinoid) or high grade are uncommonly found in the colon and rectum. Approximately 18% to 30% of intestinal carcinoids occur in the rectum or rectosigmoid, 4% to 15% occur in the colon, and 4% to 50% have been reported to occur in the appendix. They are usually discovered incidentally unless they are large. Size and depth of invasion are the best predictors of clinical behavior. Hindgut carcinoids almost never produce the carcinoid syndrome. Although large tumors may present with bleeding, obstruction, or constipation, tumors less than 2 cm are frequently asymptomatic. Diagnosis is made by endoscopic biopsy. In general, tumors less than 1 cm rarely metastasize, whereas those greater than 2 cm have increased metastatic potential; in the 1- to 2-cm range, 10% to 20% will metastasize. This makes treatment decisions for tumors in the 1- to 2-cm range problematic. Small lesions (<1 cm) are commonly well differentiated and can be adequately treated with endoscopic excision. Lesions less than 2 cm can be treated with full-thickness local excision. High-grade tumors have a poorer overall prognosis, and multidisciplinary management with or without neoadjuvant chemo/chemoradiation therapy is recommended followed by radical resection.

ANAL CANCER

Epidemiology and Etiology

An estimated 5,290 new cases and 710 deaths from anal cancer (involving the anus, anal canal, and anorectum) will occur in the United States in 2009. Although anal carcinoma has been considered an uncommon cancer, the incidence in the United States has increased by approximately 1.6 fold for men and 1.5 fold for women from the time period 1973–1979 to 1994–2000. In the HIV-infected population, the standardized incidence rate of anal carcinoma estimated to be 19/100,000 in the time period 1992–1995 has increased to 78.2 during the time period 2000–2003. Other causes of immunocompromise such as transplantation or immunotherapy for autoimmune diseases are additional risk factors. Kidney transplant patients have at least a fourfold increased incidence of the disease. In the general population, elderly women and men in their sixties are at the highest risk for anal cancer, with women having the greater risk.

Population-based evidence has established that anal cancer is a sexually transmitted disease (STD) in much the same way that cervical cancer is an STD. Women with anal cancer are more likely to have had a history of genital warts or other STDs and men with anal cancer are more likely to have reported homosexual activity or to have a history of genital warts or gonorrhea. As with cervical cancer, anal cancer has been linked to human papillomavirus (HPV-16 and HPV-18) infection. Studies have shown that 40% to 95% of anal cancers harbor HPV DNA, with the strongest association seen with nonkeratinizing squamous cell types originating from the squamous mucosa of the anal canal. This association has proven to be even stronger with advances in HPV detection techniques showing the presence of HPV-16 and HPV-18 in up to 88% of patients with anal carcinoma.

The national cancer registries in Denmark and Sweden identified 417 patients with anal cancer between 1991 and 1994 and compared them with 534 controls with rectal adenocarcinoma and 554 population controls. Using multivariate analysis while adjusting for smoking and education, this study found that the lifetime number of sexual partners, history of anal intercourse, a history of anogenital warts, gonorrhea, or cervical neoplasia, testing for HIV, and a history of partners with STDs were all associated with a significantly increased risk for anal cancer in women. Risk factors for men included lifetime number of sexual partners, homosexuality, history of anal warts or syphilis, and being unmarried with or without a current sexual partner. The associations were similar when data from Denmark and Sweden were considered separately or together. When polymerase chain reaction for HPV DNA was performed on archived tissue specimens from these patients, 88% of patients overall were positive for HPV, and HPV-16 was identified in 83% of those with HPV. This compares to cervical cancer where HPV-16 is responsible for about 50% of cases, HPV 18, 31, and 45 is responsible for an additional 30%, and additional HPV types account for the remaining 20% of cases. Analysis of the data from the SEER program revealed that the relative risks of anal cancer and vaginal cancer in women who had been diagnosed with invasive cervical cancer were 4.6 and 5.6, respectively. This increased risk for anal cancer in women with cervical dysplasia or cancer, and their sexual partners, is likely through autoinoculation by the virus that caused the cervical dysplasia.

Anal cancers can be located within the anal canal or in the perianal skin (anal margin). Anal canal cancers are three to four times more common in women than in men. Anal margin cancers (tumors of the hair-bearing perianal skin) are more common in males. There are significantly more cases of anal margin cancers in homosexual males.

Pathological Characteristics
More than 60% of malignant anal lesions are histologically SCCs. With the exception of melanoma, small cell carcinoma, and anal adenocarcinoma, all other histologic subtypes behave similarly and are treated according to their anatomical location. Basaloid carcinoma (basal cell carcinoma with a massive squamous component), mucoepidermoid carcinoma (originating in anal crypt glands), and cloacogenic carcinoma are all variants of squamous carcinoma. As with cervical cancer, SCC of the anus may be preceded by or coexist with premalignant dysplasia or anal intraepithelial neoplasia (AIN).

The prognosis of anal margin cancers is favorable. The rate of local recurrence is higher than the rate of distant metastases, which are rare. When they do occur, metastases are most commonly found in the superficial inguinal lymph nodes (approximately 15% of cases). It is unusual for anal margin cancers to metastasize to mesenteric or internal iliac nodes.

Anal canal cancers are associated with aggressive local growth and if untreated will extend to the rectal mucosa and submucosa, subcutaneous perianal tissue and perianal skin, ischiorectal fat, local skeletal muscle, perineum, genitalia, lower urinary system, and even the pelvic peritoneum and the broad ligament. Historically, mesenteric lymph node metastases have been detected in 30% to 50% of surgical specimens. More than 50% of patients will present with locally advanced disease. The most common sites of distant metastases are the liver, lung, and abdominal cavity. However, most cancer-related deaths are due to uncontrolled pelvic or perineal disease.

Diagnosis
The initial symptoms of anal cancer include bleeding, pain, and local fullness. These symptoms are similar to those caused by the common benign anal diseases, which accompany anal cancer in more than 50% of cases. A detailed history, including previous anal pathology and sexual habits, should precede a meticulous physical examination. Physical examination should attempt to identify the lesion, its size and anatomical boundaries, and any associated scarring or condylomata. It is also important to determine the resting and voluntary anal sphincter tone. Occasionally, an examination under general anesthesia may be necessary to complete the local evaluation. Pelvic and abdominal CT scans and a chest radiograph are important in assessing extent of local disease and distant spread. Proctosigmoidoscopy is essential to assess the proximal extent of disease and to obtain tissue for biopsy. Palpable inguinal lymph nodes should be evaluated by fine-needle aspiration. PET–CT may be helpful in the workup for lesions in the anal canal to evaluate for distant metastases.

Staging
The current American Joint Committee on Cancer (AJCC) staging system for anal margin and anal canal cancers is depicted in Tables 11.8 and 11.9.

TABLE 11.8	American Joint Committee on Cancer Staging of Anal Canal Cancer

Primary Tumor (T)

TX	Primary tumor cannot be assessed
T0	No evidence of primary tumor
Tis	Carcinoma in situ
T1	Tumor ≤2 cm in greatest dimension
T2	Tumor >2 cm but not >5 cm in greatest dimension
T3	Tumor >5 cm in greatest dimension
T4	Tumor of any size invades adjacent organ(s)

Lymph Nodes (N)

NX	Regional lymph nodes cannot be assessed
N0	No regional lymph node metastasis
N1	Metastasis in perirectal lymph node(s)
N2	Metastasis in unilateral internal iliac and/or inguinal lymph node(s)
	Metastasis in perirectal and inguinal lymph nodes and/or bilateral internal iliac and/or inguinal lymph nodes

Distant Metastasis (M)

MX	Presence of distant metastasis cannot be assessed
M0	No distant metastasis
M1	Distant metastasis

Stage Grouping

0	Tis	N0	M0
I	T1	N0	M0
II	T2	N0	M0
	T3	N0	M0
IIIA	T1	N1	M0
	T2	N1	M0
	T3	N1	M0
	T4	N0	M0
IIIB	T4	N1	M0
	Any T	N2	M0
	Any T	N3	M0
IV	Any T	Any N	M1

Treatment

Anal Canal

Until the 1980s, APR with permanent colostomy was the recommended treatment for all SCCs of the anal canal. This treatment, however, was associated with low survival rates as a result of distant failure. Radiation therapy in the range of 50 to 60 Gy was also used as definitive treatment of these cancers, with recurrence and survival rates similar to those seen using APR. The pioneering chemoradiation protocol developed by Nigro et al. (1974), which has since been confirmed and modified by others, has radically changed the approach to this disease. Currently, surgery with local excision is reserved for well-differentiated anal margin lesions characterized as T1N0 and APR for (a) salvage treatment in patients with persistent disease

TABLE 11.9	AJCC Staging of Anal Margin Cancer

Primary Tumor (T)

TX	Primary tumor cannot be assessed
T0	No evidence of primary tumor
Tis	Carcinoma in situ
T1	Tumor ≤2 cm in greatest dimension
T2	Tumor >2 cm but not >5 cm in greatest dimension
T3	Tumor >5 cm in greatest dimension
T4	Tumor invades deep extradermal structures (i.e., cartilage, skeletal muscle, or bone)

Lymph Nodes (N)

NX	Regional lymph nodes cannot be assessed
N0	No regional lymph node metastasis
N1	Regional lymph node metastasis

Distant Metastasis (M)

MX	Presence of distant metastasis cannot be assessed
M0	No distant metastasis
M1	Distant metastasis

Stage Grouping

0	Tis	N0	M0
I	T1	N0	M0
II	T2	N0	M0
	T3	N0	M0
III	T4	N0	M0
	Any T	N1	M0
IV	Any T	Any N	M1

(within 6 months of chemoradiation) or recurrent disease (after 6 months); (b) severely symptomatic patients (perineal sepsis, intractable urinary or fecal fistulae, and intolerable incontinence); (c) inguinal lymph node dissection for persistent inguinal disease, recurrent inguinal disease (treated first with radiation therapy unless associated with local recurrence), or primary disease in the inguinal basin, where the disease is bulky or fungating; and (d) temporary fecal diversion in patients with nearly obstructing lesions.

Since the initial work of Nigro et al. (1974), studies have been performed to dissect out the vital components and doses of the chemoradiation in order to optimize treatment. There is evidence that (a) higher doses of radiation produce better local control rates using a constant mitomycin-C dose (Rich, 1997); (b) 5-FU and mitomycin-C with radiation therapy produces better local control rates than radiation therapy alone; (c) 5-FU and mitomycin-C with radiation therapy produces better local control rates than 5-FU with radiation therapy; and (d) cisplatin with 5-FU and radiation therapy produces local control and survival rates similar to 5-FU, mitomycin-C, and radiation therapy with less toxicity. The randomized intergroup RTOG 98-11 trial investigated the use of mitomycin or cisplatin with 5-FU-based chemoradiation therapy in patients with SCC of the anus. Patients were randomly assigned to receive either induction chemotherapy with 5-FU and cisplatin for two cycles followed by concurrent chemoradiation therapy with 5-FU/cisplatin or concurrent chemoradiation therapy with 5-FU/mitomycin. No significant differences

TABLE 11.10	Current and Classic Treatment Protocols for Anal Canal Cancer
Current	External-beam radiation therapy 5 d/wk for total dose of 45–55 Gy
	5-FU, 250 mg/m^2/day, M–F for the entire duration of radiation
	Cis-platin, 4 g/m^2/day, M–F for the entire duration of radiation
Classic	
Days 1–4	5-FU, 750–1,000 mg/m^2 over 24-h continuous IV infusion
Day 1	Mitomycin C, 10–15 mg/m^2, IV bolus
Days 1–35	Radiation therapy 5 d/wk for total dose of 45–55 Gy; boosts of up to 60 Gy may be given to the anus and/or inguinal basins
Days 29–32	5-FU, 750–1,000 mg/m^2 over 24-h continuous IV infusion

5-FU, 5-fluorouracil; IV, intravenous.

were seen in disease-free survival or 5-year overall survival. Moreover, the colostomy rate was significantly increased in the cisplatin-containing arm. However, this study compared mitomycin with radiation therapy to induction chemotherapy with cisplatin and radiation therapy and therefore has been criticized with respect to its generalizability to all cisplatin-based strategies. Results from the phase III UK ACT 11 trial comparing 5-FU/mitomycin to 5-FU/cisplatin with concurrent continuous radiation of 50.4 Gy showed that at a median follow-up of 3 years, no differences were observed in complete response rate or recurrence-free survival. Furthermore, rate of colostomy was not different based on the chemotherapeutic regimen.

The current regimen for primary treatment of SCC of the anal canal is chemoradiation therapy (Table 11.10). At MDACC we utilize a 5-FU and cisplatin-based chemoradiation protocol because of decreased toxicity and similar response, survival, and colostomy data. Complete responses with this treatment can be expected in up to 90% of patients, with 5-year survival rates approaching 85%.

The presence of a persistent mass on examination 12 to 14 weeks after chemoradiation is an indication for biopsy because a persistent mass after therapy will demonstrate cancer on biopsy in 18% to 34% of cases. There are reports of positive biopsy specimen results 6 to 8 weeks after therapy (persistent disease), which will revert to negative biopsy results in patients who have refused surgery. This implies that there may be a delayed radiation effect for up to several months after treatment. At MDACC, we do not routinely obtain a biopsy specimen of the treated tumor site unless obvious disease persistence exists; instead, we wait for clinical evidence of locally recurrent disease in follow-up visits.

Patients with local recurrence or persistent disease are salvaged with APR, with a resultant 50% 5-year survival. However, cisplatin-based chemotherapy with additional radiation therapy has been used successfully to salvage up to one-third of patients with locally recurrent disease and is currently under investigation.

Anal Margin

SCC of the anal margin is defined currently by the AJCC as a lesion originating in an area between the anal margin and 5 cm in any direction onto the perianal skin and is classified with skin tumors. The terms anal margin and perianal skin are often used synonymously. Note that the data supporting the treatment of these uncommon, heterogeneous lesions derive from small, single-institution, mostly retrospective studies. Moreover, many of these studies include lesions of the lower anal canal (dentate to anal verge) that were included previously in older definitions of the anal margin. The rationale for any modality of therapy derives from the proportional increase in chance of metastases with increasing tumor size; in tumors less than 2 cm, lymph node metastases are rarely found. For lesions between 2 and 5 cm, and those greater than 5 cm, the rates are 24% and 25% to 67%, respectively.

Small (<2 cm), superficial T1, well-differentiated anal margin cancers that do not invade the sphincter complex can be treated by a negative-margin wide local excision alone, with a 5-year survival rate greater than 80%. Wide local excision may include parts of the superficial internal and external anal sphincters without compromising anal continence. Positive margins can be re-excised or consideration given to radiation therapy with or without 5-FU-based chemotherapy.

Larger T2-T4 or N-positive lesions are best treated with multimodality therapy using chemoradiation, as in anal canal cancers, given the higher local recurrence rate. Inclusion of bilateral inguinal/low pelvic nodal regions in the radiation field should be considered for more advanced cancers. Lymph node dissection is reserved for those patients with residual or recurrent disease. It is not known whether the treatment of inguinal disease translates into improved survival. Patients with T3 to T4 and poor sphincter function may require APR. For all patients, the 5-year disease-specific survival is 71% to 88%, and the local control rate after initial therapy is 70% to 100%. Platinum-based chemotherapy is recommended for metastatic disease.

Surveillance

Patients should be followed for detection of local and systemic failures and treatment complications. Local inspection, digital examination, and anoscopy are recommended between 8 and 12 weeks after chemoradiation treatment and every 3 to 6 months for 5 years thereafter. A biopsy is performed only if presence of disease is suspected after serial digital examinations. Biopsy-proven persistent disease should be re-evaluated in 4 weeks and if regression is seen continued observation and re-evaluation in 3-month intervals with yearly CT scans is appropriate. If there is no regression or there is progression of disease, the patient should be restaged and APR offered if the disease is locoregional. Distant failures of epidermoid cancer are responsive to radiation therapy, and up to 30% of patients respond to second-line chemotherapy. Therefore, chest radiography, LFTs, and pelvic CT are recommended every 6 to 12 months for 2 to 3 years after initial therapy. Patients with anal margin cancers should have careful, close follow-up, given the indolent nature of these tumors and the benefits of further local therapy.

Anal Intraepithelial Neoplasia

AIN is a term used to describe squamous intraepithelial lesions (SILs) of the anus. This is an increasingly prevalent condition associated with HPV infection and condylomata that can occur both externally on the perianal skin and internally in the anal canal. Dysplasia in squamous intraepithelial lesions may be low grade or high grade (HSIL); the latter, an intermediate stage in the malignant transformation to SCC of the anus. Anal HSIL represents cytopathological and histopathological findings that have been referred to as AIN II/III, severe dysplasia, carcinoma in situ, or Bowen disease. The presence of HPV infection is the principal risk factor for anal neoplasia. Cofactors include anal-receptive intercourse and immunocompromise. Paralleling observations in the cervix (cervical cancer and cervical intraepithelial neoplasia), infection by oncogenic strains of HPV are causally related to the development of anal cancer and to the development of the precursor lesion, HSIL. Under the microscope, cervical SIL and anal SIL are virtually indistinguishable. The anatomical region at risk includes the anal transition zone and the distal rectum extending up to 8 cm proximal to the dentate line where immature squamous metaplastic cells are the most susceptible to oncogenic HPV, although the nonkeratinizing and keratinizing squamous epithelium of the surrounding tissues are also susceptible. There is also morphologic and histologic similarity between cervical and anal cancer.

The populations at greatest risk for AIN are the same as for anal cancer. Natural history studies have demonstrated that in HIV-negative men who have sex with men (MSM), the 4-year incidence of HSIL was 17%. It is higher in HIV-positive men, with receptive anal intercourse, the presence of condylomata, multiplicity of HPV serotype infections, injection drug abuse, cigarette smoking, depressed host immunity, and the presence of cervical, vulvar, or penile neoplasia.

Treatment
Patients with anal SIL often present with minor complaints related to anal condylomata, hemorrhoids, or pruritus ani. Physical examination may reveal anything from typical condylomatous lesions to normal-appearing anal and rectal mucosa. The perianal skin and the entire surgical anal canal, as defined by the AJCC and by the World Health Organization, as extending through the length of the internal anal sphincter from the anal verge (2 to 4 cm in women, up to 6 cm in men), should be thoroughly examined.

Patients with low volume disease and no history of dysplasia may be treated with topical agents in the office, regardless of risk factors, with surveillance anal Pap smears. Patients with large volume disease are treated in the operating room with a combination of excisional biopsy or incisional biopsy and cautery destruction under monitored anesthetic care with a standard perianal block. Patients with a history of dysplasia, either from previous biopsy or Pap smear, may be "mapped" in the operating room with the operating microscope, acetic acid, and Lugol solution or may be treated in the office if the lesions are readily visualized. HSIL demonstrates various characteristic vascular patterns allowing otherwise occult premalignant disease to be identified. The tissues may subsequently be painted selectively with Lugol solution, but the Lugol solution may obscure some of the acetic acid findings. The nonkeratinizing high-grade lesions of the anal canal do not readily take up Lugol solution and stain either mahogany or yellow. HSIL may be destroyed with electrocautery by superficially "painting" the lesion and a small 2- to 10-mm rim of tissue trying to avoid injury that extends deep into the submucosa if a tissue diagnosis has been made. This strategy is safe and well tolerated and has been shown to eradicate HSIL in HIV-negative patients. In HIV-positive patients, recurrence is high and treatment may need to be repeated; however, with close follow-up, transformation to invasive cancer can be prevented.

Bowen Disease
Bowen disease is an intraepithelial SCC (carcinoma in situ or intraepithelial high-grade dysplasia) that develops most commonly in middle-age women and is often discovered during histologic evaluation of an anal specimen obtained for an unrelated diagnosis. The lesion is raised, irregular, scaly, and plaquelike, with eczematoid features. Histologically, large atypical haloed cells (Bowenoid cells) are seen that stain periodic acid-Schiff negative. Although it has previously been believed to have an association with other invasive carcinomas, the evidence for this is weak. The risk of progression to invasive cancer has been reported to be approximately 10%. Bowen disease has traditionally been treated with random biopsies and wide excision with flap reconstruction. However, even if normal tissue is sacrificed to obtain clear margins, the recurrence rate is 23%, and the patient may still be at risk for cancer development. This aggressive approach is associated with complications such as anal stenosis and fecal incontinence.

Bowen disease is histologically and immunohistochemically indistinguishable from anal HSIL and has also been associated with HPV infection. There is increasing agreement that Bowen disease and anal HSIL should be treated in a similar fashion. Local recurrence may occur, but re-excision provides excellent local control. Other therapeutic modalities include topical 5-FU cream, topical imiquimod, photodynamic therapy, radiation therapy, laser therapy, and combinations of these. The reports are generally small series with limited follow-up, but there has been anecdotal success with each approach, and the options should be kept in mind for challenging cases.

Paget Disease

Paget disease is an intraepithelial adenocarcinoma that occurs mostly in elderly women. The lesion (a well-demarcated, eczematoid plaque) is usually characteristic; however, morphologic variations can occur, making the diagnosis difficult by inspection alone. The diagnosis is made histologically by the presence of large, vacuolated Paget cells, which stain periodic acid-Schiff positive (from high mucin content). There is some evidence for the association of perianal Paget disease with other invasive carcinomas, but this relationship is not as strong as that seen with Paget disease of the breast. Invasion can develop in these lesions, and the prognosis is poor in those cases. Perianal Paget disease should be treated with wide local excision.

Anal Melanoma

Primary melanoma of the anus or rectum is a rare tumor, accounting for 0.4% to 1.6% of all melanomas and less than 1.0% of all anal canal tumors. The overall prognosis for patients with anorectal melanoma is very poor. Several reports in the literature have shown 5-year survival rates that are less than 25% and the median survival time is about 15 months. Mucosal melanoma is further discussed elsewhere in this text. This discussion focuses on anal melanoma.

Pathological Characteristics

The primary tumor may arise from the skin of the anal verge or the transitional epithelium of the anal canal. Inguinal nodal metastases are common at presentation. Prognosis is related to tumor thickness, as with cutaneous melanomas.

Diagnosis

Patients most commonly present with rectal bleeding. The incidental finding of a mass on digital examination may also lead to a workup that establishes the diagnosis. Melanoma may be an incidental pathological finding after hemorrhoidectomy. Physical examination should include evaluation of the rectal mass and palpation of the inguinal nodes. Radiographic staging should be performed as for melanomas elsewhere.

Treatment

Historically, APR has been the treatment of choice, but high failure rates have questioned the role for this radical approach. Wide local excision with at least 2 cm of normal surrounding tissue and sentinel lymph node biopsy of the inguinal lymph nodes is now performed whenever possible, reserving APR for large bulky tumors that cannot be locally excised. Therapeutic inguinal node dissection or external radiation therapy is indicated for nodal disease. Using this approach with hypofractionated adjuvant radiation therapy (30 Gy in five fractions) to the primary site and nodal beds, MDACC has reported a 5-year actuarial survival of 31%, local control rate of 74%, and a nodal control rate of 84% in 23 patients after a median follow-up of 32 months. Unresectable disease can be treated with neoadjuvant chemo/immunotherapy. Responders can be offered transanal excision or APR with postoperative radiation therapy with or without chemotherapy. Nonresponders can be offered palliative surgery.

Anal Adenocarcinoma

Adenocarcinoma of the anal canal is a rare malignancy representing less than 20% of all anal cancers with limited data regarding treatment and outcomes. In a recent retrospective consecutive cohort study at MDACC, 34 patients identified with anal adenocarcinoma were identified and overall survival and recurrence outcomes were evaluated. Six patients underwent palliative treatment and in the remaining 28 patients, 13 (46%) were treated with local excision followed by radiotherapy or chemoradiotherapy. Fifteen patients (54%) underwent radical surgery and neoadjuvant or adjuvant chemoradiotherapy. Median disease-free survival was 13 months after local excision and 32 months after radical surgery. Overall survival at five years was 43% for patients treated with local excision and 63% for patients treated with radical surgery. High risk for distant failure emphasizes the need for effective adjuvant therapeutic regimens.

Recommended Readings

Abdalla EK, Vauthey JN, Ellis LM, et al. Recurrence and outcomes following hepatic resection, radiofrequency ablation, and combined resection/ablation for colorectal liver metastases. *Ann Surg.* 2004;239 (6):818–825, discussion 825–827.

Ajani JA, Winter KA, Gunderson LL, et al. Fluorouracil, mitomycin and radiotherapy vs. fluorouracil, cisplatin and radiotherapy for carcinoma of the anal canal. A randomized controlled trial. *JAMA.* 2008;299:1714–1721.

Ajani JA, Winter KA, Gunderson LL, et al. US Intergroup Anal Carcinoma Trial: tumor diameter predicts for colostomy. *J Clin Oncol.* 2009;27:1116–1121.

Al-Tassan N, Chmiel NH, Maynard J, et al. Inherited variants of MYH associated with somatic G:C→T:A mutations in colorectal tumors. *Nat Genet.* 2002;30(2): 227–232.

Ballo MT, Gershenwald JE, Zagars GK, et al. Sphincter-sparing local excision and adjuvant radiation for anal-rectal melanoma. *J Clin Oncol.* 2002;20(23):4555–4558.

Bedrosian I, Rodriguez-Bigas MA, Feig B, et al. Predicting the node-negative mesorectum after preoperative chemoradiation for locally advanced rectal carcinoma. *J Gastrointest Surg.* 2004;8(1): 56–62, discussion 62–63.

Bertagnolli M, Miedema B, Redston M, et al. Sentinel node staging of resectable colon cancer: results of a multicenter study. *Ann Surg.* 2004;240(4):624–638, discussion 628–630.

Bonnen M, Crane C, Vauthey JN, et al. Longterm results using local excision after preoperative chemoradiation among selected T3 rectal cancer patients. *Int J Radiat Oncol Biol Phys.* 2004;60(4):1098–1105.

Bowne WB, Lee B, Wong WD, et al. Operative salvage for locoregional recurrent colon cancer after curative resection: an analysis of 100 cases. *Dis Colon Rectum.* 2005; 48(5):897–909.

Burt RW. Colon cancer screening. *Gastroenterology.* 2000;119(3):837–853.

Callender GG, Das P, Rodriguez-Bigas MA, et al. Local excision after preoperative chemoradiation results in an equivalent outcome to total mesorectal excision in selected patients with T3 rectal cancer. *Ann Surg Oncol.* 2010;17(2):441–447.

Cawthorn SJ, Parums DV, Gibbs NM, et al. Extent of mesorectal spread and involvement of lateral resection margin as prognostic factors after surgery for rectal cancer. *Lancet.* 1990;335(8697):1055–1059.

Chang GJ, Berry JM, Jay N, et al. Surgical treatment of high-grade anal squamous intraepithelial lesions: a prospective study. *Dis Colon Rectum.* 2002;45(4):453–458.

Chang GJ, Gonzalez RJ, Skibber JM, et al. A twenty-year experience with adenocarcinoma of the anal canal. *Dis Colon Rectum.* 2009;52(8):1375–1380.

Chang GJ, Rodriguez-Bigas MA, Skibber JM, et al. Lymph node evaluation and survival after curative resection of colon cancer: systematic review. *J Natl Cancer Inst.* 2007;99(6):433–441.

Chau I, Allen MJ, Cunningham D, et al. The value of routine serum carcino-embryonic antigen measurement and computed tomography in the surveillance of patients after adjuvant chemotherapy for colorectal cancer. *J Clin Oncol.* 2004; 22(8):1420–1429.

Church J, Simmang C. Practice parameters for the treatment of patients with dominantly inherited colorectal cancer (familial adenomatous polyposis and hereditary nonpolyposis colorectal cancer). *Dis Colon Rectum.* 2003;46(8): 1001–1012.

COLOR II Study Group, Buunen M, Bonjer HJ, et al. Color II. A randomized trial comparing laparoscopic and open surgery for rectal cancer. *Dan Med Bull.* 2009;56:89–91.

Compton C, Fenoglio-Preiser CM, Pettigrew N, et al. American Joint Committee on Cancer Prognostic Factors Consensus Conference: Colorectal Working Group. *Cancer.* 2000;88(7):1739–1757.

Cooper HS. Pathologic issues in the treatment of endoscopically removed malignant colorectal polyps. *J NCCN.* 2007;5: 991–996.

Cotton PB, Durkalski VL, Pineau BC, et al. Computed tomographic colonography (virtual colonoscopy): a multicenter comparison with standard colonoscopy for detection of colorectal neoplasia. *JAMA.* 2004;291(14):1713–1719.

Crane CH, Skibber JM, Birnbaum EH, et al. The addition of continuous infusion 5-FU to preoperative radiation therapy increases tumor response, leading to increased sphincter preservation in locally advanced rectal cancer. *Int J Radiat Oncol Biol Phys.* 2003;57(1):84–89.

Crane CH, Skibber JM, Feig BW, et al. Response to preoperative chemoradiation increases the use of sphincter-preserving surgery in patients with locally advanced low rectal carcinoma. *Cancer.* 2003;97(2):517–524.

Das P, Crane CH. Staging, prognostic factors, and therapy of localized rectal cancer. *Curr Oncol Rep.* 2009;11(3):167–174.

de Gramont A, Figer A, Seymour M, et al. Leucovorin and fluorouracil with or without oxaliplatin as first-line treatment in advanced colorectal cancer. *J Clin Oncol.* 2000;18(16):2938–2947.

Di Nicolantonia F, Martini M, Molinari F, et al. Wild-type BRAF is required for response to panitumumab or cetuximab in metastatic colorectal cancer. *J Clin Oncol.* 2008;26:5705–5712.

Enker WE. Sphincter-preserving operations for rectal cancer. *Oncology.* 1996;10(11): 1673–1684, 1689, discussion 1690–1692.

Farouk R, Nelson H, Gunderson LL. Aggressive multimodality treatment for locally advanced irresectable rectal cancer. *Br J Surg.* 1997;84(6):741–749.

Fisher B, Wolmark N, Rockette H, et al. Postoperative adjuvant chemotherapy or radiation therapy for rectal cancer: results from NSABP protocol R-01. *J Natl Cancer Inst.* 1988;80(1):21–29.

Frisch M, Glimelius B, Van Den Brule AJ, et al. Sexually transmitted infection as a cause of anal cancer. *N Engl J Med.* 1997;337(19): 1350–1358.

Garcia-Aguilar J, Mellgren A, Sirivongs P, et al. Local excision of rectal cancer without adjuvant therapy: a word of caution. *Ann Surg.* 2000;231(3):345–351.

Gastrointestinal Tumor Study Group. Prolongation of the disease-free interval in surgically treated rectal carcinoma. *N Engl J Med.* 1985;312(23):1465–1472.

Gerard A, Buyse M, Nordlinger B, et al. Preoperative radiotherapy as adjuvant treatment in rectal cancer. Final results of a randomized study of the European Organization for Research and Treatment of Cancer (EORTC). *Ann Surg.* 1988;208(5): 606–614.

Gill S, Sinicrope FA. Colorectal cancer prevention: is an ounce of prevention worth a pound of cure? *Semin Oncol.* 2005;32(1): 24–34.

Guillem JG, Chessin DB, Cohen AM, et al. Long-term oncologic outcome following preoperative combined modality therapy and total mesorectal excision of locally advanced rectal cancer. *Ann Surg.* 2005; 241(5):829–836, discussion 836–838.

Gunderson LL, Nelson H, Martenson JA, et al. Locally advanced primary colorectal cancer: intraoperative electron and external beam irradiation ± 5-FU. *Int J Radiat Oncol Biol Phys.* 1997;37(3):601–614.

Habr-Gama A, Perez RO, Nadalin W, et al. Operative versus nonoperative treatment for stage 0 distal rectal cancer following chemoradiation therapy: long-term results. *Ann Surg.* 2004;240(4):711–717, discussion 717–718.

Haggitt RC, Glotzbach RE, Soffer EE, et al. Prognostic factors in colorectal carcinomas arising in adenomas: implications for lesions removed by endoscopic polypectomy. *Gastroenterology.* 1985;89(2): 328–336.

Hahnloser D, Haddock MG, Nelson H. Intraoperative radiotherapy in the multimodality approach to colorectal cancer. *Surg Oncol Clin N Am.* 2003;12(4):993–1013, ix.

Harewood GC. Assessment of publication bias in the reporting of EUS performance in staging rectal cancer. *Am J Gastroenterol.* 2005;100(4):808–816.

Havenga K, Enker WE. Autonomic nerve preserving total mesorectal excision. *Surg Clin North Am.* 2002;82(5):1009–1018.

Heald RJ, Ryall RD. Recurrence and survival after total mesorectal excision for rectal cancer. *Lancet.* 1986;1(8496):1479–1482.

Hida J, Yasutomi M, Maruyama T, et al. Lymph node metastases detected in the mesorectum distal to carcinoma of the rectum by the clearing method: justification of total mesorectal excision. *J Am Coll Surg.* 1997;184(6):584–588.

Hoots BE, Palefsky JM, Pimentz JM, et al. Human papillomavirus type distinction in anal cancer and anal intraepithelial lesions. *Int J Cancer.* 2009;124:2375–2383.

Improved survival with preoperative radiotherapy in resectable rectal cancer. Swedish Rectal Cancer Trial. *N Engl J Med.* 1997;336(14):980–987.

James R, Wan S, Glynne-Jones D, et al. A randomized trial of chemoradiation using mitomycin or cisplatin with or without maintenance cisplatin/5-FU in squamous cell carcinoma of the anus. ACT II. *J Clin Oncol.* 2009;27:LBA4009.

Jasperson KW, Tuohy TM, Neklason DW, et al. Hereditary and familial colon cancer. *Gastroenterology.* 2010;138:2044–2058.

Jemal A, Murray T, Ward E, et al. Cancer statistics, 2005. *CA Cancer J Clin.* 2005; 55(1):10–30.

Johnson CD, Chen MH, Toledano AY, et al. Accuracy of CT colonography for detection of large adenomas and cancers. *N Engl J Med.* 2008;359(12):1207–1217.

Kikuchi R, Takano M, Takagi K, et al. Management of early invasive colorectal cancer. Risk of recurrence and clinical guidelines. *Dis Colon Rectum.* 1995;38(12): 1286–1295.

Korner H, Soreide K, Stokkeland PJ, et al. Systematic follow-up after curative surgery for colorectal cancer in Norway: a population-based audit of effectiveness, costs, and compliance. *J Gastrointest Surg.* 2005;9(3):320–328.

Koura AN, Giacco GG, Curley SA, et al. Carcinoid tumors of the rectum: effect of size, histopathology, and surgical treatment on metastasis-free survival. *Cancer.* 1997; 79(7):1294–1298.

Kuebler JP, Wieand HS, O'Connell MJ, et al. Oxaliplatin combined with weekly bolus fluorouracil and leucovorin as surgical adjuvant chemotherapy for stage II and III colon cancer: results from NSABP C-07. *J Clin Oncol.* 2007;25:2198–2204.

Le Voyer TE, Sigurdson ER, Hanlon AL, et al. Colon cancer survival is associated with increasing number of lymph nodes analyzed: a secondary survey of intergroup trial INT-0089. *J Clin Oncol.* 2003;21(15): 2912–2919.

Libutti SK, Alexander HR Jr, Choyke P, et al. A prospective study of 2-[18 F] fluoro-2-deoxy-D-glucose/positron emission tomography scan, 99mTc-labeled arcitumomab (CEA-scan), and blind second-look laparotomy for detecting colon cancer recurrence in patients with increasing carcinoembryonic antigen levels. *Ann Surg Oncol.* 2001;8(10):779–786.

Lowy AM, Rich TA, Skibber JM, et al. Preoperative infusional chemoradiation, selective intraoperative radiation, and resection for locally advanced pelvic recurrence of colorectal adenocarcinoma. *Ann Surg.* 1996;223(2):177–185.

Mamounas E, Wieand S, Wolmark N, et al. Comparative efficacy of adjuvant chemotherapy in patients with Dukes' B versus Dukes' C colon cancer: results from four National Surgical Adjuvant Breast and Bowel Project adjuvant studies (C-01, C-02, C-03, and C-04). *J Clin Oncol.* 1999; 17(5):1349–1355.

Mendenhall WM, Zlotecki RA, Vauthey JN, et al. Squamous cell carcinoma of the anal margin. *Oncology (Huntingt).* 1996; 10(12):1843–1848, discussion 1848, 1853–1854.

MERCURY Study Group. Diagnostic accuracy of preoperative magnetic resonance imaging in predicting curative resection of rectal cancer: prospective observational study. *BMJ.* 2006;333:779–785.

Merg A, Lynch HT, Lynch JF, et al. Hereditary colon cancer-part I. *Curr Probl Surg.* 2005;42(4):195–256.

Merg A, Lynch HT, Lynch JF, et al. Hereditary colorectal cancer-part II. *Curr Probl Surg.* 2005;42(5):267–333.

Meterissian SH, Skibber JM, Giacco GG, et al. Pelvic exenteration for locally advanced rectal carcinoma: factors predicting improved survival. *Surgery.* 1997;121(5):479–487.

Meyerhardt JA, Mayer RJ. Systemic therapy for colorectal cancer. *N Engl J Med.* 2005; 352(5):476–487.

Meyerhardt JA, Tepper JE, Niedzwiecki D, et al. Impact of hospital procedure volume on surgical operation and long-term outcomes in high-risk curatively resected rectal cancer: findings from the Intergroup 0114 Study. *J Clin Oncol.* 2004;22(1):166–174.

Middleton PF, Sutherland LM, Maddern GJ. Transanal endoscopic microsurgery: a systematic review. *Dis Colon Rectum.* 2005;48(2):270–284.

Moertel CG, Fleming TR, Macdonald JS, et al. Levamisole and fluorouracil for adjuvant therapy of resected colon carcinoma. *N Engl J Med.* 1990;322(6):352–358.

Nascimbeni R, Burgart LJ, Nivatvongs S, et al. Risk of lymph node metastasis in T1 carcinoma of the colon and rectum. *Dis Colon Rectum.* 2002;45(2):200–206.

Nelson H, Petrelli N, Carlin A, et al. Guidelines 2000 for colon and rectal cancer surgery. *J Natl Cancer Inst.* 2001;93(8):583–596.

Nigro ND, Vaitkevicius VK, Considine B, Jr. Combined therapy for cancer of the anal canal: a preliminary report. *Dis Colon Rectum.* 1974;17(3): 354–356.

NIH Consensus Conference. Adjuvant therapy for patients with colon and rectal cancer. *JAMA*. 1990;264(11):1444–1450.

Nivatvongs S. Surgical management of malignant colorectal polyps. *Surg Clin North Am*. 2002;82(5):959–966.

O'Connell MJ, Martenson JA, Wieand HS, et al. Improving adjuvant therapy for rectal cancer by combining protracted-infusion fluorouracil with radiation therapy after curative surgery. *N Engl J Med*. 1994; 331(8):502–507.

Papillon J. Intracavitary irradiation of early rectal cancer for cure. A series of 186 cases. 1975. *Dis Colon Rectum*. 1994;37(1):88–94.

Patel P, Hanson DL, Sullivan PS, et al. Incidence of types of cancer among HIV-infected persons compared with the general population in the United States, 1992–2003. *Ann Intern Med*. 2008;148:728–736.

Pickhardt PJ, Choi JR, Hwang I, et al. Computed tomographic virtual colonoscopy to screen for colorectal neoplasia in asymptomatic adults. *N Engl J Med*. 2003; 349(23):2191–2200.

Pignone M, Rich M, Teutsch SM, et al. Screening for colorectal cancer in adults at average risk: a summary of the evidence for the U.S. Preventive Services Task Force. *Ann Intern Med*. 2002;137(2):132–141.

Quirke P, Durdey P, Dixon MF, et al. Local recurrence of rectal adenocarcinoma due to inadequate surgical resection. Histopathological study of lateral tumour spread and surgical excision. *Lancet*. 1986;1(2):996–999.

Rabkin CS, Yellin F. Cancer incidence in a population with a high prevalence of infection with human immunodeficiency virus type 1. *J Natl Cancer Inst*. 1994; 86(22):1711–1716.

Repici A, Pellicano R, Strangio G, et al. Endoscopic mucosal resection for early colorectal neoplasia: pathologic basis, procedures, and outcome. *Dis Colon Rectum*. 2009;52:1502–1515.

Rodriguez-Bigas MA, Boland CR, Hamilton SR, et al. A National Cancer Institute Workshop on Hereditary Nonpolyposis Colorectal Cancer Syndrome: meeting highlights and Bethesda guidelines. *J Natl Cancer Inst*. 1997;89(23):1758–1762.

Rodriguez-Bigas MA, Chang GJ, Skibber JM. Surgical implications of colorectal cancer genetics. *Surg Oncol Clin N Am*. 2006; 15(1):51–66.

Rodriguez-Bigas MA, Stoler DL, Bertario L, et al. Colorectal cancer: how does it start? How does it metastasize? *Surg Oncol Clin*

N Am. 2000;9(4):643–652, discussion 653–654.

Rosen M, Chan L, Beart RW Jr, et al. Follow-up of colorectal cancer: a meta-analysis. *Dis Colon Rectum*. 1998;41(9):1116–1126.

Roth AD, Tejpar S, Delorenzi M, et al. Prognostic role of KRAS and BRAF in stage II and III resected colon cancer: results of the translational study on the PETACC-3, EORTC 40993, SAKK 60-00 trial. *J Clin Oncol*. 2010;28:466–474.

Saltz LB, Cox JV, Blanke C, et al. Irinotecan plus fluorouracil and leucovorin for metastatic colorectal cancer. Irinotecan Study Group. *N Engl J Med*. 2000;343(13):905–914.

Sanfilippo NJ, Crane CH, Skibber J, et al. T4 rectal cancer treated with preoperative chemoradiation to the posterior pelvis followed by multivisceral resection: patterns of failure and limitations of treatment. *Int J Radiat Oncol Biol Phys*. 2001;51(1):176–183.

Sauer R, Becker H, Hohenberger W, et al. Preoperative versus postoperative chemoradiotherapy for rectal cancer. *N Engl J Med*. 2004;351(17):1731–1740.

Schaffzin DM, Wong WD. Endorectal ultrasound in the preoperative evaluation of rectal cancer. *Clin Colorectal Cancer*. 2004;4(2):124–132.

Scott N, Jackson P, al-Jaberi T, et al. Total mesorectal excision and local recurrence: a study of tumour spread in the mesorectum distal to rectal cancer. *Br J Surg*. 1995;82(8):1031–1033.

Seitz V, Bohnacker S, Seewald S, et al. Is endoscopic polypectomy an adequate therapy for malignant colorectal adenomas? Presentation of 114 patients and review of the literature. *Dis Colon Rectum*. 2004;47:1789–1797.

Silberfein EJ, Kattepogu KM, Hu CY, et al. Long-term survival and recurrence outcomes following surgery for distal rectal cancer. *Ann Surg Oncol*. 2010;17(11):2863–2869.

Skibber J, Rodriguez-Bigas MA, Gordon PH. Surgical considerations in anal cancer. *Surg Oncol Clin N Am*. 2004;13(2):321–338.

Soetikno RM, Kaltenbach T, Rouse RV, et al. Prevalence of nonpolypoid (flat and depressed) colorectal neoplasms in asymptomatic and symptomatic adults. *JAMA*. 2008;299(9):1027–1035.

Steele GD Jr, Herndon JE, Bleday R, et al. Sphincter-sparing treatment for distal rectal adenocarcinoma. *Ann Surg Oncol*. 1999;6(5):433–441.

Stuckey CC, Pockaj BA, Novotny PJ, et al. Long-term follow-up and individual item analysis of quality of life assessments related to laparoscopic-assisted colectomy in the COST trial 93–46-53 (INT 0146). *Ann Surg Oncol.* Epub ahead of print March 31, 2011.

Tepper JE, O'Connell M, Niedzwiecki D, et al. Adjuvant therapy in rectal cancer: analysis of stage, sex, and local control–final report of intergroup 0114. *J Clin Oncol.* 2002;20(7):1744–1750.

The Clinical Outcomes of Surgical Therapy Study Group. A comparison of laparoscopically assisted and open colectomy for colon cancer. *N Engl J Med.* 2004;350(20): 2050–2059.

The SCOTIA Study Group. Single-stage treatment for malignant left-sided colonic obstruction: a prospective randomized clinical trial comparing subtotal colectomy with segmental resection following intraoperative irrigation. Subtotal colectomy versus on-table irrigation and anastomosis. *Br J Surg.* 1995;82(12): 1622–1627.

Umar A, Boland CR, Terdiman JP, et al. Revised Bethesda guidelines for hereditary nonpolyposis colorectal cancer (Lynch syndrome) and microsatellite instability. *J Natl Cancer Inst.* 2004; 96(4):261–268.

U.S. Preventative Task Force. Screening for colorectal cancer: recommendation and rationale. *Ann Internl Med.* 2002;137(2): 129–131.

Van Cutsem E, Kohne CH, Hitre E, et al. Cetuximab and chemotherapy as initial treatment for metastatic colorectal cancer. *N Engl J Med.* 2009;360:1408–1417.

Vogelsang H, Haas S, Hierholzer C, et al. Factors influencing survival after resection of pulmonary metastases from colorectal cancer. *Br J Surg.* 2004;91(8):1066–1071.

Walsh JM, Terdiman JP. Colorectal cancer screening: clinical applications. *JAMA.* 2003;289(10):1297–1302.

Walsh JM, Terdiman JP. Colorectal cancer screening: scientific review. *JAMA.* 2003; 289(10):1288–1296.

Wibe A, Eriksen MT, Syse A, et al. Effect of hospital caseload on long-term outcome after standardization of rectal cancer surgery at a national level. *Br J Surg.* 2005; 92(2):217–224.

Wilson SM, Beahrs OH. The curative treatment of carcinoma of the sigmoid, rectosigmoid, and rectum. *Ann Surg.* 1976; 183(5):556–565.

Winawer SJ, Zauber AG. Colonoscopic polypectomy and the incidence of colorectal cancer. *Gut.* 2001;48(6):753–754.

Winde G, Nottberg H, Keller R, et al. Surgical cure for early rectal carcinomas (T1). Transanal endoscopic microsurgery vs. anterior resection. *Dis Colon Rectum.* 1996; 39(9):969–976.

Wolmark N, Rockette H, Fisher B, et al. The benefit of leucovorin-modulated fluorouracil as postoperative adjuvant therapy for primary colon cancer: results from National Surgical Adjuvant Breast and Bowel Project protocol C-03. *J Clin Oncol.* 1993;11(10):1879–1887.

Young-Fadok TM, Wolff BG, Nivatvongs S, et al. Prophylactic oophorectomy in colorectal carcinoma: preliminary results of a randomized, prospective trial. *Dis Colon Rectum.* 1998;41(3):277–283, discussion 283–285.

Zaheer S, Pemberton JH, Farouk R, et al. Surgical treatment of adenocarcinoma of the rectum. *Ann Surg.* 1998;227(6):800–811.

Hepatobiliary Cancers

**Carlo M. Contreras, Eugene A. Choi, and
Eddie K. Abdalla**

INTRODUCTION

The approach to patients with liver and biliary tumors is complex. Overall assessment of comorbidity and specific indications for hepatic surgery depend on both tumor factors and liver factors. Some tumors develop in otherwise normal underlying livers, while others arise in livers compromised by biliary obstruction or underlying liver disease, such as steatosis, fibrosis, or cirrhosis. The preoperative preparation, operative approach, surgical techniques, anticipated complications, and outcome relate to both the tumor and the liver factors. Careful attention to each of these issues is necessary to optimize outcome.

Advances in hepatobiliary surgery have come largely as a result of attention to these details, and data suggest that outcome can be improved by taking a multidisciplinary approach to the patient with liver or biliary cancers. In fact, both short- and long-term outcome are significantly better in "centers of excellence," where surgeons have specialized training and experience in hepatobiliary surgery and work as part of a specialized team of oncologists, radiologists, and gastroenterologists.

This chapter outlines treatment approaches to the major hepatobiliary cancers, addresses issues of anatomy, and describes preoperative preparation and the operative approach. For each disease type, the current literature is reviewed to provide an explanation of epidemiology, pathology, clinical presentation, diagnosis, staging, and issues regarding surgical therapy.

SURGICAL ANATOMY OF THE LIVER

Hepatic anatomy is highly variable. Ten separate types of hepatic arterial anatomy have been defined, and numerous portal and biliary segmental variations are important to the hepatic surgeon. A description of the major arterial variations is beyond the scope of this chapter; however, an overview of hepatic anatomy, which is essential to the discussion of resection options for hepatic tumors, is provided.

The portal and arterial vessels in the liver are the first level of complexity in the liver's anatomy. On the basis of the portal segmentation, eight separate anatomical segments of the liver can be identified, and these are termed the Couinaud segments of the liver. This predominantly portal segmentation of the liver described by Couinaud in 1957 provides the surgeon with an anatomical approach to the liver, such that any of the eight segments can be resected while preserving the vascular inflow, venous outflow, and biliary drainage of the remaining segments.

The left and right livers are not symmetric. The right liver is typically two-thirds of the total liver volume (TLV), and the left liver is about one-third. The caudate or posterior liver, which is a single anatomical unit, represents about 1% the TLV (segment 1). The right liver can be divided into the right anterior and posterior sectors, and the left liver divided into the lateral and medial sectors. The left lateral liver is subdivided into segments II and III, and the medial left liver is known as segment IV. The right anterior liver is subdivided into segment V inferiorly and segment VIII superiorly, and the right posterior liver is subdivided into segment VI inferiorly and segment VII superiorly (Fig. 12.1).

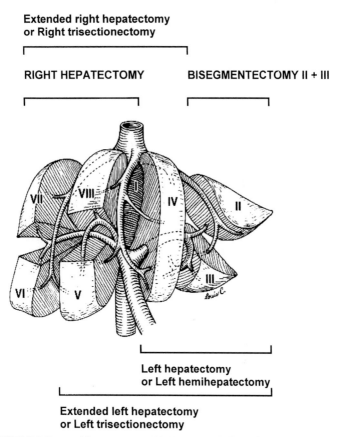

**Extended right hepatectomy
or Right trisectionectomy**

RIGHT HEPATECTOMY   **BISEGMENTECTOMY II + III**

**Left hepatectomy
or Left hemihepatectomy**

**Extended left hepatectomy
or Left trisectionectomy**

FIGURE 12.1 Segmental liver anatomy as originally described by Claude Couinaud, with the terminology that should be used to describe liver resection according to the Brisbane 2000 international consensus conference. (Adapted from Abdalla EK, Denys A, Chevalier P, et al. Total and segmental liver volume variations: implications for liver surgery. *Surgery.* 2004;135:405, with permission.)

Three major hepatic veins are typically found: the right hepatic vein, which typically drains the right liver (segments V to VIII); the middle hepatic vein, which typically drains segment IV; and the left hepatic vein, which typically drains segments II and III. The left hepatic vein crosses the left lateral liver transversely, between segments II and III. The middle hepatic vein defines the main plane, or the division between the left and right livers, which is the plane on which the right or left hepatectomy is undertaken. The caudate liver, because it arises embryologically as a separate anatomical unit from the remaining liver, has its own venous drainage, with short veins draining directly into the vena cava, and highly variable biliary and portal anatomy.

It is essential that the surgeons understand the many anatomical variations of the liver that can be identified on preoperative imaging and intraoperative ultrasound (US). Surgical techniques—including the Glissonian approach or dissection along the fibrous sheath that surrounds the portal triads—may enable the hepatic surgeon to identify important elements of the anatomy intrahepatically and thereby minimize the risk of injury to the remaining liver after resection of anatomical segments. Most liver surgeons consider intraoperative US essential for safe surgery because it permits real-time identification of the intrahepatic anatomy.

TERMINOLOGY FOR HEPATIC RESECTION

Terminology for hepatic resection has changed over time. Different definitions of the term "lobe" had been used in Europe and the United States, causing confusion. Accordingly, the Brisbane 2000 International Conference was held to establish a consensus on terminology used for liver resection. That revised terminology is used throughout this chapter (Fig. 12.1).

The terminology for hepatectomy is as follows: (a) resection of the right liver (or segments V to VIII) is termed a right hepatectomy or right hemihepatectomy; (b) resection of the left liver (or segments II to IV) is termed a left hepatectomy or left hemihepatectomy; (c) resection of the left lateral liver (or segments II and III) is termed a bisegmentectomy II + III or a left lateral sectionectomy; and (d) extended right hepatectomy, or right trisectionectomy, is the resection of segments IV to VIII, whereas extended left hepatectomy, or left trisectionectomy, is resection of segments II to V and VIII. Elimination of the term "lobe" has enabled much clearer communication among physicians worldwide when discussing and writing about hepatic resection.

PREDICTING LIVER REMNANT FUNCTION

Liver Volume Determination

Liver volume after major hepatic resection has been critically linked to liver function. Also, underlying liver disease will affect liver function so patients with normal underlying liver are treated differently than patients with diseased underlying liver. The realization that liver volume alone does not predict function leads to two additional conclusions: Large patients need large livers and small patients need small livers, and patients with diseased livers need to have a larger volume of liver preserved than patients with normal underlying livers. Careful analysis of outcome based on liver remnant volume stratified by underlying liver disease (or the absence of disease) has led to recommendations regarding the safe limits of resection. The liver remnant to be left after resection is termed the future liver remnant (FLR). For patients with normal underlying liver, complications, extended hospital stay, admission to the intensive care unit, and hepatic insufficiency are rare when the standardized FLR is >20% of the TLV as compared to when it is ≤20%. For patients with tumor-related cholestasis or marked underlying liver disease, a 40% liver remnant is necessary to avoid cholestasis, fluid retention, and liver failure. Patients with normal underlying liver and a small remnant have a greater complication rate but rarely die of those complications, whereas patients with cirrhosis and a small remnant are at risk for a cascade of complications that may culminate in liver failure and death.

When the liver remnant is normal or has only mild disease, the volume of liver remnant can be measured directly and accurately with three-dimensional computed tomography (CT) volumetry. However, CT volumetry is frequently not appropriate for determining the total functional liver volume when the goal is to use this volume to estimate the functionality of the FLR after resection. Inaccuracy may arise because the liver *to be resected* is often diseased, particularly in patients with cirrhosis or biliary obstruction; the total liver size can be large, normal, or small, or when multiple or large tumors occupy a large volume of the liver to be resected, subtracting tumor volumes from liver volume further decreases accuracy of CT volumetry. The calculated TLV, which has been derived from the close association between patient size and liver size (specifically the association between body surface area [BSA] and liver size), provides a standardizing estimate of the TLV. The following formula is used:

$$\text{TLV (cm}^3\text{)} = -794.41 + 1267.28 \times \text{BSA (square meters)}$$

Thus, the standardized FLR volume calculation uses the *measured* FLR volume from CT volumetry as the numerator and the *calculated* TLV as the denominator:

$$\text{Standardized FLR (sFLR)} = \text{measured FLR volume/TLV}$$

Calculating the standardized TLV corrects the actual liver volume to the individual patient's size and provides an individualized estimate of that patient's postresection liver function. This approach has been validated and used at The University of Texas M. D. Anderson Cancer Center, where 301 consecutive extended hepatectomies have been performed with minimal mortality. Furthermore, use of this standardized approach to liver volume measurement enables the systematic use of preoperative liver preparation to increase the liver remnant volume prior to major resection when indicated based on the criteria described previously. In the event of an inadequate FLR, preoperative liver preparation may include dietary and lifestyle modifications or portal vein embolization. Portal vein embolization will be discussed in detail in the next section.

Several other tests have been used to evaluate liver function, including the urea–nitrogen synthesis rate, galactose elimination capacity, bromsulphalein and aminopyrine breath tests, and indocyanine green (ICG) clearance. ICG is a dye that is cleared from the circulation by the liver, and its clearance is an indicator of hepatocyte function. ICG clearance is the most studied test used to select cirrhotic patients for hepatic resection, although it is used mostly in Asia. Makuuchi et al. advocated selection of cirrhotic patients for *minor* resection based on the presence or absence of ascites, stratification according to the total serum bilirubin level and ICG 15 value (i.e., the percentage of dye clearance in 15 minutes). Patients with high bilirubin levels and low hepatic clearance of ICG are considered for limited resection or alternative locoregional ablative treatments. These studies are of limited value in selecting patients for major resection because they assess global hepatic function. Standardized FLR volume remains our sole approach at the M. D. Anderson Cancer Center because it is a validated approach to assessment of liver remnant volume and guides treatment planning. The following section discusses strategies to increase the volume and function of an inadequate FLR prior to major hepatectomy.

Portal Vein Embolization

Portal vein embolization (PVE) is a preoperative procedure designed to increase the safety of major liver resections. The portal flow is diverted from the liver segments to be resected to the liver that will remain (the FLR) resulting in an increased size and improved function of the FLR before resection. PVE was refined by Makuuchi after Kinoshita observed that embolization of the portal vein to prevent tumor extension led to hypertrophy of the contralateral liver. Since then, PVE techniques and indications have been standardized to increase the safety of major hepatectomy in patients with normal and diseased livers.

The indications for PVE are the same as those predicting postresection liver function as described in the previous section. Although several different approaches to embolization have been proposed, at the M. D. Anderson Cancer Center we use the percutaneous ipsilateral approach to avoid puncturing or otherwise injuring the liver remnant. Then, using small particles followed by larger coils, the portal branches supplying the entire tumor-bearing liver, including segment IV (if this is to be resected), are occluded. This procedure diverts portal flow to the FLR. Studies have shown that hypertrophy-inducing factors are carried in the portal vein and not the hepatic artery, and so PVE leads to FLR hypertrophy. Hypertrophy occurs quite rapidly, and the normal liver can be reassessed by volumetry within 3 or 4 weeks.

Evaluation of the degree of sFLR hypertrophy following PVE is crucial. Compared to patients with a <5% increase in sFLR, patients with ≥5% hypertrophy are less likely to experience hepatic dysfunction after liver resection. While a ≥5% degree of hypertrophy is sufficient for a patient with normal underlying liver function, patients with chronic liver injury probably require a greater degree of hypertrophy. Ogata et al. suggest that patients with advanced fibrosis require ≥10% hypertrophy following PVE. Hypertrophy may occur more slowly in cirrhotic, diabetics, and patients with other types of chronic liver injury; therefore, an interval of 5 or 6 weeks may be required to achieve the desired degree of hypertrophy.

Attention to the liver remnant, systemic volumetry for major resection, and use of PVE based on carefully prescribed indications has enabled very safe extended hepatic resection in patients with normal liver function and major hepatectomy in patients with underlying liver disease. Kishi et al. reviewed 301 consecutive patients who underwent extended right hepatectomy and showed that in patients with normal underlying liver and a standardized FLR volume ≤20% of the TLV, PVE is indicated to increase the volume and function of the FLR. In patients with cirrhotic and fibrotic livers and a standardized FLR volume ≤40% of the TLV, PVE is also indicated. For patients who have undergone extensive chemotherapy, PVE should be considered when the standardized FLR is ≤30%. In addition to sFLR ≤20%, the other predictors of hepatic insufficiency following extended right hepatectomy are body mass index >25 kg/m^2, and intraoperative blood transfusion.

PRIMARY HEPATOCELLULAR CARCINOMA

Epidemiology

Worldwide, hepatocellular carcinoma (HCC) is the fifth most common malignant neoplasm in men and the ninth most common in women, accounting for 500,000 to 1 million cancer cases annually. In the United States, HCC is comparatively rare, with an annual incidence of fewer than 5 cases per 100,000 persons, making it the 22nd most common type of cancer. However, the incidence of HCC in the United States is rising because of the increasing prevalence of hepatitis B (HBV) and hepatitis C (HCV) infection.

HCC occurs with greater frequency in regions of the world where viral hepatitis is endemic. There is, however, considerable variation in the prevalence of HCC, HBV, and HCV, depending on the patient's country of origin. It is estimated that one-fourth of patients with HCC in the United States have evidence of HCV infection, and HBV and HCV infections together account for no more than 40% of HCC cases. In contrast, in many Eastern countries where both HBV and HCV infections are endemic, the vast majority of HCC patients are seropositive for either HBV or HCV. Even within Eastern countries, however, there are geographic variations. For example, in contrast to Taiwan, China, and Korea, where HBV infection rates are high, HCV and HBV + HCV infections are predominant in Japan. Patients from the West (the United States and France) are more likely than patients from the East (Hong Kong and Japan) to have negative hepatitis serology.

Several other risk factors have been implicated in the development of HCC. Alcohol-related cirrhosis is the leading cause of HCC in the United States, Canada, and Western Europe. Chemicals such as nitrites, hydrocarbons, and polychlorinated biphenyls have also been associated with HCC. Dietary intake of aflatoxins is high in several countries with a high incidence of HCC. The common etiologic factor may be recurrent chronic hepatocellular injury and/or cirrhosis. HCC has also been reported in association with several metabolic disorders, such as hemochromatosis, Wilson disease, hereditary tyrosinemia, type I glycogen storage disease, familial polyposis coli, alpha-1 antitrypsin deficiency, and Budd–Chiari syndrome. HCC is more likely to develop in men than in women. In high-incidence areas, the male-to-female ratio is approximately 8:1, and in low-incidence areas, the ratio is 4:1. HCC develops early in life in the high-incidence areas, whereas it occurs predominantly in the elderly in low-incidence areas. More important than the patient's age is the chronicity of the infection or cirrhosis. Patients with HCV infections are often older and present with active chronic hepatitis and larger tumors.

Pathology

The histologic variations of HCC are of little importance in determining treatment and prognosis, with two exceptions: fibrolamellar carcinoma is found in younger patients without cirrhosis and carries a better prognosis than standard HCC, and adenomatous hyperplasia is a premalignant lesion that can be cured by resection. HCC frequently spreads by local extension to the diaphragm and adjacent organs and into the portal and hepatic veins. Metastatic spread occurs most often to the lungs, bone, adrenal glands, and brain.

Clinical Presentation

Presentation depends on the stage of disease. In countries with systematic screening programs, HCC may be detected at an earlier stage. In the United States, where there is no systematic screening for HCC, patients usually present at a late stage, often with upper abdominal pain or discomfort, a palpable right upper quadrant mass, weight loss, ascites, or other sequelae of portal hypertension. Jaundice is relatively uncommon but ominous. The triad of abdominal pain, weight loss, and an abdominal mass is the most common clinical presentation in the United States. In fewer than 5% of cases, patients present with tumor rupture. In Eastern countries, including Taiwan, Hong Kong, Japan, and Korea, HCC is often diagnosed by surveillance abdominal US, helical CT scan, magnetic resonance imaging (MRI), or routine screening of blood for features such as elevated serum alpha-fetoprotein (AFP) before clinical symptoms are apparent. Numerous paraneoplastic complications have been described, including hypoglycemia, hypercalcemia, erythrocytosis, and hypertrophic pulmonary osteoarthropathy. Patients with HCV infection are more often screened and thus tend to present with signs and symptoms of cirrhosis and earlier-stage HCC tumors. Patients with HBV infection or no serological evidence of hepatitis infection tend to present with larger tumors and less cirrhosis.

Diagnosis

AFP is increased in 50% to 90% of all patients with HCC, with levels greater than 400 ng/mL usually found in those with large or rapidly growing tumors. Despite these general correlations, AFP is neither sensitive nor specific for HCC. A patient with a small HCC tumor may have minimal or no elevation of AFP. Moreover, transient increases in AFP may be seen with inflammatory hepatic disease or cirrhosis. Several studies have reported a correlation between AFP elevation, advanced tumor stage, and poor patient prognosis, or an association between highly elevated AFP and metastatic disease; AFP >200 ng/mL in association with characteristic imaging findings is nearly 100% sensitive for HCC.

Several imaging modalities can be used to diagnose HCC, including helical CT scanning, percutaneous US, and MRI. Both CT and MRI permit dynamic contrast-enhanced imaging. Each imaging modality has advantages and disadvantages. US is an inexpensive screening tool, but its sensitivity and specificity are low, with an overall false-negative rate of more than 50%.

At the M. D. Anderson Cancer Center, helical thin-slice CT scanning is the preferred imaging technique. These CT scans have the advantage of speed when compared with MRI, and they effectively image the entire abdomen and the liver in four phases of contrast enhancement: precontrast, early vascular or arterial phases, a portal phase, and a delayed phase. HCCs, hepatic adenomas, and metastatic disease demonstrate arterial phase enhancement. Enhancement during the portal-dominant phase reveals hypovascular tumors, such as metastatic adenocarcinoma or cholangiocarcinoma (CCA). Multiphasic MRI is used selectively at our institution to provide additional information concerning the benign or malignant nature of a hepatic lesion or the anatomic relationship between a tumor and major vessels. MRI has an advantage over CT in that it does not require the use of contrast agents for detecting lesions, although HCC protocols typically use dynamic contrast enhancement. Many institutions prefer MRI to CT, but data that demonstrate the superiority of one modality are lacking. In some regions, lipiodol, an oily derivative of the poppy seed, is combined with iodine contrast medium; the mixture is retained by the tumor and has been used with CT scanning to evaluate small HCCs.

More invasive imaging techniques are also used in the diagnosis of HCC, including CT with arterial portography (CTAP), CT hepatic arteriography (CTHA), and angiography. In CTAP, a contrast agent is injected into the superior mesenteric artery or the splenic artery prior to the scan. Delayed images are obtained when the contrast material has entered the portal venous system. Because it is not well perfused by the portal system, HCC appears as a low-density area against the surrounding liver parenchyma. Angiography of the hepatic artery is performed to further delineate aberrant blood supply to the liver or, more infrequently, prior to the placement of a hepatic artery infusion pump.

Diagnostic laparoscopy (DL), although invasive, may have a role in the workup for some patients with HCC. Patients most likely to benefit from DL are those with large or ruptured tumors, advanced cirrhosis, or indeterminate nodules in the FLR.

When the diagnosis of HCC is uncertain (e.g., when imaging findings are equivocal and AFP is normal), the histologic diagnosis of HCC can be obtained by US-guided percutaneous needle biopsy or fine-needle aspiration (FNA) biopsy of the mass. Tumor seeding along the biopsy needle track rarely occurs when using modern techniques (<1% of cases). The risks of significant bleeding are low. The risks associated with major resection or transplantation for benign disease may be outweighed by the benefit of FNA biopsy in cases where the diagnosis is uncertain.

Staging

The seventh edition American Joint Committee on Cancer (AJCC) staging system for HCC is shown in Table 12.1. This system is unified with the Union Internationale Contre le Cancer (UICC) system and is derived from the analysis by Vauthey et al. of an international group of patients from the United States, France, and Japan, who underwent complete resection of HCC. Tumor size per se has no effect on survival in patients who have solitary tumors without vascular invasion. The new system recognizes that the prognosis for T1 tumors >10 cm in greatest diameter is the same as that for smaller T1 tumors (T1 = any size, without vascular invasion). Tumors having evidence of microvascular invasion or multiple tumors less than 5 cm in diameter are designated as T2 disease. HCC with major vascular invasion or with multiple tumors, with at least one measuring 5 cm, are designated T3. Most important, the presence of severe fibrosis of the underlying liver has a negative impact on overall survival, regardless of the T classification. For stage I disease, the 5-year survival rate is 64% when there is no fibrosis (F0) and 49% when fibrosis is present (F1). For stage II disease, the 5-year survival rate is 46% for F0 disease and 30% for F1 disease. For stage IIIA disease, the 5-year survival rate is 17% for F0 disease and 9%

	American Joint Commission on Cancer Staging System for Liver Tumors (Excluding Intrahepatic Cholangiocarcinoma)

Primary Tumor (T)

TX	Primary cannot be assessed
T0	No evidence of primary tumor
T1	Solitary tumor without vascular invasion
T2	Solitary tumor with vascular invasion or multiple tumors, none more than 5 cm
T3a	Multiple tumors more than 5 cm
T3b	Single tumor or multiple tumors of any size involving a major branch of the portal or hepatic vein(s)
T4	Tumor(s) with direct invasion of adjacent organs other than the gallbladder or with perforation of visceral peritoneum

Regional Lymph Nodes (N)

NX	Regional lymph nodes cannot be assessed
N0	No regional lymph node metastasis
N1	Regional lymph node metastasis

Distant Metastasis (M)

MX	Distant metastasis cannot be assessed
M0	No distant metastasis
M1	Distant metastasis

Stage Groupings

Stage I	T1	N0	M0
Stage II	T2	N0	M0
Stage IIIA	T3a	N0	M0
Stage IIIB	T3b	N0	M0
Stage IIIC	T4	N0	M0
Stage IVA	Any T	N1	M0
Stage IVB	Any T	Any N	M1

Histological Grade (G)

GX	Grade cannot be assessed
G1	Well differentiated
G2	Moderately differentiated
G3	Poorly differentiated
G4	Undifferentiated

Fibrosis Score (F)

F0	Fibrosis score 0–4 (no fibrosis to moderate fibrosis)
F1	Fibrosis score 5–6 (severe fibrosis to cirrhosis)

Adapted from Edge SB. *AJCC Cancer Staging Manual.* 7th ed. New York, NY: Springer; 2009, with permission.

for F1 disease. The AJCC staging manual recommends notation of fibrosis but has not yet formally incorporated the F classification into the staging system.

The majority of patients analyzed in the international study by Vauthey et al. had HCV-related HCC rather than HBV-related HCC; thus, Poon et al. undertook validation of the staging system with HBV-infected patients from Hong Kong. Despite the different clinicopathological features of patients with HCV and HBV, Poon et al. demonstrated that the new staging system provides reliable prognostic information for patients with hepatitis B, and showed that the new system is simpler to use than the previous AJCC staging system. Appropriate emphasis is placed on the most important prognostic features: vascular invasion within the tumor, and fibrosis of the nontumoral liver. Several other authors from Taiwan and Europe have independently validated the AJCC/UICC system, confirming its prognostic accuracy.

Patient Selection for Surgical Treatment

HCC typically occurs in the background of cirrhosis. Thus, after assessment of a patient's candidacy for surgery based on overall health and comorbidity, assessment of liver function is necessary.

The most widely used classification system for the assessment of liver function is the Child–Pugh (sometimes called the Child–Pugh–Turcotte) system. The parameters measured in this classification system are the total bilirubin and albumin levels, presence or absence of ascites, presence or absence of encephalopathy, and prothrombin time/international normalized ratio; together, these parameters give a rough estimate of the gross synthetic and detoxification capacity of the liver. Numerous studies have validated this system as an overall predictor of survival after surgery in cirrhotic patients (Table 12.2). Patients with Child–Pugh class A liver function generally tolerate hepatic resection. Patients with class B liver function may tolerate minor resection, but generally do not tolerate major resection. Patients with class C liver function are at significant risk from anesthesia and laparotomy.

Several other clinical staging systems have been developed to guide initial therapy for HCC. The Okuda staging system, developed in Japan, incorporates tumor size, ascites status, and albumin and bilirubin levels, accounting for both liver function and tumor extension. The Cancer of the Liver Italian Program (CLIP) group derived a system from a retrospective study of 435 patients diagnosed with HCC that incorporates the Child–Pugh score, data on tumor morphology and extension, presence or absence of portal vein thrombosis, and serum level of AFP. The Barcelona Clinic Liver Cancer (BCLC) system uses a clinical staging system based on tumor progression and liver function. The CLIP and Okuda systems may be useful to predict prognosis in patients who have advanced tumors and liver disease but are not useful for treatment selection. The BCLC system is highly criticized and has not been widely accepted because it allocates palliative treatment to patients who are candidates for curative resection. The BCLC system is generally considered to be more of a treatment algorithm than a staging system.

For anatomically resectable HCC without extrahepatic metastases, our approach to patient selection for major hepatectomy is first based on clinical parameters (performance status, Child–Pugh classification) and degree of portal hypertension. We require a platelet count ≥100,000 and exclude patients with gastric or esophageal varices. Next, systematic determination of the FLR volume, as described previously, is necessary. PVE is considered on the basis of the previous criteria. We do not use ICG clearance or other tests of liver function in this assessment.

TABLE 12.2   Child–Pugh Classification of Hepatic Functional Reserve

Clinical or Laboratory Feature	1 Point	2 Points	3 Points
Encephalopathy (grade)	0 (absent)	1–2	3–4
Ascites	Absent	Slight	Marked
Bilirubin (mg/dL)	<2.0	2.0–3.0	>3.0
Albumin (g/dL)	>3.5	2.8–3.5	<2.8
International normalized ratio	<1.7	1.7–2.2	>2.2

Each feature is assigned 1, 2, or 3 points.
Class A: 5–6 points; Class B: 7–9 points; Class C: 10–15 points.

This approach enables resection in cirrhotics with low incidences of liver failure and death. In patients with normal livers, this approach enables extended hepatectomy with <1% mortality and very low morbidity. The systematic evaluation of patients using standardized volumetry is the key to low morbidity and mortality, allowing extensive and aggressive hepatic surgery in our center.

Surgical Resection

The standard treatment for HCC is surgical resection or orthotopic liver transplantation (OLT). However, not all patients with HCC are candidates for surgical resection; of those presenting with HCC, only 10% to 30% will be eligible for surgery, and of those patients who undergo exploratory surgery, only 50% to 70% will have a resection with curative intent. Patients with cirrhosis may be candidates for limited surgical resection, OLT, or locoregional ablative treatment, depending on the severity of the cirrhosis.

The only absolute criterion that initially renders a tumor unresectable is the presence of extrahepatic disease (and even this exclusion has caveats in highly selected cases). Other relative contraindications to resection are evidence of severe hepatic dysfunction, an inadequate FLR, and tumor involvement of the portal vein or vena cava. Patients with normal liver parenchyma are usually eligible for extensive resection. Patients with compensated cirrhosis may be candidates for minor or major hepatectomy in selected cases. As previously described, when indicated, PVE can be a useful preoperative maneuver in patients with HCC. Palavecino et al. compared the outcomes of patients who did and did not undergo PVE prior to major hepatic resection for HCC. The patients who underwent PVE had equivalent overall- and disease-free survival, and were less likely to experience major complications. No deaths occurred in the PVE group compared to 18% in the non-PVE group, re-emphasizing the importance of FLR volume analysis.

Once the tumor has been determined to be resectable, the next decision is the extent of liver resection to be done. The extent of surgery will depend, in part, on the size of the mass, the number of nodules, the tumor's proximity to vascular structures, and as discussed previously, the severity of any underlying liver disease. Formerly, a 1-cm surgical margin was believed to be necessary to ensure long-term survival after resection. However, Poon et al. analyzed outcome based on resection margins in 288 patients who underwent hepatectomy for HCC and found that recurrence rates were similar between groups with narrow (<1 cm) and wide (≥1 cm) margins; only patients with histologically positive margins or satellite nodules separate from the main tumor had relatively high recurrence rates. The authors noted that patients with margins positive for HCC had a higher incidence of intratumoral microvascular invasion than other patients. In addition, recurrences did not necessarily occur at the margin, but also sometimes appeared in the remaining liver, distant from the margin, reflecting tumor biology that was more likely to lead to a positive margin.

The operative approach to the patient with a potentially resectable HCC should begin with a thorough surgical exploration of the abdomen, searching for evidence of extrahepatic disease. In particular, care should be taken to evaluate the periportal lymph nodes in addition to the nodes in the hepatoduodenal ligament. The liver then should be completely mobilized to allow full examination of the organ. Intraoperative US should be used to define both the size of the tumor and its relationship to the major vascular and biliary structures. DL should be considered in patients with ruptured tumors, indeterminate nodules, or possible extrahepatic disease.

Anatomical resections are preferred over segmental resections, when feasible, based on the extent of underlying liver disease and because of the tendency of HCC to spread along portal tracts. In addition, portal-oriented resections have been shown to be associated with lower morbidity, mortality, and blood loss, as well as higher survival rates, than segmental resections. Regimbeau et al. demonstrated that the overall 5-year survival rate in patients who underwent anatomical resections (54%) exceeded that of those who had segmental resections (35%). Extended hepatectomy is generally not feasible in patients with cirrhosis, but major hepatectomy can be considered when PVE is used appropriately, as described previously, following systematic volumetry of the FLR.

A major pattern of recurrence after hepatic resection is intrahepatic failure with development of new disease. The concept of the field of cancerization—that is, the tendency of the remaining liver to generate new HCCs—partially explains the 30% to 70% recurrence rate after hepatic resection. Recurrence risk and survival vary, based on two dominant factors and several other minor factors. The most potent predictors of poor survival and high-risk recurrence of HCC are vascular invasion in the tumor and severe fibrosis in the underlying liver. Other correlates with poor outcome are absence of a tumor capsule and high-grade or poor tumor differentiation.

A study from our International Liver Tumor Study Group examined the risk factors for recurrence <1 year after resection. We identified tumor size greater than 5 cm, multiple tumors, and histology revealing more than five mitoses per ten high-power fields as being associated with risk of early death due to recurrence. We stress that these are not exclusion criteria—that is, the presence of multiple or large tumors that are resectable should not exclude patients from consideration for potentially curative resection. Rather, these factors help us move forward in identifying patients whose HCCs are likely to recur and who might benefit from adjuvant therapy, when effective agents are developed.

Hepatitis serology has also been proposed as a factor related to the risk of HCC, but in another large study from our institution, we demonstrated that hepatitis serology, per se, is not a predictor of survival. Analysis of 446 patients in our international database who underwent complete resection for HCC demonstrated that patients with HBV infection or no infection tended to have larger tumors than patients with HCV or HBV + HCV infection. In addition, the serology-negative and HBV-infected patients had a higher incidence of vascular invasion; in contrast, they had lower incidence of severe, underlying liver fibrosis, which was predominant in the other two groups. However, the final analysis revealed that status of vascular invasion and fibrosis were equally predictive of poor outcome and that the other putative risk factors were not independent; that is, patients with HBV or no infection have larger tumors with vascular invasion but no fibrosis, whereas patients with HCV infection who are screened regularly tend to have smaller tumors and a lower incidence of vascular invasion but established cirrhosis.

Major vascular invasion, that is, invasion of a main portal trunk or hepatic vein, even extending to the vena cava, presents a difficult problem. Survival in patients with this feature has generally been poor; however, selected patients can derive a significant palliative benefit from hepatectomy with extraction of tumor thrombi or hepatectomy in the presence of segmental portal vein thrombosis. Specific indications for such extensive surgery are beyond the scope of this chapter, but selected patients in this group can be treated with major hepatectomy, which can provide significantly better survival than other treatment options.

In the event of recurrence after resection, selected patients can be considered for repeat resection, depending on the pattern of recurrence. Both focal, intrahepatic, recurrent tumors and certain adrenal metastases can be resected. Solitary extrahepatic metastases at sites such as the lung, diaphragm, and abdominal wall can also be resected. In all these cases, median survival may be as high as 50 months, compared with survival on the order of 10 months for those treated without surgery.

Although some classification systems, such as the BCLC system, and some groups in the United States propose that patients with large tumors should not be considered for surgery, many authors recognize that tumor size alone does not predict biology. In fact, multiple studies have shown that patients with T1 tumors >10 cm in diameter have exactly the same survival pattern after resection as those with tumors <3 cm. We analyzed 300 patients undergoing resection for tumors >10 cm and found that, for the entire group, including some patients with vascular invasion, the 5-year survival was 27% and the 10-year survival was 18%. Perioperative mortality was 5%. There were long-term (≥10 years) survivors among patients who had more than one tumor in which the largest exceeded 10 cm in diameter. As would be expected, the best survival was achieved in patients who had tumors without vascular invasion and who did not have severe fibrosis. We also analyzed the utility of a clinical scoring system to select patients with large HCCs for resection, using AFP, tumor number, and presence or absence of major vascular invasion and fibrosis as the factors placed into the scoring system. Patients with no risk factors (high AFP, multiple tumors, major vascular invasion or fibrosis) had a 5-year survival rate of nearly 50%. Those with any risk factor had a 5-year survival rate in the 20% range, but even in the group of patients with three risk factors, there were 10-year survivors. AJCC T classification clearly stratifies survival; this has been validated in many studies, including that of Yamanaka et al. who found that resection of T1 tumors yielded a 5-year survival rate as high as 78%.

Orthotopic Liver Transplantation

Even after margin-negative resection of HCC, recurrence remains a problem. Most published series report a median survival of 30 to 40 months with a 5-year survival rate of 30% to 40%, as well as a high incidence of recurrence, ranging from 30% to 70%. It has been suggested that the liver fibrosis and necrosis associated with chronic, active hepatitis caused by HBV and HCV provides a potential field for further HCC development (a field of cancerization); imaging studies of patients with chronic liver disease have led to the early detection of small HCCs (<5 cm). For these reasons, some have proposed that the only definitive treatment for HCC is orthotopic liver transplantation (OLT) to remove both the HCC tumors and the damaged liver parenchyma.

Once liver transplantation was established as a safe treatment for cirrhosis, it began to be considered as a treatment option for unresectable tumors of the liver, but early recurrence was the rule. The outcome following transplantation for liver failure in patients found *incidentally* to have small HCC suggested that better selection criteria might reinsert liver transplantation into the treatment strategy for HCC. These criteria were formalized after analysis of a study by Mazzaferro et al. who evaluated patients with cirrhosis and either a single tumor ≤5 cm or three tumors ≤3 cm in maximum diameter, who underwent liver transplantation. Survival at 5 years after transplantation exceeded 60%, with disease-free survival exceeding 50%. These criteria, based on the Milan Meeting, were then adopted as the criteria for appropriate selection of patients for OLT for HCC, although the study was small (48 patients) and no tumor had vascular invasion.

On the basis of 70 cirrhotic patients who underwent OLT for HCC during a 12-year period at the University of California–San Francisco (UCSF), some groups now advocate OLT for solitary tumors <6.5 cm, or 3 nodules with the largest lesion ≤4.5 cm and total tumor diameter ≤8 cm, commonly referred to as the "UCSF criteria." Future refinements in selection criteria should emphasize biological selection criteria (e.g., tumor grade, AFP level, and gene-expression profile) over simple morphologic criteria such as tumor size and number. Finally, the effect of chronic immunosuppression on the course of recurrent cancer after transplantation is unclear.

Nonresectional Locoregional Therapies

For selected patients with HCC confined to the liver whose disease is not amenable to surgical resection or OLT, locoregional ablative therapies can be considered. Although these therapies may also be used in patients with resectable HCC, their efficacy has not been established as equivalent to resection. A discussion of ablation treatments follows.

The advantages of ablation techniques include destruction of tumors and preservation of a maximal volume of nontumorous liver, and the potential to combine ablation of small lesions with resection of larger lesions. The major disadvantages of any ablation technique are the limited ability to evaluate treatment margins and the need to obtain negative treatment margins in three dimensions. All ablation techniques have higher local recurrence rates than resection for virtually all tumors. Percutaneous ablation is particularly attractive for treatment of patients with severe underlying liver disease, for treatment of patients with a contraindication to laparotomy, or as a bridge to more definitive therapy, such as OLT.

Percutaneous Ethanol Injection

Percutaneous ethanol injection (PEI) is a treatment administered under US guidance through a fine (22-gauge) needle. Absolute ethanol (8 to 10 mL) induces cellular dehydration, necrosis, and vascular thrombosis, causing tumor cell death. Outpatient treatments are repeated once or twice a week, for up to 6 weeks. PEI is most effective for tumors <3 cm in diameter. Studies have demonstrated 100% necrosis in HCCs <2 cm in diameter. The treatment-related death rate has been reported to be 0.09% to 0.1% and the complication rate 1.7% to 3.2%. PEI is contraindicated in patients with gross ascites, coagulopathy, and obstructive jaundice, as well as in patients with large tumors, thrombosis in the main portal or hepatic vein, and extrahepatic metastasis. Complications that can occur with this method include minor adverse effects, such as pain and fever, as well as hemorrhage, liver abscess and failure, and cholangitis.

Several studies have documented post-PEI survival rates similar to those obtained with hepatic resection for extremely small tumors in well-selected patients, but HCC recurrence in the liver is frequent, with an incidence of 50% at 2 years; the majority of recurrences are new lesions in distant segments of the liver. Randomized trials suggest PEI is appropriate for tumors ≤2 cm in diameter because it has lower rates of morbidity but equivalent efficacy when compared with other ablation techniques, such as radiofrequency ablation (RFA).

Cryotherapy

Cryotherapy is no longer commonly used as an ablation technique. Serious complications that can occur with this method include intraoperative hemorrhage from the probe tract, bile duct fistula, freezing injury to adjacent structures, and renal failure related to myoglobinuria. For these reasons, cryotherapy has largely been supplanted by newer ablation techniques.

Radiofrequency Ablation

RFA uses heat to destroy tumors. Using US or CT guidance, a needle electrode with an uninsulated tip is inserted into the tumor. The electrode delivers a high-frequency alternating current, generating rapid vibration of ions, which leads to frictional heat and, ultimately, coagulative tissue necrosis. RFA can be performed percutaneously, laparoscopically, or through an open incision and is most effective in tumors <3 cm in diameter. Larger tumors generally require several insertions of the electrode.

RFA complications are rare but may include pneumothorax, pleural effusion, hemorrhage, subcapsular hematoma, hemobilia, biliary stricture, and liver abscess. The treatment-related death rate has been reported to be 0% to 1% and the complication rate 0% to 12%. Early tumor recurrence after RFA treatment is associated with large tumor size, poor histological differentiation, advanced stage of presentation, elevated serum AFP, and the presence of hepatitis. RFA may be more effective in patients with cirrhosis because the fibrotic liver permits a "baking effect" by confining the heat to the tumor. The safety and efficacy of RFA for HCC in cirrhotic patients were largely established at the M. D. Anderson Cancer Center.

Several studies have suggested that RFA may be effective for unresectable tumors. Two reports have directly compared percutaneous RFA and surgery for treatment of HCC. Despite having higher rates of local recurrence, patients treated with RFA had overall survival and recurrence-free survival rates similar to those of patients undergoing surgical resection. Hong et al. reported a series of 148 patients who presented with solitary small (<4 cm diameter) HCCs and either no evidence of cirrhosis or Child–Pugh class A hepatic function. The patients selected for RFA either refused surgery or were predicted to have insufficient postoperative hepatic reserve to justify the high operative risks, and were significantly older than those in the comparative resection group. The overall recurrence rates for RFA and surgery were 41.8% and 54.8%, respectively, but the rate of local recurrence (defined as occurring near the margin of the ablation) was higher in the RFA group (7.3%) than in the surgery group (0.0%). The rates of remote recurrence (defined as distant metastasis or intrahepatic metastasis in the hepatic parenchyma, but somewhere other than the original tumor site) and of simultaneous local and remote recurrence were similar between the two treatment groups. The 1- and 3-year overall survival rates were 97.9% and 83.9%, respectively, in the surgery group and 100% and 72.7%, respectively, in the RFA group.

Vivarelli et al. reported 158 patients who underwent either RFA or surgical resection. The majority of patients in the surgery group had Child–Pugh class A liver function, whereas most patients treated with RFA had class B function. The RFA group did have a few patients with Child–Pugh class A liver function with a single potentially resectable nodule. Furthermore, in both the RFA and surgery groups, a majority of patients had chronic hepatitis caused by HBV, HCV, or HCV + HBV infection. The overall and disease-free survival rates were significantly higher for patients treated with resection. One- and 3-year rates of overall survival were 78% and 33%, respectively, for surgical patients and were 60% and 20%, respectively, for RFA patients. Patients with Child–Pugh class A liver function and with solitary lesions, as well as lesions <3 cm in maximum diameter, had significantly higher rates of survival with surgery (overall 3-year survival = 79%) than with RFA (overall 3-year survival = 50%).

The high rate of HCC recurrence following RFA is supported by studies which evaluate the explanted liver following OLT. Mazzaferro et al. observed that among a group of patients with HCC and cirrhosis who underwent RFA followed by OLT, 45% had evidence of residual HCC in the explanted liver. Likewise, Pompili et al. studied a similar cohort and found that 53% of the ablated HCC nodules showed incomplete necrosis. Consequently, RFA is unattractive as the sole modality for treatment of HCC in patients without evidence of underlying cirrhosis. RFA may play a role in the therapy of other HCC-subgroups. RFA may be the preferred treatment for small HCCs in patients whose tumor cannot be resected safely due to tumor location or due to underlying cirrhosis. In the cirrhotic population, the increased risk of HCC recurrence with RFA is tolerable when considering the high risk of major morbidity or mortality associated with resection. Either resection or ablation can be employed as a means of preventing tumor growth/spread prior to transplantation in selected patients. For patients who have a tumor recurrence after treatment and who are not candidates for resection, RFA is a satisfactory "salvage technique" and may enable remission. Therefore, ablation techniques such as RFA clearly have an important role in the treatment of this HCC patient subset.

Chemotherapy
In general, systemic chemotherapy has little activity against HCC. Single-agent chemotherapy with 5-fluorouracil (5-FU), doxorubicin, cisplatin, vinblastine, etoposide, and mitoxantrone provides response rates of 15% to 20%, and the responses are usually transient. Combination chemotherapy does not seem to improve these results. The most active agent appears to be doxorubicin, with an overall response rate pooled from several trials of 19%.

Investigational regimens for unresectable HCC combine conventional chemotherapy (specifically 5-FU) with immunomodulatory agents, such as alpha-interferon. Preclinical and clinical studies have demonstrated that the two drugs have synergistic activity against colorectal cancer. Despite its considerable toxic effects, including myelosuppression, the combination of doxorubicin, 5-FU, and alpha-interferon (PIAF) downstaged initially unresectable tumors to a size amenable for resection, and increased the overall median survival rate in an important study conducted in Hong Kong. The same investigators have reported sufficient tumor regression for subsequent resection, enabling long-term survival after PIAF.

A recent phase III trial demonstrated that in patients with advanced HCC and preserved liver function (Childs A status), the oral multikinase inhibitor sorafenib was associated with a 3-month increase in median overall survival compared to placebo. Sorafenib is currently being studied in the adjuvant setting; a phase III study is investigating its effect on recurrence-free survival after surgical resection or local ablation, and a phase I trial is investigating effect of adjuvant sorafenib after liver transplantation.

Transcatheter Arterial Embolization and Transarterial Chemoembolization
Transarterial chemoembolization (TACE) is a combination of intra-arterially infused chemotherapy and hepatic artery occlusion, whereas transcatheter arterial embolization (TAE) omits doxorubicin, the most common chemotherapeutic agent. Chemotherapeutic agents may be either infused into the liver before embolization or impregnated in the gelatin sponges used for the embolization. Lipiodol also has been used in conjunction with TACE because this agent will remain selectively in HCCs for an extended period, allowing the delivery of locally concentrated therapy.

Two randomized control trials have shown that TACE provides a survival advantage for patients with unresectable HCC; thus, TACE is the standard of care for patients who are not candidates for resection, transplantation, or ablation. Furthermore, TACE can be used in combination with ablation or resection or as a bridge to transplantation.

Despite the favorable results of TACE therapy, this treatment modality has limitations. Morbidity rates have been reported to be as high as 23%, especially among patients with HCCs >10 cm in diameter. Moreover, postembolization syndrome, including fever, nausea, and pain, is common. Other adverse reactions, such as fatal hepatic necrosis and liver failure, have rarely been reported. TACE is generally contraindicated in patients with ascites.

Lo et al. presented a randomized controlled trial of TACE and Lipiodol for unresectable HCC in patients with compensated liver failure and in patients with advanced disease (including segmental portal invasion). The chemotherapeutic agent was an emulsion of cisplatin in Lipiodol and gelatin-sponge particles, which was injected through the hepatic artery. The chemoembolization group (40 patients) received a median of 4.5 courses per patient and showed significant tumor response. For the chemoembolization group, the 1-, 2-, and 3-year survival rates were 57%, 31%, and 26%, respectively, while for the control group the rates were 32%, 11%, and 3%, respectively ($P = 0.005$).

Another investigator from the BCLC group performed a randomized trial comparing either TAE or TACE with symptomatic treatment in a much more selected group of patients, who had favorable characteristics compared with those studied by Lo et al. The 112 nonsurgical candidates with HCC and cirrhosis had Child–Pugh class A or B liver functional reserve. The TACE group received doxorubicin combined with Lipiodol and Gelfoam. The trial was stopped when data review demonstrated that chemoembolization yielded survival rates significantly higher than those of conservative treatment. One- and two-year survival rates were, respectively, 75% and 50% for the embolization group, 82% and 63% for the chemoembolization group, and 63% and 27% for the control group. Since publication of these trials, TACE has secured a role in the treatment of selected patients with HCC.

Radiation Therapy
External-beam radiation therapy has limited utility in the treatment of HCC. The dose that can be safely delivered to the liver is approximately 30 Gy; higher doses cause radiation hepatitis. More recently, radioembolization with yttrium-90-labeled microspheres has emerged as a local therapy. The advantage of this modality compared to external-beam radiation relates to the delivery of a higher radiation dose that is confined within a more precise liver volume. The target lesion is identified and isolated using catheter-based techniques identical to TACE. The radiolabeled particles are delivered into tumoral arterial feeding vessels. The 25 μm spheres lodge at the distal arteriolar level and the emitted radiation penetrates approximately 10 mm, delivering a dose of about 150 Gray. Data are limited describing the long-term outcomes of this therapy. Although this modality is generally reserved for patients who are not candidates for ablation, resection, or transplantation, radioembolization might also be used to bridge or downstage patients with advanced HCC.

Multimodality Therapy
Combinations of surgical and nonsurgical therapies are the state-of-the-art for HCC. Some unresectable tumors can be rendered resectable by transarterial chemotherapy, portal vein embolization, radioembolization, or systemic chemotherapy. Various chemotherapeutic agents have been studied in the neoadjuvant setting, including doxorubicin, 5-FU, mitomycin C, and cisplatin. Furthermore, tumor recurrence may be prevented by the administration of adjuvant intra-arterial chemotherapy after surgical resection or PEI.

Two small series describe strategies implementing sequential TACE and PVE in patients with HCC and marginal liver function. TACE inhibits tumor progression because HCCs derive the majority of their blood supply from hepatic artery branches. Subsequent PVE induces hypertrophy of the contralateral liver without diverting blood through the tumor's arterial blood supply. Both series showed that this sequential approach is associated with a high degree of complete pathologic tumor necrosis, and a degree of FLR hypertrophy greater than would be expected after PVE alone. Consequently, this approach may enable a broader range of patients to undergo resection. This combined treatment modality may be particularly important for HCCs with vascular invasion of the portal or major hepatic vein.

METASTASES TO THE LIVER

Nearly all malignant tumors can metastasize to and proliferate in the liver. Most metastases originate from gastrointestinal primary tumors, and of these, most are from the colon and rectum. In general, 5-year survival is rare among patients who undergo resection for noncolorectal metastases to the liver. The exceptions are selected patients with, in particular, neuroendocrine tumors, Wilm's tumor, and to a lesser extent, renal cell carcinoma; 5-year survival rates of 40% to >70% have been reported after resection of their metastases. Hepatic resection may provide excellent endocrinopathy palliation in selected patients with hormone-secreting neuroendocrine tumors. Given that the vast majority of liver metastases that are considered for resection are from colorectal primary tumors, the remainder of this discussion is concerned with their management.

Epidemiology and Etiology

Colorectal cancer represents the third most common type of cancer for both men and women in the United States, with an estimated incidence of 150,000 cases per year. Approximately 85% of the patients will have malignancies that are amenable to surgical cure, but half of the resected cancers will recur within 5 years. Only 20% of these recurrences will be solely or predominantly in the liver, and fewer still will be amenable to surgical resection a second time. It has been estimated that 15,000 to 20,000 patients per year are potential candidates for resection of their liver metastases.

Clinical Presentation and Diagnosis

Symptoms or clinical signs suggesting metastatic disease in the liver usually are late occurrences. Consequently, findings such as ascites, jaundice, right upper quadrant pain, and increases in serum levels of factors associated with liver function are associated with a poor prognosis. In the vast majority of patients, metastases to the liver are found during routine postoperative carcinoembryonic antigen (CEA) screening or radiologic imaging after resection of a colorectal primary tumor. Patients with increasing CEA levels should undergo thorough diagnostic evaluation, including chest radiography and contrast-enhanced CT scan of the abdomen and pelvis. A slowly increasing CEA level usually indicates local or regional recurrence, whereas a rapidly increasing CEA level suggests hepatic metastases. Overall, 75% to 90% of patients with hepatic colorectal cancer metastases have an increased CEA level. In addition, colonoscopy should be performed to exclude a local recurrence or metachronous colon or rectal primary tumor as the source of the increasing CEA value.

Determining Resectability

When all hepatic disease can be extirpated with a negative margin, leaving an adequate FLR (20% of the standardized TLV) with adequate vascular inflow, hepatic venous outflow, and biliary drainage, metastases from colorectal cancer should be deemed resectable. Specific recommendations with regard to response to chemotherapy are difficult to make, although progression of liver metastasis during systemic chemotherapy should prompt selection of alternate chemotherapy agents rather than hepatic resection due to the poor outcomes observed in these patients. Clinical criteria such as CEA level, number of tumors, size of tumors, and location of the primary tumor, although prognostic, cannot be used to exclude patients from resection and a potential cure. The planned hepatic resection should encompass all metastases detectable on the prechemotherapy imaging. Benoist et al. showed that a complete radiographic response cannot be equated with a complete pathologic response; in fact, 83% of metastases suggestive of a complete radiographic response harbor viable tumor cells or develop early intrahepatic recurrence. Conversely, patients with imaging suggestive of viable tumor after preoperative chemotherapy may demonstrate evidence of a complete pathologic response at the time of resection. In a series of 767 patients, Adam et al. observed that 4% of patients had a complete pathologic response, but *none* of these patients had a complete radiographic response.

In cases of bilateral disease, multistage approaches to surgery should be considered. At the first stage, wedge or limited resection clears the planned FLR, preserving the major portion of the parenchyma in preparation for resection of the remaining liver. At the second stage, major hepatectomy or extended hepatectomy removes all remaining disease. Resection of dominant lesions and RFA of residual disease may be considered, but this approach yields poor survival compared with staged resection. Staged resection requires a certain level of excellence, an integrated multidisciplinary approach to disease management, and usually, interval PVE to increase the volume and function of the FLR after the first-stage resection. Chun et al. recently showed that the two-stage approach can be undertaken with equivalent morbidity, mortality, and survival compared to the single stage approach. High tumor number, large tumor size, presence of limited extrahepatic disease, and extensive resection are no longer absolute barriers to resection. Systemic chemotherapy can reduce the size and volume of tumors such that all tumor sites can be resected safely and provide long-term survival. Highly selected patients with extrahepatic disease—whether limited peritoneal carcinomatosis, minimal hilar lymphadenopathy, or metastatic disease to the lung—can undergo resection with acceptable survival.

The notion that a 1-cm margin is necessary to ensure long-term survival has been dispelled. Analysis of nearly 500 patients in a multi-institutional database showed that the pattern and probability of disease recurrence and the rates of disease-free and overall survival were identical in patients with 1-mm and 1-cm resection margins. Thus, determining whether metastases from colorectal cancer are resectable requires a multidisciplinary approach and the participation of an experienced hepatic surgeon; otherwise, patients who have metastases that would otherwise be considered resectable will be relegated to noncurative therapy, such as systemic chemotherapy. A 1-cm margin remains the goal, but close margin-negative resection is also oncologically acceptable with close postoperative surveillance.

Evaluation of Operative Risk

Most patients with colorectal liver metastases (CRLM) have a normal underlying liver, although some will have injury due to prior therapy or more important patient factors (e.g., obesity and diabetes, which are associated with steatosis). Although some studies suggest that hepatic resection in patients with steatosis is associated with increased operative risk, blood loss, and complications, we have not found an increase in operative or postoperative complications related to chemotherapy. Most agree that mortality is equivalent to that for resection in patients without significant steatosis.

Patients who require extended hepatectomy should undergo systematic volumetry as described previously and if the FLR volume is <20% of the standardized TLV, they should undergo PVE of the entire tumor-bearing liver before resection. Some investigators have proposed that a larger remnant (e.g., 30% of the TLV) is necessary for patients who have received intensive chemotherapy; however, this group has not been studied systematically.

Unique to patients with metastases is the concern that tumor growth may be incited by the embolization. We have shown that complete embolization of the tumor-bearing liver is not associated with changes in tumor size that affect resectability; thus, we stress the importance of complete embolization of the liver to be resected and complete hepatic resection when this approach is used.

Other Methods of Preoperative Staging

High-quality imaging is critical to assessment of CRLM resectability. We favor CT scanning almost exclusively at our institution; our published survival rates are equal to the best reported for resection of metastases from colorectal cancer, validating this approach. CT not only permits assessment of extrahepatic structures, but also accurately provides for liver volumetry, accurate localization of the tumors within the liver, and accurate lesion detection. Multiphase, thin-cut, spiral, hepatic

CT is our modality of choice, and the information thus gained has been superior to that afforded by MRI and other approaches, resulting in our high rates of survival. MRI is useful in patients with metastases poorly visualized on CT and in patients with a significant degree of underlying steatosis.

DL has a limited role in staging of CRLM; mainly because imaging is sensitive, full exploration by means of DL is often limited due to prior surgery, and additional findings at DL may change aspects the operative approach, but typically do not lead to abandonment of resection.

Careful prelaparotomy staging must include colonoscopy to rule out local recurrence, plain radiography of the chest, and CT of the chest when indicated by the radiographic findings.

Although [^{18}F]fluoro-2-deoxy-D-glucose PET has been proposed by Fernandez et al. as necessary for staging, no study (including that by Fernandez et al. which did not use high-quality CT) has shown that PET improves outcome when high-quality cross-sectional imaging is used. However, false-negative PET is the rule after chemotherapy, limiting the utility of this technique alone. PET is likely to improve detection of extrahepatic disease, but has not yet become the standard of care.

Surgical Therapy

At exploratory laparotomy, a careful search for extrahepatic disease should be undertaken, and detection of enlarged portal and celiac lymph nodes may prompt biopsy. The colon and rectum should be examined for any local recurrence of the primary tumor. The liver is examined by visual inspection and palpation, and then by intraoperative US. US will help define the relationship of the tumor(s) to the portal veins, hepatic veins, and vena cava. In addition, it can identify small lesions that were not palpable or demonstrable on preoperative imaging studies. Suspicious areas can be sampled by FNA under US guidance. The goal of the resection is to remove all disease and obtain microscopically disease-negative margins. Anatomically oriented resection is favored over wedge resection because it is associated with less blood loss and lower likelihood of positive margins; this technique is often mandatory for patients with multiple lesions. However, it should be recognized that there is no oncologic indication for which anatomical resection is preferred to wedge resection, as long as the resection margin is tumor-free.

Survival After Resection of Colorectal Liver Metastases

Modern reports on series of patients undergoing hepatic resection for CRLM reveal that the 5-year survival rate is 53% to 58%. The 5-year survival rate has improved from earlier reported rates of 25% to 40%, despite the expansion of criteria, including resection of larger, more numerous, and bilobar tumors, as well as resection of synchronous CRLM, and resection with CRLM in the presence of limited extrahepatic disease. In select cases, it may be possible to resect synchronous liver metastases at the same time as the primary tumor. The complexity of the operation necessary to remove the primary tumor and the extent of hepatic resection required for the liver metastases will affect decision making because the risk of adverse events from hepatic resection increases when the procedure is associated with extrahepatic surgery. Earlier studies demonstrated by univariate analysis that synchronous metastases were a predictor of poor prognosis. Solitary, small, peripherally located lesions in a healthy, hemodynamically stable patient that can be excised adequately by non-anatomical resection or segmentectomy may be resected at the same time as the primary tumor. Lesions that are larger or that will require a major hepatic resection are best approached during a second operation, after further evaluation and staging. A delay of weeks or months between surgeries has not been shown to negatively affect survival. At the time of the initial operation, a thorough exploration should be conducted to rule out the presence of extrahepatic metastases.

Prognostic Factors After Resection

Several modern studies have highlighted the improvement in survival over time with the use of improved operative techniques, anesthesia, patient selection, imaging, and probably chemotherapy. Figueras et al. who deemed all CRLMs resectable in patients who had an adequate FLR, regardless of tumor size or number, and who included patients with resectable extrahepatic disease, reported a 5-year survival rate of 53%. Choti et al. reported on a series of patients treated between 1984 and 1992 and compared the outcome with that of patients treated at the same institution between 1993 and 1999. They demonstrated a significant increase in the rate of 5-year overall survival, which was 31% in the early group and 58% in the later group, despite reductions in the hospitalization duration and the rate of perioperative blood transfusion and similar rates of morbidity and mortality. It is noteworthy that PET scanning was not routinely used in this study; <10% of the patients underwent PET scanning, although more patients received pre- or postoperative chemotherapy.

We subsequently published a report on the largest modern series of patients who underwent resection of CRLMs. Most patients required a major resection (64% underwent a hemihepatectomy or extended hepatectomy), and nearly one-fourth of the patients required a procedure in addition to the hepatic resection. Survival in our series was 58%, identical to that seen in the Choti et al. series. Fernandez et al. used PET rather than high-quality CT, and the outcome for the 100 patients in their series was similar, with survival of 58% at 5 years. Thus, despite an expansion in the indications for resection, clearly a new gold standard of 58% 5-year survival can be achieved because this rate has been validated in several series from different institutions around the world.

Despite the progressive improvement in survival after resection of CRLM, most patients (50% to 70%) will have a tumor recurrence after hepatic resection. Several important studies have outlined the key prognostic factors.

The first is from Scheele et al. who analyzed 654 patients treated between 1960 and 1998. This is an important study because none of the patients received chemotherapy. The 5-, 10-, and 20-year survival rates were 39%, 28%, and 24%, respectively. In this series, patients with only one tumor had the same survival rate as patients with three or more tumors despite the absence of chemotherapy. Scheele et al. appropriately emphasized the importance of margin-negative (R0) resection.

The second and most widely quoted study to outline prognostic factors is from Fong et al. who evaluated a series of 1,001 consecutive patients who underwent hepatic resection for metastatic colorectal cancer at the Memorial Sloan-Kettering Cancer Center. Seven independent factors were associated with poor outcome, including disease at the surgical margin, presence of extrahepatic disease, metastatic disease in the lymph nodes of the primary lesion, a short disease-free interval from resection of the primary tumor to detection of metastases, the number of hepatic tumors, hepatic tumor diameter >5 cm, and the elevation of the CEA level. These factors contribute to outcome in different degrees, and scoring of these factors is helpful in predicting prognosis after resection, but not in selecting patients for surgery.

A study from the M. D. Anderson Cancer Center clarified the importance of a margin-negative resection by examining the site of recurrence after resection for CRLM based on surgical margin status in a multi-institutional database. Patients with surgical margins positive for tumor cells had an overall recurrence rate of 52%, compared with 39% for patients with negative margins. Margin width (whether > or <1 cm) did not affect recurrence frequency, location, or overall survival. The overall recurrence rate for all 557 patients was 40%. The majority of patients who had recurrences developed them at an extrahepatic site (66%), whether alone (30%) or with simultaneous intrahepatic recurrence (36%). Only 3.8% of patients had a recurrence at the surgical margin. The recurrence rates were similar in patients with negative margins of 1 and 4 mm (39%), 5 and 9 mm (41%), and ≥1 cm (39%). This multi-institutional study confirmed the previously published 58% 5-year survival rate after resection of CRLM.

In addition to margin status, the pathologic response to preoperative chemotherapy has emerged as an important prognostic factor after resection of colorectal liver metastases. Blazer et al. showed that the 5-year overall survival for patients with no residual tumor cells in the resected specimen is 75% versus 33% for patients whose resected specimens contain ≥50% residual tumor cells.

Ablative Therapy

RFA is used widely as a treatment for CRLM. Unfortunately, its use was widespread before consistent indications for ablation were established. Initial, well-designed studies proved the safety, excellent side effects profile, and efficacy of RFA for CRLM. Initial studies from our institution and later from Europe and the Cleveland Clinic suggested a 78% 1-year survival rate could be attained by RFA, with 3-year survival at 46%. Unfortunately, >12% of patients had disease recurrence at 1 year. Although RFA provides a modest survival benefit over chemotherapy alone for CRLM at 4 years (22% vs. 7%), the outcome after RFA is vastly inferior to that after resection in terms of both overall and disease-free survival, whether single or multiple tumors are treated and regardless of tumor size. Furthermore, the overall recurrence rate after RFA (84%) in our study was much greater than that after resection (52%); intrahepatic-only recurrence was four times higher with RFA (44%) than with resection (11%), and the frequency of true local recurrences at the RFA site (9%) was 4.5 times that of margin recurrences after resection (2%). Although we ablated only unresectable tumors, these data strongly suggest RFA is inferior to resection as a treatment for CRLM.

Subsequent studies have supported these findings. In 2003, Livraghi et al. reported on percutaneous RFA of potentially resectable CRLMs. Despite the investigators' experience with RFA, they reported a 40% treatment failure rate and a 70% recurrence rate in the 88 treated patients. This result can be contrasted with the 10% or less rate of recurrence in the case of positive-margin resection, and the 50% or less recurrence rate among patients who undergo hepatic resection with much more aggressive tumors, larger tumors, more lesions, and even patients with extrahepatic disease, suggesting that RFA is not equivalent to resection in patients with potentially resectable lesions.

The next important study compared RFA with resection in patients with solitary CRLMs, and was reported by Oshowo et al. in 2003. They, too, showed that RFA is inferior to resection as a treatment modality for the group of patients with probably the best prognosis—that is, those with solitary lesions. Although these investigators claimed that the RFA outcome was equivalent to that of resection, they reported only a 55% 3-year survival rate for patients with solitary metastases after resection (compared with 53% with RFA), which is inferior to the survival rate achieved by resection in virtually every other series, including our own (which yielded a 5-year survival rate >60%).

RFA may be used as an adjunct to resection, as proposed by Elias et al. and further analyzed by our group. Resection of dominant lesions may be supplemented with RFA of small, residual tumors in the FLR. Unfortunately, our series reveals that this approach is no more effective than RFA alone, and 5-year survival will be <20%. Furthermore, mortality rates are higher with this approach (2.3%) than with extended hepatectomy (0.8% in our series). Finally, several studies examining two-stage approaches to resection with PVE have demonstrated survival rates of 40% at 5 years, again proving the superiority of complete resection over ablation of CRLM.

Ablation may be used to treat disease that is unresectable because the patient is not a candidate for laparotomy (because of comorbidity) or because removal of the tumor-bearing liver with a negative margin would leave an insufficient FLR, particularly in patients with underlying liver disease. An alternative to RFA in some patients is staged hepatic resection and portal vein embolization. RFA may also have a role in treatment of the ill-placed recurrence after major hepatectomy when repeat resection is not safe.

The potential for ablation may be limited by a tumor's proximity to the confluence of the bile ducts because thermal injury to the bile ducts can lead to biloma and bile fistula; a 1-cm distance is required. Furthermore, the effect of thermal damage on the FLR can be more significant than that identified at the time of treatment; ablation at the time of resection must be performed with care.

RFA is safe. Curley et al. reported a treatment-related mortality rate of 0.5% and an early (<30 days) treatment-related complication rate of 7.1%. The late (>30 days) complication rate was 2.4%. The two most common early complications were symptomatic pleural effusion and perihepatic and RFA lesion abscesses. Late complications included bilomas in the RFA lesion or biliary fistulas. Open or laparoscopic RFA is contraindicated for lesions within 2 cm of the biliary confluence, in the presence of bilioenteric anastomosis, and near critical portal structures in the liver remnant after resection or at the time of combined resection and ablation. Close proximity to bowel or the diaphragm is a relative contraindication. Mullen et al. reported successful RFA using a transthoracic approach for a postresection recurrence adjacent to the diaphragm. Contraindications for percutaneous RFA include not only those for the open/laparoscopic approach, but also inability to adequately image or access the lesion percutaneously. Percutaneous RFA is associated with treatment failure and, consequently, a higher recurrence rate.

Thus, as for assessment of the resectability of CRLM, assessment for RFA of CRLM should be made jointly by an experienced multidisciplinary team that includes a hepatic surgeon.

Chemotherapy

Recent advances in chemotherapy for colorectal cancer have dramatically changed the outlook for patients with stage IV disease. The former standard was a combination of 5-FU and leucovorin (LV), which provided response rates from 12% to 40% and median survival of 10 to 17 months. Two new drugs that have shown promise are irinotecan (CPT-11) and oxaliplatin. Various combination therapies using these agents (5-FU or LV, with or without oxaliplatin, FOLFOX [5-FU, LV, folinic acid, and oxaliplatin], and FOLFIRI [5-FU, LV, folinic acid, and irinotecan]) have yielded overall response rates >50% and median survival times >20 months in the general population of patients with stage IV disease. Prior to the development of contemporary agents, regional chemotherapy via hepatic arterial infusion (HAI) was explored as a method to increase the efficacy of the previous generation of chemotherapy agents. The best reported response rates using HAI chemotherapy are 50% to 62% in studies that date from the late 1980s. Two recent European trials using 5-FU in patients with unresectable liver disease failed to demonstrate an improvement in survival and had a high complication rate. HAI therapy for unresectable disease has failed to keep pace with improving systemic chemotherapy including the emergence of new agents such as irinotecan and oxaliplatin that can yield high response rates (54% to 56%) and median survival of 22 months with acceptable toxicity. The addition of biological agents (including bevacizumab and cetuximab) has increased response rates by 10% and increased median survival to 25 to 27 months. As an adjuvant to liver resection, prospective randomized studies of HAI showed no survival advantage. Furthermore, the treatment failed in the majority of patients, with extrahepatic disease as a component of recurrence. This locoregional strategy fails to address occult metastases, which are supplied by the portal vein, and distant extrahepatic disease, which occurs in the majority of patients with CRLM.

Use of the new chemotherapeutic and biological drugs has made it possible to downstage unresectable tumors to the point where surgical resection is possible. HAI therapy alone enables only 2% to 3% of patients with unresectable CRLM to downstage such that resection is possible; the rate is significantly lower than that obtained using preoperative systemic chemotherapy. At our institution, we have all but abandoned HAI therapy in any form for CRLM. Given the response rates of contemporary chemotherapy agents, systemic administration effectively addresses all metastatic sites, including hepatic. Historically, chemotherapy has been administered after liver resection, but recent data demonstrate the advantages of a preoperative strategy.

One of these advantages is the potential for rendering unresectable tumors resectable with chemotherapy. Giacchetti et al. and subsequently Adam et al. showed that about 13% of patients who present with unresectable CRLM, with or without extrahepatic disease, can undergo resection after chemotherapy. Adam has shown a 33% rate of overall survival and a 22% rate of disease-free survival after resection in patients with previously unresectable disease treated using this approach. In contrast to administering chemotherapy after all measurable tumor has been resected, the efficacy of a given chemotherapy regimen can be ascertained while the patient is receiving preoperative therapy. Patients in the EORTC 40983 trial who received preoperative chemotherapy were less likely to have the planned resection aborted than patients who had not received preoperative chemotherapy. More importantly, in the EORTC 40983 trial the use of perioperative chemotherapy was associated with a statistically significant improvement in progression-free survival in the subset of patients who underwent resection.

In spite of their oncologic benefits, specific chemotherapy agents have been linked to three types of hepatotoxicity. Steatosis is manifested by a grossly yellow appearance to the liver, and is associated with the use of 5-FU. This type of parenchymal injury does not appear to increase postoperative morbidity. On the other hand, steatohepatitis has been associated with the use of irinotecan and shown to result in an increase in 90-day mortality following liver resection (15% vs. 2% in patients without steatohepatitis). Consequently, major hepatic resection in the setting of steatohepatitis is a relative contraindication. This type of injury is characterized by inflammatory features such as hepatocyte ballooning and lobular inflammation. Sinusoidal injury is associated with oxaliplatin treatment, which results in a grossly blue hue to the liver surface. Histologically these changes can be recognized by the presence of hepatic sinusoidal congestion and dilatation. Sinusoidal injury may increase the risk of hepatic resection, but the conflicting nature of the published data probably indicates that this entity is of lesser clinical concern than steatohepatitis.

As discussed previously, the biological agents such as bevacizumab and cetuximab that target angiogenesis generally increase the response rates of standard chemotherapy regimens by about 10%. Ribero et al. investigated the effect of bevacizumab on the outcome of patients receiving a fluoropyrimidine plus oxaliplatin regimen prior to resection and showed that bevacizumab is associated with an improvement in the rate of pathologic response. In patients who receive bevacizumab-based regimens, the degree of pathologic response in the resected specimen is related to the radiographic appearance of lesions after completion of chemotherapy. The three features that indicate effective chemotherapy-induced tumor death include (a) a homogenous hypo-attenuating lesion with (b) a sharp tumor-liver interface, and (c) no residual rim of enhancement surrounding the tumor. Finally, bevacizumab is associated with a decrease in the incidence of sinusoidal dilatation when used with oxaliplatin-based regimens. The molecular mechanism of this protective effect on sinusoidal dilatation has not been characterized.

CANCER OF THE EXTRAHEPATIC BILE DUCT

Epidemiology and Etiology

Cancer of the extrahepatic bile duct (CCA) is extremely rare, comprising 2% of all cancers in the United States. In 2004, 3,000 new cases of CCA were diagnosed in the United States. In most reported series, males and females have nearly equal incidence (with the male:female incidence ratio at 1.2 to 1.5:1), and patients were ≥60 years old. The incidence of CCA is 1 case per 100,000 people in the United States, 5.5 cases to per 100,000 in Japan, and 7 cases per 100,000 in Israel. People of Asian descent are affected almost twice as often as whites and blacks, probably because of endemic chronic parasitic infestation.

The etiology of CCA is unknown. Several diseases are associated with an increased risk of such tumors—sclerosing cholangitis, ulcerative colitis, and choledochal cysts or Caroli disease (a congenital disease characterized by multiple intrahepatic biliary cysts). Exposure to Thorotrast and chronic typhoid carrier status has also been shown to increase risk. No strong evidence implicates gallstones or parasitic infection with *Opisthorchis viverrini* or *Clonorchis sinensis* in CCA carcinogenesis, but there is an increased risk of CCA in patients who have parasitic infestation or hepatolithiasis. The common cancer-causing factor in these conditions is unclear, although chronic inflammation of the bile duct probably plays a role.

Pathological Characteristics

Adenocarcinoma is the most common histological type of biliary cancer; morphologically, CCA can be classified as papillary (<5% of cases), nodular (20%), or sclerosing (70%). Most papillary tumors are well differentiated and present with multiple lesions within the duct. Virtually all long-term survivors have papillary-type CCA. Conversely, most sclerosing-type CCAs are poorly differentiated, and this type is often associated with a poor prognosis. A tumor arising at the confluence of the right and left hepatic ducts is termed Klatskin's tumor, following the description of 13 such lesions by Klatskin in 1965.

CCAs are slow growing and most often spread by local intrabiliary ductal extension, peritoneal metastasis, or intrahepatic metastasis. Metastasis to regional lymph nodes occurs less frequently (30% to 50% of cases), and perineural extension occurs as well. Distant metastases are present in approximately 25% to 30% of patients at the time of diagnosis, but hematogenous spread is rare. Lesions of the proximal and middle thirds of the extrahepatic bile duct can compress, constrict, or invade the underlying portal vein or hepatic artery. In addition, proximal tumors can invade the liver parenchyma. Hilar CCAs will involve the parenchyma of the caudate lobe in as many as 36% of patients; their appearance at this site usually occurs by means of biliary extension through the short caudate ducts that drain to the confluence, although they may emanate from a tumor located near the biliary confluence.

Intrahepatic Cholangiocarcinoma

Intrahepatic CCA is a different entity than hilar CCA, and forms of intrahepatic CCA can be grouped according to their growth patterns. These cancers can be mass-forming (MF), periductal-infiltrating (PI), or can grow within the duct lumens (intraductal growth). The MF type presents as a round mass within the liver parenchyma and can recur in the remnant liver after hepatic resection. The PI type of intrahepatic CCA grows longitudinally along the bile duct, often causing an obstruction or stricture. Several pathological findings are important in predicting the outcome of patients with CCA; poorer outcome is associated with tumor infiltration of the bile duct serosa, lymph node metastases, and vascular and perineural invasion. Intrahepatic CCAs have a higher propensity to metastasize to lymph nodes than hilar CCAs.

Clinical Presentation

The most common presenting symptoms in patients with hilar CCA are obstructive jaundice (which occurs in 90% of patients) and itching. Rarely, a very proximal tumor may block a segmental or lobar bile duct without causing jaundice. Other symptoms that may occur are weight loss (29% of cases), vague abdominal pain (20%), fatigue, and nausea. A patient may also present with cholangitis and sepsis resulting from bacterial contamination of the obstructed bile. In the case of middle or distal duct obstruction, a distended gallbladder may be palpable on abdominal examination; conversely, hilar CCA is typically associated with a nondistended gall-bladder. In addition to having elevated serum total bilirubin, patients with CCA will present with elevated alkaline phosphatase, gamma-glutamyltransferase, and possibly elevated tumor markers (carbohydrate antigen 19-9 [CA19-9] and CEA).

Diagnosis

The first radiologic test that should be performed when extrahepatic bile duct obstruction is suspected is US, which can provide information about the level and nature of an obstructing lesion. US can also give information regarding the morphology of the lesions, possible dilation of extrahepatic and intrahepatic bile ducts, portal vein and hepatic artery obstruction, and the presence of gallstones and gall-bladder dilation.

Further imaging is necessary to delineate the cross-sectional and longitudinal (intrabiliary) extent of the tumor. Some centers use a combination of MRI and color or spectral Doppler US. At the M. D. Anderson Cancer Center, multiphase helical thin-cut CT scanning is used in combination with pre-referral endoscopic retrograde cholangiopancreatography (ERCP). Helical CT scanning has an overall accuracy of 76% to 100%, and MRI has an overall accuracy of 89% for staging CCA. We prefer CT because patients usually present to us after ERCP; also, the CT permits assessment of vascular encasement, cross-sectional assessment of tumor extent, and accurate delineation of the tumor's biliary extent in a single study.

CT is as sensitive as US in demonstrating biliary dilation, but in addition CT can give information about the local, regional, and distant extent of the disease. CT also gives information about the relationship between the tumor and surrounding structures (including the hepatic artery and portal vein and hepatic lobar atrophy), and may be used in the search for metastatic spread. If distant disease is demonstrated on CT, palliative percutaneous or endoscopic stent placement can be performed during cholangiography.

In the absence of distant disease, the actual location of the tumor and its proximal and distal extent must be defined before any intervention is planned. This information can be obtained using ERCP, magnetic resonance cholangiopancreatography (MRCP), or percutaneous transhepatic cholangiography (PTC). To evaluate lesions in the distal bile duct, ERCP is superior to the other techniques because it images both the bile and the pancreatic ducts. MRCP can also image the bile duct and provides information about surrounding vascular structures. MRCP usually has an advantage over ERCP because it is noninvasive. Both ERCP and MRCP overestimate the extent of bile duct involvement in about 40% of cases. Both imaging modalities may fail to define the extent of intrabiliary tumor proximally. If the point of obstruction is believed to be proximal to the perihilar region, PTC is the preferred method for defining the biliary tract. PTC also allows brush biopsies of the tumor, external drainage of obstructed biliary ducts, and palliative stent placement when indicated. The workup for a suspected CCA rarely requires visceral angiography or portography to assess vascular involvement because of the high quality of modern CT and MRI, with or without three-dimensional reconstruction.

Despite improved prelaparotomy imaging, 25% to 40% of patients are found to have unresectable disease at the time of surgery. DL is considered in most patients with large or extensive hilar tumors because of the frequency of metastases in the peritoneal cavity and because its use in selected cases results in fewer non-therapeutic laparotomies and shorter hospital stays.

For resectable CCA, obtaining tissue to confirm the diagnosis of bile duct cancer is not essential and may be difficult. In most instances, the decision to operate is based on the preoperative radiologic findings, not histologic confirmation. The sensitivity of brush biopsies is poor (well below 50%), although newer techniques such as fluorescence in situ hybridization assay and endoscopic US-guided FNA of the bile duct may improve diagnostic accuracy. Treatment is guided by anatomical findings (e.g., biliary obstruction, enhancing hilar mass, vascular encasement, liver atrophy).

Staging and Anatomical Classification

The seventh edition AJCC staging system for hepatobiliary cancers is now subdivided. Consequently, intrahepatic cholangiocarcinoma, perihilar cholangiocarcinoma, extrahepatic cholangiocarcinoma, and gallbladder cancer are each considered separately. Intrahepatic cholangiocarcinoma now has its own staging system which is largely based on a study by Nathan et al., which analyzed a 598-patient SEER cohort (Table 12.3). The AJCC subdivided the schema for extrahepatic cholangiocarcinoma into perihilar (Table 12.4) and distal bile duct (Table 12.5) varieties. Gallbladder cancer is considered in the section that follows.

TABLE 12.3	American Joint Commission on Cancer Staging System for Cancer of the Intrahepatic Bile Duct

Primary Tumor (T)

TX	Primary tumor cannot be assessed
T0	No evidence of primary tumor
T1	Solitary tumor without vascular invasion
T2a	Solitary tumor with vascular invasion
T2b	Multiple tumors, with or without vascular invasion
T3	Tumor perforating the visceral peritoneum or involving local extrahepatic structures by direct invasion
T4	Tumor with periductal invasion

Regional Lymph Nodes (N)

NX	Regional lymph nodes cannot be assessed
N0	No regional lymph node metastasis
N1	Regional lymph node metastasis

Distant Metastasis (M)

MX	Distant metastasis cannot be assessed
M0	No distant metastasis
M1	Distant metastasis

Stage Groupings

Stage 0	Tis	N0	M0
Stage IA	T1	N0	M0
Stage II	T2	N0	M0
Stage III	T3	N0	M0
Stage IVA	T4	N0	M0
	Any T	N1	M0
Stage IVB	Any T	Any N	M1

Adapted from Edge SB. *AJCC Cancer Staging Manual.* 7th ed. New York, NY: Springer; 2009, with permission.

	American Joint Commission on Cancer Staging System for Cancer of the Perihilar Bile Ducts

Primary Tumor (T)

TX	Primary cannot be assessed
T0	No evidence of primary tumor
Tis	Carcinoma in situ
T1	Tumor confined to bile duct, with extension up to the muscle layer or fibrous tissue
T2a	Tumor invades beyond the wall of the bile duct to surrounding adipose tissue
T2b	Tumor invades adjacent hepatic parenchyma
T3	Tumor invades unilateral branches of the portal vein or hepatic artery
T4	Tumor invades main portal vein or its branches bilaterally; or the common hepatic artery; or the second-order biliary radicals bilaterally; or unilateral second-order biliary radicals with contralateral portal vein or hepatic artery involvement

Regional Lymph Nodes (N)

NX	Regional lymph nodes cannot be assessed
N0	No regional lymph node metastasis
N1	Regional lymph node metastasis (including nodes along the cystic duct, common bile duct, hepatic artery, and portal vein)
	Metastases to periaortic, pericaval, superior mesenteric artery and/or celiac artery lymph nodes

Distant Metastasis (M)

MX	Distant metastasis cannot be assessed
M0	No distant metastasis
M1	Distant metastasis

Stage Groupings

Stage 0	Tis	N0	M0
Stage I	T1	N0	M0
Stage II	T2a-b	N0	M0
Stage IIIA	T3	N0	M0
Stage IIIB	T1–T3	N1	M0
Stage IVA	T4	N0–1	M0
Stage IVB	Any T	N2	M0
	Any T	Any N	M1

Adapted from Edge SB. *AJCC Cancer Staging Manual.* 7th ed. New York, NY: Springer; 2009, with permission.

The anatomical classification of CCA is subdivided by the site of origin: intrahepatic (6%), distal extrahepatic (27%), or perihilar (67%). Extrahepatic CCA is typically classified according to the Bismuth–Corlette classification, which describes the common patterns of hilar CCA within the biliary tree, defines the surgical strategy, and provides the language used to describe such tumors (Fig. 12.2). Type I tumors obstruct the biliary confluence but do not touch the "roof" of the biliary confluence. Type II tumors are similar to type I tumors but *do* touch the roof. Type III lesions extend through the intrahepatic bile ducts to involve second-order ducts to the right (type IIIa) or left (type IIIb) only, sparing contralateral ducts. Type IV tumors extend to second-order ducts on both the right and the left. Treatment is defined by location due to the fact that the liver drained by all involved ducts must be resected for cure.

TABLE 12.5	American Joint Commission on Cancer Staging System for Cancer of the Distal Bile Duct

Primary Tumor (T)

TX	Primary cannot be assessed
T0	No evidence of primary tumor
Tis	Carcinoma in situ
T1	Tumor confined to bile duct histologically
T2	Tumor invades beyond the wall of the bile duct
T3	Tumor invades the gallbladder, pancreas, duodenum, or other adjacent organs without involvement of the celiac axis, or the superior mesenteric artery
T4	Tumor involves the celiac axis, or the superior mesenteric artery

Regional Lymph Nodes (N)

NX	Regional lymph nodes cannot be assessed
N0	No regional lymph node metastasis
N1	Regional lymph node metastasis

Distant Metastasis (M)

MX	Distant metastasis cannot be assessed
M0	No distant metastasis
M1	Distant metastasis

Stage Groupings

Stage 0	Tis	N0	M0
Stage IA	T1	N0	M0
Stage IB	T2	N0	M0
Stage IIA	T3	N0	M0
Stage IIB	T1–T3	N1	M0
Stage III	T4	Any N	M0
Stage IV	Any T	Any N	M1

Adapted from Edge SB. *AJCC Cancer Staging Manual.* 7th ed. New York, NY: Springer; 2009, with permission.

RESECTABILITY CRITERIA

The definitive therapy for all extrahepatic bile duct carcinomas is complete resection. Overall resectability rates range from 10% to 85%, depending on whether distal cancers are present. Lesions of the lower third of the bile duct have the best rates of resectability by pancreaticoduodenectomy (considered in Chapter 13); middle-third obstructions of the bile duct are almost always due to gallbladder cancer, which is considered separately. Hilar CCAs and Klatskin's tumors are technically more challenging to resect, giving them the lowest rate of resectability among bile duct tumors. Standard criteria used to determine resectability relate to the biliary extent and vascular encasement by the tumor. Involvement of secondary bile ducts necessitates hepatic resection on the side involved. Vascular involvement of the portal vein or hepatic artery necessitates hepatic resection of the anatomical side involved as well. Thus, if secondary biliary extension and vascular encasement occur unilaterally, these tumors can be resected along with the hepatic resection. If secondary bile ducts are involved on one side and vascular encasement occurs on the opposite side, complete resection is not possible. Lymph node involvement outside the hepatic pedicle (N2) and distant metastases also preclude resection. Intrahepatic CCAs are treated by hepatic resection with tumor-free margins.

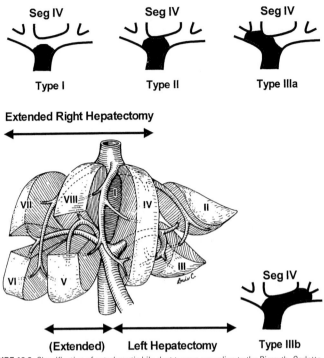

FIGURE 12.2 Classification of extrahepatic bile duct tumors according to the Bismuth–Corlette system, which describes the common patterns of hilar CCA within the biliary tree. The figure displays the surgical strategy for each tumor type and provides the language used to describe such tumors. Types I, II, and IIIa are treated by extended right hepatectomy, whereas type IIIb is treated by left or extended left hepatectomy.

Surgical treatment of hilar CCA is subject to several controversies, which are described briefly: biliary drainage, extent of hepatic and caudate resections, and portal vein resection. Other factors in selecting patients for resection, such as patient performance status, are common between this disease and any others, and assessment of the FLR volume is a mandatory part of CCA treatment because most patients require major or extended hepatectomy with resection of the extrahepatic bile duct. This is not controversial.

Studies from our own institution, as well as that of the largest series of patients in the world (from Nagino and Nimura in Japan), show that FLR volume must be considered and PVE used to increase the FLR volume prior to extended hepatectomy for hilar CCA. Because the confluence of the bile ducts sits at the base of segment IV, this segment must usually be resected, regardless of whether the tumor is central, to the left, or to the right. Hepatic resection is usually to the right, to include extended right hepatectomy, because 97% of the described variations in biliary anatomy include preservation of a long left hepatic duct. Thus, hilar disease extending even slightly to the left or significantly to the right can be cleared by means of extended right hepatectomy, taking advantage of this long left duct.

Clearly, disease to the left requires a left hepatectomy, which necessarily includes resection of segment IV or extended left hepatectomy. On the basis of these principles, we next discuss the four controversial issues and provide our recommendations, which attend closely to the principles of preoperative preparation of the patient and liver for surgery.

Biliary Drainage

The need for preoperative biliary drainage has been debated at length in the literature, but most consider resolution of jaundice as a critical element in preparing the patient and liver for major hepatectomy. Prior studies evaluating stent placement and its associated morbidity and mortality, including six randomized studies (conducted during 1985–1994), reported only a single patient who subsequently underwent hepatectomy. Moreover, only one retrospective review demonstrated that stent placement was associated with an increase in infectious complications. At the M. D. Anderson Cancer Center, routine placement of preoperative biliary drainage catheters is done for several reasons. The effect of hyperbilirubinemia is well known: It impairs liver regeneration and reduces resistance to systemic infection. Hepatic resection in a jaundiced patient is associated with increased rates of mortality (36% vs. 16% for those with bilirubin <2 mg/dL) and complications (50% vs. 15%). Cameron et al. advocated routine preoperative placement of biliary drainage catheters to facilitate identification and dissection of the bile duct during surgery and to aid the intraoperative placement of larger, softer transhepatic Silastic stents. In a Japanese series of 160 patients with hilar CCA, percutaneous intrahepatic biliary drainage was performed in 50 of the 52 patients who underwent combined liver and portal vein resection without complications. At the M. D. Anderson Cancer Center, we universally drain the FLR, but drain the liver to be resected only if necessary to resolve jaundice, and do not leave transanastomotic biliary drains. The degree of cholestasis in the FLR impacts not only the need for preoperative biliary drainage, but also may impact the threshold to pursue PVE. Although an sFLR ≥20% is usually adequate in a patient without cirrhosis, the presence of significant cholestasis may justifiably decrease the threshold to pursue PVE as patients with hilar cholangiocarcinoma often require a larger remnant.

Extent of Hepatic Resection

In terms of outcome for surgical treatment of hilar CCA, patients in centers where major hepatic resection is performed (rather than duct excision) have the best prognosis. Resection of hilar CCA should be performed only when negative surgical margins (R0) can be achieved. The necessity of resecting the caudate lobe (segment I) en bloc with the bile duct is also a point of controversy. Anatomically, resection of hilar cholangiocarcinoma should be considered to include the caudate for two reasons. First, preoperative imaging inadequately defines the precise caudate drainage, which is quite variable among the general population. Second, the boundary between the posterior caudate and the anterior right or left hepatic lobes is often difficult to appreciate intraoperatively. Attempts at preserving the caudate parenchyma may unintentionally result in incomplete tumor resection. Pathological examination of resected specimens demonstrates direct invasion of tumor into the liver parenchyma or bile ducts of the caudate lobe in as many as 35% of patients. In addition, the caudate lobe is often the site of tumor recurrence following bile duct resection. Despite this, some believe the caudate lobe should be removed only if it has been invaded by the tumor, noting that survival data for those who had caudate resection are similar to data for those with similar CCA who did not undergo this procedure.

Jarnagin et al. reported a series of 80 patients who underwent resection for CCA; the operative mortality and 5-year survival rates were 10% and 27%, respectively. However, the 5-year survival after resection including hepatectomy (28% with caudate resection) was 37% versus 0% after resection of the bile duct without hepatectomy. Ebata et al. later reported a series of 160 patients, all of whom underwent hepatic resection with caudate resection and reported a similar operative mortality (10%) and 5-year survival (37%), despite the need for portal resection in 52/160 patients. At our institution, we resect the liver including segment IV, the caudate process, and paracaval caudate lobe in all cases; Spiegel's lobe is resected when the dominant Spiegel's duct drains to the tumorous duct.

Lesions of the lower third of the bile duct do not require hepatic resection, but rather pancreaticoduodenectomy (Whipple procedure). The proximal bile duct should be resected to the point that the surgical margin is negative for tumor. Occasionally, this may require removal of most of the extrahepatic biliary tract with a high hepaticojejunostomy. The operative approach for pancreaticoduodenectomy at the M. D. Anderson Cancer Center is outlined in Chapter 13.

Lesions of the middle third of the bile duct (termed type 0 tumors by Akeeb and Pitt) are exceedingly rare. Because of these tumors' proximity to the hepatic artery and the portal vein, these structures are typically invaded. When a type 0 tumor is deemed resectable, it is best treated by either hilar resection or pancreaticoduodenectomy. Clinically, most mid-duct obstructions are due to gallbladder cancer.

Limited regional lymphadenectomy is generally indicated for hilar CCAs during extrahepatic bile duct resection so staging and stratification for postoperative therapy and prognosis can be done.

Portal Vein Resection

There are two general approaches to portal vein (PV) invasion when considering resection of hilar CCA. Although some would consider portal invasion a contraindication to resection, long-term survival can be achieved by complete resection, even including PV resection (PVR).

Neuhaus et al. in Germany proposed a systematic approach to PVR, the "no touch technique." It involves PVR in all cases of hilar CCA. Although a better 5-year survival rate was attained with PV resection (65%) than without (0%), most patients with PVR underwent right-sided margin-negative resection (which, as described previously, enables a tumor-negative margin because of the long left duct). Furthermore, the operative mortality rate was 17%, perhaps unacceptably high. A second approach was proposed by Nimura et al. and updated by their group in a report from Ebata et al. This group recommended evaluating portal adherence to the region of the tumor at surgery. They validated their selective PVR approach (used in 52/160 patients) by demonstrating that 69% of those who underwent PVR had microscopic evidence of tumor invasion in the resected PV. Those in this series who did not undergo PVR had a better 5-year survival rate (37%) than those who did (10%), which reflects the different biologies in these cases and supports a selective approach.

At the M. D. Anderson Cancer Center, the surgical approach to proximal bile duct tumors depends on their location relative to the confluence of the right and left hepatic bile ducts and on their proximal extension. Lesions in this region are assessed according to the classification described by Bismuth and Corlette. Intrahepatic CCAs are managed with hepatic resection. Resectable lesions of the lower third of the bile duct are treated with a pancreaticoduodenectomy. Lesions of the middle third (type 0) are managed by pancreaticoduodenectomy or hepatectomy, depending on their location within the mid-duct. Type I, II, and IIIa CCAs are treated with an extended right hepatectomy, along with resection of the caudate process and paracaval caudate. The Speigel lobe is resected if the duct is involved. Type IIIb CCAs are treated with a left or extended left hepatectomy, along with resection of the entire caudate liver. The PV is resected and reconstructed when the vein is inseparable from the tumor and when resection of the vein will enable a margin-negative resection. Routine PVR is not performed at our institution.

Type IV lesions are generally not considered to be resectable. Several studies have reported OLT as a treatment option for CCA as a part of a multimodality protocol-based approach. The results have been consistently disappointing, with high tumor recurrence rates and low overall survival (5-year survival rate of 23%).

The sequence of open laparotomy for staging, intensive chemoradiation, and then OLT has been investigated primarily at the Mayo Clinic (Rochester, MN). Approximately 80% of patients satisfying the strict entrance criteria eventually undergo transplantation. The 5-year survival for all patients after the start of chemoradiation therapy is 55%, and 71% for those patients who undergo transplantation. Patients entering this protocol need not have biopsy-proven cholangiocarcinoma; instead, the inclusion criteria accommodate for several other radiographic and biochemical surrogates. Consequently, the possibility that a proportion of the patients may not have definitively had cholangiocarcinoma prior to initiation of neoadjuvant therapy and subsequent transplantation remains plausible.

Despite aggressive surgical management, most patients with bile duct carcinoma will succumb to their tumors. Survival after resection of distal bile duct tumors has generally been better than that after resection of hilar CCAs. Reported 5-year survival rates range from 9% to 18% for proximal CCAs and 20% to 30% for distal lesions. Median survival is 18 to 30 months for patients without hilar involvement but only 12 to 24 months in patients with hilar involvement. Factors that are predictive of long-term survival after hepatic resection for CCA are T1 tumor stage, N0 lymph node stage, non–mass-forming histology, and R0 resection. Vascular invasion, N2 lymph node metastases, and lobar atrophy are all associated with an adverse outcome. Lymph node metastases are found in 3% to 53% of patients; no data support extended lymphadenectomy.

The optimal palliation for patients with unresectable tumors is unclear. If the tumor has been deemed unresectable before exploration, the bile duct can be drained either percutaneously or endoscopically. The use of metallic in-dwelling stents, which are more durable than traditional stents, has made this option more appealing. If the tumor has been found to be unresectable at exploration, the duct can be intubated with either transhepatic Silastic stents or a T-tube after dilation of the lesion. Operative biliary bypass, with or without palliative tumor resection, is not generally recommended. Unresectable lesions at the bile duct confluence, especially Bismuth type III and IV lesions, can be particularly difficult to palliate and usually require percutaneous stenting, although the goal of tube-free palliation may be achieved by endoscopic or percutaneous methods.

Chemotherapy

No chemotherapeutic agents are clearly effective against CCA. Single-agent trials using 5-FU have demonstrated response rates less than 15%. Other agents, such as doxorubicin, mitomycin C, and cisplatin, used alone or in combination with 5-FU, have been no more successful. Newer agents, particularly gemcitabine and oxaliplatin, are showing some promise, particularly in combination. Toxicity remains a problem in patients with biliary obstruction and stents.

Radiation Therapy

Several studies have investigated the role of adjuvant radiation therapy after bile duct resection. Two separate studies from The Johns Hopkins University found no benefit from adjuvant radiation therapy. Kamada et al. however, showed radiation to be beneficial in patients with surgical margins histologically positive for disease. At the M. D. Anderson Cancer Center, postoperative chemoradiation is given routinely to patients with resected bile duct cancers. If pathological analysis reveals positive margins or nodes, or peritoneal invasion, patients receive a continuous infusion of 5-FU concomitantly with 54 Gy of radiation to the tumor bed. Although patient numbers are small and follow-up duration is short, initial results suggest a longer survival in treated patients than in untreated, historical controls. Radiation therapy has also been found to be effective in the palliation of unresectable bile duct cancers. Doses of 40 to 60 Gy have resulted in a median survival of 12 months, as well as reduced symptoms, probably because of improved stent patency. Palliative photodynamic bile duct therapy is also emerging as a potential palliative treatment option.

GALLBLADDER CANCER

Epidemiology and Etiology

Although carcinoma of the gallbladder is rare, it was the most common malignant neoplasm among the estimated 6,950 cases of biliary tract cancer diagnosed in the United States in 2004 and is the sixth most common cancer of the gastrointestinal tract. The tumor has been reported in all age groups, but occurs most often in patients in their fifties and sixties. There is a striking difference in incidence of the tumor between the genders: females are affected three to four times as often as males. Examination of the SEER database reveals an incidence of 1.2 cases per 100,000 people per year in the United States.

The exact etiology of carcinoma of the gallbladder is not known; however, it has been associated with several conditions. Cholelithiasis is present in 75% and 92% of gallbladder carcinoma cases. Patients with larger stones (>3 cm in diameter) have a ten times greater risk of cancer than patients with small stones (<1 cm). In addition, gallbladder carcinoma can be found in 1% to 2% of all cholecystectomy specimens, a rate several times higher than that reported in autopsy studies. Chronic cholecystitis, including cases in which the gallbladder is calcified ("porcelain" gallbladder), is not associated with an increased risk of cancer, as was once believed. Towfigh et al. evaluated the pathology slides of 10,741 gallbladder specimens for evidence of calcification and gallbladder carcinoma. Among the specimens reviewed, none had gallbladder carcinoma.

The incidence of gallbladder cancer is higher in certain ethnic groups, such as Alaskan and American natives, mirroring the incidence of cholelithiasis. Other factors linked to gallbladder carcinoma include cholecystenteric fistulas, anomalous pancreaticobiliary junction, exposure to chemical carcinogens, inflammatory bowel disease, female gender, familial predisposition, chronic salmonella carrier status, and Mirizzi syndrome.

Pathological Characteristics

Adenocarcinoma of the gallbladder is a slow-growing tumor that arises from the fundus in 60% of cases. On gross examination, the gallbladder appears firm with thickened walls. The papillary adenocarcinoma subtype characteristically grows intraluminally and spreads intraductally. It is a less aggressive tumor that, consequently, carries a better prognosis when compared with other histological subtypes. Adenosquamous cancer is very rare and is treated like adenocarcinoma.

Gallbladder carcinoma spreads by metastasis to the lymph nodes and direct invasion of the adjacent liver. It can spread to the peritoneal cavity after bile spillage, and cells may be implanted in biopsy tracts or at laparoscopic port sites. Lymph node metastases are found in 56% of T2 gallbladder carcinomas and peritoneal disease has been found in 79% of patients with T4 gallbladder carcinoma. The cystic duct node, at the confluence of the cystic and hepatic ducts, is the usual initial site of regional lymphatic spread. Invasion of the liver, either by direct extension or via draining veins that empty into segments IV and V, is seen in >50% of patients. The most common site of distant extra-abdominal metastasis is the lung.

Clinical Presentation

In most series, abdominal pain is the most common presenting symptom. Nausea, vomiting, weight loss, and jaundice are other frequent symptoms. On physical examination, patients may have right upper quadrant pain with hepatomegaly or a palpable, distended gallbladder. Laboratory results are unremarkable unless the patient has developed obstructive jaundice. The tumor markers CEA and CA19-9 may be elevated in patients with gallbladder carcinoma but are neither sensitive nor specific for the disease.

Diagnosis

No laboratory or radiologic tests have shown consistent sensitivity in the diagnosis of gallbladder carcinoma. Furthermore, the paucity of clinical signs and symptoms makes preoperative diagnosis of this cancer difficult. The disease is usually diagnosed either incidentally after cholecystectomy or at an advanced stage, when presenting with a mass, jaundice, ascites, or peritoneal disease. A correct preoperative diagnosis of gallbladder carcinoma is made in fewer than 10% of cases in most series. In the Roswell Park experience, none of the 71 cases reported were diagnosed correctly preoperatively. The most common preoperative diagnoses are acute or chronic cholecystitis and malignancies of the bile duct or pancreas. Jaundice with a mid-left bile duct stricture (type 0) is almost always related to gallbladder cancer.

In the case of gallbladder carcinoma, US may demonstrate an abnormally thickened gallbladder wall or the presence of a mass. Additional imaging by contrast-enhanced CT or MRI will help determine resectability and provide information about the local extent of disease, including portal vascular invasion, the presence of lymphadenopathy, and distant metastases.

Staging

Numerous staging systems have been described for gallbladder carcinoma. The original staging system, as described by Nevin, is based on the depth of invasion and the spread of tumor. The AJCC staging system for gallbladder carcinoma was revised recently (Table 12.6). The most significant change in the AJCC staging system is that there is no longer a distinction between T3 and T4 tumors based on the depth of liver invasion; instead, T3 tumors are defined as those that directly invade the liver and/or other adjacent organs and T4 tumors as those that invade the portal vein, hepatic artery, or multiple adjacent extrahepatic organs or structures.

Laparoscopy has a clear role in prelaparotomy staging of gallbladder carcinoma because DL complements high-quality imaging in detection of peritoneal disease, which is common with this cancer. Gallbladder carcinoma also spreads locally, metastasizing to the locoregional (N1) and distant parapancreatic/periaortic lymph nodes, often encasing the portal vein and hepatic artery precluding surgical resection. Two studies demonstrated that DL could prevent nontherapeutic laparotomy in 33% to 55% of patients with metastatic disease. Laparoscopy was more accurate than CT in detecting peritoneal disease in patients with locally advanced tumors, suggesting that patients with T3 and T4 lesions may benefit from DL prior to surgery.

Surgical Therapy

Standard features that make a gallbladder tumor unresectable include (a) the presence of distant hematogenous or lymphatic metastases; (b) the presence of peritoneal implants; and (c) invasion of tumor into major vascular structures such as the celiac or superior mesenteric arteries, vena cava, or aorta. Gallbladder carcinoma in situ (Tis) and carcinoma limited to the mucosa (T1) can be treated adequately with a cholecystectomy alone, provided that the cystic duct margin is negative for

TABLE 12.6	American Joint Commission on Cancer Staging System for Gallbladder Carcinoma

Primary Tumor (T)

TX	Primary cannot be assessed
T0	No evidence of primary tumor
Tis	Carcinoma in situ
T1a	Tumor invades lamina propria
T1b	Tumor invades muscular layer
T2	Tumor invades perimuscular connective tissue; no extension beyond serosa or into liver
T3	Tumor perforates the serosa (visceral peritoneum) and/or directly invades the liver and/or one other adjacent organ or structure, such as the stomach, duodenum, colon or pancreas, omentum, or extrahepatic bile ducts
T4	Tumor invades main portal vein or hepatic artery or invades two or more extrahepatic organs or structures

Regional Lymph Nodes (N)

NX	Regional lymph nodes cannot be assessed
N0	No regional lymph node metastasis
N1	Metastases to nodes along the cystic duct, common bile duct, hepatic artery, and/or portal vein
N2	Metastases to periaortic, pericaval, superior mesenteric artery and/or celiac artery lymph nodes

Distant Metastasis (M)

MX	Distant metastasis cannot be assessed
M0	No distant metastasis
M1	Distant metastasis

Stage Groupings

Stage 0	Tis	N0	M0
Stage I	T1	N0	M0
Stage II	T2	N0	M0
Stage IIIA	T3	N0	M0
Stage IIIB	T1–T3	N1	M0
Stage IVA	T4	N0–1	M0
Stage IVB	Any T	N2	M0
	Any T	Any N	M1

Adapted from Edge SB. *AJCC Cancer Staging Manual.* 7th ed. New York, NY: Springer; 2009, with permission.

disease. This approach can give 5-year survival rates as high as 100%. When carcinoma is suspected before surgery, open cholecystectomy with hepatoduodenal lymphadenectomy is advocated because the exact T classification cannot be determined at the time of surgery and because bile spillage is a significant risk factor for peritoneal or wound recurrence. Lymphadenectomy is performed primarily for staging purposes but may also improve local control of disease.

Surgical treatment for T2 tumors is somewhat controversial. Because the incidence of lymph node spread in the case of T2 tumors is 56%, optimal surgical treatment for these patients would consist of at least an extended cholecystectomy that includes resection of the gallbladder en bloc along with the portal lymph nodes. Addition of a wedge resection of the gallbladder bed (wedge resection of segments IVb and V) is controversial. Several recent studies evaluating extended resection for T2 tumors demonstrated significant improvements in 5-year survival rates (61% to 100%) compared with simple cholecystectomy (19% to 45%). Radical second operations for T2 tumors are also associated with improved 5-year survival rates (61% to 75%). In contrast, other studies have reported similar survival rates after cholecystectomy when compared with more radical operations for T2 lesions. At the M. D. Anderson Cancer Center, we recommend extended cholecystectomy that includes a resection of the gallbladder en bloc along with the portal lymph nodes, and wedge or anatomical resection of the gallbladder bed (segments IVb and V) for T2 tumors.

Locally advanced tumors (T3 and T4) often present with lymph node metastases (75% of cases) and peritoneal metastases (79%) and are often associated with long-term (>5 year) survival rates in the range of 0% to 5%. However, recent studies have reported 5-year survival rates of 21% to 44% for series of patients with T3 and T4 tumors who underwent radical resection. The extent of hepatic resection is determined by the extent of tumor invasion into the gallbladder fossa and involvement of the right portal triad. To achieve a tumor-free margin, a right hepatectomy, extended right hepatectomy, or pancreaticoduodenectomy may be necessary. Pancreaticoduodenectomy has been proposed to optimize lymph node clearance, but it is generally not warranted unless the tumor extends into the head of the pancreas. Other studies have reported routine resection of the extrahepatic bile duct and pericholedochal and hilar lymph nodes, as well as en bloc resection of grossly involved adjacent structures to achieve R0 resections because there is a high incidence of occult, microscopic invasion of the hepatoduodenal ligament in cases of advanced gallbladder carcinoma. Tumors involving the hepatic artery or portal vein have been extirpated with en bloc vascular resection and subsequent reconstruction, but such an extensive procedure is not considered to be standard therapy because of the associated high morbidity and mortality rates. The most significant negative prognostic factor in gallbladder carcinoma is lymph node involvement, and vascular invasion has also been reported as indicative of poor prognosis. We recommend routine resection of the extrahepatic bile duct and portal lymph nodes.

Nonoperative Therapy

The use of single and multiple chemotherapeutic agents, either as primary or adjuvant therapy, has been disappointing. The response rate of locally advanced gallbladder cancer to 5-FU regimens is approximately 12%. 5-FU combined with doxorubicin has produced response rates of 30% to 40%. HAI chemotherapy produces response rates of 50% to 60% in patients with unresectable disease. These responses are short lived, however, and most patients die of progressive disease within 12 months; thus, HAI is not recommended.

Radiation therapy has shown some promise in the postoperative adjuvant setting, although most series have been small. Intraoperative radiation therapy has also been used with some success. External-beam radiation therapy at a dose of 45 Gy can reduce the tumor size in 20% to 70% of cases and relieves jaundice in up to 80% of patients. At the M. D. Anderson Cancer Center, patients with gallbladder cancer are treated postoperatively with a combination of continuous-infusion chemotherapy and external-beam radiation therapy in an approach similar to that used in patients with CCA.

CONCLUSION

Many advances have been made in the surgical treatment of diseases of the liver. Advances in imaging, patient selection, and patient preparation for major hepatectomy have translated into longer and better survival of patients who undergo surgery. In particular, careful attention to liver volume measurement prior to major resection in patients with liver disease and extended resection in patients with normal liver, using such techniques as PVE, have enabled much lower morbidity and very low mortality for liver surgery. For HCC, the spectrum of treatments reflects the spectrum of the disease and/or underlying liver disease complex. Treatments range widely, including OLT, hepatic resection, tumor ablation, and transarterial embolization. For this disease, systemic therapy has a relatively small role in a highly selected group of patients.

For patients with CRLM, criteria for resection are expanding rapidly, to include larger, multiple, and bilateral tumors. Despite these expanded indications, survival is improving. Furthermore, rapidly evolving effective chemotherapy is expanding the population of patients eligible for definitive surgical treatment.

These benefits from adjuvant therapy have, unfortunately, not extended to patients with biliary tract cancer. Although a small group of patients with hilar CCA and gallbladder carcinoma benefit from major hepatic resection, most patients present with unresectable disease and limited treatment options, despite therapeutic advances in other areas.

In summary, the multidisciplinary approach to patients with liver tumors requires the involvement of specialists in hepatobiliary surgery; surgical, medical, and radiation oncology; gastroenterology; and radiology to enable optimal treatment today and advancement of treatment in the future.

Recommended Readings

Abdalla EK, Barnett CC, Doherty D, et al. Extended hepatectomy in patients with hepatobiliary malignancies with and without preoperative portal vein embolization. *Arch Surg.* 2002;137(6):675–680.

Abdalla EK, Denys A, Chevalier P, et al. Total and segmental liver volume variations: implications for liver surgery. *Surgery.* 2004;135(4):404–410.

Abdalla EK, Hicks ME, Vauthey JN. Portal vein embolization: rationale, technique and future prospects. *Br J Surg.* 2001;88(2):165–175.

Abdalla EK, Vauthey JN. Focus on treatment of large hepatocellular carcinoma. *Ann Surg Oncol.* 2004;11(12):1035–1036.

Abdalla EK, Vauthey JN, Couinaud C. The caudate lobe of the liver: implications of embryology and anatomy for surgery. *Surg Oncol Clin N Am.* 2002;11(4):835–848.

Abdalla EK, Vauthey JN, Ellis LM, et al. Recurrence and outcomes following hepatic resection, radiofrequency ablation, and combined resection/ablation for colorectal liver metastases. *Ann Surg.* 2004; 239(6):818–825.

Adam R, Wicherts DA, de Haas RJ, et al. Complete pathologic response after preoperative chemotherapy for colorectal liver metastases: myth or reality? *J Clin Oncol.* 2008;26(10):1635–1641.

Ahmad SA, Bilimoria MM, Wang XM, et al. Hepatitis B or C virus serology as a prognostic factor in patients with hepatocellular carcinoma. *J Gastrointest Surg.* 2001;5(5):468–476.

Bartlett DL, Fong Y, Fortner JG, et al. Long-term results after resection for gallbladder cancer. Implications for staging and management. *Ann Surg.* 1996;224(5):639–646.

Belghiti J, Cortes A, Abdalla EK, et al. Resection prior to liver transplantation for hepatocellular carcinoma. *Ann Surg.* 2003;238(6):885–892.

Benoist S, Brouquet A, Penna C, et al. Complete response of colorectal liver metastases after chemotherapy: does it mean cure? *J Clin Oncol.* 2006;24(24): 3939–3945.

Bismuth H, Corlette MB. Intrahepatic cholangioenteric anastomosis in carcinoma of the hilus of the liver. *Surg Gynecol Obstet.* 1975;140(2):170–178.

Bismuth H, Nakache R, Diamond T. Management strategies in resection for hilar cholangiocarcinoma. *Ann Surg.* 1992;215(1):31–38.

Blazer DG, Kishi Y, Maru DM, et al. Pathologic response to preoperative chemotherapy: a new outcome end point after resection of hepatic colorectal metastases. *J Clin Oncol.* 2008;25(33):5344–5351.

Blumgart LH, Kelley CJ. Hepaticojejunostomy in benign and malignant high bile duct stricture: approaches to the left hepatic ducts. *Br J Surg.* 1984;71(4):257–261.

Bruix J, Castells A, Bosch J, et al. Surgical resection of hepatocellular carcinoma in cirrhotic patients: prognostic value of preoperative portal pressure. *Gastroenterology.* 1996;111(4):1018–1022.

Burke EC, Jarnagin WR, Hochwald SN, et al. Hilar cholangiocarcinoma: patterns of spread, the importance of hepatic resection for curative operation, and a presurgical clinical staging system. *Ann Surg.* 1998;228(3):385–394.

Choti MA, Sitzmann JV, Tiburi MF, et al. Trends in long-term survival following liver resection for hepatic colorectal metastases. *Ann Surg.* 2002;235(6):759–766.

Chun YS, Vauthey JN, Boonsirikamchai P, et al. Association of computed tomography morphologic criteria with pathologic response and survival in patients treated with bevacizumab for colorectal liver metastases. *JAMA.* 2009;302(21): 2338–2344.

Chun YS, Vauthey JN, Ribero D, et al. Systemic chemotherapy and two-stage hepatectomy for extensive bilateral colorectal liver metastases: perioperative safety and survival. *J Gastrointest Surg.* 2007;11(11):1498–1505.

Cillo U, Vitale A, Bassanello M, et al. Liver transplantation for the treatment of moderately or well-differentiated hepatocellular carcinoma. *Ann Surg.* 2004;239(2): 150–159.

Corvera CU, Weber SM, Jarnagin WR. Role of laparoscopy in the evaluation of biliary tract cancer. *Surg Oncol Clin N Am.* 2002; 11(4):877–891.

Curley SA, Izzo F, Delrio P, et al. Radiofrequency ablation of unresectable primary and metastatic hepatic malignancies: results in 123 patients. *Ann Surg.* 1999; 230(1):1–8.

Curley SA, Marra P, Beaty K, et al. Early and late complications after radiofrequency ablation of malignant liver tumors in 608 patients. *Ann Surg.* 2004;239(4):450–458.

Ebata T, Nagino M, Kamiya J, et al. Hepatectomy with portal vein resection for hilar cholangiocarcinoma: audit of 52 consecutive cases. *Ann Surg.* 2003;238(5):720–727.

Edge SE, Byrd DR, Compton CC, et al. *AJCC Cancer Staging Manual.* 7th ed. New York, NY: Springer; 2009.

Esnaola N, Vauthey JN, Lauwers G. Liver fibrosis increases the risk of intrahepatic recurrence after hepatectomy for hepatocellular carcinoma (*Br J Surg* 2002;89: 57–62). *Br J Surg.* 2002;89(7):939–940.

Farges O, Belghiti J, Kianmanesh R, et al. Portal vein embolization before right hepatectomy: prospective clinical trial. *Ann Surg.* 2003;237(2):208–217.

Figueras J, Jaurrieta E, Valls C, et al. Resection or transplantation for hepatocellular carcinoma in cirrhotic patients: outcomes based on indicated treatment strategy. *J Am Coll Surg.* 2000;190(5):580–587.

Figueras J, Valls C, Rafecas A, et al. Resection rate and effect of postoperative chemotherapy on survival after surgery for colorectal liver metastases. *Br J Surg.* 2001; 88(7):980–985.

Fong Y, Fortner J, Sun RL, et al. Clinical score for predicting recurrence after hepatic resection for metastatic colorectal cancer: analysis of 1001 consecutive cases. *Ann Surg.* 1999;230(3):309–318.

Gagner M, Rossi RL. Radical operations for carcinoma of the gallbladder: present status in North America. *World J Surg.* 1991;15(3):344–347.

Grobmyer SR, Fong Y, D'Angelica M, et al. Diagnostic laparoscopy prior to planned hepatic resection for colorectal metastases. *Arch Surg.* 2004;139(12):1326–1330.

Groupe d'Etude et de Traitement du Carcinome Hepatocellulaire. A comparison of lipiodol chemoembolization and conservative treatment for unresectable hepatocellular carcinoma. *N Engl J Med.* 1995; 332(19):1256–1261.

Iwatsuki S, Starzl TE, Sheahan DG, et al. Hepatic resection versus transplantation for hepatocellular carcinoma. *Ann Surg.* 1991;214(3):221–228.

Jarnagin WR, Bodniewicz J, Dougherty E, et al. A prospective analysis of staging laparoscopy in patients with primary and secondary hepatobiliary malignancies. *J Gastrointest Surg.* 2000;4(1):34–43.

Jarnagin WR, Fong Y, Dematteo RP, et al. Staging, resectability, and outcome in 225 patients with hilar cholangiocarcinoma. *Ann Surg.* 2001;234(4):507–517.

Kamada T, Saitou H, Takamura A, et al. The role of radiotherapy in the management of extrahepatic bile duct cancer: an analysis of 145 consecutive patients treated with intraluminal and/or external beam radiotherapy. *Int J Radiat Oncol Biol Phys.* 1996;34(4):767–774.

Kanematsu T, Matsumata T, Shirabe K, et al. A comparative study of hepatic resection and transcatheter arterial embolization for the treatment of primary hepatocellular carcinoma. *Cancer.* 1993;71(7):2181–2186.

Kawai S, Okamura J, Ogawa M, et al. Prospective and randomized clinical trial for the treatment of hepatocellular carcinoma—a comparison of lipiodol-transcatheter arterial embolization with and without adriamycin (first cooperative study). The Cooperative Study Group for Liver Cancer Treatment of Japan. *Cancer Chemother Pharmacol.* 1992;31(suppl):S1–S6.

Kemeny N, Huang Y, Cohen AM, et al. Hepatic arterial infusion of chemotherapy after resection of hepatic metastases from colorectal cancer. *N Engl J Med.* 1999;341(27):2039–2048.

Kishi Y, Abdalla EK, Chun YS, et al. Three hundred and one consecutive extended right hepatectomies. *Ann Surg.* 2009; 250(4):540–548.

Klatskin G. Adenocarcinoma of the hepatic duct at its bifurcation within the porta hepatis. An unusual tumor with distinctive clinical and pathological features. *Am J Med.* 1965;38:241–256.

Klempnauer J, Ridder GJ, von Wasielewski R, et al. Resectional surgery of hilar cholangiocarcinoma: a multivariate analysis of prognostic factors. *J Clin Oncol.* 1997 ;15(3):947–954.

Llovet JM, Bruix J. Systematic review of randomized trials for unresectable hepatocellular carcinoma: chemoembolization improves survival. *Hepatology.* 2003 ;37(2):429–442.

Llovet JM, Real MI, Montana X, et al. Arterial embolisation or chemoembolisation versus symptomatic treatment in patients with unresectable hepatocellular carcinoma: a randomised controlled trial. *Lancet.* 2002;359(9319):1734–1739.

Llovet JM, Ricci S, Mazzaferro V, et al. Sorafenib in advanced hepatocellular carcinoma. *N Engl J Med.* 2008;359(4): 378–390.

Lo CM, Ngan H, Tso WK, et al. Randomized controlled trial of transarterial lipiodol chemoembolization for unresectable hepatocellular carcinoma. *Hepatology.* 2002;35(5):1164–1171.

Lorenz M, Muller HH, Schramm H, et al. Randomized trial of surgery versus surgery followed by adjuvant hepatic arterial infusion with 5-fluorouracil and folinic acid for liver metastases of colorectal cancer. German Cooperative on Liver Metastases (Arbeitsgruppe Lebermetastasen). *Ann Surg.* 1998;228(6):756–762.

Madoff DC, Hicks ME, Abdalla EK, et al. Portal vein embolization with polyvinyl alcohol particles and coils in preparation for major liver resection for hepatobiliary malignancy: safety and effectiveness—study in 26 patients. *Radiology.* 2003; 227(1):251–260.

Madoff DC, Hicks ME, Vauthey JN, et al. Transhepatic portal vein embolization: anatomy, indications, and technical considerations. *Radiographics.* 2002;22(5): 1063–1076.

Mazzaferro V, Battiston C, Perrone S, et al. Radiofrequency ablation of small hepatocellular carcinoma in cirrhotic patients awaiting liver transplantation: a prospective study. *Ann Surg.* 2004;240(5):900–909.

Mazzaferro V, Regalia E, Doci R, et al. Liver transplantation for the treatment of small hepatocellular carcinomas in patients with cirrhosis. *N Engl J Med.* 1996;334(11): 693–699.

McPherson GA, Benjamin IS, Hodgson HJ, et al. Pre-operative percutaneous transhepatic biliary drainage: the results of a controlled trial. *Br J Surg.* 1984;71(5): 371–375.

Meric F, Patt YZ, Curley SA, et al. Surgery after downstaging of unresectable hepatic tumors with intra-arterial chemotherapy. *Ann Surg Oncol.* 2000;7(7): 490–495.

Mullen JT, Walsh GL, Abdalla EK, et al. Transdiaphragmatic radiofrequency ablation of liver tumors. *J Am Coll Surg.* 2004;199(5): 826–829.

Nagino M, Kamiya J, Kanai M, et al. Right trisegment portal vein embolization for biliary tract carcinoma: technique and clinical utility. *Surgery.* 2000;127(2): 155–160.

Nagino M, Kamiya J, Uesaka K, et al. Complications of hepatectomy for hilar cholangiocarcinoma. *World J Surg.* 2001;25(10): 1277–1283.

Nathan H, Aloia TA, Vauthey JN, et al. A proposed staging system for intrahepatic cholangiocarcinoma. *Ann Surg Oncol.* 2008;16(1):14–22.

Neuhaus P, Jonas S. Surgery for hilar cholangiocarcinoma—the German experience. *J Hepatobiliary Pancreat Surg.* 2000;7(2): 142–147.

Neuhaus P, Jonas S, Bechstein WO, et al. Extended resections for hilar cholangiocarcinoma. *Ann Surg.* 1999;230(6):808–818.

Neuhaus P, Jonas S, Settmacher U, et al. Surgical management of proximal bile duct cancer: extended right lobe resection increases resectability and radicality. *Langenbecks Arch Surg.* 2003;388(3):194–200.

Nevin JE, Moran TJ, Kay S, et al. Carcinoma of the gallbladder: staging, treatment, and prognosis. *Cancer.* 1976;37(1):141–148.

Nordlinger B, Sorbye H, Glimelius B, et al. Perioperative chemotherapy with FOLFOX4 and surgery versus surgery alone for resectable liver metastases from colorectal cancer (EORTC Intergroup trial 40983): a randomised controlled trial. *Lancet.* 2008;371(9617):1007–1016.

Ogata S, Belghiti J, Farges O, et al. Sequential arterial and portal vein embolizations before right hepatectomy in patients with cirrhosis and hepatocellular carcinoma. *Br J Surg.* 2006;93(9):1091–1098.

Oshowo A, Gillams A, Harrison E, et al. Comparison of resection and radiofrequency ablation for treatment of solitary colorectal liver metastases. *Br J Surg.* 2003;90(10): 1240–1243.

Parikh AA, Gentner B, Wu TT, et al. Perioperative complications in patients undergoing major liver resection with or without neoadjuvant chemotherapy. *J Gastrointest Surg.* 2003;7(8):1082–1088.

Pawlik TM, Esnaola NF, Vauthey JN. Surgical treatment of hepatocellular carcinoma: similar long-term results despite geographic variations. *Liver Transpl.* 2004; 10(2 suppl 1):S74–S80.

Pawlik TM, Poon RT, Abdalla EK, et al. Hepatectomy for hepatocellular carcinoma with major portal or hepatic vein invasion: results of a multicenter study. *Surgery.* 2005;137(4):403–410.

Pawlik TM, Poon RT, Abdalla EK, et al. Hepatitis serology predicts tumor and liver-disease characteristics but not prognosis after resection of hepatocellular carcinoma. *J Gastrointest Surg.* 2004;8(7):794–804.

Pawlik TM, Scoggins CR, Zorzi D, et al. Effect of surgical margin status on survival and site of recurrence after hepatic resection for colorectal metastases. *Ann Surg.* 2005;241(5):715–722, discussion.

Poon RT, Fan ST. Evaluation of the new AJCC/UICC staging system for hepatocellular carcinoma after hepatic resection in Chinese patients. *Surg Oncol Clin N Am.* 2003;12(1):35–50, viii.

Poon RT, Fan ST. Hepatectomy for hepatocellular carcinoma: patient selection and postoperative outcome. *Liver Transpl.* 2004;10(2 suppl 1):S39–S45.

Poon RT, Fan ST, Lo CM, et al. Improving survival results after resection of hepatocellular carcinoma: a prospective study of 377 patients over 10 years. *Ann Surg.* 2001 ;234(1):63–70.

Poon RT, Fan ST, Lo CM, et al. Long-term survival and pattern of recurrence after resection of small hepatocellular carcinoma in patients with preserved liver function: implications for a strategy of salvage transplantation. *Ann Surg.* 2002; 235(3):373–382.

Poon RT, Fan ST, Ng IO, et al. Different risk factors and prognosis for early and late intrahepatic recurrence after resection of hepatocellular carcinoma. *Cancer.* 2000 ;89(3):500–507.

Poon RT, Fan ST, Ng IO, et al. Significance of resection margin in hepatectomy for hepatocellular carcinoma: a critical reappraisal. *Ann Surg.* 2000;231(4):544–551.

Poon RT, Fan ST, O'Suilleabhain CB, et al. Aggressive management of patients with extrahepatic and intrahepatic recurrences of hepatocellular carcinoma by combined resection and locoregional therapy. *J Am Coll Surg.* 2002;195(3):311–318.

Poon RT, Fan ST, Tsang FH, et al. Locoregional therapies for hepatocellular carcinoma: a critical review from the surgeon's perspective. *Ann Surg.* 2002;235(4): 466–486.

Poon RT, Fan ST, Wong J. Selection criteria for hepatic resection in patients with large hepatocellular carcinoma larger than 10 cm in diameter. *J Am Coll Surg.* 2002; 194(5):592–602.

Poon RT, Ng IO, Fan ST, et al. Clinicopathologic features of long-term survivors and disease-free survivors after resection of hepatocellular carcinoma: a study of a prospective cohort. *J Clin Oncol.* 2001; 19(12):3037–3044.

Rea DJ, Rosen CB, Nagorney DM, et al. Transplantation for cholangiocarcinoma: when and for whom? *Surg Clin N Am.* 2009; 18(2):325–337.

Regimbeau JM, Abdalla EK, Vauthey JN, et al. Risk factors for early death due to recurrence after liver resection for hepatocellular carcinoma: results of a multicenter study. *J Surg Oncol.* 2004;85(1):36–41.

Regimbeau JM, Kianmanesh R, Farges O, et al. Extent of liver resection influences the outcome in patients with cirrhosis and small hepatocellular carcinoma. *Surgery.* 2002;131(3):311–317.

Ribero D, Wang H, Donadon M, et al. Bevacizumab improves pathologic response and protects against hepatic injury in patients treated with oxaliplatin-based chemotherapy for colorectal liver metastases. *Cancer.* 2007;110(12):2761–2767.

Sala M, Varela M, Bruix J. Selection of candidates with HCC for transplantation in the MELD era. *Liver Transpl.* 2004;10(10 suppl 2):S4–S9.

Shirabe K, Shimada M, Gion T, et al. Postoperative liver failure after major hepatic resection for hepatocellular carcinoma in the modern era with special reference to remnant liver volume. *J Am Coll Surg.* 1999;188(3): 304–309.

Shirai Y, Yoshida K, Tsukada K, et al. Inapparent carcinoma of the gallbladder. An appraisal of a radical second operation after simple cholecystectomy. *Ann Surg.* 1992;215(4):326–331.

Smith DL, Soria JC, Morat L, et al. Human telomerase reverse transcriptase (hTERT) and Ki-67 are better predictors of survival than established clinical indicators in patients undergoing curative hepatic resection for colorectal metastases. *Ann Surg Oncol.* 2004;11(1):45–51.

Townsend CM, Sabiston DC. *Sabiston Textbook of Surgery: The Biological Basis of Modern Surgical Practice.* 17th ed. Philadelphia, PA: Elsevier; 2004.

Tuttle TM, Curley SA, Roh MS. Repeat hepatic resection as effective treatment of recurrent colorectal liver metastases. *Ann Surg Oncol.* 1997;4(2):125–130.

Vauthey JN, Abdalla EK, Doherty DA, et al. Body surface area and body weight predict total liver volume in Western adults. *Liver Transpl.* 2002;8(3):233–240.

Vauthey JN, Chaoui A, Do KA, et al. Standardized measurement of the future liver remnant prior to extended liver resection: methodology and clinical associations. *Surgery.* 2000;127(5):512–519.

Vauthey JN, Lauwers GY, Esnaola NF, et al. Simplified staging for hepatocellular carcinoma. *J Clin Oncol.* 2002;20(6):1527–1536.

Vauthey JN, Pawlik TM, Lauwers GY, et al. Critical evaluation of the different staging systems for hepatocellular carcinoma. *Br J Surg.* 2004;91(8):1072.

Vauthey JN, Sobin LH. On the uniform use of the AJCC/UICC staging system for hepatocellular carcinoma. *Surgery.* 2000; 128(5):870.

Wayne JD, Lauwers GY, Ikai I, et al. Preoperative predictors of survival after resection of small hepatocellular carcinomas. *Ann Surg.* 2002;235(5):722–730.

Yamamoto J, Sugihara K, Kosuge T, et al. Pathologic support for limited hepatectomy in the treatment of liver metastases from colorectal cancer. *Ann Surg.* 1995;221(1):74–78.

Yao FY, Ferrell L, Bass NM, et al. Liver transplantation for hepatocellular carcinoma: expansion of the tumor size limits does not adversely impact survival. *Hepatology.* 2001;33(6):1394–1403.

Yigitler C, Farges O, Kianmanesh R, et al. The small remnant liver after major liver resection: how common and how relevant? *Liver Transpl.* 2003;9(9):S18–S25.

Yoo HY, Patt CH, Geschwind JF, et al. The outcome of liver transplantation in patients with hepatocellular carcinoma in the United States between 1988 and 2001: 5-year survival has improved significantly with time. *J Clin Oncol.* 2003;21(23):4329–4335.

13

Pancreatic Adenocarcinoma

Debashish Bose, Matthew H. G. Katz, and Jason B. Fleming

EPIDEMIOLOGY

Pancreatic adenocarcinoma is the most common malignancy of the exocrine pancreas. The disease is the fourth most common cause of cancer-related death in the United States, with a yearly incidence of 11.7 deaths per 100,000 people. Despite advances in the diagnosis and treatment of pancreatic adenocarcinoma, the 5-year overall survival rate remains a dismal 5%, in part because the majority of patients present with advanced disease that precludes curative therapy. The overall risk of developing pancreatic cancer rises after age 50 years, and the majority of patients with the disease are between 60 and 80 years old.

Several inherited cancer syndromes are associated with pancreatic cancer, including Peutz-Jeghers syndrome, hereditary breast–ovarian cancer syndrome (associated with *BRCA1* or *BRCA2* mutations), familial atypical multiple mole melanoma syndrome, and possibly hereditary nonpolyposis colon cancer syndrome. Up to 10% of all pancreatic cancers are familial, and a person's risk of developing pancreatic cancer appears to increase with the number of people in his or her family who have the disease.

Significant risk factors for sporadic pancreatic cancer include cigarette smoking, alcoholism, and chronic pancreatitis. One case-control study of more than 1,600 patients revealed that smoking and diabetes acted synergistically with family history to increase the risk of pancreatic cancer. Another major study revealed that diabetes and elevated insulin concentrations were associated with a twofold higher risk of pancreatic cancer.

Despite the identification of several risk factors for this disease, pancreatic cancer screening is impractical because of the low prevalence of the disease in the general population and the lack of well-defined subgroups of patients who are at a high enough risk of pancreatic cancer to justify the morbidity and/or expense associated with currently available diagnostic procedures.

CLINICAL PRESENTATION

The clinical presentation of pancreatic cancer is variable and nonspecific. The most common symptom at presentation is jaundice related to extrahepatic biliary obstruction, which occurs in up to 50% of pancreatic cancer patients and is more common in patients with cancers of the pancreatic head than in patients with cancers of the pancreatic tail. Nonspecific complaints include constitutional symptoms, weight loss, and abdominal pain that often radiates to the back. Many patients diagnosed with pancreatic cancer have been recently diagnosed with diabetes, which may be related to peripheral insulin resistance induced by a tumor-derived factor such as islet amyloid polypeptide.

Pancreatic cancer patients' symptoms are often indicative of the stage of their disease and their overall prognosis. In particular, preoperative pain may be indicative of advanced cancer. Kelsen et al. (1997) found that patients who presented with pain had a shorter median overall survival than did patients who did not, regardless of the resectability status of their tumors.

Pancreatic cancer patients may also present with physical findings that may be helpful in assessing disease stage and prognosis. One retrospective study of 227 pancreatic cancer patients with disease that was radiographically determined to be resectable revealed that patients with cachexia had a lower resection rate than patients without cachexia (77.8% vs. 48.9%) and that cachexia was associated with lower overall survival rates among patients who underwent resection and patients who received only palliative care. More subtle signs of metastatic disease include enlargement of one or more left supraclavicular lymph nodes (Virchow node) or periumbilical lymph nodes (Sister Mary Joseph node). Rectal examination may reveal a Blumer shelf, which may indicate intraperitoneal tumor deposits. Ascites, a more common finding, may indicate carcinomatosis. Rarely, patients with advanced disease present with cutaneous nodules. A palpable gallbladder (Courvoisier sign) may indicate biliary obstruction but is not generally considered a sign of metastatic disease.

PREOPERATIVE EVALUATION

The two fundamental goals of the initial evaluation of a patient with a pancreatic mass suspicious for pancreatic cancer are (a) to secure or verify the histopathologic diagnosis of cancer and then (b) to accurately determine whether the primary cancer is anatomically resectable or unresectable.

Serum CA 19-9

The serum tumor marker used most frequently in the diagnostic workup of patients with suspected pancreatic cancer is carbohydrate antigen (CA) 19-9, a ganglioside Lewis blood group–associated antigen. An elevated level of CA 19-9 in the serum has a sensitivity of about 79% and a specificity of about 82% for identifying patients who have pancreatic cancer. Because biliary obstruction from any cause can elevate CA 19-9 levels, the specificity of CA 19-9 is reduced in the setting of cholestasis; therefore, serum bilirubin levels should always be measured alongside serum CA 19-9 levels. The diagnostic specificity of CA 19-9 may increase in the presence of certain other diagnostic findings. For example, a retrospective analysis of 150 patients who underwent surgery for suspected pancreatic cancer revealed that the combination of a serum CA 19-9 level >37 U/mL, weight loss of >20 lb, and a serum bilirubin level >3 mg/dL was associated with 100% sensitivity and a 100% positive predictive value for pancreatic cancer. Overall, a rational approach to diagnosing pancreatic cancer uses CA 19-9 in conjunction with other diagnostic modalities that include an exhaustive history and thorough physical examination.

CA 19-9 is also useful as a marker of disease stage that can be used to guide initial management in patients with localized cancers. Ferrone et al. (2006) analyzed CA 19-9 levels in a series of pancreatic cancer patients with serum bilirubin levels <2 mg/dL who underwent surgery for their disease and found that preoperative CA 19-9 levels correlated with the tumors' N and T stages. We recently found that a decrease in serum CA 19-9 levels over the course of neoadjuvant therapy for patients with potentially resectable pancreatic cancer was associated with the completion of all therapy including surgery; however, CA 19-9 had a low negative predictive value in this setting—a rise in CA 19-9 did not reliably indicate tumor progression and thus preclude successful tumor resection. In another study of pancreatic cancer patients with borderline resectable disease, we found that a decline in serum CA 19-9 levels over the course of neoadjuvant chemoradiation was associated with undergoing pancreatectomy and improved overall survival.

Radiologic Studies

Computed tomography (CT) remains the most important modality in the diagnostic workup of patients with suspected pancreatic cancer. CT is highly sensitive for the detection of pancreatic masses and provides the anatomic information necessary to determine disease stage and resectability. At M. D. Anderson Cancer Center, radiologists use dual-phase multidetector CT (MDCT) to identify (a) the presence of a primary tumor in the pancreas; (b) evidence of peritoneal or hepatic metastases; (c) the patency of the confluence of the superior mesenteric vein (SMV) and portal vein (PV) and these vessels' relation to the tumor; and (d) the relationship of the tumor to the superior mesenteric artery (SMA), celiac trunk, and hepatic artery.

MDCT images are obtained at 25 and 55 seconds after injection of 150 mL of ioversol (Optiray; 300 mg iodine/mL; Mallinkrodt, St. Louis, MO, USA) at a rate of 5 mL/second and ingestion of water as an oral contrast agent. In the pancreatic parenchymal phase of contrast enhancement, images are obtained at a 2.5-mm slice thickness with a table speed of 7.5 mm/second and then reconstructed to 1.25-mm contiguous images. Images in the portal venous phase are then obtained at a 5-mm slice thickness at a table speed of 15 mm/second and then reconstructed to 2.5-mm contiguous images. At M. D. Anderson, this protocol has a sensitivity and specificity of 93% and 72%, respectively, and positive and negative predictive values of 95% and 65%, respectively, for the detection of pancreatic cancers of any size. In addition, MDCT has a sensitivity of 92% for identifying locally advanced or metastatic (unresectable) disease, with a specificity of 91% and an overall accuracy of 92%. False negatives generally reflect occult vascular involvement or small liver or peritoneal metastases.

Endoscopy

Endoscopic instrumentation of the biliary tree is often used to place a decompressive stent to manage obstructive jaundice. Simultaneous endoscopic ultrasonography (EUS) may aid in diagnosis and is particularly valuable in the evaluation of smaller pancreatic lesions: EUS has an overall sensitivity of 99% and a sensitivity of 96% for tumors <2 cm in diameter. EUS can also be used to help assess the primary tumor's relationship to the mesenteric vasculature and regional lymph node involvement. EUS-guided fine-needle aspiration biopsy may then be used to secure a tissue diagnosis of the primary tumor and any suspicious regional lymph nodes.

Staging Laparotomy

Despite clear evidence that high-quality cross-sectional imaging accurately and reliably predicts the resectability of pancreatic tumors, many patients undergo laparotomy for suspected pancreatic cancer without having undergone adequate preoperative assessment with imaging studies. As a result, some patients who do not undergo preoperative imaging studies are found to have unresectable tumors only during surgery. In the past, when imaging technologies were less advanced and could not be used to reliably predict tumor resectability, many patients in whom tumors were found to be unresectable during surgery would have undergone surgical palliation aimed at relieving biliary obstruction, gastric outlet obstruction, and pain. Currently, however, minimally invasive and endoscopic techniques can be used to provide palliation without subjecting patients to open surgical exploration. Therefore, staging laparotomy has no role in the workup of patients with suspected pancreatic cancer.

Laparoscopy

Several studies have validated the use of laparoscopy in identifying subtle hepatic and peritoneal metastases that CT may not detect. Although some studies found that laparoscopy changed the management of up to 44% of pancreatic cancer patients with radiographically resectable disease, the yield of laparoscopy for cancer staging has decreased as imaging techniques have improved. A 2001 study showed that laparoscopic findings enabled laparotomy to be avoided in only 4% to 13% of patients who had disease that was radiographically determined to be resectable. And more recently, a large study of more than 1,000 patients revealed that laparoscopy was of even less benefit, especially among patients in whom high-quality CT had been recently performed.

At M. D. Anderson, we reserve laparoscopy for patients with large primary tumors, patients with cancers in the pancreatic body or tail, patients with markedly elevated levels of CA 19-9, patients with a history of severe weight loss and hypoalbuminemia, and patients with radiographic findings equivocal for the presence of metastatic disease or carcinomatosis. We rarely perform staging laparoscopy as a separate procedure. Given the simplicity of and the low morbidity associated with laparoscopy, we perform a diagnostic laparoscopy immediately before a planned laparotomy; if we find the mass to be resectable, we proceed to open surgery—but if the mass is not resectable, we are able to avoid an unnecessary laparotomy.

DISEASE STAGING

The current American Joint Committee on Cancer (AJCC) staging system for pancreatic cancer is summarized in Table 13.1. We use MDCT findings to prospectively stage pancreatic cancers as potentially resectable (AJCC stage I or II), borderline resectable (stage III), locally advanced (stage III), or metastatic (stage IV) (Table 13.2). Potentially resectable pancreatic cancer is characterized on cross-sectional imaging by (a) the absence of extrapancreatic disease, (b) a patent SMV–PV confluence, and (c) clear tissue planes between the tumor and the celiac axis, hepatic artery, and SMA. At M. D Anderson, we define borderline resectable pancreatic cancer by the absence of extrapancreatic disease and presence of one or more of the following: (a) tumor involvement or occlusion of the SMV–PV confluence amenable to surgical resection and reconstruction; (b) tumor abutment of

TABLE 13.1	American Joint Committee on Cancer (7th Edition) Classification and Staging of Pancreatic Cancer

Primary Tumor (T)

T1	Tumor ≤2 cm confined to pancreas
T2	Tumor >2 cm confined to pancreas
T3	Tumor extends beyond pancreas
T4	Tumor invades superior mesenteric artery or celiac axis

Regional Lymph Nodes (N)

N0	No regional lymph node metastasis
N1	Regional lymph node metastasis

Distant Metastasis (M)

M0	No distant metastasis
M1	Distant metastasis

Stage Grouping

Stage IA	T1	N0	M0
Stage IB	T2	N0	M0
Stage IIA	T3	N0	M0
Stage IIB	T1–T3	N1	M0
Stage III	T4	Any N	M0
Stage IV	Any T	Any N	M1

TABLE 13.2	Clinical/Radiologic Staging of Localized Pancreatic Cancer
Resectable	No encasement of the celiac axis or SMA
	Patient SMV–PV confluence
	No extrapancreatic disease
Borderline resectable	SMV–PV occlusion with anatomy sufficient for venous reconstruction
	Short segment abutment of SMA
	Short segment abutment or encasement of hepatic artery
Locally advanced	Encasement of SMA or celiac axis

SMA, superior mesenteric artery; SMV–PV, superior mesenteric vein–portal vein.

the SMA for less than 180 degrees or less of the vessel's circumference; or (c) tumor encasement of a short segment of the hepatic artery. (Recently, the American Hepatopancreaticobiliary Association and the Society of Surgical Oncology proposed a similar set of criteria for borderline resectable pancreatic cancer.) Locally advanced pancreatic cancer is characterized by tumor encasement of the SMA or celiac axis for greater than 180 degrees of the vessel's circumference in the absence of extrapancreatic disease. Metastatic disease is defined by radiographic or clinical evidence of metastases in distant organs or the peritoneum.

BILIARY STENTING

An endobiliary stent may be placed to palliate cholestasis symptoms in patients with malignant biliary obstruction before they undergo definitive surgery for pancreatic cancer. Biliary decompression may enable patients to temporarily postpone definitive therapy, during which time neoadjuvant therapy may be administered, referral to a tertiary care center may be coordinated, or a comprehensive preoperative evaluation of comorbidities may be performed. Endobiliary stenting may be performed by gastroenterologists in the community and need not be delayed.

We routinely employ endobiliary stents to relieve biliary obstruction in patients with potentially resectable pancreatic cancer; however, the practice remains controversial. In 1998, the Eastern Cooperative Oncology Group (ECOG) reported results of a phase II trial of preoperative chemoradiation and chemotherapy in which biliary stenting caused complications requiring hospitalization in 38% of patients and two patients' deaths. However, when we evaluated 154 patients at our institution who were enrolled in a trial of a similar preoperative therapy regimen, we found a much lower rate of stent-related complications, a lower rate of hospital admissions for stent complications (15%), and no stent-related deaths. We also investigated preoperative biliary decompression in a series of 300 consecutive patients who underwent pancreaticoduodenectomy and found that preoperative biliary decompression increased the risk of postoperative wound infection but not pancreatic fistula, intra-abdominal abscess, or perioperative death. In a subsequent study, we found no difference in perioperative morbidity or mortality between patients who did and patients who did not undergo biliary decompression, and we found no increased risk of perioperative morbidity or mortality in patients in whom expanding metal stents had been placed. Moreover, a cost analysis revealed that metal stents are less expensive than plastic stents by about $285,000 per 100 patients. Thus, our cumulative experience at M. D. Anderson supports the routine use of short, metal stents for preoperative biliary decompression.

SURGICAL TREATMENT

Surgical Considerations

The majority of pancreatic adenocarcinomas arise in the proximal gland. Such lesions are optimally treated surgically with pancreaticoduodenectomy. In contrast, distal lesions are treated with distal pancreatectomy, which typically includes splenectomy. Total pancreatectomy is generally avoided because of the high morbidity associated with the procedure and its adverse effects on pancreatic endocrine function. The surgical approach should be selected with the goal of achieving microscopically negative surgical margins (R0 resection).

Pancreaticoduodenectomy

Patients with potentially resectable pancreatic cancer as determined radiographically and with good performance status are eligible for resection. If diagnostic laparoscopy does not reveal extrapancreatic disease, the surgeon makes either a midline or bilateral subcostal incision and carefully inspects the liver and the peritoneum for evidence of radiographically occult metastatic disease. At M. D. Anderson, we do not routinely perform intraoperative frozen section analysis of regional lymph nodes in pancreatic cancer patients. Instead, the decision about frozen section analysis is made on an individual basis. For example, intraoperative frozen section analysis of regional lymph nodes is often performed in high-risk patients (patients with advanced age, significant medical comorbidities, high CA 19-9 serum levels, etc.). In such patients, the finding of metastatic disease in regional lymph nodes might suggest that pancreaticoduodenectomy is unjustified, even in the absence of visceral metastases.

To help organize a complex operation, minimize operative time, and provide a clear operative plan, we divide pancreaticoduodenectomy into six well-defined steps (Fig. 13.1).

1. A Cattell-Braasch maneuver is performed by mobilizing the right colon and incising the visceral peritoneum to the ligament of Treitz, which facilitates retraction of the right colon and small bowel, thereby exposing the duodenum. (Optimal duodenal exposure may not require a full Cattell-Braasch maneuver, and if vein resection is to be performed, excessive mobilization of the mesentery can cause unwanted axial motion that can twist and narrow venous anastomoses.) Access to the omental bursa is

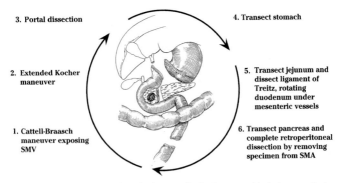

FIGURE 13.1 Six surgical steps of standard pancreaticoduodenectomy (clockwise resection). SMV, superior mesenteric vein; SMA, superior mesenteric artery. (From Tyler DS, Evans DB. Reoperative pancreaticoduodenectomy. *Ann Surg.* 1994;219:214, reprinted with permission.)

gained by separating the greater omentum from the transverse colon in the avascular plane. The infrapancreatic SMV is identified by following the course of the middle colic vein to the root of the mesentery.

2. The Kocher maneuver is performed to mobilize the duodenum and head of the pancreas to the level of the left renal vein.

3. Portal dissection is performed to expose the common hepatic artery both proximal and distal to the origin of the gastroduodenal artery. The gastroduodenal artery is then ligated and divided. The gallbladder is dissected from the liver, and the common hepatic duct is transected just cephalad to its junction with the cystic duct. The PV is exposed by dividing the common hepatic duct and performing cephalad retraction of the common hepatic artery; during this step, any variant hepatic artery anatomy must be identified to avoid hepatic injury and complications such as biliary fistulae (see later).

4. If the pylorus is to be preserved, the duodenum is transected 1 to 2 cm distal to the pylorus to preserve a cuff for anastomosis. Otherwise, a standard antrectomy is performed.

5. The jejunum is transected approximately 10 cm distal to the ligament of Treitz. The jejunal and duodenal mesenteries are sequentially ligated and divided to the level of the aorta. The duodenum and jejunum are then rotated beneath the mesenteric vessels.

6. The pancreas is transected using electrocautery at the level of the PV. The specimen is separated from the SMV by ligating and dividing the small venous tributaries to the uncinate process and the pancreatic head. The SMA is completely exposed, and the lateral aspect of the vessel is skeletonized in the periadventitial plane to its origin at the aorta. This step is crucial for achieving a negative SMA margin, which is one of the main drivers of good oncologic outcome. The specimen is then removed from the abdomen.

Reconstruction is initiated in a similar, but reverse, stepwise fashion (Fig. 13.2). The four steps of reconstruction are (a) end-to-side pancreaticojejunostomy; (b) end-to-side choledochojejunostomy; (c) end-to-side duodenojejunostomy or gastrojejunostomy; and (d) placement of a gastrostomy tube, a jejunostomy tube, and drains according to surgeon's preference. We do not routinely place a gastrostomy tube, and we reserve jejunostomy tubes for patients at high risk of nutritional deficiency following surgery.

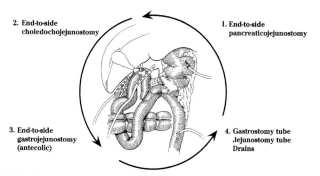

FIGURE 13.2 Four surgical steps of counterclockwise reconstruction following standard pancreaticoduodenectomy. (From Tyler DS, Evans DB. Reoperative pancreaticoduodenectomy. *Ann Surg.* 1994;219:214, reprinted with permission.)

Pylorus Preservation

We perform pylorus-preserving pancreaticoduodenectomy (PPPD) in many pancreatic cancer patients. PPPD is especially beneficial in patients who are at high risk of postoperative nutritional depletion, which may occur as a result of rapid gastrointestinal transit through the gastrojejunostomy after standard pancreaticoduodenectomy. PPPD may facilitate controlled gastric emptying, reduce intestinal transit time, and enhance intestinal absorption. For example, Klinkenbijl et al. (1999) reported that 47 patients who underwent PPPD had better weight gain during follow-up than 44 patients who underwent standard pancreaticoduodenectomy. While the nutritional advantage afforded by PPPD does not appear to confer a survival benefit, it may improve patients' quality of life. Han et al. (2007) reported that 44 patients who underwent PPPD had a better quality of life and higher nutritional status than 23 patients who underwent standard pancreaticoduodenectomy. In addition, one small series suggested that patients who underwent PPPD had better physical, but not necessarily mental, quality of life than patients who underwent standard pancreaticoduodenectomy. Relatively large trials and case series have not provided evidence that pylorus preservation increases delayed gastric emptying. We generally do not perform PPPD in patients with bulky neoplasms in the pancreatic head, patients with duodenal neoplasms involving the first portion of the duodenum, or patients with lesions associated with grossly positive pyloric or peripyloric lymph nodes.

Vascular Anatomic Variants

Important surgical issues may arise as a consequence of variant vascular anatomy, which can typically be identified on preoperative imaging studies. The most common arterial variant, which is observed in approximately 11% of patients who undergo surgery for pancreatic adenocarcinoma, is a replaced right hepatic artery (RRHA) that arises from the SMA rather than the proper hepatic artery. An RRHA typically courses posteriorly and superiorly from the SMA into the porta hepatis behind the uncinate and head of the pancreas, where it may be encased by tumor. The consequences of sacrifice of the RRHA include poor liver perfusion, compromise of the hepaticojejunostomy, and biliary fistula. Although an RRHA may be reconstructed, dissection of the vessel from the adjacent tumor is often successful. In some patients, an RRHA may actually represent an accessory vessel, be occluded by the tumor, or contribute little perfusion because of its diminutive size; in these rare cases, the vessel may be resected with little consequence. However, because approximately 2.5% of patients have a replaced common hepatic artery that originates at the SMA and follows the same posterior course as an RRHA, great care must be taken to clearly dissect the portal vasculature to ensure the hepatic arterial blood supply before contemplating removal. We also assess back bleeding from the distal vessel to determine whether we need to reconstruct an RRHA that has been removed to achieve tumor extirpation.

One patient in 10 has a replaced left hepatic artery, which typically arises from the left gastric artery. In rare instances, a vessel thought to be a replaced left hepatic artery may actually be an accessory vessel or a replaced common hepatic artery. The preservation of such rostral vessels does not typically present a challenge unless the tumor is bulky and/or involves the arteries directly.

A small number of other variations in hepatic arterial supply—typically variations at the celiac axis or hepatic arteries deriving directly from the aorta—have been reported. Surgeons planning pancreaticoduodenectomy should be alert to these possibilities and attempt to identify anomalous vascular anatomy on preoperative imaging studies.

Vascular Resection

Vascular involvement, particularly involvement of the SMV–PV, no longer represents an absolute contraindication to pancreatic tumor resection. Preoperative imaging can predict the need for vascular resection in approximately 84% of patients who will need it. We found that resecting and reconstructing the SMV–PV confluence at pancreaticoduodenectomy is both safe and associated with an overall survival rate similar to that of patients who do not require venous resection to achieve negative surgical margins. Although procedures requiring venous resection may result in a positive retroperitoneal margin, this does not translate into shorter overall survival. Others have reported similar results. At our institution, most patients with tumors that involve the SMV or PV receive preoperative chemotherapy and/or chemoradiation. Venous resection should be attempted only to achieve a negative resection margin and not as part of an en bloc regional pancreatectomy.

Unlike venous resection and reconstruction, arterial resection is generally unjustified during pancreaticoduodenectomy. The exception is the resection and reconstruction of the common hepatic artery, which may be performed in certain circumstances to achieve negative surgical margins. When common hepatic artery involvement is evident on MDCT, we usually offer patients preoperative chemoradiation before attempting tumor resection.

ADJUVANT THERAPY

In the first study of adjuvant chemoradiation for patients with resectable pancreatic cancer, the Gastrointestinal Study Group reported in 1985 that patients who were treated postoperatively with 5-FU–based chemoradiation had significantly longer median overall survival (21.0 months) than patients who underwent surgery alone (10.9 months), thus establishing 5-FU as the standard for postoperative chemoradiation. However, subsequent trials conducted by the European Organization for Research and Treatment of Cancer (EORTC) and the European Study Group for Pancreatic Cancer (ESPAC) did not confirm that a clear survival advantage was associated with the use of chemoradiation. Indeed, the ESPAC-1 trial suggested that chemoradiation was actually harmful.

More recently, the Charite Onkologie and the Radiation Therapy Oncology Group evaluated the role of adjuvant systemic gemcitabine after pancreatic cancer resection. The Charite Onkologie trial found that postoperative gemcitabine was associated with significantly increased disease-free and overall survival relative to surgery alone. To examine the relative efficacy of systemic gemcitabine and 5-FU, the Radiation Therapy Oncology Group trial randomized patients to receive either gemcitabine or 5-FU for 3 weeks, followed by 5-FU–based chemoradiation and then 12 weeks of continued chemotherapy. Patients treated with gemcitabine had a median overall survival of 20.5 months, whereas patients who received 5-FU had a median overall survival of 16.9 months. This difference was different on multivariate ($P = 0.05$) but not on univariate ($P = 0.09$) analysis. Based on the results of these studies, the National Comprehensive Cancer Network currently recommends either chemotherapy alone or chemotherapy followed by chemoradiation as adjuvant treatments for pancreatic cancer patients who have undergone tumor resection.

Interferon-based chemoradiation has also been used as an adjuvant therapy in pancreatic cancer patients who have undergone tumor resection. Picozzi et al. (2003) found interferon-based chemoradiation to be associated with favorable survival, reporting 1-, 2-, and 5-year overall survival rates of 95%, 64%, and 55%, respectively. An ACOSOG trial of interferon-based adjuvant chemoradiation demonstrated a median overall survival duration of 25.4 months but was closed early because of the regimen's unacceptable toxicity. In a recent randomized phase III trial, patients treated with interferon-based chemoradiation had a lower risk of local recurrence than patients treated with 5-FU/folinic acid chemotherapy alone; however, the difference between the two groups' median overall survival durations was not significant (32.1 months vs. 28.5 months), and 68% of the patients in the interferon arm developed grade 3 or 4 toxicities. Nevertheless, given the poor outcomes with current 5-FU–based adjuvant therapy, interferon-based adjuvant therapy warrants further investigation in pancreatic cancer patients.

NEOADJUVANT THERAPY

Resectable Tumors

We routinely offer preoperative adjuvant—that is, neoadjuvant—therapy to patients with resectable or borderline resectable pancreatic cancer. Our overall management algorithm is depicted in Fig. 13.3. In five neoadjuvant chemoradiation trials that were conducted at our institution, the longest median overall survival duration was 34 months for patients who received neoadjuvant gemcitabine-based chemoradiation and underwent tumor resection. In the most recent study, the addition of systemic gemcitabine and cisplatin prior to gemcitabine-based chemoradiation did not appear to improve the survival duration.

Neoadjuvant therapy is offered to all patients with resectable pancreatic cancer in part because the disease recurs in 80% to 90% of patients who undergo potentially curative resection. In addition, 25% to 30% of pancreatic cancer patients who undergo disease resection ultimately do not receive preoperative adjuvant therapy for reasons related to the surgery (e.g., complications, nutritional impairment) and the disease itself (e.g., disease progression, decline in performance status). Delivering adjuvant therapy before surgery enables patients to receive systemic therapy immediately and ensures that all patients who undergo resection receive systemic therapy. Neoadjuvant therapy also facilitates the selection of patients for surgery who are most likely to benefit; patients with clinically occult but progressive systemic disease can often be identified during the preoperative therapy period and spared the potential morbidity associated with pancreatic resection.

A number of studies' findings support the use of neoadjuvant treatment in patients with resectable pancreatic cancer. White et al. (2001) found that

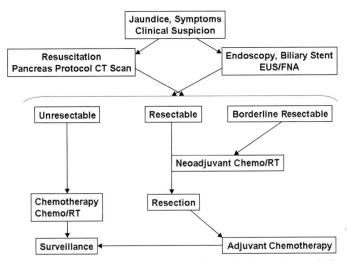

FIGURE 13.3 Simplified algorithm for the management of pancreatic adenocarcinoma at M. D. Anderson. CT, computed tomographic; EUS/FNA, endoscopic ultrasonography with fine-needle aspiration; RT, radiation therapy.

neoadjuvant therapy with 5-FU–based chemoradiation was associated with a significantly higher rate of R0 resection (70%) than postoperative adjuvant therapy (36%). In a retrospective study of 116 pancreatic cancer patients who underwent disease resection, Sasson et al. (2003) found that the patients who received neoadjuvant 5-FU plus mitomycin C or neoadjuvant gemcitabine, given concurrently with external-beam radiation therapy (50.4 Gy), had a longer median survival duration (23 months) than the 55 patients who did not receive neoadjuvant therapy (16 months); the longer survival in the neoadjuvant therapy group may have been due to the group's lower rate of margin positivity. Another retrospective review revealed that the median overall survival of 19 patients who had R0 resections after neoadjuvant gemcitabine-based chemoradiation (54 months) was longer than that of 45 patients who had R0 resections alone (23 months). A recent analysis of Surveillance, Epidemiology, and End Results registry data revealed that the median overall survival durations for patients who received neoadjuvant radiation therapy, patients with resectable pancreatic cancer who received adjuvant radiation therapy, and patients who did not receive radiation therapy were 23, 17, and 12 months, respectively. A phase II trial in the United Kingdom demonstrated that neoadjuvant chemotherapy with gemcitabine and cisplatin was associated with a high rate of R0 resection. Taken together, these studies' findings and our own experience suggest that neoadjuvant therapy helps optimize patient selection for surgery and may increase rates of R0 resection.

Borderline Resectable Tumors

We employ neoadjuvant therapy when treating pancreatic cancer patients with borderline resectable disease. In a series of 160 pancreatic cancer patients with borderline resectable disease who were evaluated and treated at our center, 125 patients (78%) were able to complete preoperative treatment and testing. The median overall survival duration of the 66 patients (41%) who were able to undergo resection was 40 months. Although various regimens were used to treat the patients in this series, systemic chemotherapy followed by chemoradiation was the most frequently used strategy. Ideally, pancreatic cancer patients with borderline resectable disease should be treated in the setting of a clinical trial in centers with multidisciplinary expertise.

Treatment Outcomes

In 2009, we published our cumulative institutional experience with the surgical treatment of patients with localized pancreatic cancer. Three hundred twenty-nine patients treated between 1990 and 2002 were evaluated. Two hundred fifty-three (77%) patients received neoadjuvant chemotherapy and/or chemoradiation. Most patients (302, 92%) underwent pancreaticoduodenectomy. A total of 108 (33%) patients underwent vascular resection and reconstruction. Involved regional lymph nodes were identified in 157 (48%) of patients and margins were microscopically positive in 52 (16%) patients. The median overall survival was 23.9 months and 88 (27%) patients survived a minimum of 5 years.

Other specialist centers have reported similar results for patients who underwent pancreaticoduodenectomy for pancreatic adenocarcinoma. Of 1,175 patients who underwent pancreatic adenocarcinoma resection at Johns Hopkins, 42% had positive resection margins and 78% had nodal disease; the median overall survival was 18 months. Among 696 patients who underwent resection for pancreatic adenocarcinoma at Memorial Sloan-Kettering Cancer Center, patients without nodal disease had a longer median overall survival duration (27 months) than patients with nodal disease (16 months). At the Mayo Clinic, 466 patients who underwent pancreaticoduodenectomy had a median overall survival of 21.6 months, and patients who received postoperative adjuvant chemoradiation had a median overall survival of 25.2 months; positive lymph node status and tumor grade were significant negative predictors of overall survival.

SURVEILLANCE

We typically see patients every 4 months for the first 2 years following potentially curative resection with a computed tomographic scan of the abdomen, chest x-ray, and CA 19-9 level. Visits are spread out to every 6 months after 2 years and yearly after 5 years.

Recommended Readings

Abrams RA, Lowy AM, O'Reilly EM, et al. Combined modality treatment of resectable and borderline resectable pancreas cancer: expert consensus statement. *Ann Surg Oncol.* 2009;16(7):1751–1756.

Bachmann J, Heiligensetzer M, Krakowski-Roosen H, et al. Cachexia worsens prognosis in patients with resectable pancreatic cancer. *J Gastrointest Surg.* 2008;12(7): 1193–1201.

Balachandran A, Darden DL, Tamm EP, et al. Arterial variants in pancreatic adenocarcinoma. *Abdom Imaging.* 2008;33(2):214–221.

Bold RJ, Charnsangavej C, Cleary KR, et al. Major vascular resection as part of pancreaticoduodenectomy for cancer: radiologic, intraoperative, and pathologic analysis. *J Gastrointest Surg.* 1999;3(3): 233–243.

Breslin TM, Hess KR, Harbison DB, et al. Neoadjuvant chemoradiotherapy for adenocarcinoma of the pancreas: treatment variables and survival duration. *Ann Surg Oncol.* 2001;8(2):123–132.

Callery MP, Chang KJ, Fishman EK, et al. Pretreatment assessment of resectable and borderline resectable pancreatic cancer: expert consensus statement. *Ann Surg Oncol.* 2009;16(7):1727–1733.

Corsini MM, Miller RC, Haddock MG, et al. Adjuvant radiotherapy and chemotherapy for pancreatic carcinoma: the Mayo Clinic experience (1975-2005). *J Clin Oncol.* 2008;26(21):3511–3516.

Diener MK, Heukaufer C, Schwarzer G, et al. Pancreaticoduodenectomy (classic Whipple) versus pylorus-preserving pancreaticoduodenectomy (pp Whipple) for surgical treatment of periampullary and pancreatic carcinoma. *Cochrane Database Syst Rev.* 2008(2):CD006053.

Evans DB, Farnell MB, Lillemoe KD, et al. Surgical treatment of resectable and borderline resectable pancreas cancer: expert consensus statement. *Ann Surg Oncol.* 2009;16(7):1736–1744.

Evans DB, Multidisciplinary Pancreatic Cancer Study Group. Resectable pancreatic cancer: the role for neoadjuvant/preoperative therapy. *HPB (Oxford).* 2006;8(5): 365–368.

Evans DB, Rich TA, Byrd DR, et al. Preoperative chemoradiation and pancreaticoduodenectomy for adenocarcinoma of the pancreas. *Arch Surg.* 1992;127(11): 1335–1339.

Evans DB, Varadhachary GR, Crane CH, et al. Preoperative gemcitabine-based chemoradiation for patients with resectable adenocarcinoma of the pancreatic head. *J Clin Oncol.* 2008;26(21):3496–3502.

Ferrone CR, Finkelstein DM, Thayer SP, et al. Perioperative CA 19-9 levels can predict stage and survival in patients with resectable pancreatic adenocarcinoma. *J Clin Oncol.* 2006;24(18):2897–2902.

Goonetilleke KS, Siriwardena AK. Systematic review of carbohydrate antigen (CA 19-9) as a biochemical marker in the diagnosis of pancreatic cancer. *Eur J Surg Oncol.* 2007;33(3):266–270.

Hassan MM, Bondy ML, Wolff RA, et al. Risk factors for pancreatic cancer: case-control study. *Am J Gastroenterol.* 2007; 102(12):2696–2707.

Han SS, Kim SW, Jang JY, et al. A comparison of the long-term functional outcomes of standard pancreatoduodenectomy and pylorus-preserving pancreatoduodenectomy. *Hepatogastroenterology.* 2007; 54(78):1831–1835.

Hoffman JP, Lipsitz S, Pisansky T, et al. Phase II trial of preoperative radiation therapy and chemotherapy for patients with localized, resectable adenocarcinoma of the pancreas: an Eastern Cooperative Oncology Group Study. *J Clin Oncol.* 1998;16(1):317–323.

Hruban RH, Canto MI, Yeo CJ. Prevention of pancreatic cancer and strategies for management of familial pancreatic cancer. *Dig Dis.* 2001;19(1):76–84.

Iqbal N, Lovegrove RE, Tilney HS, et al. A comparison of pancreaticoduodenectomy with pylorus preserving pancreaticoduo-denectomy: a meta-analysis of 2822 patients. *Eur J Surg Oncol.* 2008;34(11): 1237–1245.

Jemal A, Siegel R, Xu J, Ward E. Cancer statistics, 2010. *CA Cancer J Clin.* 2010;60(5): 277–300.

Kalser MH, Ellenberg SS. Pancreatic cancer. Adjuvant combined radiation and chemotherapy following curative resection. *Arch Surg.* 1985;120(8):899–903.

Katz MH, Pisters PW, Evans DB, et al. Borderline resectable pancreatic cancer: the importance of this emerging stage of disease. *J Am Coll Surg.* 2008;206(5):833–846; discussion 846–848.

Katz MH, Varadhachary GR, Fleming JB, et al. Serum CA 19-9 as a marker of resectability and survival in patients with potentially resectable pancreatic cancer treated with neoadjuvant chemoradiation. *Ann Surg Oncol.* 2010;17(7): 1794–1801.

Katz MH, Wang H, Fleming JB, et al. Long-term survival after multidisciplinary management of resected pancreatic adenocarcinoma. *Ann Surg Oncol.* 2009;16(4):836–847.

Kelsen DP, Portenoy R, Thaler H, et al. Pain as a predictor of outcome in patients with operable pancreatic carcinoma. *Surgery.* 1997;122(1):53–59.

Klinkenbijl JH, Jeekel J, Sahmoud T, et al. Adjuvant radiotherapy and 5-fluorouracil after curative resection of cancer of the pancreas and periampullary region: phase III trial of the EORTC gastrointestinal tract cancer cooperative group. *Ann Surg.* 1999;230(6):776–782; discussion 782–784.

Klinkenbijl JH, Van Der Schelling GP, Hop WC, et al. The advantages of pylorus-preserving pancreatoduodenectomy in malignant disease of the pancreas and periampullary region. *Ann Surg.* 1992; 216(2):142–145.

Marten A SJ, Debus J, Harig S, et al. CapRI: final results of the open-label, multicenter, randomized phase III trial of adjuvant chemoradiation plus interferon-a2b (CRI) versus 5-FU alone for patients with resected pancreatic adenocarcinoma (PAC). *J Clin Oncol.* 2010;28(suppl 18).

Mullen JT, Lee JH, Gomez HF, et al. Pancreaticoduodenectomy after placement of endobiliary metal stents. *J Gastrointest Surg.* 2005;9(8):1094–1104; discussion 1104–1105.

Neoptolemos JP, Stocken DD, Friess H, et al. A randomized trial of chemoradiotherapy and chemotherapy after resection of pancreatic cancer. *N Engl J Med.* 2004; 350(12):1200–1210.

Neuhaus P, Riess H, Post S, et al. CONKO-001: Final results of the randomized, prospective, multicenter phase III trial of adjuvant chemotherapy with gemcitabine versus observation in patients with resected pancreatic cancer (PC). *J Clin Oncol.* 2008;26(suppl).

Nukui Y, Picozzi VJ, Traverso LW. Interferon-based adjuvant chemoradiation therapy improves survival after pancreaticoduodenectomy for pancreatic adenocarcinoma. *Am J Surg.* 2000;179(5):367–371.

Oettle H, Post S, Neuhaus P, et al. Adjuvant chemotherapy with gemcitabine vs observation in patients undergoing curative-intent resection of pancreatic cancer: a randomized controlled trial. *JAMA.* 2007;297(3):267–277.

Pancreatic Adenocarcinoma. NCCN Clinical Practice Guidelines in Oncology, 2009 [Available from: NCCN.org].

Picozzi VJ, Kozarek RA, Traverso LW. Interferon-based adjuvant chemoradiation therapy after pancreaticoduodenectomy for pancreatic adenocarcinoma. *Am J Surg.* 2003;185(5):476–480.

Pingpank JF, Hoffman JP, Ross EA, et al. Effect of preoperative chemoradiotherapy on surgical margin status of resected adenocarcinoma of the head of the pancreas. *J Gastrointest Surg.* 2001;5(2):121–130.

Pisters PW, Hudec WA, Hess KR, et al. Effect of preoperative biliary decompression on pancreaticoduodenectomy-associated morbidity in 300 consecutive patients. *Ann Surg.* 2001;234(1):47–55.

Pisters PW, Hudec WA, Lee JE, et al. Preoperative chemoradiation for patients with pancreatic cancer: toxicity of endobiliary stents. *J Clin Oncol.* 2000;18(4):860–867.

Pisters PW, Lee JE, Vauthey JN, et al. Laparoscopy in the staging of pancreatic cancer. *Br J Surg.* 2001;88(3):325–337.

Pisters PW, Wolff RA, Janjan NA, et al. Preoperative paclitaxel and concurrent rapid-fractionation radiation for resectable pancreatic adenocarcinoma: toxicities, histologic response rates, and event-free outcome. *J Clin Oncol.* 2002;20(10): 2537–2544.

Raut CP, Tseng JF, Sun CC, et al. Impact of resection status on pattern of failure and survival after pancreaticoduodenectomy for pancreatic adenocarcinoma. *Ann Surg.* 2007;246(1):52–60.

Regine WF, Winter KA, Abrams RA, et al. Fluorouracil vs gemcitabine chemotherapy before and after fluorouracil-based chemoradiation following resection of pancreatic adenocarcinoma: a randomized controlled trial. *JAMA.* 2008;299(9): 1019–1026.

Sasson AR, Wetherington RW, Hoffman JP, et al. Neoadjuvant chemoradiotherapy for adenocarcinoma of the pancreas: analysis of histopathology and outcome. *Int J Gastrointest Cancer.* 2003;34(2–3):121–128.

Smeenk HG, van Eijck CH, Hop WC, et al. Long-term survival and metastatic pattern of pancreatic and periampullary cancer after adjuvant chemoradiation or observation: long-term results of EORTC trial 40891. *Ann Surg.* 2007;246(5):734–740.

Stessin AM, Meyer JE, Sherr DL. Neoadjuvant radiation is associated with improved survival in patients with resectable pancreatic cancer: an analysis of data from the surveillance, epidemiology, and end results (SEER) registry. *Int J Radiat Oncol Biol Phys.* 2008;72(4):1128–1133.

Tamm EP, Loyer EM, Faria SC, et al. Retrospective analysis of dual-phase MDCT and follow-up EUS/EUS-FNA in the diagnosis of pancreatic cancer. *Abdom Imaging.* 2007;32(5):660–667.

Tamm EP, Loyer EM, Faria S, et al. Staging of pancreatic cancer with multidetector CT in the setting of preoperative chemoradiation therapy. *Abdom Imaging.* 2006; 31(5):568–574.

Tseng JF, Raut CP, Lee JE, et al. Pancreaticoduodenectomy with vascular resection: margin status and survival duration. *J Gastrointest Surg.* 2004;8(8):935–949; discussion 949–950.

Varadhachary GR, Tamm EP, Abbruzzese JL, et al. Borderline resectable pancreatic cancer: definitions, management, and role of preoperative therapy. *Ann Surg Oncol.* 2006;13(8):1035–1046.

Varadhachary GR, Wolff RA, Crane CH, et al. Preoperative gemcitabine and cisplatin followed by gemcitabine-based chemoradiation for resectable adenocarcinoma of the pancreatic head. *J Clin Oncol.* 2008;26(21):3487–3495.

White RR, Hurwitz HI, Morse MA, et al. Neoadjuvant chemoradiation for localized adenocarcinoma of the pancreas. *Ann Surg Oncol.* 2001;8(10):758–765.

White RR, Xie HB, Gottfried MR, et al. Significance of histological response to preoperative chemoradiotherapy for pancreatic cancer. *Ann Surg Oncol.* 2005;12(3):214–221.

White R, Winston C, Gonen M, et al. Current utility of staging laparoscopy for pancreatic and peripancreatic neoplasms. *J Am Coll Surg.* 2008;206(3):445–450.

Winter JM, Cameron JL, Campbell KA, et al. 1423 pancreaticoduodenectomies for pancreatic cancer: a single-institution experience. *J Gastrointest Surg.* 2006; 10(9): 1199–1210; discussion 1210–1211.

Yekebas EF, Bogoevski D, Cataldegirmen G, et al. En bloc vascular resection for locally advanced pancreatic malignancies infiltrating major blood vessels: perioperative outcome and long-term survival in 136 patients. *Ann Surg.* 2008;247(2): 300–309.

14

Pancreatic Endocrine Tumors and Multiple Endocrine Neoplasia

Christine S. Landry and Jeffrey E. Lee

SPORADIC PANCREATIC ENDOCRINE TUMORS

Pancreatic endocrine tumors (PETs), which arise from pancreatic islet cells, account for 1.3% to 3% of pancreatic malignancies. PETs may be functional or nonfunctional, and the clinical manifestations are dependent on the specific hormones produced (Table 14.1). There is no generally accepted international staging system for PETs. The behavior of these tumors ranges from benign and indolent to malignant and aggressive. Recent series have suggested that metastatic disease, tumor size, neurovascular invasion, mitotic index, Ki-67 protein index, nuclear atypia, tumor grade, and associated clinical syndromes may impact overall survival.

Nonfunctioning Pancreatic Endocrine Tumors

Fifty-eight to eighty-five percent of PETs are nonfunctional, and they occur more commonly in the pancreatic head. PETs are often diagnosed late in the course of the disease because symptoms do not become evident until they grow large enough to compress adjacent structures. Patients with nonfunctioning PETs usually present with abdominal pain, weight loss, obstructive jaundice, or other obstructive symptoms. The median overall survival duration among all patients with nonfunctioning PETs is approximately 3.2 years; 7.1 years in patients with localized disease who have a potentially curative resection; 5.2 years in patients with locally advanced, unresectable nonmetastatic disease; and 2.1 years in patients with unresectable metastatic disease.

Diagnosis

Nonfunctioning PETs are usually diagnosed with computed tomography (CT) or magnetic resonance imaging (MRI). They have a hypervascular appearance on radiographic images. CT, MRI, and ultrasonography detect: 20% of PETs <1 cm in size, 30% to 40% of PETs 1 to 3 cm in size, and 75% of PETs >3 cm in size. The most sensitive technique for identifying small PETs is endoscopic ultrasound (EUS), which can detect neoplasms as small as 0.3 cm in size. Because PETs and pancreatic adenocarcinomas have similar radiographic features, EUS may be needed to obtain a pathologic diagnosis before treatment is initiated. EUS can also be helpful in defining the extent and distribution of multiple PETs often associated with patients who have inherited endocrine tumor syndromes (e.g., multiple endocrine neoplasia type 1 [MEN1]). Octreotide imaging may be useful when planning surgical intervention because this modality assists with tumor localization and occasionally identifies occult regional lymph node metastases.

Nonfunctioning PETs may secrete a variety of hormones whose effects are not clinically apparent. For instance, as many as 75% of patients with nonfunctioning PETs have elevated fasting pancreatic polypeptide levels. Chromogranin A levels are elevated in 60% to 100% of patients with PETs. However, chromogranin A levels may be falsely elevated in older patients, alcoholic patients, patients with inflammatory conditions, patients with renal failure, and patients consuming proton pump inhibitors (PPIs).

TABLE 14.1 Functional Pancreatic Endocrine Tumors

Pancreatic Endocrine Tumor	Hormone	Pancreatic Cell Type	Clinical Manifestation	Diagnostic Test	Unique Tumor Localization Tests
Gastrinoma	Gastrin	D	Peptic ulcer disease	• Fasting serum gastrin level • Basal acid output to maximal acid output ratio • Basal acid output >15 mEq/h • Nocturnal (12 h) gastric acid secretion test • Secretin stimulation test	Abdominal angiography with selective arterial secretin injection
Insulinoma	Insulin	Beta	Hypoglycemia with symptom relief after glucose administration	Monitored 72-h fast	Intra-arterial calcium stimulation test
VIPoma	Vasoactive intestinal polypeptide	A–D	Watery diarrhea, hypokalemia, achlorhydria, dehydration	Fasting plasma vasoactive intestinal polypeptide level	None
Glucagonoma	Glucagon	Alpha	Diabetes, necrolytic migratory erythema, weight loss, depression, psychosis, venous thrombosis	Fasting plasma glucagon level	None
Somatostatinoma	Somatostatin	Delta	Mild diabetes, cholelithiasis, steatorrhea, weight loss, anemia, diarrhea	Fasting plasma somatostatin level	None

Treatment

Surgical resection with regional lymph node dissection is the only potentially cura-tive therapy for patients with localized nonfunctioning PETs. The anatomic consid-erations for determining the resectability of and the surgical approaches for nonfunctioning PETs are the same as those for pancreatic adenocarcinomas. (Please see Chapter 13, Pancreatic Adenocarcinoma, for specific information about the pre-operative radiographic evaluation of pancreatic tumors that determine resectability and the surgical strategies for patients with resectable disease.) As patients with locally advanced nonfunctioning PETs often have favorable survival durations, incomplete resection or tumor debulking of nonfunctioning PETs is not recom-mended because of the potential considerable morbidity associated with palliative pancreatic resection. There is no standard adjuvant systemic therapy for patients who undergo potentially curative surgical resection. Careful follow-up after surgery is essential; up to 50% of patients who undergo complete resection develop meta-chronous liver metastasis. Distant metastatic disease (e.g., solitary liver metastasis) should be resected if possible. Patients with unresectable hepatic metastases may benefit from radiofrequency ablation or Yttrium-90 radioembolization.

Since effective systemic treatment options for patients with unresectable locally advanced or metastatic PETs remain limited, and since PETs are often bio-logically indolent, initial observation without specific systemic therapy is an acceptable strategy for selected patients, particularly in the absence of symptoms. Patients with unresectable locally advanced or metastatic PETs who have symp-toms or evidence of disease progression on serial imaging may be considered for systemic therapy. Systemic treatment options include streptozocin-based chemo-therapy, octreotide (long-acting release form, LAR), and protocol-based therapies. At M. D. Anderson, streptozocin, doxorubicin, and 5-fluorouracil have elicited a tumor response in up to 39% of patients with nonfunctioning PETs. Alternatively (especially for patients with relatively indolent tumors), octreotide LAR has recently been demonstrated to lengthen time to progression in patients with metastatic neuroendocrine tumors. Lanreotide, another somatostatin analogue, has been shown to have some antiproliferative effects on metastatic PETs when used alone or in combination with interferon-alpha. Other promising therapies for patients with metastatic PETs include mammalian target of Rapamycin (mTOR) inhibitors, vascular endothelial growth factor (VEGF) inhibitors, and hepatic chemoemboliza-tion or radionuclide embolization.

Functioning Pancreatic Endocrine Tumors

Insulinoma

In 1935, Whipple and Frantz first described the clinical manifestations of insulinoma as a triad of hypoglycemic symptoms while fasting, blood glucose levels <50 mg/dL, and symptomatic relief after glucose administration (Whipple's triad). Insulinomas are the most common type of functioning PET; approximately 10% exhibit malignant behavior, 10% are associated with MEN1, and 10% are multiple. Insulinomas overse-crete insulin, and the resultant hypoglycemic episodes are exacerbated during peri-ods of fasting or exercise. During an insulin surge, patients may develop a sympathetic overdrive characterized by sweating, weakness, tremors, hyperphasia, and palpitations. Neuroglycopenic symptoms including confusion, visual changes, altered consciousness, and convulsions have also been associated with insulinomas.

Diagnosis. The most reliable test for diagnosing insulinomas is a monitored 72-hour fast, during which the patient's plasma glucose, C-peptide, proinsulin, and insulin levels are measured every 4 to 6 hours. The test is continued until the plasma glucose level is <45 mg/dL and the patient develops hypoglycemic symptoms; 33% of patients become symptomatic within 12 hours, 80% within 24 hours, 90% within 48 hours, and 100% within 72 hours. The diagnosis of insulinoma is established by a serum insulin concentration ≥6 μU/mL, an insulin-to-glucose ratio >0.3, a C-peptide level ≥0.2 nmol/L, a proinsulin level ≥5 pmol/L, and a documented absence of plasma sulfonylurea. Patients who self-administer exogenous forms of insulin usually have low C-peptide and proinsulin levels because commercial insulin does not contain insulin precursor or cleavage fragments. Patients who consume oral hypoglycemic agents may have elevated C-peptide and proinsulin levels; however, these patients can be differentiated from insulinoma patients in that only insulinoma patients will have an absence of plasma sulfonylurea.

Depending on the size of the tumors, insulinomas may be visualized by CT, MRI, or EUS. Octreotide imaging is of limited use because many insulinomas (especially smaller ones) do not express somatostatin receptor-2. Although rarely necessary nowadays because of improvements in cross-sectional abdominal imaging and EUS, selective intra-arterial calcium injection of major pancreatic arteries with hepatic venous sampling (calcium arterial stimulation test) has been reported to successfully regionalize tumors in more than 80% of patients with insulinomas. A twofold increase in insulin after intra-arterial calcium infusion (0.025 mEq/kg) identifies the arterial distribution supplying the tumor. Lesions in the head and neck of the pancreas are characterized by elevated insulin levels in the superior mesenteric artery or gastroduodenal artery, whereas lesions in the pancreatic tail are characterized by elevated insulin levels in the splenic artery. Liver metastases demonstrate a response after calcium injection into the hepatic artery.

Treatment. The primary treatment for sporadic insulinoma is surgical resection. The median disease-free survival after resection of malignant insulinoma is approximately 5 years.

Before surgery, glucose levels should be controlled with frequent small meals and diazoxide, a drug that inhibits insulin release and promotes glycogenolysis. The operation is directed by the results of preoperative imaging; intraoperative ultrasound can be used to definitively localize small tumors deep in the pancreatic parenchyma as well as liver metastases. When possible, enucleation should be performed. Larger lesions require pancreatic resection (pancreaticoduodenectomy, distal pancreatectomy, or, in selected patients, central pancreatectomy) depending on the location of the neoplasm. Pancreatic resection is also indicated if there are signs of malignancy (i.e., lymph node metastasis and/or local invasion). If no tumor can be localized at the time of operative intervention, the surgeon may perform a pancreatic biopsy to rule out beta cell hyperplasia or adult nesidioblastosis. Blind distal pancreatectomy is no longer recommended when a tumor cannot be localized. Instead, the surgeon should abandon attempts at resection and perform postoperative repeat biochemical testing, repeat imaging, and regionalization studies, including consideration for selective arterial injection-hepatic vein sampling as described earlier.

Unresectable or metastatic disease may be treated using strategies similar to those recommended for patients with nonfunctioning PETs, for example, streptozocin in combination with doxorubicin or 5-fluorouracil. Hepatic metastases should be resected if possible.

Gastrinoma
In 1955, Zollinger and Ellison first described a new clinical triad consisting of atypical peptic ulcerations, gastric hypersecretion with hyperacidity, and a noninsulin producing islet tumor of the pancreas. Later referred to as Zollinger–Ellison syndrome, gastrinomas secrete gastrin, a hormone that induces hyperchlorhydria and parietal cell hyperplasia. Patients with sporadic gastrinoma often present around

45 years of age with abdominal pain (75% to 100%), diarrhea (35% to 73%), heartburn (44% to 64%), duodenal and prepyloric ulcers (71% to 91%), and complications associated with ulcer disease. Gastrinomas account for <1% of all cases of peptic ulcer disease. Approximately 75% of gastrinomas are sporadic; the remaining 25% are associated with MEN1 (described later in this chapter). Most gastrinomas are located in the duodenum and the pancreas (63% of pancreatic tumors are in the head) in a 3:1 ratio, but tumors have been identified in other sites such as the stomach, jejunum, peripancreatic tissue, ovaries, and liver. The majority (60% to 90%) of gastrinomas are malignant, and the most important predictor of survival is the presence of hepatic metastasis.

Diagnosis. Patients with a suspected gastrinoma should be evaluated with a fasting gastrin level and gastric pH 1 to 2 weeks after discontinuation of PPIs. Withdrawing PPIs among patients with gastrinoma should be done carefully because perforation can occur if not closely monitored. A fasting gastrin level >1000 pg/mL with a gastric pH of <2.5 is highly suggestive of gastrinoma.

Other causes of hypergastrinemia include PPI use, autoimmune pernicious anemia, vagotomy, fundectomy, gastric outlet obstruction, resection of the large bowel, chronic renal failure, and *Helicobacter pylori* gastritis with atrophy.

The majority of patients with gastrinomas have a basal acid output to maximal acid output ratio ≥0.6, or a 12-hour nocturnal gastric acid secretion >100 mEq of hydrochloric acid. To establish the diagnosis in the setting of occult (nonimageable) disease, a basal acid output >15 mEq/hour and a positive secretin stimulation test has traditionally been used; such testing is now rarely employed. The secretin stimulation test involves administering 2 units/kg of intravenous secretin after an overnight fast. Serum gastrin levels are obtained at 15 and 2 minutes prior to secretin injection and again at 0, 2, 5, 10, and 20 minutes after infusion. The test is positive for gastrinoma when there is a paradoxical increase in serum gastrin by more than 200 pg/mL over baseline levels.

Tumor localizing studies are usually deferred until the diagnosis of gastrinoma is established. CT and MRI are beneficial in localizing larger tumors; esophagogastroduodenoscopy (EGD) with EUS is necessary to identify smaller tumors (<1 cm). CT and MRI are the most sensitive imaging modalities for identifying liver metastasis from gastrinoma. Octreotide imaging may be helpful in localizing the tumor and determining the extent of the disease. Although 80% to 100% of gastrinomas may be detected by a combination of selective abdominal angiography and selective arterial secretin injection, this invasive imaging strategy is rarely necessary in the current era.

Treatment. Patients with gastrinoma should first be treated with a PPI or a histamine (H2) antagonist to control acid hypersecretion. Somatostatin may help decrease the secretion of gastrin and other hormones.

Because resection has been shown to increase overall survival in patients with sporadic gastrinomas, surgical treatment is recommended even if a tumor cannot be identified on preoperative localization studies. If a tumor is identified on imaging, then enucleation or resection along with regional lymph node dissection is recommended. Thirty to fifty percent of gastrinoma patients have regional lymph node metastasis at the time of operative intervention. If enucleation is not possible, distal pancreatectomy is appropriate for lesions in the pancreatic tail, and pancreaticoduodenectomy with periduodenal lymphadenectomy is appropriate for lesions in the pancreatic head.

Surgical exploration should include the following: intraoperative ultrasound of the liver and pancreas; exploration of the lesser sac to evaluate the pancreatic body and tail; a Kocher maneuver to inspect the pancreatic head; duodenotomy with digital palpation to identify small duodenal wall tumors; periduodenal, peripancreatic head, portal, and hepatic arterial lymph node dissection; and exploration of extrapancreatic locations including the ovary, stomach wall, small bowel, omentum, and bowel mesentery. Intraoperative endoscopy with transillumination may help localize duodenal wall tumors; if done, it should be performed prior to duodenotomy. Total gastrectomy may be considered for patients in whom medical therapy has failed, who are noncompliant, or who have recurrent complications from peptic ulcer disease. However, patients who undergo total gastrectomy must be followed up after surgery to monitor for disease progression.

The strongest predictor of long-term survival in patients with gastrinomas is the presence of liver metastasis. Isolated liver metastases should be resected when possible, because there have been long-term survivors reported even when the primary tumor was not identified. When hepatic resection is not possible, hepatic artery embolization may be considered. Patients who have unresectable disease or diffuse metastasis may be treated with systemic chemotherapy or protocol-based therapies; streptozocin-based chemotherapy with doxorubicin or 5-fluorouracil has been shown to have some activity in these patients.

Vasoactive Intestinal Polypeptidoma

Vasoactive intestinal polypeptide (VIP)-secreting tumors (VIPomas; also referred to as Verner–Morrison syndrome or watery diarrhea–hypokalemia–achlorhydria (WDHA) syndrome) are very rare tumors characterized by large-volume secretory diarrhea that persists when fasting, electrolyte imbalances (hypokalemia and hypercalcemia), dehydration, hypochlorhydria or achlorhydria hyperglycemia, and flushing. Sixty to eighty percent of VIPomas are metastatic at presentation. The 5-year overall survival rate for patients with VIPomas (all stages) is 69%. The 5-year survival rate for patients with metastatic disease is 60%, and 94% for patients without metastasis. More than 80% of VIPomas are isolated to the pancreas; 75% involve the pancreatic body and tail. Extrapancreatic primary tumors that secrete VIP have been identified in the chest and retroperitoneum and have included such tumors as ganglioneuroblastomas, ganglioneuromas, and neuroblastomas.

Diagnosis. Even if not visualized on imaging, fasting plasma vasoactive intestinal polypeptide levels >500 pg/mL along with high volume diarrhea is suggestive of a VIPoma. Concomitant elevation of serum pancreatic polypeptide helps to confirm the diagnosis. These tumors are usually identified on CT, MRI, EUS, or octreotide scans. Other options for tumor localization include mesenteric arteriography and portal venous sampling.

Treatment. VIPomas are usually treated with surgical resection. Before operative intervention, patients should be hydrated, their electrolytes should be normalized, and they should receive octreotide to control the diarrhea. Given the malignant potential of VIPomas, surgical resection should include regional lymph node dissection. As with other functioning PETs, streptozocin-based systemic chemotherapy is appropriate for unresectable tumors or metastatic disease that cannot be debulked. Somatostatin analogues may also be effective. The treatment of liver metastases is the same as previously described for other functioning metastatic PETs.

Glucagonoma

Glucagonomas, which arise from the alpha cells of the pancreas, are characterized by excess glucagon secretion that results in glucose intolerance (occurring in >90% of patients), weight loss, neuropsychiatric disturbances (usually depression or psychosis), and venous thrombosis. Approximately 70% of glucagonoma patients develop necrolytic migratory erythema, a rash that occurs on the lower abdomen, perineum, perioral area, and/or feet. The majority (70%) of glucagonomas are malignant; patients frequently present with metastasis.

Diagnosis. Inappropriately elevated fasting glucagon level >500 to 1000 pg/mL is diagnostic of a glucagonoma. However, elevated glucagon levels may also be apparent in patients with cirrhosis, pancreatitis, diabetes mellitus, prolonged fasting, renal failure, burns, sepsis, familial glucagonemia, and acromegaly. A diagnosis of glucagonoma can be confirmed with a biopsy of the necrolytic migratory erythema. Glucagonomas are most often easily identified with CT and/or MRI because they are typically large (>5 cm in diameter) at diagnosis. Octreotide scanning is also helpful for localizing and staging glucagonomas. Although venous sampling has been used to localize glucagonomas, this modality is rarely necessary.

Treatment. When possible, glucagonoma treatment should include surgical resection with regional lymph node dissection. Metastatic disease should be resected when possible to provide potential symptomatic relief. Like other functioning PETs, metastatic and unresectable glucagonomas have been treated with systemic streptozocin with doxorubicin or 5-fluorouracil, or dacarbazine based chemotherapy. Necrolytic migratory erythema secondary to glucagonoma can usually be effectively treated with somatostatin.

Somatostatinoma

Somatostatinomas, which arise from the delta cells of the pancreas, are extremely rare and have an estimated incidence of 1 in 40 million. To date, only about 200 cases of somatostatinomas have been reported. Ninety percent of somatostatinomas are malignant. The majority (90%) of somatostatinomas are sporadic, and approximately 7% have been linked to familial disorders such as neurofibromatosis type 1 (NF1), MEN1, and Von Hippel–Lindau (VHL) disease.

Somatostatinomas are most frequently located in the pancreas or duodenum; however, there have been reports of somatostatinomas occurring in other locations such as the jejunum. Patients with duodenal somatostatinomas commonly present with symptoms of obstruction, whereas patients with pancreatic somatostatinomas frequently present with diabetes mellitus, cholelithiasis, steatorrhea, weight loss, anemia, and/or diarrhea. In their literature review, Soga and Yakuwa found that the 5-year overall survival rate for patients with somatostatinomas (all stages) was 75%, 100% for patients with localized disease, and 60% for patients with distant metastatic disease.

Diagnosis. Patients with somatostatinomas are often diagnosed late in the course of the disease because the lesions are extremely rare and the symptoms are often mild and nonspecific. A somatostatin level >100 pg/mL and a tumor identified on CT, MRI, octreotide scan, and/or EUS suggest a diagnosis of somatostatinoma. Pancreatic somatostatinomas are typically solitary, large, and located in the head of the pancreas. Duodenal somatostatinomas, which are generally smaller than pancreatic somatostatinomas, can usually be identified on EGD.

Treatment. Somatostatinoma patients frequently present with metastatic disease; nevertheless, these patients should undergo surgical resection of the primary tumor and regional lymph node dissection when possible. Given the high incidence of cholelithiasis in somatostatinoma patients, cholecystectomy should be performed at the time of surgery. Tumor debulking may be performed for palliation.

MULTIPLE ENDOCRINE NEOPLASIA AND OTHER HEREDITARY SYNDROMES ASSOCIATED WITH PANCREATIC ENDOCRINE TUMORS

Even though the majority of PETs are sporadic, several hereditary syndromes are associated with an increased incidence of PETs. As with sporadic PETs, treatment generally involves surgical resection when possible. However, a unique aspect of PETs in the setting of an inherited tumor syndrome is their multiplicity. Therefore, surgical management of patients with inherited PETs may be complicated by the desire to preserve pancreatic parenchyma and avoid diabetes, particularly when the identified tumors are small and distributed throughout the pancreas.

Multiple Endocrine Neoplasia Type 1

MEN1, also known as Wermer syndrome, is an autosomal dominant disorder caused by germline mutations in the *MEN1* gene. Located on chromosome 11q13, *MEN1* is a tumor suppressor gene that encodes menin, a protein involved in DNA replication, repair, transcription, and chromatin modification.

Individuals with MEN1 most commonly develop tumors in the anterior pituitary gland, parathyroid glands, and endocrine pancreas. More than 20 other endocrine tumors (e.g., foregut carcinoids and adrenocortical and medullary lesions) and nonendocrine tumors (e.g., facial angiofibromas and collagenomas) have been described in patients with MEN1. Thyroid nodules, meningiomas, ependymomas, leiomyomas, and lipomas are also more common in MEN1 patients.

Parathyroid Tumors

Frequently the first clinical manifestation, primary hyperparathyroidism (PHPT) is the most common endocrinopathy associated with MEN1. The age at PHPT onset ranges from 20 to 25 years, which is approximately 30 years earlier than that for sporadic PHPT. Nearly all MEN1 patients develop multiglandular PHPT by the age of 50 years. Therefore, all patients younger than 40 years who are diagnosed with multiglandular PHPT should be considered for genetic counseling and/or testing. Patients with PHPT may be completely asymptomatic or they may develop nephrolithiasis, osteoporosis, myopathy, fatigue, peptic ulcer disease, and/or neurocognitive deficits (such as depression and difficulty sleeping).

Screening high-risk individuals or patients with a *MEN1* mutation may begin at 8 years of age by obtaining annual serum calcium and parathyroid hormone (PTH) levels. An elevated serum calcium level with an inappropriately elevated PTH level confirms the diagnosis of PHPT. The timing of surgical intervention is the same in patients with MEN1-associated PHPT as patients with sporadic PHPT. (For more information, please refer to the parathyroid chapter 16.)

Two major operative strategies for MEN1 patients with PHPT have been described: subtotal parathyroidectomy and total parathyroidectomy. Because MEN1 patients are at increased risk for thymic carcinoid and because supernumerary parathyroid glands are often located in the thymus, cervical thymectomy is recommended as a component of both strategies. At M. D. Anderson, we prefer subtotal parathyroidectomy (3.5-gland resection) with cervical thymectomy and parathyroid cryopreservation. In the event of recurrent hyperparathyroidism, which occurs in 30% to 40% of patients who undergo subtotal parathyroidectomy, we recommend performing completion (total) parathyroidectomy with autografting and cryopreservation of the remaining parathyroid tissue. An alternative operative strategy, favored by some as the initial operation, is total parathyroidectomy with cervical thymectomy, autografting, and consideration for cryopreservation. A disadvantage of this approach is that up to one-third of patients will develop permanent postoperative hypoparathyroidism due to autograft failure.

Pituitary Tumors

More commonly identified in women, anterior pituitary adenomas are diagnosed in 10% to 60% of MEN1 patients at an average age of 35 years (the same age as seen in sporadic tumors). Pituitary adenomas are the first clinical manifestations of MEN1 in approximately 10% of patients. The most common pituitary adenomas are prolactinomas (60%), nonfunctioning pituitary tumors (15%), somatotropinomas (10% to 15%), and corticotropin-secreting tumors (5%). Up to 85% of MEN1-associated pituitary tumors are macroadenomas that often present with symptoms of local compression such as headache, visual field deficits, hypopituitarism, temporal lobe epilepsy, mild hyperprolactinemia from stalk compression, and cranial nerve III or VI dysfunction. Pituitary adenomas are best detected by MRI with and without gadolinium at 3 mm intervals. Surgical resection is indicated for symptomatic or growing tumors.

Women with prolactinomas may present with amenorrhea and/or galactorrhea, whereas men with prolactinomas may present with sexual dysfunction and/or gynecomastia. A serum prolactin level >200 ng/mL and an associated adenoma on MRI confirm the diagnosis of prolactinoma. Patients with an adenoma on MRI and who have an elevated prolactin level that is <100 ng/mL most likely have a nonfunctional tumor that is producing mildly increased amounts of prolactin from stalk compression. The treatment of prolactinomas begins with long-acting dopamine agonists such as cabergoline or bromocriptine; if medical therapy fails, resection is warranted. Patients with MEN1-associated prolactinomas have a poorer response to treatment than patients with sporadic tumors.

Somatotropinomas produce excess insulin-like growth factor (IGF-1) and/or growth hormone (GH), leading to gigantism in prepubescent children and acromegaly (frontal bossing; coarse facial features; enlargement of the hands, feet, and lower jaw; dental malocclusion; carpal tunnel syndrome; osteoarthritis; diabetes; hypertension; nephrolithiasis; skin tags; and colon polyps) in adults. The diagnosis is rendered with an elevated IGF-1 and a tumor on MRI; serum GH levels may or may not be elevated. Inability to suppress GH levels to <5 ng/dL after administering 1.75 g/kg (max 100 g) of oral glucose is diagnostic of a somatotropinoma. The treatment of choice is surgical resection. High-risk patients for surgical intervention may be treated with dopamine agonists, somatostatin analogues, or pegvisomant, a GH receptor blocker. Focused irradiation after surgical debulking may be beneficial in some cases.

Corticotropin-secreting pituitary tumors lead to the development of Cushing's disease. The clinical manifestations of corticotropin-secreting tumors include central weight gain, mood changes, thinning of the skin, easy bruising, diabetes, hypertension, and osteoporosis. Excess cortisol production can be detected by measuring the urinary free cortisol level. The diagnosis may also be confirmed by obtaining a plasma adrenocorticotrophic hormone (ACTH) level, a midnight salivary cortisol level, or by performing the dexamethasone suppression test. Inferior petrosal sinus sampling is the most invasive but also the most definitive test. Corticotropin-secreting tumors are treated with surgical resection. Other treatment modalities include focused irradiation and bilateral adrenalectomy. Drugs that inhibit adrenal steroid production, such as ketoconazole and metyrapone, may be used for short-term symptom control; unfortunately, long-term ketoconazole use has been associated with liver toxicity.

Screening for pituitary tumors in patients with MEN1 (or at increased risk of MEN1) begins with annual serum prolactin and IGF-1 levels as early 5 years of age. Brain MRI every 2 to 3 years may also be considered.

Pancreatic Endocrine Tumors

PETs develop in 50% to 75% of patients with MEN1, and metastatic PETs are the most frequent cause of death among MEN1 patients. PETs associated with MEN1 are usually diagnosed at an earlier age than sporadic PETs. These tumors usually become clinically apparent during the fourth or fifth decade of life, but hormonal symptoms from functioning PETs may be recognized earlier. Asymptomatic MEN1 patients have been diagnosed with nonfunctioning PETs before 20 years of age. As in patients with sporadic PETs, the vagueness of the clinical manifestations associated with hormone overproduction may delay the diagnosis of PETs even in patients with functioning tumors.

PETs may be solitary or multifocal, functional or nonfunctional (>50%), and solid or cystic. Like sporadic PETs, MEN1-associated PETs usually stain positive for chromogranin A, synaptophysin, and neuron-specific enolase. Microscopically, the pancreas in MEN1 patients demonstrates multiple microadenomas, islet cell hypertrophy, hyperplasia, and dysplasia. Tumor localization strategies in patients with MEN1-associated PETs are the same as in patients with sporadic PETs: CT, MRI, EUS, and octreotide scanning. In general, early diagnosis and surgical excision of MEN1-associated PETs improves overall survival, although treating MEN1 patients who have relatively small, nonfunctioning PETs remains controversial (see later).

Although several types of functioning PETs can occur within the same patient, one hormonal syndrome usually dominates. Gastrinoma, which has been identified in as many as 60% of MEN1 patients, is the most common functioning PET or duodenal endocrine tumor in MEN1 patients. More than 80% of MEN1-associated gastrinomas are located in the duodenum. Duodenal gastrinomas are usually very small tumors that are not readily apparent on standard imaging modalities or upper endoscopy. Therefore, in MEN1 patients with an elevated gastrin level and PET, it should not be assumed that their PET is the source of the elevated gastrin level. Patients with MEN1 develop gastrinomas approximately 10 years earlier than their sporadic counterparts (35 vs. 45 years). The clinical manifestations and the diagnosis of MEN1-associated gastrinoma are the same as those of the sporadic form.

Because gastrinomas recur frequently after surgical resection and symptoms are often controlled with PPIs, the surgical management of gastrinoma in MEN1 patients is controversial. Patients with MEN1-associated gastrinomas and concomitant PHPT should undergo parathyroidectomy first because achieving normocalcemia may decrease serum gastrin levels. Patients with locoregionally advanced gastrinomas who undergo surgical resection have been shown to have survival rates similar to those of patients with localized disease. However, unlike patients with sporadic gastrinoma, patients with MEN1-associated gastrinoma are unlikely to be cured with surgical resection. As in patients with sporadic gastrinoma, surgical intervention in patients with MEN1-associated gastrinoma should involve an extensive abdominal exploration, including regional lymph node dissection and transillumination and opening of the duodenum for manual palpation, as described previously in this chapter for sporadic gastrinomas.

MEN1-associated insulinomas, which are diagnosed in 10% to 20% of patients with MEN1, are often multifocal, present earlier than sporadic insulinomas, and may be located throughout the pancreas. Eighty-five to ninety-five percent of MEN1-associated insulinomas are benign; however, they have a higher recurrence rate after surgical resection than do sporadic insulinomas. Because medical therapy is not effective, surgical resection is the primary treatment for insulinoma.

As many as 5% of MEN1 patients with PETs have other functioning tumors such as glucagonomas, VIPomas, or somatostatinomas. The diagnosis and treatment of these rare tumors is identical to that of their sporadic counterparts.

High-risk patients or patients diagnosed with MEN1 should undergo yearly serum fasting glucose, insulin, gastrin, chromogranin-A, glucagon, and proinsulin levels. Surveillance for nonfunctioning PETs may be achieved by obtaining CT or MRI of the abdomen every 1 to 3 years.

Surgical Considerations for Nonfunctioning Pancreatic Endocrine Tumors in MEN1 Patients

Selecting the appropriate time for surgical intervention in MEN1 patients with PETs can be extremely challenging. MEN1 patients frequently develop multiple PETs during their lifespan. Because surgery is generally not curative, PETs often exhibit an indolent tumor biology, and total pancreatectomy is associated with severe insulin-dependent diabetes, the primary objective of surgical intervention is to delay total pancreatectomy as long as possible. These considerations must be balanced against the desire to remove identified PETs before a significant risk of metastasis develops.

Consensus statements on the management of patients with inherited PETs endorse surgical resection for radiographically visible PETs, even for tumors <1 cm in size. However, treatment decisions for patients with MEN1-associated PETs must still be individualized based on the size, multiplicity, distribution and functional status of the tumors, any existing comorbidities that may impact the overall operative risk, and available information regarding the overall rate of tumor progression in the individual patient. For example, one operative strategy that is ideal for patients with disease primarily involving the pancreatic body and tail and concomitant hypergastrinemia includes distal pancreatectomy, enucleation of any palpable or ultrasound-visible tumors in the pancreatic head, regional lymphadenectomy, and duodenotomy to identify occult gastrinomas (Thompson procedure).

Other Manifestations of MEN1

Adrenocortical abnormalities such as nonfunctional nodular hyperplasia or adenomas have been identified in as many as 55% of patients with MEN1. Functioning tumors, including aldosterone-secreting tumors, cortisol-secreting tumors, pheochromocytomas, and adrenocortical carcinomas, have also been described in MEN1 patients. The diagnosis and treatment of adrenal disease in MEN1 patients is the same as in patients with sporadic adrenal disease. (For more information, please refer to the adrenal chapter 15.)

Five to ten percent of MEN1 patients are diagnosed with foregut (i.e., bronchial, thymic, gastric, or duodenal) carcinoid tumors, which are the second most common cause of MEN1-specific death. Similar to the sporadic form, foregut carcinoids present at an average age of 35 years. The most aggressive carcinoid tumor arises from the thymus and patients with thymic carcinoids have a poor prognosis. Prophylactic thymectomy as part of an operative intervention for PHPT does not necessarily eliminate the risk of the future development of thymic carcinoids. Duodenal and gastric carcinoids are often multifocal and malignant. Gastric carcinoids may develop from MEN1-related gastrinoma(s). In such patients, lowering the gastrin level may cause gastric carcinoid tumors to regress. Hepatic metastasis from carcinoids is best treated with surgical resection, but other modalities such as radiofrequency ablation and chemoembolization may safely be performed.

Diagnosis of MEN1 and the Role of Genetic Testing

An accurate family history is the key to identifying MEN1 patients. Patients are clinically diagnosed with MEN1 if they develop two or more of the classic MEN1-associated tumors—pituitary, parathyroid, or endocrine tumors of the pancreas or duodenum—or have one of the classic tumors and at least one close relative with a clinical diagnosis of MEN1. Genetic counseling and the option of genetic testing should be offered to all patients with a clinical diagnosis of MEN1, to patients with one classic feature and a nonclassic tumor such as a foregut carcinoid or lipoma, and to patients with one of the classic tumors plus a family history of a classic tumor.

Multiple mutations have been identified within the *MEN1* gene, and specific mutations may be unique to each family. As many as 90% of MEN1 patients have an identifiable *MEN1* mutation. Negative genetic testing does not rule out a diagnosis of MEN1. One study found that as many as 10% of *MEN1* mutations (i.e., 5/47 mutations among 63 unrelated kindreds) arose de novo. Unlike patients with multiple endocrine neoplasia type 2 (MEN2), no genotype–phenotype correlations have been identified in patients with MEN1.

Using genetic testing to identify patients with MEN1 before symptoms become clinically apparent may prevent some of the complications associated with long-term hormonal excess. Genetic testing may also identify asymptomatic patients with pancreatic and duodenal tumors so that they can be treated earlier, thus improving overall survival. Patients may show biochemical evidence of MEN1 as early as 10 years before clinical manifestations develop. In addition, MEN1 patients who are diagnosed by genetic testing early in the disease process are able to consider preimplantation or prenatal genetic testing to assist in family planning. Genetic testing also allows mutation-negative relatives to be spared unnecessary clinical screening.

Multiple Endocrine Neoplasia Type 2

Overview
MEN2 is an autosomal dominant disorder associated with the development of medullary thyroid carcinoma (MTC), pheochromocytomas, and PHPT. MEN2 is divided into three different subtypes: MEN2A, familial medullary thyroid carcinoma (FMTC), and MEN2B. Roughly 95% of MEN2 patients have germline activating missense mutations of the *RET* (rearranged during transfection) proto-oncogene. The *RET* gene encodes a tyrosine kinase receptor that is expressed in neuroendocrine and neural cells and consists of 21 exons located on chromosome 10q11.2. The specific RET mutation in MEN2 patients can be used to predict the MEN2 subtype as well as the aggressiveness of MTC. MTC is usually the first manifestation of MEN2, and the time of presentation varies from younger than 10 years of age to the fourth decade of life.

MEN2A
MEN2A comprises at least 75% of MEN2 patients and is associated with the presence of MTC in 90%, PHPT in 20% to 30%, and pheochromocytoma in up to 50% of patients. *RET* mutations are identified in more than 95% of MEN2A patients. Patients who test negative for a *RET* mutation may be diagnosed with MEN2A if at least two of the classic features of the disease (i.e., MTC, pheochromocytoma, and PHPT) are present.

Recently, FMTC has been classified as a clinical variant of MEN2A, in which MTC is the only manifestation. Even though these patients are at low risk for the development of pheochromocytoma and PHPT, families once thought to have FMTC have later developed clinical manifestations of MEN2A and, therefore, must be monitored for the development of these tumors.

MEN2B
Less common than MEN2A, MEN2B is a condition characterized by MTC (nearly 100%), a marfanoid habitus; medullated corneal nerve fibers; ganglioneuromatosis; and pheochromocytoma (50% of patients). PHPT is not associated with MEN2B. Patients with MEN2B typically develop MTC approximately 10 years earlier than patients with MEN2A. MEN2B patients commonly have an elongated face with enlarged, nodular lips; thickened and everted eyelids; and neuromas of the tongue and oral mucosa. Patients may also develop skeletal abnormalities such as genu valgum, pes cavus, club foot, and kyphoscoliosis. Neuromas are frequently identified in the gastrointestinal tract but may also occur in organs with a submucosa, such as the bronchi and bladder. In addition, abdominal distention, megacolon, constipation, and diarrhea may develop in MEN2B patients as a result of the ganglioneuromatosis of the GI tract.

Medullary Thyroid Carcinoma in MEN2

MTC develops from the parafollicular cells (C-cells) of the thyroid gland that produce calcitonin, a hormone that decreases plasma calcium levels by inhibiting osteoclastic bone absorption and stimulating urinary excretion of calcium and phosphate. In MEN2 patients, MTC is preceded by the development of C-cell hyperplasia, leading to an increase in serum calcitonin levels. Because the majority of C-cells are located in the superior one-third of the thyroid gland, MTC is most commonly concentrated in this location. MTC in patients with MEN2 is usually bilateral and multicentric. A serum calcitonin level >1000 pg/mL and an elevated carcinoembryonic antigen (CEA) level suggest MTC; a positive pentagastrin stimulation test and the identification of a thyroid mass with positive cytologic evidence of MTC on ultrasonography-guided fine-needle aspiration biopsy renders the definitive diagnosis.

MTC is a relatively aggressive disease. Patients may present with neck pain, a palpable neck mass, or diarrhea due to elevated serum calcitonin levels. Patients who have dysphagia and/or hoarseness probably have advanced disease. Metastasis first develops in cervical or mediastinal lymph nodes, followed by the lungs, liver, and bones. Surgical resection is the treatment of choice for MTC; the disease is generally resistant to chemotherapy, and radioactive iodine is ineffective. The timing and extent of surgery should be individualized according to the patients' specific *RET* mutation to achieve the best overall outcome (Table 14.2).

TABLE 14.2 Aggressiveness of MTC Based on *RET* Mutation

American Thyroid Association Level	RET Mutation	Aggressiveness of MTC	Timing of Prophylactic Thyroidectomy
A	768, 790, 791, 804, 891	Lowest risk of aggressiveness (lower serum calcitonin, lower tumor stage, and higher rate of cure than level B tumors)	May be delayed beyond 5 years of age if serum *calcitonin* and neck ultrasound are normal[a]
B	609, 611, 618, 620, 630	Lower risk of aggressiveness	Consider prophylactic thyroidectomy before age 5 years (may be delayed beyond 5 years of age if serum calcitonin and neck ultrasound are normal[a])
C	634	High risk of aggressiveness	Before 5 years of age
D	883, 918	Highest risk of aggressiveness and youngest age at onset	Within the first year of life

[a]Must be screened with annual serum calcitonin levels and cervical ultrasonography; if abnormal, thyroidectomy is indicated at that time.
MTC, medullary thyroid carcinoma; RET, rearranged during transfection.

The initial evaluation of patients diagnosed with MTC includes performing cervical neck ultrasonography and measuring serum CEA, serum calcium, and serum calcitonin levels. Prior to operative intervention, serum calcium, PTH, and plasma metanephrines and/or normetanephrines should be measured to rule out pheochromocytoma and PHPT. If a pheochromocytoma is present, it should be resected before thyroidectomy to prevent a hypertensive crisis. Total thyroidectomy with prophylactic central neck dissection is recommended for patients with no evidence of local invasion or lymph node metastasis. In patients who have calcitonin levels >400 pg/mL or evidence of lymph node metastasis, a three-phase CT of the neck, chest, and liver is necessary to rule out distant metastasis. In patients with disease in the central neck, treatment includes total thyroidectomy and therapeutic central neck lymph node dissection. The role of lateral neck dissection in patients without evidence of lateral cervical lymph node metastasis is unknown. However, patients who demonstrate lateral cervical lymph node metastasis should undergo a lateral neck dissection of levels IIA, III, IV, and V on the affected side. In patients with established distant metastatic disease, a limited surgical resection to preserve speech and swallowing may be considered.

Thyroid hormone suppression therapy is not effective for patients with MTC, so patients should be provided only thyroid hormone replacement therapy following total thyroidectomy. Baseline serum calcitonin and CEA levels should be measured 2 to 3 months following operative intervention and every 6 to 12 months thereafter. Cervical ultrasonography should be performed 6 months after surgical resection.

The detection of calcitonin after total thyroidectomy indicates that residual or persistent disease is present. Patients in whom serum calcitonin and CEA levels are undetectable may be followed with biochemical assessments alone. However, patients who have an elevated postoperative calcitonin up to 150 pg/mL should undergo a neck ultrasonography to evaluate for persistent or recurrent disease. Additional imaging such as CT or MRI of the neck, chest, and abdomen (three-phase CT or MRI of liver) is recommended if the serum calcitonin is >150 pg/mL. The effectiveness of chemotherapy and external beam radiation in patients with unresectable disease has not been established; therefore, the use of these treatments should be considered on an individual basis. There is considerable current interest in targeted therapeutic options for patients with advanced and metastatic MTC, especially in therapies that target RET and VEGF.

Recommendations for the timing of prophylactic thyroidectomy are determined by the biologic behavior of each *RET* mutation. In an attempt to improve overall survival, the American Thyroid Association has established specific guidelines for thyroidectomy according to the aggressiveness of each *RET* mutation (Table 14.2). Prophylactic thyroidectomy should be performed by experienced surgeons at a tertiary care center.

Primary Hyperparathyroidism in MEN2A
Most commonly associated with a 634 mutation, PHPT occurs in 10% to 35% of patients with MEN2A. PHPT has also been identified in patients with mutations in codons 609, 611, 618, 620, 790, and 791. The diagnosis and the clinical presentation of PHPT in MEN2A patients are the same as those in patients with sporadic PHPT and patients with MEN1-associated PHPT. However, unlike MEN1, PHPT associated with MEN2A is milder and ranges from a single adenoma to four-gland hyperplasia.

Surgical intervention for MEN2A-associated PHPT is different than for MEN1-associated PHPT. MEN2A patients who have PHPT at the time of initial thyroidectomy should undergo resection of visibly enlarged parathyroid glands with possible forearm autograft, subtotal parathyroidectomy (leaving one or a piece of one gland in situ), or total parathyroidectomy with forearm autograft. Because the risk of permanent hypoparathyroidism is significant, most surgeons avoid total parathyroidectomy unless all four glands are abnormal. In patients who develop PHPT after initial thyroidectomy, surgical intervention should be guided by the identification of abnormal parathyroid glands on preoperative imaging, and the use of forearm autografting should be considered.

During thyroidectomy for patients with MEN2, the potential for devascularization of parathyroid glands during future operations for recurrent disease must be considered. Devascularized parathyroid glands in MEN2B patients may be reimplanted in the sternocleidomastoid muscle. However, devascularized normal parathyroid glands in MEN2A patients with a strong family history of PHPT should be implanted into the forearm. MEN2A patients with a low risk of developing PHPT according to family history and their *RET* mutation may have devascularized parathyroid glands implanted into the sternocleidomastoid muscle or the forearm.

Pheochromocytoma

Pheochromocytomas—catecholamine-secreting tumors of the adrenal medulla—develop in up to 50% of MEN2A patients during their lifespan. Patients with pheochromocytomas typically present with headache, sweating, palpitations, hypertension, and anxiety. MEN2 patients may develop hyperplasia of the adrenal medulla before pheochromocytomas become evident. Most commonly associated with codons 634 and 918, pheochromocytomas may be unilateral or bilateral and synchronous or metachronous. These tumors often develop 10 to 20 years earlier in MEN2 patients than in patients with sporadic pheochromocytoma. Elevated plasma-free metanephrines and normetanephrines or urinary metanephrines are necessary for the diagnosis. Once biochemical diagnosis is established, CT or MRI of the abdomen should be performed to identify an adrenal tumor. Metaiodobenzylguanidine (MIBG) scanning may be used to help localize the tumor before surgery.

The treatment of choice for pheochromocytomas is surgical resection. At least 1 to 2 weeks before operation, patients should be well hydrated and treated with an alpha antagonist. The recommended initial dose of phenoxybenzamine is 10 mg twice a day with a goal to achieve a blood pressure of 130/80 mm Hg while sitting and 100 mm Hg systolic when standing. When needed, beta blockers may be used to obtain a target heart rate of 60 to 70 beats per minute while sitting and 70 to 80 beats per minute while standing. Beta-1 blockers (atenolol 12.5 to 25 mg three times per day, or metoprolol 25 to 50 mg two to three times per day) are preferred and must always be used with alpha adrenergic blockade. Beta blockers should never be used alone or prior to the initiation of alpha blockade, due to the risk of exacerbating hypertension in these patients. The benefit of a specialized team consisting of a dedicated anesthesiologist, endocrinologist, endocrine surgeon, internist, and cardiologist to minimize the risks of complications during operative intervention should not be underestimated.

The most common operative approach in patients with a unilateral pheochromocytoma is laparoscopic adrenalectomy. At M. D. Anderson, we prefer retroperitoneoscopic adrenalectomy (PRA) for patients with modestly sized, clinically benign pheochromocytomas. PRA avoids intra-abdominal solid organ mobilization, and patients with bilateral tumors do not require repositioning during the procedure. If possible, cortical sparing adrenalectomy should be performed in patients with bilateral pheochromocytomas because the procedure can avoid postoperative corticosteroid dependence in up to 65% of patients. Otherwise, patients who undergo bilateral adrenalectomy require lifelong corticosteroid supplementation to avoid adrenal insufficiency.

Genetic Testing

Genetic counseling and testing is recommended for patients who are diagnosed with MTC, primary C-cell hyperplasia, cutaneous lichen amyloidosis, early-onset adrenergic pheochromocytoma, or MEN2. *RET* genetic testing should also be suggested to patients who have a positive family history of MEN2 or FMTC. Patients at risk for developing MEN2A should begin genetic testing before 5 years of age, and patients at risk for MEN2B should be tested shortly after birth. If possible, all first degree relatives should be offered genetic testing before the age of recommended prophylactic thyroidectomy if a specific *RET* mutation is identified within a family.

Von Hippel–Lindau Disease

VHL disease, an autosomal dominant disease characterized by mutations of the VHL gene, is associated with pancreatic involvement in 20% to 75% of patients. VHL patients most commonly develop pancreatic cysts, but 10% to 17% of patients develop PETs. Other characteristics of this disease include hemangioblastomas of the nervous system, retinal angiomas, clear cell renal carcinomas, pheochromocytomas, and endolymphatic sac tumors. PETs associated with VHL may be multiple in number, located anywhere in the pancreas, and are diagnosed younger than their sporadic counterparts.

Tuberous Sclerosis

Another disorder associated with the development of PETs is tuberous sclerosis, a rare, autosomal dominant disorder. Tuberous sclerosis is associated with mutations in the *TSC1* gene on the 9q34 chromosome or the *TSC2* gene on the 16p13.3 chromosome. Tuberin, a *TSC2* gene product associated with cell growth and proliferation, has been associated with the development of malignant PETs in tuberous sclerosis patients.

Von Recklinghausen's Disease

Von Recklinghausen's disease, also known as NF1, has also been associated with the development of PETs. Associated with a mutation of the *NF1* tumor suppressor gene, NF1 is manifested by the development of neurofibromas, café-au-lait macules, optic gliomas, Lisch nodules, bony lesions, short stature, learning disabilities, and macroencephaly. Malignant pheochromocytomas are the most common endocrine malignancy associated with NF1. A few case reports of pancreatic insulinomas and duodenal somatostatinomas in NF1 patients have been published. To date, only 34 patients with both NF1 and duodenal somatostatinomas have been reported.

Recommended Readings

Abood GJ, Go A, Malhotra D, et al. The surgical and systemic management of neuroendocrine tumors of the pancreas. *Surg Clin North Am.* 2009;89(1):249–266, x.

Agarwal SK, Lee BA, Sukhodolets KE, et al. Molecular pathology of the MEN1 gene. *Ann N Y Acad Sci.* 2004;1014:189–198.

Altimari AF, Badrinath K, Reisel HJ, et al. DTIC therapy in patients with malignant intra-abdominal neuroendocrine tumors. *Surgery.* 1987;102(6):1009–1017.

Bartsch DK, Fendrich V, Langer P, et al. Outcome of duodenopancreatic resections in patients with multiple endocrine neoplasia type 1. *Ann Surg.* 2005;242(6):757–764, discussion.

Bassett JH, Forbes SA, Pannett AA, et al. Characterization of mutations in patients with multiple endocrine neoplasia type 1. *Am J Hum Genet.* 1998;62(2): 232–244.

Beckers A, Daly AF. The clinical, pathological, and genetic features of familial isolated pituitary adenomas. *Eur J Endocrinol.* 2007;157(4):371–382.

Brandi ML, Gagel RF, Angeli A, et al. Guidelines for diagnosis and therapy of MEN type 1 and type 2. *J Clin Endocrinol Metab.* 2001;86(12):5658–5671.

Callender GG, Rich TA, Perrier ND. Multiple endocrine neoplasia syndromes. *Surg Clin North Am.* 2008;88(4):863–895, viii.

Clark OH, Ajani JA, Benson AB III, et al. NCCN Clinical Practice Guidelines in Oncology: neuroendocrine tumors. *J Natl Compr Canc Netw.* 2009;7(7):712–747.

Coker LH, Rorie K, Cantley L, et al. Primary hyperparathyroidism, cognition, and health-related quality of life. *Ann Surg.* 2005;242(5):642–650.

Dackiw AP, Cote GJ, Fleming JB, et al. Screening for MEN1 mutations in patients with atypical endocrine neoplasia. *Surgery.* 1999;126(6):1097–1103.

Danforth DN Jr, Gorden P, Brennan MF. Metastatic insulin-secreting carcinoma of the pancreas: clinical course and the role of surgery. *Surgery.* 1984;96(6): 1027–1037.

Doherty GM, Olson JA, Frisella MM, et al. Lethality of multiple endocrine neoplasia type I. *World J Surg.* 1998;22(6):581–586.

Doherty GM, Thompson NW. Multiple endocrine neoplasia type 1: duodenopancreatic tumours. *J Intern Med.* 2003;253(6): 590–598.

Elaraj DM, Skarulis MC, Libutti SK, et al. Results of initial operation for hyperparathyroidism in patients with multiple endocrine neoplasia type 1. *Surgery.* 2003;134(6):858–864.

Evans DB, Skibber JM, Lee JE, et al. Nonfunctioning islet cell carcinoma of the pancreas. *Surgery.* 1993;114(6):1175–1181.

Faiss S, Pape UF, Bohmig M, et al. Prospective, randomized, multicenter trial on the antiproliferative effect of lanreotide, interferon alfa, and their combination for therapy of metastatic neuroendocrine gastroenteropancreatic tumors–the International Lanreotide and Interferon Alfa Study Group. *J Clin Oncol.* 2003;21(14):2689–2696.

Fendrich V, Langer P, Waldmann J, et al. Management of sporadic and multiple endocrine neoplasia type 1 gastrinomas. *Br J Surg.* 2007;94(11):1331–1341.

Fendrich V, Ramaswamy A, Slater EP, et al. Duodenal somatostatinoma associated with Von Recklinghausen's disease. *J Hepatobiliary Pancreat Surg.* 2004;11(6): 417–421.

Ferolla P, Falchetti A, Filosso P, et al. Thymic neuroendocrine carcinoma (carcinoid) in multiple endocrine neoplasia type 1 syndrome: the Italian series. *J Clin Endocrinol Metab.* 2005;90(5):2603–2609.

Figueiredo FA, Giovannini M, Monges G, et al. Pancreatic endocrine tumors: a large single-center experience. *Pancreas.* 2009; 38(8):936–940.

Francalanci P, Diomedi-Camassei F, Purificato C, et al. Malignant pancreatic endocrine tumor in a child with tuberous sclerosis. *Am J Surg Pathol.* 2003;27(10): 1386–1389.

Gauger PG, Scheiman JM, Wamsteker EJ, et al. Role of endoscopic ultrasonography in screening and treatment of pancreatic endocrine tumours in asymptomatic patients with multiple endocrine neoplasia type 1. *Br J Surg.* 2003;90(6): 748–754.

Guettier JM, Kam A, Chang R, et al. Localization of insulinomas to regions of the pancreas by intraarterial calcium stimulation: the NIH experience. *J Clin Endocrinol Metab.* 2009;94(4):1074–1080.

Hausman MS Jr, Thompson NW, Gauger PG, et al. The surgical management of MEN-1 pancreatoduodenal neuroendocrine disease. *Surgery.* 2004;136(6):1205–1211.

Imamura M, Takahashi K, Adachi H, et al. Usefulness of selective arterial secretin injection test for localization of gastrinoma in the Zollinger-Ellison syndrome. *Ann Surg.* 1987;205(3):230–239.

Ito T, Sasano H, Tanaka M, et al. Epidemiological study of gastroenteropancreatic neuroendocrine tumors in Japan. *J Gastroenterol.* 2010;45(2):234–243.

Jensen RT, Berna MJ, Bingham DB, et al. Inherited pancreatic endocrine tumor syndromes: advances in molecular pathogenesis, diagnosis, management, and controversies. *Cancer.* 2008;113(7, Suppl):1807–1843.

Kindmark H, Sundin A, Granberg D, et al. Endocrine pancreatic tumors with glucagon hypersecretion: a retrospective study of 23 cases during 20 years. *Med Oncol.* 2007;24(3):330–337.

Kloos RT, Eng C, Evans DB, et al. Medullary thyroid cancer: management guidelines of the American Thyroid Association. *Thyroid.* 2009;19(6):565–612.

Kouvaraki MA, Shapiro SE, Cote GJ, et al. Management of pancreatic endocrine tumors in multiple endocrine neoplasia type 1. *World J Surg.* 2006;30(5):643–653.

Kouvaraki MA, Solorzano CC, Shapiro SE, et al. Surgical treatment of nonfunctioning pancreatic islet cell tumors. *J Surg Oncol.* 2005;89(3):170–185.

Kulke MH, Lenz HJ, Meropol NJ, et al. Activity of sunitinib in patients with advanced neuroendocrine tumors. *J Clin Oncol.* 2008;26(20):3403–3410.

Kulke MH, Stuart K, Enzinger PC, et al. Phase II study of temozolomide and thalidomide in patients with metastatic neuroendocrine tumors. *J Clin Oncol.* 2006; 24(3):401–406.

Kvols LK, Buck M, Moertel CG, et al. Treatment of metastatic islet cell carcinoma with a somatostatin analogue (SMS 201–995). *Ann Intern Med.* 1987;107(2): 162–168.

Lairmore TC, Piersall LD, DeBenedetti MK, et al. Clinical genetic testing and early surgical intervention in patients with multiple endocrine neoplasia type 1 (MEN 1). *Ann Surg.* 2004;239(5):637–645.

Lambert LA, Shapiro SE, Lee JE, et al. Surgical treatment of hyperparathyroidism in patients with multiple endocrine neoplasia type 1. *Arch Surg.* 2005;140(4): 374–382.

Lam ET, Ringel MD, Kloos RT, et al. Phase II clinical trial of sorafenib in metastatic medullary thyroid cancer. *J Clin Oncol.* 2010;28(14):2323–2330.

Landry CS, Scoggins CR, McMasters KM, et al. Management of hepatic metastasis of gastrointestinal carcinoid tumors. *J Surg Oncol.* 2008;97(3):253–258.

Landry CS, Waguespack SG, Perrier ND. Surgical management of nonmultiple endocrine neoplasia endocrinopathies: state-of-the-art review. *Surg Clin North Am.* 2009;89(5):1069–1089.

La RS, Klersy C, Uccella S, et al. Improved histologic and clinicopathologic criteria for prognostic evaluation of pancreatic endocrine tumors. *Hum Pathol.* 2009; 40(1):30–40.

McGevna L, McFadden D, Ritvo J, et al. Glucagonoma-associated neuropsychiatric and affective symptoms: diagnostic dilemmas raised by paraneoplastic phenomena. *Psychosomatics.* 2009;50(5):548–550.

Melmed S. Update in pituitary disease. *J Clin Endocrinol Metab.* 2008;93(2):331–338.

Metz DC, Jensen RT. Gastrointestinal neuroendocrine tumors: pancreatic endocrine tumors. *Gastroenterology.* 2008;135(5): 1469–1492.

Miller CR, Ellison EC. Multiple endocrine neoplasia type 2B. In: Clark OH, Duh QY, Kebebew E, eds. *Textbook of Endocrine Surgery.* 2nd ed. Philadelphia: Elsevier Saunders; 2005:757–763.

Mittendorf EA, Wefel JS, Meyers CA, et al. Improvement of sleep disturbance and neurocognitive function after parathyroidectomy in patients with primary hyperparathyroidism. *Endocr Pract.* 2007;13(4):338–344.

Modlin IM, Oberg K, Chung DC, et al. Gastroenteropancreatic neuroendocrine tumours. *Lancet Oncol.* 2008;9(1):61–72.

Moertel CG, Lefkopoulo M, Lipsitz S, et al. Streptozocin-doxorubicin, streptozocin-fluorouracil or chlorozotocin in the treatment of advanced islet-cell carcinoma. *N Engl J Med.* 1992;326(8):519–523.

Nesi G, Marcucci T, Rubio CA, et al. Somatostatinoma: clinico-pathological features of three cases and literature reviewed. *J Gastroenterol Hepatol.* 2008; 23(4):521–526.

Newey PJ, Jeyabalan J, Walls GV, et al. Asymptomatic children with multiple endocrine neoplasia type 1 (MEN1) mutations may harbour non-functioning pancreatic neuroendocrine tumors. *J Clin Endocrinol Metab.* 2009;94(10): 3640–3646.

Norton JA, Alexander HR, Fraker DL, et al. Comparison of surgical results in patients with advanced and limited disease with multiple endocrine neoplasia type 1 and Zollinger-Ellison syndrome. *Ann Surg.* 2001;234(4):495–505.

Norton JA, Alexander HR, Fraker DL, et al. Does the use of routine duodenotomy (DUODX) affect rate of cure, development of liver metastases, or survival in patients with Zollinger-Ellison syndrome? *Ann Surg.* 2004;239(5):617–625.

Norton JA, Fraker DL, Alexander HR, et al. Surgery increases survival in patients with gastrinoma. *Ann Surg.* 2006;244(3): 410–419.

Norton JA, Fraker DL, Alexander HR, et al. Surgery to cure the Zollinger-Ellison syndrome. *N Engl J Med.* 1999;341(9):635–644.

Norton JA, Jensen RT. Current surgical management of Zollinger-Ellison syndrome (ZES) in patients without multiple endocrine neoplasia-type 1 (MEN1). *Surg Oncol.* 2003;12(2):145–151.

Okauchi Y, Nammo T, Iwahashi H, et al. Glucagonoma diagnosed by arterial stimulation and venous sampling (ASVS). *Intern Med.* 2009;48(12):1025–1030.

Pacak K. Preoperative management of the pheochromocytoma patient. *J Clin Endocrinol Metab.* 2007;92(11):4069–4079.

Perrier ND, Kennamer DL, Bao R, et al. Posterior retroperitoneoscopic adrenalectomy: preferred technique for removal of benign tumors and isolated metastases. *Ann Surg.* 2008;248(4):666–674.

Rich TA, Perrier ND. Risk assessment and genetic counseling for multiple endocrine neoplasia type 1 (MEN1). *Community Oncol.* 2008;5(9):502–514.

Rinke A, Muller HH, Schade-Brittinger C, et al. Placebo-controlled, double-blind, prospective, randomized study on the effect of octreotide LAR in the control of tumor growth in patients with metastatic neuroendocrine midgut tumors: a report from the PROMID Study Group. *J Clin Oncol.* 2009;27(28):4656–4663.

Saxena A, Chua TC, Bester L, et al. Factors predicting response and survival after yttrium-90 radioembolization of unresectable neuroendocrine tumor liver metastases: a critical appraisal of 48 cases. *Ann Surg.* 2010;251(5):910–916.

Schlumberger MJ, Elisei R, Bastholt L, et al. Phase II study of safety and efficacy of motesanib in patients with progressive or symptomatic, advanced or metastatic medullary thyroid cancer. *J Clin Oncol.* 2009;27(23):3794–3801.

Schuffenecker I, Billaud M, Calender A, et al. RET proto-oncogene mutations in French MEN 2A and FMTC families. *Hum Mol Genet.* 1994;3(11):1939–1943.

Soga J, Yakuwa Y. Somatostatinoma/inhibitory syndrome: a statistical evaluation of 173 reported cases as compared to other pancreatic endocrinomas. *J Exp Clin Cancer Res.* 1999;18(1):13–22.

Soga J, Yakuwa Y. Vipoma/diarrheogenic syndrome: a statistical evaluation of 241 reported cases. *J Exp Clin Cancer Res.* 1998;17(4):389–400.

Solorzano CC, Lee JE, Pisters PW, et al. Nonfunctioning islet cell carcinoma of the pancreas: survival results in a contemporary series of 163 patients. *Surgery.* 2001; 130(6):1078–1085.

Thompson GB, Young WF. Multiple endocrine neoplasia type 1. In: Clark OH, Duh QY, Kebebew E, eds. *Textbook of Endocrine Surgery.* 2nd ed. Philadelphia: Elsevier Saunders; 2005:673–690.

Thom AK, Norton JA, Doppman JL, et al. Prospective study of the use of intraarterial secretin injection and portal venous sampling to localize duodenal gastrinomas. *Surgery.* 1992;112(6):1002–1008.

Tomassetti P, Migliori M, Caletti GC, et al. Treatment of type II gastric carcinoid tumors with somatostatin analogues. *N Engl J Med.* 2000;343(8):551–554.

Tonelli F, Marcucci T, Fratini G, et al. Is total parathyroidectomy the treatment of choice for hyperparathyroidism in multiple endocrine neoplasia type 1? *Ann Surg.* 2007;246(6):1075–1082.

Vance ML. Pituitary adenoma: a clinician's perspective. *Endocr Pract.* 2008;14(6): 757–763.

Verges B, Boureille F, Goudet P, et al. Pituitary disease in MEN type 1 (MEN1): data from the France-Belgium MEN1 multicenter study. *J Clin Endocrinol Metab.* 2002;87(2):457–465.

Waldmann J, Bartsch DK, Kann PH, et al. Adrenal involvement in multiple endocrine neoplasia type 1: results of 7 years prospective screening. *Langenbecks Arch Surg.* 2007;392(4):437–443.

Wells SA Jr, Gosnell JE, Gagel RF, et al. Vandetanib for the treatment of patients with locally advanced or metastatic hereditary medullary thyroid cancer. *J Clin Oncol.* 2010;28(5):767–772.

Whipple AO, Frantz VK. Adenoma of islet cells with hyperinsulinism: a review. *Ann Surg.* 1935;101(6):1299–1335.

Wiedenmann B, Jensen RT, Mignon M, et al. Preoperative diagnosis and surgical management of neuroendocrine gastroenteropancreatic tumors: general recommendations by a consensus workshop. *World J Surg.* 1998;22(3):309–318.

Wilson SD. Gastrinoma. In: Clark OH, Duh QY, Kebebew E, eds. *Textbook of Endocrine Surgery.* 2nd ed. Philadelphia: Elsevier; 2005:745–756.

Yao JC. Neuroendocrine tumors. Molecular targeted therapy for carcinoid and islet-cell carcinoma. *Best Pract Res Clin Endocrinol Metab.* 2007;21(1):163–172.

Yao JC, Eisner MP, Leary C, et al. Population-based study of islet cell carcinoma. *Ann Surg Oncol.* 2007;14(12):3492–3500.

Yao JC, Lombard-Bohas C, Baudin E, et al. Daily oral everolimus activity in patients with metastatic pancreatic neuroendocrine tumors after failure of cytotoxic chemotherapy: a phase II trial. *J Clin Oncol.* 2010;28(1):69–76.

Yip L, Cote GJ, Shapiro SE, et al. Multiple endocrine neoplasia type 2: evaluation of the genotype-phenotype relationship. *Arch Surg.* 2003;138(4):409–416.

Yip L, Lee JE, Shapiro SE, et al. Surgical management of hereditary pheochromocytoma. *J Am Coll Surg.* 2004;198(4):525–534.

Yu F, Venzon DJ, Serrano J, et al. Prospective study of the clinical course, prognostic factors, causes of death, and survival in patients with long-standing Zollinger-Ellison syndrome. *J Clin Oncol.* 1999;17(2):615–630.

Zhou J, Enewold L, Stojadinovic A, et al. Incidence rates of exocrine and endocrine pancreatic cancers in the United States. Cancer Causes Control. 2010;21(6): 853–861.

Zollinger RM, Ellison EH. Primary peptic ulcerations of the jejunum associated with islet cell tumors of the pancreas. *Ann Surg.* 1955;142(4):709–723.

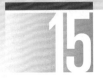

Adrenal Tumors

Jula Veerapong and Jeffrey E. Lee

INTRODUCTION

Proper evaluation and treatment of adrenal tumors can be rather complex and includes the application of appropriate imaging, selective endocrine hormone testing, and, when indicated, either minimally invasive or open surgery. Advances in diagnostic imaging have facilitated detection and accurate surgical treatment planning, whereas advances in minimally invasive and open surgical techniques have improved the surgeon's ability to minimize surgical morbidity while maximizing surgical outcomes. Evaluation of the patient presenting with an adrenal mass requires a thorough understanding of adrenal endocrine physiology. Appropriate biochemical evaluation and radiographic assessment of an identified adrenal mass are crucial before surgical intervention, as biochemical evaluation determines the functional status of the tumor, helps dictate management, and aids in the determination of the role for surgical intervention. Common functioning adrenal tumors include aldosteronomas, cortisol-producing adrenal adenomas, pheochromocytomas, and many adrenal cortical carcinomas. Nonfunctioning tumors include nonfunctioning adrenal adenomas or "incidentalomas," nonfunctioning carcinomas, and metastases to the adrenal gland.

ANATOMY

The adrenal glands are paired, pyramid-shaped structures located in the retroperitoneum that sit atop the superior-medial aspect of each kidney. The normal adult adrenal gland weighs approximately 4 to 5 g, with dimensions spanning approximately 4 to 5 cm vertically, 3 cm transversely, and 1 cm in the anteroposterior plane. The adrenal glands are soft and highly vascular structures that are completely surrounded by perirenal fat. The adrenal glands have two major discrete embryologic, anatomic, and functional layers: the cortex (outer) and the medulla (inner). The cortex is a thin (1 to 2 mm), bright yellow layer which produces steroid hormones. From superficial to deep, it is subdivided into the zona glomerulosa which produces the mineralocorticoid aldosterone, the zona fasciculata which produces the glucocorticoid cortisol, and the zona reticularis which produces the sex steroids, primarily androgens. The medulla is a dark reddish gray layer which produces norepinephrine and epinephrine.

The arterial blood supply to the adrenal glands is derived from branches of the inferior phrenic artery, the renal artery, and contributions directly from the aorta. Nutrient arteries coalesce and form a capsular arterial plexus that sends capillaries throughout the cortex, which subsequently combine to form a venous portal system that drains into the adrenal medulla. In the medulla, the vessels come together to join the central adrenal vein. The adrenal medulla is also supplied by arteriae medullae that penetrate directly into the medullary substance. Although there are some small veins draining the surface of the adrenal cortex, the central vein drains most of the blood from the medulla stemming from the cortex via the capsular plexus. The right adrenal vein is short and wide as it exits the gland and immediately enters the posterolateral aspect of the inferior vena cava. The left adrenal vein exits anteriorly and usually drains into the left renal vein, although it occasionally may enter the inferior vena cava directly. It is therefore easier to obtain vascular control of the left adrenal vein. Vascular control of the right adrenal vein can become more challenging with increasing size of the adrenal tumor.

ALDOSTERONOMA

Introduction

Primary hyperaldosteronism was first described by J. W. Conn in 1955 in the setting of an aldosterone hypersecreting adenoma in association with hypertension and hyperkalemia (Conn syndrome). Since then, it has been understood that primary hyperaldosteronism may have multiple etiologies. The two major causes are unilateral aldosterone-producing adenoma (60%) and bilateral adrenal hyperplasia or idiopathic hyperaldosteronism (40%). Other rare causes of primary aldosteronism include unilateral primary adrenal hyperplasia, aldosterone-producing adrenocortical carcinoma, familial hyperaldosteronism (glucocorticoid-suppressible and idiopathic hyperaldosteronism), and aldosterone-secreting ovarian tumors. Primary hyperaldosteronism is responsible for approximately 0.5% to 2.0% of all cases of hypertension and accounts for the most common cause of secondary hypertension. Moreover, it represents 5% to 10% of surgically correctable cases of hypertension.

Clinical Manifestations

Symptoms of primary hyperaldosteronism are usually mild and nonspecific. The most common symptoms are headache, muscle weakness, fatigue, polydipsia, polyuria, and nocturia. Hypertension is almost always present but is frequently mild, with diastolic blood pressures less than 120 mm Hg in more than 70% of cases.

Diagnosis

Initial findings that support a diagnosis of primary hyperaldosteronism include hypertension and spontaneous hypokalemia. Electrolyte abnormalities may include hypernatremia and a hypochloremic metabolic alkalosis. Prior to endocrine evaluation, diuretics should be discontinued for at least 2 weeks. A plasma aldosterone/plasma renin ratio greater than 30 (ng/dL : ng/mL/h) along with a plasma aldosterone level greater than 20 ng/dL is sensitive and specific in the screening and diagnosis of primary hyperaldosteronism. If aldosterone and renin determination is equivocal, confirmation of hyperaldosteronism can be obtained using the saline suppression test or the 3-day sodium loading test; in the straightforward situation, these are unnecessary. In the saline suppression test, 2 L of normal saline is infused intravenously over 4 hours and plasma aldosterone is measured. Confirmation of hyperaldosteronism is obtained when the plasma aldosterone level is greater than 10 ng/dL. In the 3-day sodium loading test (100 mmol NaCl per day), a 24-hour urine collection is obtained in the third day of the test to measure aldosterone, sodium, and potassium, and serum is obtained to measure sodium and potassium. Confirmation of hyperaldosteronism is obtained when the urinary aldosterone is greater than 14 μg per 24 hours. In the latter test, it is important to demonstrate adequate salt loading; therefore urinary sodium should be greater than 200 mEq per 24 hours.

Once the diagnosis of hyperaldosteronism is established, it is critical to differentiate unilateral adrenal adenoma (60% of cases) from bilateral hyperplasia of the zona glomerulosa (idiopathic hyperaldosteronism, 40% of cases). In patients with aldosterone-producing adenoma, unilateral adrenalectomy corrects the hypokalemia and decreases the blood pressure in 70% of surgically treated patients. However, surgery is of little value in patients with idiopathic hyperaldosteronism. Patients with unilateral adenoma usually have more severe hypertension, higher plasma aldosterone levels, and therefore more profound hypokalemia. However, these findings alone cannot accurately differentiate patients with unilateral adenoma from those with idiopathic hyperaldosteronism. Computed tomography (CT) and magnetic resonance imaging (MRI) can help confirm the presence of a unilateral adrenal nodule while selective venous sampling for aldosterone determination can localize the hyperfunctioning adrenal tissue to the right or left side. The high frequency of nonfunctioning adenomas in the normal population (2% to 8%) means that the finding of a small adrenal mass on CT or MRI is not necessarily diagnostic of a unilateral aldosterone-producing adenoma.

Selective venous sampling is an invasive test that requires special expertise to perform. Furthermore, difficulty in cannulating the short right adrenal vein in particular can lead to results that are difficult or impossible to interpret. Finally, complications such as adrenal vein thrombosis with adrenal infarction may occasionally result, particularly on the right side. However, selective venous sampling has been helpful in selecting the appropriate patients for surgical intervention and confirming the side of the functioning tumor, especially in patients with no nodules, small nodules, or bilateral nodules. In a study at the Mayo Clinic, Young et al. (2004) selected 203 patients with primary hyperaldosteronism and prior CT imaging for selective venous sampling. An infusion of 50 μg of cosyntropin per hour was initiated 30 minutes before catheterization of the adrenal veins by the percutaneous femoral approach. Venous samples were obtained from both adrenal veins (the left-sided sample was obtained from the inferior phrenic vein near the entrance of the adrenal vein) and inferior vena cava below the level of the renal veins. Concentrations of cortisol and aldosterone were measured. Sampling was considered successful if the plasma level of cortisol in the adrenal vein was greater than five times that of the inferior vena cava. Aldosterone concentrations of each adrenal vein were divided by the respective cortisol concentrations to correct for an asymmetric dilutional effect between the adrenal veins. Bilateral adrenal cannulation was successful in 194 of the 203 patients. Of these 194 patients, CT correctly identified unilateral or bilateral disease in 53%. On the basis of CT findings alone, 21.7% of patients may have been incorrectly bypassed as candidates for surgery, while 24.7% may have had an unnecessary adrenalectomy. Therefore, selective venous sampling may be useful in localization and in guiding therapeutic management. Our current approach to the evaluation of patients suspected of having primary hyperaldosteronism is shown in Fig. 15.1.

Treatment

The treatment of primary hyperaldosteronism depends on the etiology. Bilateral adrenal hyperplasia is best managed medically using the aldosterone antagonist spironolactone. Most patients can achieve adequate control of their blood pressure with this medication alone or in conjunction with other antihypertensives. When an aldosterone-producing adenoma is diagnosed, the appropriate therapy remains surgical resection. Preoperatively, patients should be placed on spironolactone and given potassium supplementation to help normalize fluid and electrolyte balance over a 3- to 4-week period.

Surgical resection can be performed either through an open, a transabdominal laparoscopic, or a retroperitoneoscopic approach. Since nearly all patients with aldosteronomas have relatively small tumors which are universally benign, they are usually excellent candidates for a minimally invasive approach. Minimally invasive adrenalectomy has become the standard surgical approach for patients with aldosterone-producing adenomas due to its lower morbidity, lower rate of postoperative complications, and equal cure rates compared to open adrenalectomy. Nearly all patients with aldosteronoma will have resolution of hypokalemia following adrenalectomy, and 70% will have resolution of hypertension, while 30% will require continued management with antihypertensive medications. Even those patients who

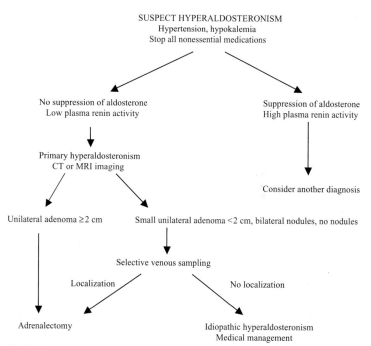

SUSPECT HYPERALDOSTERONISM
Hypertension, hypokalemia
Stop all nonessential medications

No suppression of aldosterone
Low plasma renin activity

Suppression of aldosterone
High plasma renin activity

Primary hyperaldosteronism
CT or MRI imaging

Consider another diagnosis

Unilateral adenoma ≥2 cm

Small unilateral adenoma <2 cm, bilateral nodules, no nodules

Selective venous sampling

Localization

No localization

Adrenalectomy

Idiopathic hyperaldosteronism
Medical management

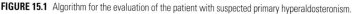

FIGURE 15.1 Algorithm for the evaluation of the patient with suspected primary hyperaldosteronism.

require continued antihypertensive therapy will usually require fewer medications for adequate blood pressure control compared to the preoperative period.

Approximately 2% or less of adrenocortical carcinomas cause isolated hyperaldosteronism. In the very rare situation of a patient presenting with hyperaldosteronism and a large adrenal mass, an open anterior approach should be used to facilitate complete resection (see Adrenal Cortical Carcinoma).

CORTISOL-PRODUCING ADRENAL ADENOMA

Introduction

Cushing syndrome is the term used to refer to the state of hypercortisolism that can result from a number of different pathologic processes (Table 15.1). Cortisol regulation involves feedback loops through the pituitary gland and hypothalamus. The most common cause of Cushing syndrome is exogenous steroid administration. After exclusion of patients taking exogenous steroids, approximately 70% of the remaining cases of hypercortisolism are secondary to hypersecretion of adrenocorticotropic hormone (ACTH) from the pituitary gland, a condition known as Cushing disease. Cushing disease is usually caused by a small pituitary adenoma. Ectopic secretion of ACTH, referred to as ectopic ACTH syndrome, is the cause of approximately 15% of cases of Cushing syndrome. Ectopic ACTH syndrome is usually caused by malignant tumors, with carcinoma of the lung, carcinoma of the pancreas, carcinoid tumors, and malignant thymoma accounting for 80% of such cases. Ectopic secretion of corticotropin-releasing factor is exceedingly rare but has been reported in a few cases.

TABLE 15.1 Causes of Cushing Syndrome

Exogenous steroids
Cushing disease (due to pituitary adenoma)
Adrenal tumors
   Adrenal cortical adenoma
   Adrenal cortical carcinoma
Primary adrenal cortical hyperplasia
Ectopic adrenocorticotropin syndrome
Ectopic corticotropin-releasing factor syndrome

Hypersecretion of cortisol from the adrenal glands accounts for approximately 10% to 20% of cases of Cushing syndrome. The underlying cause is adrenal adenoma 50% to 60% of the time and adrenocortical carcinoma 20% to 25% of the time. Bilateral adrenal hyperplasia accounts for the remaining 20% to 30% of cases.

Clinical Manifestations
Weight gain is the most common feature of hypercortisolism and occurs predominantly in the truncal area. This so-called centripetal obesity combined with muscle wasting in the extremities, fat deposition in the head and neck region ("moon facies"), and dorsal kyphosis ("buffalo hump") gives the patient a characteristic habitus. Abdominal striae, hypertension, and hyperglycemia are three other common findings. In some patients with Cushing syndrome due to an adrenal cortical tumor, these signs may be subtle or even absent altogether ("subclinical Cushing").

Diagnosis
The evaluation for Cushing syndrome should be aimed at establishing the diagnosis first and then determining the etiology. To establish the diagnosis, a state of hypercortisolism must be documented. The adult adrenal glands secrete on average 10 to 30 mg of cortisol each day. The secretion follows a diurnal variation: cortisol levels tend to be high early in the morning and low in the evening. The most sensitive initial screening test for hypercortisolism in patients with an adrenal mass is an overnight 1 mg dexamethasone suppression test (described below). Documentation of lack of cortisol suppression following 1 mg of dexamethasone should be followed by measurement of 24-hour urinary-free cortisol; the normal level is generally below 80 µg/day. In addition, to determine the etiology of elevated cortisol level, plasma ACTH levels must be checked. Secretion of ACTH also follows a diurnal variation, preceding that of cortisol by 1 to 2 hours. Suppressed levels of ACTH are seen in patients with adrenal adenomas, adrenocortical carcinomas, or autonomously functioning adrenal hyperplasia. In such cases, autonomous secretion of cortisol by the pathologic process within the adrenal gland inhibits pituitary ACTH release. Patients with Cushing disease (i.e., a pituitary adenoma-secreting ACTH) usually have plasma ACTH levels that are elevated or within the upper limits of normal. When there is an ectopic source of ACTH secretion, for example a metastatic tumor process, the plasma ACTH level is usually markedly increased.

The most sensitive method for detecting hypercortisolism is the overnight low-dose dexamethasone suppression test. One milligram of dexamethasone is taken orally at 10:00 or 11:00 p.m. The vast majority of normal individuals will suppress their cortisol levels to less than 5 µg/dL at 8:00 a.m. by the following morning. Failure to suppress the 8:00 a.m. cortisol level to less than 5 µg/dL is consistent with hypercortisolism. This test has a false-negative rate of only 3% but unfortunately a false-positive rate of 30%. While a normal overnight dexamethasone suppression test excludes clinically significant hypercortisolism, an abnormal test result does not necessarily establish the presence of hypercortisolism but does require further investigation. Some experts propose further testing even in patients with serum cortisol values between 1.8 and 5 µg/dL to increase the detection of subclinical hypercortisolism. Naturally, when lower cutoffs are used, specificity decreases, yielding more false positives. Since false-positive results are common, patients with elevated cortisol levels following overnight testing should undergo further evaluation by obtaining 8 a.m. cortisol and ACTH levels along with 24-hour urine collection for urinary-free (unmetabolized) cortisol. The 24-hour urinary-free cortisol is somewhat less sensitive than overnight dexamethasone suppression but more specific. In patients who have obvious signs or symptoms of hypercortisolism, a timed urinary collection should be obtained for cortisol determination.

In equivocal cases, a formal 2-day low-dose dexamethasone test may be performed to detect the presence of slight cortisol overproduction by an adrenal tumor. A dose of 0.5 mg of dexamethasone is administered every 6 hours for 2 days with pre- and postdexamethasone 24-hour urinary-free cortisol levels. Alternatively, individuals with failure of suppression after the 1-mg overnight dexamethasone test may be subjected to a higher dose (3 or 8 mg overnight suppression). Patients with true autonomous secretion should continue to exhibit nonsuppression with these higher doses of dexamethasone. Of note, dehydroepiandrosterone sulfate levels will be low in patients with ACTH suppression from autonomous cortisol secretion by an adrenal mass.

All patients with an incidentally identified adrenal mass should undergo an evaluation to exclude Cushing syndrome. Initial screening involves the 1-mg overnight dexamethasone suppression test. Patients with suppressed cortisol levels do not have Cushing syndrome and do not require further evaluation for this condition. Patients without suppressed cortisol levels should undergo a 24-hour urine collection for measurement of free cortisol.

Treatment

The appropriate management of Cushing syndrome depends on the underlying etiology. Patients with Cushing disease should undergo transsphenoidal hypophysectomy of the pituitary adenoma when it is believed to be resectable. Bilateral adrenalectomy is rarely indicated for patients with Cushing syndrome and should be reserved for those patients who fail to respond to standard management, including medical therapy and transsphenoidal hypophysectomy, and who experience end-organ injury from the consequences of overt hypercortisolism. If bilateral adrenalectomy is performed, patients require not only perioperative steroid coverage (Tables 15.2 and 15.3) but also lifelong replacement of both glucocorticoids and mineralocorticoids. Patients with autonomously functioning bilateral adrenal hyperplasia usually require bilateral adrenalectomy. Patients with ectopic ACTH syndrome should have the underlying malignant condition identified and treated. Bilateral adrenalectomy in this setting should be reserved for the small group of patients whose primary tumor is unresectable and whose symptoms of cortisol excess cannot be controlled medically. Bilateral adrenalectomy can be performed laparoscopically, retroperitoneoscopically, via an open posterior retroperitoneal approach, or via open laparotomy. Our current preferred approach to the majority of these patients is via a minimally invasive retroperitoneoscopic approach when body habitus and adrenal size will permit.

Patients with a cortisol-producing neoplasm of the adrenal gland, whether adenoma or carcinoma, should undergo resection of the involved side. Although almost all adenomas can be resected, adrenocortical carcinomas that secrete cortisol are resectable in only 25% to 35% of patients. Chemotherapy has been

TABLE 15.2 Recommendations for Perioperative Glucocorticoid Coverage

Surgical Stress	Examples	Hydrocortisone Equivalent (mg)	Duration (d)
Minor	Inguinal herniorrhaphy	25	1
Moderate	Open cholecystectomy Lower-extremity revascularization Segmental colon resection Total joint replacement Abdominal hysterectomy	50–75	1–2
Major	Pancreaticoduodenectomy Esophagogastrectomy Total proctocolectomy Cardiac surgery with cardiopulmonary bypass	100–150	2–3

disappointing in patients with unresectable or metastatic adrenocortical carcinoma. Symptoms related to hypercortisolism in patients with metastatic or unresectable functioning tumors can sometimes be minimized with various agents that are toxic to adrenal tissue or interfere with steroid hormone synthesis, including mitotane, aminoglutethimide, metyrapone, or ketoconazole.

PHEOCHROMOCYTOMA

Introduction

Pheochromocytomas represent a potentially curable form of endocrine hypertension that, if undetected, places patients at high risk for morbidity and mortality, particularly during surgery and pregnancy. The estimated incidence is between 0.005% and 0.1% of the general population and between 0.1% and 0.2% of the adult hypertensive population. These neuroectodermal tumors arise from the chromaffin cells of the adrenal medulla. Approximately 10% of pheochromocytomas are bilateral, with some patients presenting with multiple tumors. Ten percent of pheochromocytomas can be found in extra-adrenal sites, where they are more appropriately called paragangliomas because of their close association with ganglia of the

TABLE 15.3 Comparison of Steroid Preparations

Steroid	Half-Life (h)	Glucocorticoid Activity (Relative to Cortisol)	Mineralocorticoid Activity (Relative to Cortisol)
Cortisol	8–12	1	1
Cortisone	8–12	0.8	0.8
Prednisone	12–36	4	0.25
Prednisolone	12–36	4	0.25
Methylprednisolone	12–36	5	0
Triamcinolone	12–36	5	0
Betamethasone	36–72	25	0
Dexamethasone	36–72	30–40	0

sympathetic nervous system. The most common extra-adrenal sites include the organ of Zuckerkandl (located between the inferior mesenteric artery and the aortic bifurcation), the urinary bladder, the thorax, and the renal hilum.

Histologic evidence of malignancy in pheochromocytomas can be demonstrated approximately 10% of the time; malignancy is more commonly seen with extra-adrenal lesions than with those arising in the adrenal glands. Documenting malignancy can be difficult because invasion of adjacent organs or metastatic disease must be present. Furthermore, both benign and malignant lesions may show tumor penetration of the gland's capsule, invasion of veins draining the gland, cellular pleomorphism, mitoses, and atypical nuclei.

Familial pheochromocytomas have been estimated to account for approximately 10% of cases; however, recent data suggest that up to 25% of unselected cases of apparently sporadic pheochromocytomas are in fact hereditary. Hereditary pheochromocytomas are almost always benign. The familial syndromes associated with pheochromocytomas include multiple endocrine neoplasia (MEN) types IIA and IIB, in which bilateral tumors are common, as well as the neuroectodermal dysplasias consisting of neurofibromatosis, tuberous sclerosis, Sturge–Weber syndrome, and von Hippel–Lindau disease. The risk for inherited pheochromocytomas is very low in neurofibromatosis type 1 (<1%) and MEN 1 syndrome (<1%). Pheochromocytoma can also occur in hereditary paraganglioma syndrome (mutations in *SDHD*, *SDHB*, and *SDHC* genes). Hereditary paraganglioma syndrome predisposes to both extra-adrenal and adrenal paragangliomas. Patients with familial pheochromocytoma syndromes require follow-up and periodic screening for pheochromocytoma, especially before any planned surgical procedure.

Clinical Manifestations

The clinical manifestations of pheochromocytoma can be varied and at times quite dramatic. Hypertension, sustained or paroxysmal, is the most common clinical presentation. Paroxysmal elevations in blood pressure can vary markedly in frequency and duration and can be initiated by a variety of events, including heavy physical exertion and eating foods high in tyramine (e.g., chocolate, cheese, red wine). Other common symptoms include excessive sweating, palpitations, tremulousness, anxiety, and chest pain. More than half of patients with pheochromocytomas have impaired glucose tolerance and may have symptoms of diabetes mellitus, including polydipsia or polyuria. These signs and symptoms are secondary to the excess catecholamine secretion by the tumors and resolve with tumor resection. Patients with functioning tumors are rarely asymptomatic; an exception is patients with hereditary pheochromocytomas. Nonfunctioning pheochromocytomas are rare; extra-adrenal paragangliomas, however, may be nonfunctioning.

Diagnosis

The diagnosis of pheochromocytoma is made by documenting excess secretion of catecholamines. Plasma-free metanephrine determination is a very sensitive screen for the presence of catecholamine elevation and is more convenient than timed urine collection. Twenty-four-hour urine collection for free catecholamine levels (dopamine, epinephrine, and norepinephrine) and their metabolites (nor-metanephrine, metanephrine, vanillylmandelic acid) should be used to confirm suspected catecholamine elevation identified by plasma screen. Increased levels of catecholamines or their metabolites are seen in more than 90% of patients with pheochromocytoma. The adrenal glands and the organ of Zuckerkandl produce the enzyme phenylethanolamine-*N*-methyl-transferase, which converts norepinephrine to epinephrine. Pheochromocytomas that arise elsewhere do not contain this enzyme and thus do not produce much, if any, epinephrine. As a result, extra-adrenal pheochromocytomas (paragangliomas) secrete predominantly dopamine and norepinephrine.

Once the diagnosis of pheochromocytoma is made, localization studies can be carried out. A review of preoperative imaging in a large series of histologically confirmed pheochromocytomas found that MRI was the most sensitive modality (98%), followed by CT imaging (89%) and ^{131}I-metaiodobenzylguanidine (MIBG) scanning (81%). Our experience indicates that high-quality spiral CT can detect up to 95% of adrenal masses larger than 6 to 8 mm and is usually the initial imaging study of choice; it is rare for a clinically significant primary pheochromocytoma to not be imaged by CT. Magnetic resonance imaging may be useful in selected cases because the T2-weighted images can identify chromaffin tissue; the T2-weighted adrenal mass-to-liver ratio of pheochromocytomas or paragangliomas is usually more than 3. This ratio is higher than that of adrenal cortical adenomas, adrenal cortical carcinomas, or metastases to the adrenal gland. Thus the MRI may provide potentially useful functional or biochemical information. The MIBG scan is another procedure that is helpful in localizing extra-adrenal, metastatic, or bilateral pheochromocytomas. This radiolabeled amine is selectively picked up by chromaffin tissue and can identify the majority of pheochromocytomas, regardless of their location. Therefore, MIBG scanning is useful in patients with biochemical evidence of pheochromocytoma whose tumors cannot be localized by CT or MRI and in the follow-up evaluation of patients with suspected or documented recurrent or metastatic disease. Using these techniques, it is rare to have a patient whose pheochromocytoma cannot be localized preoperatively.

Treatment

After diagnosis and localization of the pheochromocytoma, careful preoperative preparation is required to prevent a cardiovascular crisis during surgery caused by excess catecholamine secretion. The main focus of preoperative preparation is adequate alpha-adrenergic blockade and restoration of fluid and electrolyte balance. Phenoxybenzamine is the alpha-adrenergic blocking agent of choice and is usually begun at a dose of 10 mg twice a day. The dosage is gradually increased over a 2- to 3-week period until adequate blockade is reached to the point of postural hypotension and/or nasal stuffiness. The total dose used should not exceed 1 to 2 mg per kg per day. Beta blockade following alpha blockade may help prevent tachycardia and other arrhythmias. Beta blockade should not be instituted unless alpha blockade has been established; otherwise, the beta-blocker will inhibit epinephrine-induced vasodilation, leading to more significant hypertension and left heart strain. In addition to requiring pharmacologic preparation, patients with pheochromocytoma require correction of fluid volume depletion as well as any concurrent electrolyte imbalances.

The perioperative management of patients with pheochromocytoma can be difficult. Rarely is alpha-adrenergic blockade complete. The anesthesiologist should be prepared to treat a hypertensive crisis with sodium nitroprusside and tachyarrhythmias with either a beta-blocker or anti-arrhythmics. Commonly used preoperative and perioperative medications are listed in Table 15.4. If preoperative imaging suggests a modestly-sized, benign-appearing unilateral pheochromocytoma with a radiographically normal contralateral gland, we currently prefer a unilateral laparoscopic or posterior retroperitoneoscopic approach. A minimally invasive approach is also appropriate for patients with MEN II or von Hippel–Lindau disease with a small, unilateral pheochromocytoma less than 6 cm in size. For patients with MEN II or von Hippel–Lindau disease with bilateral disease, a bilateral minimally invasive approach may also be appropriate. Cortical-sparing adrenalectomy, either open or laparoscopic, has been performed successfully in patients with MEN II or von Hippel–Lindau disease with bilateral pheochromocytomas, avoiding chronic steroid hormone replacement and the risk of Addisonian crisis in most patients. For tumors greater than 6 cm in size, open adrenalectomy is preferred due to the increased risk of malignancy as high as 25%. Whatever the operative approach,

TABLE
15.4

Common Medications in the Management of Pheochromocytoma

Medication	Standard Dosage	Contraindication	Main Drug Interaction	Main Side Effects	Comments
Phenoxybenzamine (nonselective α-blocker)	10 mg BID-TID	Conditions compromised by hypotension	Reports of hypertensive episodes when used in combinations with β-blockers	Dosing endpoints to postural hypotension and/or nasal stuffiness to ensure adequate α-blockade. Tachycardia, hypoglycemia, miosis, sexual dysfunction.	May be increased to 20–40 mg/d to total dose of 1–2 mg/kg/d BID-TID
Prazosin (selective α1-blocker)	0.5–1.0 mg dosed at bedtime, titrated up to 3–20 mg/d, as QD-BID	Hypersensitivity to product or quinazolines	β-blockers, verapamil	Hypotension, tachycardia, dizziness	Rarely used
Metyrosine (tyrosine hydroxylase inhibitor)	250 mg TID-QID, with doses titrated by 250–500 mg to maximum of 1.5–4 g/d	Hypersensitivity to metyrosine products	Minimal	Crystalluria, extrapyramidal effects, diarrhea, anxiety, drowsiness, se dation, depression, nightmares. Long-term use can result in heart failure.	Best used for epinephrine-only secreting tumors, or in patients with contraindications to β-blockade. Best to limit use to the peri-operative period due to cardiac toxicity. Given as a half dose the morning of surgery.
Propranolol (nonselective β-blocker)	10–40 mg BID-TID	Lack of α-blockade, second or third degree atrioventricular block, congestive heart failure, myocarditis, hypersensitivity, asthma	Can interact with other cardiac medications, anti-diabetic medications, cimetidine, fentanyl, rifampin, theophylline	Bradycardia, bronchospasm, depression, diarrhea	May be added to the preoperative medical preparation, especially if tachycardia develops after α-blockade

(continued)

TABLE 15.4 Common Medications in the Management of Pheochromocytoma (*continued*)

Medication	Standard Dosage	Contraindication	Main Drug Interaction	Main Side Effects	Comments
Nitroprusside (direct vasodilator)	2–4 µg/kg/min	Hypersensitivity, anemia, optic atrophy, head trauma, tobacco amblyopia	Sildenafil (a phosphodies- terase inhibitor, which potentiates hypotensive effects)	Hypotension, headache, methemoglobinemia, cyanide toxicity	Dilute in D5W only. With prolonged infusion (>24 h), patients can develop cyanide toxicity. Dose reduced in patients with liver or renal impairment
Esmolol (β-blocker)	Titrate to effect (12–200 µg/kg/min)	Hypersensitivity, bradycardia, atrioventricular block, and cardiogenic shock	Fentanyl, cardiac medications	Hypotension, bradycardia	Short duration of action (half-life 10 min)
Norepinephrine (α-agonist)	4–16 µg/min as an infusion	Hypovolemia	Tricyclic antidepressants, cardiac medications	Hypertension, decreased visceral perfusion, anxiety, nausea, vomiting, urinary retention, cardiac arrhythmias	Avoid subcutaneous extravasation
Epinephrine (β-agonist)	0.1–0.2 mg/kg	Hypersensitivity, cardiac dilative cardiomyopathy, coronary artery disease, narrow angle glaucoma, hypovolemic shock, intra- arterial injection, labor	Cardiac medications, halothane, tricyclic antidepressants	Hypertension, nausea, vomiting, headache, cardiac arrhythmias, tachycardia	Limited utility

the surgeon should manipulate the tumor as little as possible and ligate the tumor's venous outflow via the adrenal vein as early in the procedure as possible.

Postoperatively, patients should be monitored carefully for 24 hours so that they can be observed for arrhythmias, as well as hypotension secondary to compensatory vasodilation. Occasionally, hypertension remains a problem postoperatively, especially in those patients who had sustained hypertension preoperatively. Following surgical treatment for pheochromocytoma, all patients should undergo yearly evaluation to include plasma-free metanephrine level or timed urine collection for catecholamine determination to exclude recurrence.

The most common sites of metastases from malignant pheochromocytoma are bone, liver, and lungs and less commonly, regional lymph nodes. Patients with known or suspected malignant pheochromocytoma should be staged with standard imaging studies as well as MIBG scanning. Therapy should be individualized based upon the extent of disease. Palliative therapy may include treatment with alpha-methyltyrosine, as well as α- and β-blockade. Resection of malignant pheochromocytoma, including resection of metastases, may be considered in good-risk individuals if the metastases are limited in extent. The most commonly used chemotherapy regimens for pheochromocytoma are high-dose streptozocin and a combination of cyclophosphamide, vincristine, and dacarbazine. The overall response rates with these regimens are approximately 50%. Radiation therapy has been effective only for bony metastases. There has been some interest in treating metastatic lesions with therapeutic doses of ^{131}I-MIBG. Unfortunately, a high percentage of metastatic pheochromocytomas do not take up ^{131}I-MIBG; therefore, the response rate, as manifested by a reduction in urinary catecholamines, is only approximately 50%. Objective responses as determined by imaging studies are seen even less frequently. The 5-year survival rate for patients with malignant pheochromocytoma is approximately 43%, as compared with a 97% 5-year survival rate for benign lesions.

ADRENAL CORTICAL CARCINOMA

Introduction

Adrenal cortical carcinoma is a rare endocrine malignancy with an incidence of 0.5 to 2 cases per 1 million people each year in the United States. There is a bimodal age distribution, with incidence peaking in young children less than 5 years old and then again between 40 and 50 years of age. Prognosis tends to be poor because diagnosis is usually delayed, and there is dearth of effective systemic chemotherapy. Surgical resection remains the mainstay of curative therapy.

Clinical Manifestations

Patients with adrenal cortical carcinoma usually present with vague abdominal symptoms secondary to an enlarging retroperitoneal mass or with clinical manifestations of overproduction of one or more adrenal cortical hormones. Most of these tumors are functional as measured by biochemical parameters. Up to 50% secrete cortisol, producing Cushing syndrome. The workup and treatment of patients with Cushing syndrome are described under section Cortisol-Producing Adrenal Adenoma above. Another 10% to 20% of adrenocortical carcinomas produce androgens, estrogens, or aldosterone, which can cause virilization in females, feminization in males, or hypertension, respectively.

Diagnosis

The preoperative evaluation of these patients involves biochemical screening for cortisol overproduction as detailed above. The results of this screening serve to guide perioperative replacement therapy. Screening to exclude pheochromocytoma should also be performed. Standard preoperative staging in patients with suspected adrenal cancer includes high-resolution abdominal CT or MRI. MRI may be especially helpful in delineating tumor extension into the inferior vena cava. Positron emission tomography when combined with CT imaging may be helpful in detecting metastasis or recurrence in patients with adrenal cortical cancer. Chest radiography may be helpful in ruling out pulmonary metastasis. The various staging systems for adrenocortical carcinomas are shown in Table 15.5.

Treatment

Complete surgical resection is currently the only potentially curative therapy for localized adrenal cortical cancer. Approximately 50% of the tumors are localized to the adrenal gland at the time of initial presentation. We recommend an open transabdominal approach to facilitate adequate exposure to ensure complete resection, minimize the risk of tumor spillage, and allow for vascular control of the inferior vena cava, aorta, and renal vessels when necessary. Radical en bloc resection that includes adjacent organs, if necessary, provides the only chance for long-term survival. Patients who undergo a complete resection of their tumor have a 5-year survival rate of approximately 40% and a median survival of 43 months; those who undergo incomplete resection have a median survival duration of less than 12 months. Therefore, the strongest predictor of outcome in this disease is the ability to perform a complete resection. Laparoscopic resection of adrenal cortical carcinoma, while technically potentially feasible in the rare patient with a small, localized adrenal cortical carcinoma, has been associated with a very high rate of tumor recurrence and peritoneal carcinomatosis, presumably due to tumor fracture and peritoneal contamination. For this reason, we continue to prefer open adrenalectomy for patients with known or suspected adrenal cortical carcinoma, including most patients with an adrenal incidentaloma (see Adrenal Incidentaloma).

Common sites of metastasis of adrenal cortical carcinoma include lungs, lymph nodes, liver, peritoneum, and bone. Complete resection of recurrent disease, including pulmonary metastases, is associated with prolonged survival in some patients and can help control symptoms related to excess hormone production. After a potentially curative resection, patients whose tumors were hormonally active should be monitored with interval steroid measurement as well as abdominal CT and chest radiograph.

Radiation therapy can provide palliation for bone metastasis from adrenal cancer. No chemotherapeutic agent or combination of agents has been shown to be consistently effective against unresectable or metastatic adrenal cortical cancer. Mitotane has been one of the most commonly used systemic agents because of its ability to palliate the endocrine effects of the tumor. This drug is an isomer of dichlorodiphenyltrichloroethane and not only inhibits steroid production but also leads to atrophy of adrenocortical cells. Mitotane is associated with a number of side effects, most notably gastrointestinal and neuromuscular symptoms. In addition, the drug has a relatively narrow therapeutic range, and it requires close monitoring of serum levels as well as provision of exogenous steroid hormone replacement to avoid symptoms associated with adrenal insufficiency due to suppression of cortisol production by the normal contralateral adrenal gland. Other systemic treatment options for patients with unresectable local recurrence or distant metastases include suramin, ketoconazole, and systemic chemotherapy regimens containing cisplatin, etoposide, doxorubicin, or vincristine.

The role of mitotane in the adjuvant setting after radical resection of adrenocortical carcinoma is still somewhat controversial. A recent nonrandomized retrospective study by Terzolo et al. (2007) examined the role of adjuvant mitotane postoperatively with respect to overall and recurrence-free survival. The authors examined 177 patients with adrenocortical carcinoma who had undergone resection in 55 centers in Italy and Germany over a period of 20 years. The study included a

TABLE 15.5

Staging Systems for Adrenal Cortical Carcinoma

Stage	Macfarlane (1958)	Sullivan (1978)	Icard (1992)	Lee (1995)	American Joint Committee on Cancer 7 (2010)
I	T1 (≤5 cm), N0, M0	T1 (≤5 cm), N0, M0	T1 (≤5 cm), N0, M0	T1 (≤5 cm), N0, M0	T1 (≤5 cm), N0, M0
II	T2 (>5 cm), N0, M0	T2 (>5 cm), N0, M0	T2 (>5 cm), N0, M0	T2 (>5 cm), N0, M0	T2 (>5 cm), N0, M0
III	T3 (local invasion without involvement of adjacent organs) or mobile positive lymph nodes, M0	T3 (local invasion), N0, M0 or T1–2, N1 (positive lymph nodes), M0	T3 (local invasion) and/or N1 (positive regional lymph nodes), M0	T3/T4 (local invasion as demonstrated by histologic evidence of adjacent organ invasion, direct tumor extension to IVC, and/or tumor thrombus within IVC or renal vein) and/or N1 (positive regional lymph nodes), M0	T1/T2, N1 (positive regional lymph nodes), M0 T3 (local invasion, but not invading adjacent organs), N0, M0
IV	T4 (invasion of adjacent organs) or fixed positive lymph nodes or M1 (distant metastasis)	T4 (local invasion), N0, M0; or T3, N1, M0; or T1–4, N0–1, M1 (distant metastasis)	T1–4, N0–1, M1 (distant metastasis)	T1–4, N0–1, M1 (distant metastasis)	T3/T4, N1, M0 T4, N0, M0 Any T, Any N, M1 (distant metastasis)

IVC, inferior vena cava.

group of 47 Italian patients treated at a single center who had received adjuvant mitotane and compared these patients to a group of 55 Italian patients and another group of 75 German patients who had not received adjuvant mitotane. While there was no significant difference in overall survival, recurrence-free survival was prolonged in the mitotane group (median 42 months) compared to the Italian (10 months) and German (25 months) controls. The recurrence rates were 49% in the mitotane group, 91% in the Italian control group, and 73% in the German control group. Limitations of the study included lack of details regarding the mitotane regimen and potential inconsistencies in surgery and follow-up evaluation among the various institutions over the span of two decades, resulting in an ascertainment and lead-time bias in the detection of recurrences. Importantly, the high recurrence rate of the Italian control group suggests that some patients may not have had a complete resection.

The importance of complete resection has been highlighted in a study of 113 patients treated for adrenocortical cancer at Memorial Sloan-Kettering Cancer Center. Patients with complete primary resections had improved 5-year survival rates compared to patients with incomplete resections (55% vs. 5%). Moreover, the benefit of complete resection was demonstrated in patients with repeat surgery. Patients with a complete second resection demonstrated improved 5-year survival rates compared to patients with incomplete second resection (57% vs. 0%).

Our group has examined 218 patients with adrenocortical carcinoma who underwent primary resection either at our (index) institution (28 patients) or an outside institution (190 patients). After a median follow-up of 7.3 years, patients who had undergone surgery at the index institution had superior overall survival compared with outside patients (median not reached vs. 44 months) as well as superior disease-free survival (median 25 vs. 12 months). The overall survival rates were 68% versus 32%, and the recurrence rates were 50% versus 86% for the index and outside patients, respectively. Twenty-two of the 218 patients (10%) in this series received adjuvant mitotane. A subanalysis demonstrated a prolonged disease-free survival in the mitotane group (median of 30 months vs. 12 months) without a benefit in overall survival. The outcomes of the index and outside patients in our study fare comparably to the outcomes of the mitotane and control groups in the Terzolo et al. (2007) study. Based on these results, it appears that differences in outcomes between the patient groups in the European mitotane study may be related at least partly to quality and completeness of surgery rather than adjuvant mitotane. We therefore advocate individualizing adjuvant mitotane therapy in the postoperative management of patients with resected adrenal cortical carcinoma; we generally favor adjuvant mitotane in the postoperative management of relatively young healthy patients with a good performance status.

ADRENAL INCIDENTALOMA

With the widespread use of abdominal CT imaging, asymptomatic adrenal lesions are being discovered with increasing frequency. These lesions, termed incidentalomas, are seen in up to 4% of routinely performed abdominal imaging studies and in up to 9% of autopsy series. Although most of these lesions are benign adenomas, some are hormonally active, and a small minority represents an invasive malignancy.

Patients identified with an incidental adrenal mass >1 cm in size should be screened to rule out a hormonally active adenoma or pheochromocytoma. Evaluation of patients with an incidentally identified adrenal mass includes measurement of serum electrolyte levels, an overnight 1-mg dexamethasone suppression test (described previously), and measurement of plasma metanephrine levels (Fig. 15.2). Any hormonally active lesion, regardless of size, should be resected. Furthermore, surgery is indicated if the adrenal mass demonstrates radiographic characteristics suggestive of malignancy or if the tumor enlarges during follow-up.

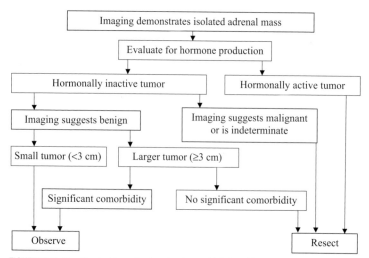

FIGURE 15.2 Algorithm for the evaluation of patients with isolated, incidentally identified adrenal tumors.

If the incidentaloma is nonfunctioning, the risk of malignancy is related to its size and radiographic characteristics. Size is the single best clinical indicator of malignancy in patients who present with incidental adrenal mass. Adrenal cortical carcinoma accounts for 2%, 6%, and 35% of incidentalomas smaller than 4 cm, 4.1 to 6 cm, and greater than 6 cm in size, respectively. In general, lesions larger than 6 cm should be resected, because of the high risk of malignancy. Observation and follow-up is generally recommended for nonfunctioning lesions smaller than 3 cm in diameter, but the management of tumors between 3 and 6 cm is more controversial. Data from our own institution and elsewhere have identified patients with adrenal cortical carcinomas arising in tumors smaller than 5 cm. The majority of these small tumors had CT or MRI characteristics suspicious for carcinoma such as heterogeneity and irregular borders. Based on individual experience and a review of the literature, recent recommendations for resection of nonfunctioning adrenal masses have ranged from 5 cm down to 3 cm. The recent success and advantages of laparoscopic adrenalectomy has led some investigators to suggest operative removal of even relatively small incidentalomas.

At M. D. Anderson, we recommend adrenalectomy for all biochemically confirmed functioning adrenal tumors and those with suspicious radiographic findings regardless of size. A recent study comparing the incidence of carcinomatosis and local recurrence in patients managed with open versus laparoscopic adrenalectomy identified a much higher rate of carcinomatosis in the laparoscopic group (83%) when compared to open adrenalectomy (8%). Because of the risk of capsular fracture and resultant peritoneal carcinomatosis, we reserve the laparoscopic approach for lesions without worrisome radiographic features on cross-sectional imaging (CT and/or MRI), and lesions that are less than 4 cm in greatest transverse diameter, while an open transabdominal approach is used for all lesions that do not meet these criteria. Nonfunctioning tumors between 3 and 6 cm in diameter are most appropriately managed on an individual basis with respect to patient age and general health. For example, a 3 cm tumor in an otherwise healthy 40-year-old patient is probably most appropriately managed by adrenalectomy, whereas the same tumor in a 75-year-old patient with multiple comorbidities might be observed. The following may be helpful in evaluating such patients with intermediate-size nonfunctioning adrenal masses: MRI, a more thorough endocrine evaluation, and consideration of age and comorbidity. Figure 15.3 provides an overview of our approach to patients with adrenal incidentalomas.

ADRENAL METASTASES

Cancer metastasis to the adrenal glands is relatively common. Based on autopsy studies, 42% of lung cancers, 16% of gastric cancers, 58% of breast cancers, 50% of malignant melanomas, and a high percentage of renal and prostate cancers have metastasized to the adrenal glands by the time of death. However, only rarely are clinical problems related to these adrenal metastases, such as adrenal insufficiency, encountered. In general, more than 90% of normal adrenal cortical tissue must be replaced before clinically detectable adrenal cortical hypofunction is appreciated. When adrenal insufficiency does occur, it is usually in the setting of gross enlargement of the adrenal glands as detected by CT.

Surgery for isolated metastases to the adrenal gland may be considered in highly selected patients. Appropriate selection criteria include good-risk individuals in whom there is a prolonged disease-free interval and evidence of favorable underlying tumor biology. Favorable tumor biology is implied in those who have had a significant progression-free interval, those who have responded to systemic therapy, and those who have had a history of isolated metachronous metastases. In particular, a longer disease-free interval from the time of primary cancer therapy to adrenal metastasis is associated with a survival advantage following adrenalectomy. Primary tumor site also appears to affect survival, in that longer median survival times are observed following resection of metastases from primary kidney, melanoma, colon, and lung cancers, and poorer survival in patients with esophageal, liver, unknown primary tumors, and high-grade sarcomas.

Evaluation of the patient with an adrenal mass and a history of malignancy includes an evaluation for hormone production, since as many as 50% of these patients will have occult, functioning adrenal tumors unrelated to their prior malignancy, for example pheochromocytoma (Fig. 15.3). Fine-needle aspiration biopsy may be helpful in selected patients when the results would influence the treatment plan; for example, to confirm a diagnosis of metastasis, particularly in those who are not surgical candidates and in those patients who have not yet had their primary cancer resected. In a study of patients with operable nonsmall cell lung cancer and an adrenal mass, 40% had nonfunctioning adenomas by CT-guided biopsy. In selected patients, however, surgical therapy may be planned solely based on the patient's history and on noninvasive studies and without preoperative needle biopsy. A history of a malignancy that commonly metastasizes to the adrenal glands, with favorable tumor biology, negative biochemical screening for hormone production, and a mass that either fulfills size criteria for surgical excision or is radiographically suspicious for metastasis, may be considered for resection without preoperative tissue diagnosis.

At the University of Texas M. D. Anderson Cancer Center, we investigated the incidence of adrenal metastasis in patients with either a known concurrent extra-adrenal malignancy or a prior extra-adrenal malignancy. One hundred and ninety-six patients were referred for adrenalectomy, and of these, 81 had a prior or concurrent extra-adrenal malignancy. Of the 81 patients, 42 patients (52%) had metastatic disease to the adrenal gland. The three most common primary malignancies were from renal, melanoma, and colorectal primaries. Cross- sectional imaging (CT and/or MRI) was suggestive of metastatic disease in 17 patients (40%),

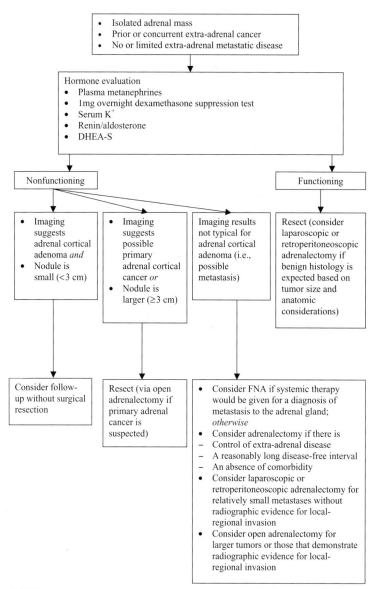

FIGURE 15.3 Algorithm for the evaluation and surgical treatment of patients with extra-adrenal cancer presenting with an adrenal mass. VMA, vanillylmandelic acid.

while FNA was used in 18 patients (43%) and supported a diagnosis of cancer in 16 (89%) of these patients. The median actuarial survival of these patients was 3.4 years after adrenalectomy. Thus, in selected patients with a long disease-free interval, acceptable performance status, and controlled extra-adrenal disease, long-term palliation may be achieved with adrenalectomy as seen in patients who undergo metastasectomy in other organs. In another retrospective review examining patients with melanoma metastasis to the adrenal gland, patients who underwent adrenalectomy with or without a concomitant metastasectomy had improved survival compared to patients managed nonoperatively. Therefore, surgical treatment of cancer metastasis to the adrenal gland, including melanoma metastasis, can be considered in highly selected patients.

We emphasize that we do not recommend routine fine-needle aspiration of incidentally identified adrenal tumors in patients without a previous diagnosis of cancer. In the absence of signs or symptoms of a solid tumor malignancy, unilateral adrenal metastases are uncommon. Our experience with over 1,600 patients found that the incidence of metastasis from an occult primary cancer was 0.2% (4 of 1,639). In all four of these patients, malignancy was suspected on the basis of tumor size, bilateral involvement, or symptoms. Therefore, we do not routinely biopsy patients with small nonfunctioning adrenal tumors searching for occult metastatic disease.

SURGICAL APPROACH

Introduction

When choosing an operative approach for a patient with an adrenal tumor, several factors must be considered: the size and site of the tumor, the malignant potential of the disease, the laterality or bilaterality of the disease, the presence of multiple or extra-adrenal tumors, the presence of additional intra-abdominal disease or extra-abdominal extension, history of prior abdominal surgery, the patient's body habitus, and the surgeon's experience. As a general rule, large tumors and tumors with malignant potential are best approached with open operation.

Open Adrenalectomy

An open adrenalectomy is indicated for known or suspected primary adrenal cancer, large tumors, recurrent disease, and for tumors that involve adjacent viscera. Open adrenalectomy can be performed by four approaches: anterior, posterior, lateral (flank), and thoracoabdominal. The anterior approach is the preferred method for resection of most adrenocortical carcinomas. The patient is placed in a supine or semi-lateral position. Access is accomplished via a midline incision, a bilateral subcostal incision, or a Makuuchi (hockey stick-shaped) incision.

For open adrenalectomy of the left adrenal gland, the splenic flexure and descending colon are mobilized inferiorly and the retroperitoneum is entered by incising along the inferior border of the pancreas. Medial visceral rotation of the spleen and tail of pancreas is usually helpful and necessary when dealing with large tumors. The adrenal gland can be visualized by exposing the renal hilum and then following the left renal vein to the junction of the adrenal vein. The left adrenal gland lies lateral to the aorta, just above the left renal vein. The adrenal vein should be ligated early in the procedure if possible to limit the release of catecholamines when dealing with pheochromocytoma. Small arterial perforators from the aorta, inferior phrenic, and renal arteries are identified and ligated.

Open adrenalectomy of the right adrenal gland is approached similarly; on the right side, mobilization of the right triangular ligament of the liver allows antero-medial rotation of the liver and access to the right adrenal gland. A Kocher maneuver facilitates exposure of the right kidney and vena cava and is helpful when the adrenal tumor is large. The right adrenal vein generally drains directly into the vena cava and is very short. Care is taken to control it appropriately, and the arterial supply to the adrenal gland is then ligated. Drains are usually unnecessary.

The open posterior approach, formerly commonly used in the resection of small, benign adrenal tumors (e.g., aldosteronomas) is now rarely employed. The procedure begins with the patient in a prone position with the table flexed about 35°. An oblique incision is made over the 12th rib with retraction of sacrospinalis medially, resection of the 12th rib, and reflection of the pleura superiorly. On the left, the superior extent of the dissection is the diaphragm. The perirenal fat and soft tissues are reflected down with diaphragm exposed superomedially. Medially, a vertically coursing inferior phrenic vein can be encountered indicating the adrenal gland is nearby, laterally. On the right, care is taken to preserve the subcostal nerve and exposure is facilitated by transecting the free edge of the diaphragm medially to the spine. The adrenal gland is located against the bare area of the liver with exposure of the liver delineating the superior extent of the dissection.

The thoracoabdominal approach provides the broadest exposure and is useful for tumors that may require en bloc resection of adjacent organs or extensive lymph node dissection. The patient is placed in the decubitus position and the incision is carried over the 10th rib on the right or over the 11th rib on the left, followed by resection of the rib. For tumors with significant extension into the IVC, the hepatic veins, or the right atrium, a median sternotomy may be necessary.

In the lateral (flank) approach, the patient is placed in a lateral decubitus position with an extraperitoneal approach to the involved side. The lateral approach can be helpful in obese patients with gravity assisting the retraction. This approach can obviate the need to perform extensive adhesiolysis in a patient with previous abdominal surgery. However, vascular control of large vessels may be difficult.

Laparoscopic Adrenalectomy

Since the first description of laparoscopic adrenalectomy in 1992, this approach has been expanded and is considered now the standard approach for modestly sized benign adrenal tumors. Patients who undergo laparoscopic adrenalectomy have a more rapid recovery, less discomfort, faster return to preoperative activity level, and better cosmetic results compared to patients who undergo open adrenalectomy. Patients who are good candidates for laparoscopic adrenalectomy include those with aldosterone-producing adenomas, other small (<4 cm) functioning cortical neoplasms, those with unilateral, benign-appearing sporadic pheochromocytomas, MEN II or Von Hippel-Lindau Syndrome patients with a unilateral pheochromocytoma, and selected patients with adrenal metastasis. Bilateral laparoscopic adrenalectomy can be performed in selected patients with bilateral adrenal hyperplasia. Laparoscopic cortical-sparing partial adrenalectomy has been successfully performed in patients with bilateral pheochromocytomas in the familial setting. Surgeons should be aware, however, that an open anterior approach may still maximize the opportunity for adrenal cortical preservation in these patients. We continue to urge caution in the use of laparoscopic adrenalectomy for patients with malignant or potentially malignant primary adrenal tumors. This includes the occasional patient with sporadic pheochromocytoma in whom radiographic imaging raises suspicion for malignancy, patients with hereditary paraganglioma syndrome, and those with cortical neoplasms (functioning or nonfunctioning) 4 cm in size or greater, or those with radiographic evidence of malignancy. It is emphasized that the reason for operating on patients with nonfunctioning adrenal tumors (incidentalomas) is that they are potentially malignant cortical neoplasms. Therefore, we specifically do not recommend laparoscopic adrenalectomy for patients in whom adrenal cortical carcinoma is part of the preoperative differential diagnosis.

For a left adrenalectomy, the patient is placed in the right lateral decubitus position, with the table appropriately padded and flexed. The abdomen and chest are prepped from the nipple to below the iliac crest, and from the right of the umbilicus to the vertebral column. An infracostal port, 10 to 15 cm anterior to the anterior axillary line, is placed using the open technique, abdominal insufflation achieved, and the 30-degree laparoscope is inserted. Three additional 10 mm trocars are then placed under direct vision. One is placed at the anterior axillary line, one is placed at the posterior axillary line, and one is placed 5 cm posterior to the posterior axillary port, just medial to the left kidney. Dissection begins by mobilizing the splenic flexure of the colon, and gravity is used to carry it inferiorly and medially. Mobilization of the spleen is performed by incising the peritoneum lateral to the spleen. This incision is developed around to the level of the short gastric vessels. This allows the spleen to rotate medially. It is often helpful to move the laparoscope to the posterior port as dissection proceeds to maximize visualization of the adrenal bed. The adrenal gland is dissected from the retroperitoneal fat; the Harmonic Scalpel (Ethicon Endo-Surgery, Inc.) works well for this dissection. In contrast to the open approach, technical considerations in laparoscopic adrenalectomy often result in delaying ligation of the adrenal vein to the penultimate step in the procedure, following complete mobilization of the tumor and the adrenal gland, and just prior to specimen removal. Vein division on the left side can be safely accomplished with either the vascular stapler or with two to three titanium clips placed on the proximal side of the vein. The specimen is removed in a sterile plastic retrieval bag through the umbilical port site. Right laparoscopic adrenalectomy is performed with similar positioning in the left lateral decubitus position. Abdominal access is obtained through placement of four 10-mm ports, placed similar to those on the left side. The most medial port is used to assist in retraction of the liver. The surgeon begins the operation through the two lateral ports; the right lateral hepatic attachments and the right triangular ligament of the liver are divided to allow for medial retraction of the liver. The adrenal gland is then dissected inferiorly along the renal vein and medially along the vena cava. The right adrenal vein is usually short and wide, and drains directly into the vena cava. Titanium clips may not adequately secure the vein on the right side, and therefore a laparoscopic vascular stapler is preferred.

Posterior Retroperitoneoscopic Adrenalectomy

The posterior retroperitoneoscopic adrenalectomy (PRA) has become the preferred technique at our institution for resection of small, benign adrenal masses and isolated metastases to the adrenal gland. The technique of PRA was first reported by Mercan et al. in 1995 and further modified by Walz et al. (1996) in Essen, Germany. This method offers the advantage of a minimally invasive approach to the adrenal glands obviating the need for adhesiolysis while minimizing hemodynamic or respiratory instability from CO_2 insufflation. In addition, this approach allows the surgeon to address bilateral disease without the need for patient repositioning. Contraindications include suspicion of adrenocortical carcinoma or malignant pheochromocytoma, adjacent organ invasion, lesions greater than 6 cm, morbid obesity, and limited distance between the ribs and iliac crest.

With the patient placed in a prone jackknife position on a Cloward table saddle (Fig. 15.4), the 12th rib is palpated and a 1.5 cm transverse incision is made just beneath the tip of the rib. This will be the eventual site of the middle (12 mm) trocar. The soft tissues are divided sharply and retroperitoneal space is entered. Using the index finger, a small space is created, and the index finger is then used to guide the placement of the medial (10 mm) and lateral (5 mm) trocars into this space. The medial trocar is placed approximately 5 cm medial to the middle trocar site, just lateral to the paraspinal musculature. This trocar is angled at 45° and aimed slightly

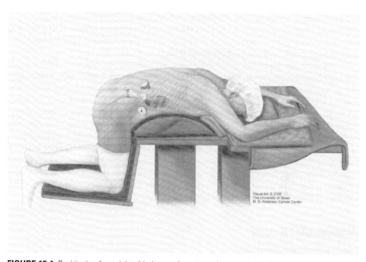

FIGURE 15.4 Positioning for a right-sided posterior retroperitoneoscopic adrenalectomy.

laterally toward the adrenal gland. The lateral trocar is placed approximately 5 cm lateral to the middle trocar site, beneath the 11th rib, and aimed medially. The blunt 12 mm middle trocar with an inflatable balloon and an adjustable sleeve is then placed into the retroperitoneal space through the remaining incision. Pneumoretroperitoneum is then created with CO_2 insufflation to a pressure of 20 to 24 mm Hg.

A 30° 10-mm videoscope is inserted through the middle trocar, allowing for a combination of blunt and sharp dissection to establish the retroperitoneal space beneath the diaphragm. The videoscope is then inserted into the medial trocar, and middle and lateral trocars become the working ports. Gerota fascia is entered and the superior pole of the kidney is identified. The paraspinous muscles, the posterior surface of the liver or spleen which is visible through the peritoneum, and the superior pole of the kidney serve as landmarks. On the right side, the inferior vena cava is a key landmark.

The adrenal gland is retracted superiorly with gentle downward retraction on the kidney. Division of the tissue along the superior border of the kidney is performed using the Harmonic Scalpel, the EnSeal device (Ethicon Endo-Surgery, Inc.), or laparoscopic scissors. It is critical to dissect the adrenal gland from the kidney before dividing the superior and medial attachments of the adrenal. This maneuver minimizes direct manipulation of the fragile adrenal gland and allows the gland to be suspended from its superior attachments until late in the procedure, greatly facilitating dissection.

On the left side, the adrenal vein drains inferiorly into the renal vein. On the right side, the adrenal vein is identified coursing medially to drain into the inferior vena cava. The inferior vena cava must be carefully identified. Due to high insufflation pressures, it loses its normal tubular appearance and its lateral border appears as a flat white line. The adrenal vein is dissected and divided between clips, whilst retracting the gland with a "Walz grasper" on the distal side of the adrenal vein. Bleeding tends to be very modest due in part to the high insufflation pressures.

The adrenal gland is then completely mobilized medially and superiorly. A retrieval bag is used to remove the specimen through the middle trocar site. The retroperitoneal space is then inspected for hemostasis. Insufflation is gradually decreased to pressures of 8 to 12 mm Hg, facilitating visualization of any venous bleeding that may have been tamponaded by the high insufflation pressures. Ports are then removed, and the skin is closed with absorbable suture.

We recently reported our experience with posterior retroperitoneoscopic adrenalectomies performed at our institution between 2005 and 2008. Sixty-eight PRAs were performed on a total of 62 patients for indications which included functioning tumors (pheochromocytomas, Cushing syndrome, failure of medical management of Cushing disease, etc), nonfunctioning cortical adenomas, and isolated adrenal metastasis. Mean tumor size was 3.4 cm. Median operating time was 121 minutes, with six conversions (three open and three video-assisted). Complications occurred in 16% with no perioperative mortality. Of note, 36% of the patients had a body mass index greater than 30. We have found the PRA to be a safe and preferred approach for resection of benign tumors and small adrenal metastases, generally bypassing the difficulties encountered in patients with obese habitus or extensive adhesions secondary to previous abdominal surgery.

Recommended Readings

Primary Hyperaldosteronism

Blumenfeld JC, Sealey JE, Schlussel Y, et al. Diagnosis and therapy of primary hyperaldosteronism. *Ann Intern Med.* 1994; 121:877.

Lo CY, Tam PC, Kung AWC, et al. Primary aldosteronism: results of surgical treatment. *Ann Surg.* 1996;224:125.

Rossi H, Kim A, Prinz RA, et al. Primary hyperaldosteronism in the era of laparoscopic adrenalectomy. *Am Surg.* 2002; 68:253.

Sawka AM, Young WF Jr, Thompson GB, et al. Primary aldosteronism: factors associated with normalization of blood pressure after surgery. *Ann Intern Med.* 2001; 135(4): 258–261.

Vallotton MB. Primary aldosteronism. Parts I and II. *Clin Endocrinol.* 1996;45:47.

Weigel RJ, Wells SA, Gunnells JC, et al. Surgical treatment of primary hyperaldosteronism. *Ann Surg.* 1994;219:347.

Weinberger MH, Fineberg NS. The diagnosis of primary aldosteronism and separation of two major subtypes. *Arch Intern Med.* 1993;153:2125.

Young WF, Stanson AW, Thompson GB, et al. Role for adrenal venous sampling in primary aldosteronism. *Surgery.* 2004;136(6): 1227–1235.

Cushing Syndrome

Lacroix A, Bolte E, Tremblay J, et al. Gastric inhibitory polypeptide-dependent cortisol hypersecretion: a new cause of Cushing's syndrome. *N Engl J Med.* 1992;327: 974.

Orth DN. Cushing's syndrome. *N Engl J Med.* 1995;332:791.

van Heerden JA, Young WF Jr, Grant CS, et al. Adrenal surgery for hypercortisolism: surgical aspects. *Surgery.* 1995;117:466.

Zieger MA, Pass HI, Doppman JD, et al. Surgical strategy in the management of non-small cell ectopic adrenocorticotropic hormone syndrome. *Surgery.* 1992; 112:994.

Pheochromocytoma

Baghi M, Thompson GB, Young WF, et al. Pheochromocytomas and paragangliomas in Von Hippel-Lindau disease: a role for laparoscopic and cortical-sparing surgery. *Arch Surg.* 2002;137:682–689.

Gagner M, Breton JG, Pharand D, et al. Is laparoscopic adrenalectomy indicated for pheochromocytomas? *Surgery.* 1996; 120:1076.

Jalil ND, Pattou FN, Combemale F, et al. Effectiveness and limits of preoperative imaging studies for the localization of pheochromocytomas and paragangliomas: a review of 282 cases. *Eur J Surg.* 1998;164:23–28.

Lee JE, Curley SA, Gagel RF, et al. Cortical-sparing adrenalectomy for patients with bilateral pheochromocytoma. *Surgery.* 1995;120:1064.

Mittendorf EA, Evans DB, Lee JE, et al. Pheochromocytoma: advances in genetics, diagnosis, localization, and treatment. *Hematol Oncol Clin North Am.* 2007;21(3): 509–525; ix.

Neuman HPH, Bausch B, McWhinney SR, et al. Germ-line mutations in nonsyndromic pheochromocytoma. *N Engl J Med.* 2002;346:1459–1466.

Orchard T, Grant CS, van Heerden JA, et al. Pheochromocytoma: continuing evolution of surgical therapy. *Surgery.* 1993; 114:1153.

Pederson LC, Lee JE. Pheochromocytoma. *Curr Treat Options Oncol.* 2003;4:329–337.

Peplinski GR, Norton JA. The predictive value of diagnostic tests for pheochromocytoma. *Surgery.* 1994;116:1101.

Perrier ND, Kennamer DL, Bao R, et al. Posterior retroperitoneoscopic adrenalectomy: preferred technique for removal of benign tumors and isolated metastases. *Ann Surg.* 2008;248(4):666–674.

Werbel SS, Ober KP. Pheochromocytoma: update on diagnosis, localization, and management. *Med Clin North Am.* 1995; 79:131.

Yip L, Lee JE, Shapiro S, et al. Surgical management of hereditary pheochromocytoma. *J Am Coll Surg.* 2004;198:525.

Adrenocortical Masses and Carcinoma

Baba S, Ito K, Yanaihara H, et al. Retroperitoneoscopic adrenalectomy by a lumbodorsal approach: clinical experience with solo surgery. *World J Urol.* 1999;17: 54–58.

Baba S, Miyajima A, Uchida A, et al. A posterior lumbar approach for retroperitoneoscopic adrenalectomy: assessment of surgical efficacy. *Urology.* 1997;50: 19–24.

Barnett CC, Varma DG, El-Naggar AK, et al. Limitations of size as a criterion in the evaluation of adrenal tumors. *Surgery.* 2000;128:973–982.

Bornstein SR, Stratakis CA, Chrousos GP. Adrenocortical tumors: recent advances in basic concepts and clinical management. *Ann Intern Med.* 1999;130:759–771.

Dackiw AP, Lee JE, Gagel RF, et al. Adrenal cortical carcinoma. *World J Surg.* 2001;25:914–926.

Demeter JG, De Jong SA, Brooks MH, et al. Long-term results of adrenal autotransplantation in Cushing's disease. *Surgery.* 1990;108:1117.

Doppman JL, Reinig JW, Dwyer AJ, et al. Differentiation of adrenal masses by magnetic resonance imaging. *Surgery.* 1987;102:1018.

Gagner M, Lacroix A, Bolte E. Laparoscopic adrenalectomy in Cushing's syndrome and pheochromocytoma. *N Engl J Med.* 1992;327:1033.

Gonzalez RJ, Shapiro S, Sarlis N, et al. Laparoscopic resection of adrenal cortical carcinoma: a cautionary note. *Surgery.* 2005;138(6):1078–1085; discussion 1085–1086.

Gonzalez RJ, Tamm EP, Ng C, et al. Response to mitotane predicts outcome in patients with recurrent adrenal cortical carcinoma. *Surgery.* 2007;142(6):867–875; discussion 867–875.

Graham DJ, McHenry CR. The adrenal incidentaloma: guidelines for evaluation and recommendations for management. *Surg Oncol Clin North Am.* 1998;7: 749–764.

Grubbs EG, Callender GG, Xing Y, et al. Recurrence of adrenal cortical carcinoma following resection: surgery alone can achieve results equal to surgery plus mitotane. *Ann Surg Oncol.* 2010;17(1): 263–270.

Herrera MF, Grant CS, van Heerden JA, et al. Incidentally discovered adrenal tumors: an institutional perspective. *Surgery.* 1991;110:1014.

Icard P, Chapuis Y, Andreassian BA, et al. Adrenocortical carcinoma in surgically treated patients: a retrospective study on 156 cases by the French Association of Endocrine Surgery. *Surgery.* 1992;112: 972.

Lee JE. Adjuvant mitotane in adrenocortical carcinoma. *N Engl J Med.* 2007; 357(12): 1258; author reply 1259.

Lee JE, Berger DH, El-Naggar AK, et al. Surgical management, DNA content, and patient survival in adrenal cortical carcinoma. *Surgery.* 1995;118:1090.

Lee JE, Evans DB, Hickey RC, et al. Unknown primary cancer presenting as an adrenal mass: frequency and implications for diagnostic evaluation of adrenal incidentalomas. *Surgery.* 1998;124:115–122.

Lenert JT, Barnett CC, Kudelka AP, et al. Evaluation and surgical resection of adrenal masses in patients with a history of extraadrenal malignancy. *Surgery.* 2001;130: 1060–1064.

Luton JP, Cerdas S, Billaud L, et al. Clinical features of adrenocortical carcinoma, prognostic factors, and the effect of mitotane therapy. *N Engl J Med.* 1990;322:1195.

McFarlane DA. Cancer of the adrenal cortex: the natural history, prognosis and treatment in a study of fifty-five cases. *Ann R Coll Surg Engl.* 1958;23:155.

Mercan S, Seven R, Ozarmagan S, et al. Endoscopic retroperitoneal adrenalectomy. *Surgery.* 1995;118:1071–1075; discussion 1075–1076.

Mittendorf EA, Lim SJ, Schacherer CW, et al. Melanoma adrenal metastasis: natural history and surgical management. *Am J Surg.* 2008;195(3):363–368; discussion 368–369.

Paul CA, Virgo KS, Wade TP, et al. Adrenalectomy for isolated adrenal metastases from non-adrenal cancer. *Int J Oncol.* 2000;17(1):181–187.

Pommier RF, Brennan MF, An eleven-year experience with adrenocortical carcinoma. *Surgery.* 1992;112:963.

Ross NS, Aron DC. Hormonal evaluation of the patient with an incidentally discovered adrenal mass. *N Engl J Med.* 1990;323:1401.

Salem M, Tainsh RE, Bromberg J, et al. Perioperative glucocorticoid coverage: a reassessment 42 years after emergence of a problem. *Ann Surg.* 1994;4:416.

Schteingart DE. Adjuvant mitotane therapy of adrenal cancer—use and controversy. *N Engl J Med.* 2007;357(12):1257–1258; author reply 1259.

Schulick RD, Brennan MF. Long-term survival after complete resection and repeat resection in patients with adrenocortical carcinoma. *Ann Surg Oncol.* 1999;6(8):719–726.

Shen WT, Lim RC, Siperstein AE, et al. Laparoscopic vs open adrenalectomy for the treatment of primary hyperaldosteronism. *Arch Surg.* 1999;134:628–631; discussion 631–632.

Siperstein AE, Berber E, Engle KL, et al. Laparoscopic posterior adrenalectomy: technical considerations. *Arch Surg.* 2000; 135:967–971.

Siren J, Tervahartiala P, Sivula A, et al. Natural course of adrenal incidentalomas: seven-year follow-up study. *World J Surg.* 2000; 24:579–582.

Smith CD, Weber CJ, Amerson JR. Laparoscopic adrenalectomy: new gold standard. *World J Surg.* 1999;23:389–396.

Sullivan M, Boileau M, Hodges CV. Adrenal cortical carcinoma. *J Urol.* 1978;120: 660.

Terzolo M, Angeli A, Fassnacht M, et al. Adjuvant mitotane treatment for adrenocortical carcinoma. *N Engl J Med.* 2007; 356(23):2372–2380.

Vassilopoulou-Sellin R, Guinee VF, Klein MJ, et al. Impact of adjuvant mitotane on the clinical course of patients with adrenocortical cancer. *Cancer.* 1993;71:3119.

Walz MK, Peitgen K, Hoermann R, et al. Posterior retroperitoneoscopy as a new minimally invasive approach for adrenalectomy: results of 30 adrenalectomies in 27 patients. *World J Surg.* 1996;20(7): 769–774.

16

Well-Differentiated Carcinoma of the Thyroid and Neoplasms of the Parathyroid Glands

Ryan M. Thomas, Mouhammed A. Habra, Nancy D. Perrier, and Elizabeth G. Grubbs

THYROID CANCER

Introduction

The incidence of thyroid carcinoma has been increasing steadily since the mid-1990s with an estimated incidence of 44,670 cases in 2010. This cancer represents the most common endocrine malignancy and accounts for approximately 3% of all human malignancies, with 75% of cases occurring in women. The death rate for thyroid cancer has remained stable for women but has increased at a rate of approximately 1% per year since 1983 for men and will be responsible for an estimated 1,690 deaths in 2010. The relatively low death rate compared to the incidence is due, in part, to the indolent nature of most thyroid cancers. While a small percentage of cases are due to the aggressive anaplastic variety, more than 90% of thyroid cancers are well differentiated, and follow an indolent, protracted course. Patients with differentiated thyroid cancer (DTC) usually have an excellent long-term prognosis, with a 5-year survival rates approaching 100% for localized disease.

The screening and diagnosis of both primary and recurrent DTC has evolved over the years with increased utilization of thyroid ultrasound, fine-needle aspiration (FNA), molecular testing, and measurement of the serum marker thyroglobulin. This evolution has led to increased controversy regarding the appropriate medical and surgical management of DTC. The extent of surgical resection, role of lymphadenectomy, and adjuvant medical treatment for DTC are currently debated and present unique challenges in treatment of these patients.

Risk Factors

A thorough understanding of the factors that increase a patient's risk of developing thyroid cancer is necessary when evaluating someone with complaints related to a thyroid mass or nodule, change in voice, or symptoms of dyspnea or dysphagia. These risk factors include a personal or family history of thyroid cancer, certain diseases with a genetic predilection toward the development of thyroid cancer, and prior radiation exposure.

A past history of radiation exposure accounts for approximately 9% of all cases of thyroid carcinoma and the risk is inversely related to age at exposure but directly related to radiation dose, with the risk of cancer increasing linearly up to a dose of 20 Gy. When thyroid cancer develops as a result of ionizing radiation, it invariably is the papillary type and behaves similarly to sporadic papillary thyroid cancer (PTC), although evidence from the Chernobyl nuclear disaster suggests that radiation dosage may be linked to the aggressiveness or dedifferentiation of thyroid cancer. Children exposed to the Chernobyl disaster had a higher proportion of thyroid cancers that were less well differentiated and of the solid-variant papillary subtype than patients who did not have any history of radiation exposure. The type of radiation, along with radiation dose, has been associated with the aggressiveness of thyroid cancer. Different forms of radiation have been linked to different genetic

TABLE 16.1	Hereditary Syndromes Associated with Increased Risk of Thyroid Cancer

- Familial adenomatous polyposis (PTC; inactivating mutations of *APC*)
- Cowden's disease (FTC; *PTEN* mutation)
- Werner's syndrome (PTC, FTC, ATC; *WRN* mutation)
- Carney's complex (PTC, FTC; *PRKAR1α* mutation)
- Multiple endocrine neoplasia 2A and 2B (MTC; *RET* proto-oncogene mutations)
- Familial medullary thyroid cancer (MTC; *RET* proto-oncogene mutations)

alterations associated with thyroid carcinoma, resulting in variable aggressiveness. Radiation exposure therefore plays a critical role in the development of thyroid cancer, especially in patients younger than 15 years old, and may play a role in its aggressiveness based on genetic alterations and dose exposure.

A personal history of thyroid cancer increases one's risk of developing future or recurrent thyroid tumors. Evidence also exists for a familial predisposition, with several inherited syndromes demonstrating increased risk for the development of thyroid cancer (Table 16.1). The mechanisms underlying these associations are not well understood.

Over the past decade, significant progress has been made in the identification of genes linked to the pathogenesis of thyroid cancer. Studies of the patterns of genetic alterations present in thyroid tumors suggest that there are differences in the pathogenesis of the different thyroid tumor types, which most likely account for the range in biological behavior observed among thyroid cancers. The initiation of PTC is usually the result of one of several mutational events. In approximately 50% of cases, a constitutive activation of the BRAF kinase, a member of the *Ras/MAPK* pathway, is present and results from a V600E amino acid substitution. BRAF is normally dependent on *Ras* activation in order to propagate extracellular signal transduction. In certain scenarios, activation of the *Ras* oncogene, upstream of BRAF, has also been implicated as an initiating event in PTC, as well as follicular thyroid cancer. Somatic mutations in the *Ras* oncogene have been found in both benign and malignant thyroid tumors, and thus seem to be an early event in thyroid tumorigenesis. Some reports suggest that *Ras* mutations are more prevalent in follicular thyroid cancers (FTCs), follicular variant of PTC, and follicular adenomas. Mutations in *Ras* may result in allelic loss or in chromosomal rearrangements leading to increased rates of follicular thyroid cancer formation. Chromosomal rearrangements have also been observed in RET/PTC oncogene formation and portend an unfavorable prognosis. Although other mutational events may be responsible for the initiation and progression of papillary and follicular thyroid cancer, such as DNA hypermethylation, histone deacetylation, and constitutive activation of other cell-cycle regulators, further work is still needed to elucidate such pathways.

The *RET* proto-oncogene is a tyrosine kinase receptor that is mainly expressed in tumors of neural crest origin, explaining the high incidence of mutations in medullary thyroid cancers (MTC) which originate from the parafollicular cells (C cells). The *RET* gene is located on chromosome 10 and germline mutations result in missense activating mutations which are responsible for 95% of inherited MTC, including those associated with multiple endocrine neoplasia 2A and 2B (MEN2A/B) and familial medullary thyroid cancer (FMTC). In 80% of cases of MTC, the disease is sporadic, without an inherited etiology but a somatic mutation in *RET* is identified in 40% to 70% of these sporadic cases. In these sporadic cases, mutations are most often found in codon 918 which results in constitutive activation of the *RET* tyrosine kinase receptor. Nearly all patients with autosomal dominant MEN 2A or MEN 2B will develop MTC and screening for germline *RET* mutations has been invaluable in the early identification of patients who have a genetic basis for their disease. Even in patients with sporadic MTC, 6% to 10% of these patients will have a *RET* proto-oncogene germline mutation, thus revealing a new kindred of patients with previously undiagnosed MTC. The discovery of the *RET* proto-oncogene has had significant clinical impact, affecting the screening and prophylactic treatment of patients who are members of the MEN and familial MTC kindreds.

Anaplastic thyroid cancer (ATC) develops from the dedifferentiation of thyroid tumors although no specific inciting event has been elucidated to cause the transformation. Mutations in the *p53* tumor-suppressor gene are frequently found in ATC and are absent in well-differentiated thyroid neoplasms. This observation suggests that *p53* mutations play a role later in thyroid tumor pathogenesis—specifically, in the dedifferentiating transition to the anaplastic phenotype. A myriad of mutations in other pathways including the PI3K/Akt and Ras/MAPK pathways have also been implicated in the formation of ATC.

Despite the tremendous work that has been performed to solidify the role of the *RET* tyrosine kinase receptor in medullary thyroid tumor initiation, as well as the role of *Ras* and BRAF in papillary and follicular thyroid carcinomas, much work is still needed to detail the signaling pathways that lead to tumor progression and aggressiveness and that will ultimately translate into improved clinical management for patients who suffer from this disease.

Pathology

Papillary, follicular, medullary, and anaplastic thyroid cancers make up the vast majority of all thyroid cancers (90%) with the remaining proportion represented by lymphoma, squamous cell carcinoma, sarcoma, melanoma, or metastatic disease (breast, renal cell, lung, colon, and gastric carcinomas). PTC and FTC are broadly categorized as DTCs but can be further subclassified based on their histological appearance or biological behavior (Table 16.2). PTC accounts for 80% of all thyroid malignancies and is the predominate histology seen in patients exposed to radiation. The mean age at presentation is 30 to 40 years and females are more often affected than males (2:1 ratio). Macroscopically, the tumors tend to be sharply

TABLE 16.2 Pathological Classification of Thyroid Malignancies

Subtype	Variants	Incidence
Papillary (80%)	Conventional	65–85%
	Follicular	15–20%
	Tall cell	5–10%
	Solid	1–3%
	Diffuse sclerosing	1–2%
	Columnar	<1%
Follicular (10%)	Hürthle	
Poorly differentiated	Insular	
Medullary (5%)		
Anaplastic (1–5%)		
Other	Lymphoma	
	Metastatic	

Incidence is representative for each variant of a particular subtype.

circumscribed and white in color. Unlike normal thyroid or benign colloid lesions that bulge upon sectioning, PTC remains flat. Diagnosis is made by microscopic evaluation and can be made on the basis of FNA. Lesions often have papillary projections although a mixed papillary/follicular and pure follicular variant can sometimes be seen. A definitive diagnosis is made on the basis of cellular and nuclear characteristics with cells adopting a cuboidal shape with nuclear "grooving" and cytoplasmic inclusions. These characteristic findings are described as the pathognomonic "Orphan Annie" nuclei. Psammoma bodies, present in 50% of specimens, help to secure the diagnosis of PTC and represent calcified deposits of sloughed cells that have been deposited in the stroma or lymphatics. PTC is characterized by multifocality in 80% to 85% of patients and is associated with an increased risk of lymph node metastasis. Cervical lymph node metastases are fairly common in patients with PTC at presentation with a frequency ranging from 30% to 80% in some series. Despite this high incidence, the 10-year survival rate is still 95%.

The second most common thyroid cancer is FTC which represents approximately 10% of all thyroid cancers. These tumors are most often found in iodine-deficient areas and like PTC, have a female predominance with a 3:1 (female : male) ratio. FTC is often found in association with benign thyroid disorders, such as endemic goiter and a relationship between TSH stimulation and follicular carcinoma has been suggested because of the greater incidence of FTC in iodine-deficient areas. The mean age at diagnosis is approximately 10 years later than those with PTC, presenting in the fifth to sixth decade of life. Patients usually present with a history of a solitary nodule, often with a rapid increase in size. FTCs are usually unifocal, well-encapsulated lesions containing highly cellular follicles, and are easily confused with benign follicular adenomas on FNA. Pathological diagnosis of this malignancy can only be made by permanent sectioning, demonstrating the presence of capsular or vascular invasion. Metastasis to the cervical lymph nodes is uncommon with FTC, being present in 5% to 10% of cases at initial presentation. Distant spread is more common at initial presentation and is seen in 10% to 33% of patients, most often presenting with hematological spread to the lungs or bone. Ten-year survival rates for FTC are 70% to 95%, slightly worse than those for PTC, which is possibly due to later presentation and presence of distant metastases at the initial diagnosis.

Hürthle cell carcinomas, although considered a variant of FTC, deserve special discussion as they comprise 5% of all thyroid malignancies and have a biological behavior and natural history that makes them distinct from FTC. These tumors are consisted of sheets of polygonal, hyperchromatic cells that contain many mitochondria. As with FTC, Hürthle cell carcinoma requires permanent sectioning in order to identify vascular or capsular invasion. In contrast to FTC, Hürthle cell carcinomas are often multifocal (30%), present with lymph node metastasis (25%), and often fail to concentrate radioactive iodine. In part due to these factors, patients with Hürthle cell carcinoma have higher tumor recurrence rates and lower survival rates when compared to patients with PTC or FTC.

Five percent of thyroid malignancies are MTCs. Although the majority of cases are sporadic, 15% to 20% of cases are part of an autosomal dominant hereditary syndrome. The sporadic form of MTC typically presents as a unilateral solitary nodule in the fifth decade of life. Familial forms, such as MEN 2A/B and familial MTC, present in the fourth decade and are typically multifocal. Because MTC arises from the C cells, these tumors are localized to the upper poles of the thyroid gland where C cells reside. The presence of C cell hyperplasia is thought to be a harbinger for the development of hereditary MTC. These lesions are nonencapsulated and ill-defined, consisting of a heterogeneous mix of spindle-shaped or round cells. The cells are separated by fibrous septa and amyloid, the latter of which aids in the diagnosis of MTC by immunohistochemical (IHC) staining as does IHC for calcitonin and carcinoembryonic antigen (CEA). Although these tumors grow slowly, they have a propensity to metastasize early, usually before the primary tumor has reached 2 cm. Cervical and upper mediastinal lymph nodes are typically the first areas involved with metastatic disease and 50% of patients will have regional metastases at the time of diagnosis. The survival for patients with MTC lies between that of differentiated and undifferentiated (anaplastic) thyroid cancers. When disease is confined to the thyroid gland, the 10-year survival rate is 90% versus patients with distant metastatic disease having a 10-year survival of only 20%.

In comparison to the DTCs and MTC, anaplastic thyroid cancers are highly aggressive and considered one of the deadliest malignancies. It is thought that these tumors arise from an area of DTC but over time dedifferentiation may occur. This tumor is rare, comprising only 1% to 5% of all thyroid malignancies with a peak incidence in the seventh decade of life and incidence that is similar between men and women. Patients usually present with a rapidly growing mass and symptoms of dysphagia, dysphonia, or dyspnea secondary to compressive symptoms from the mass which is often fixed to underlying structures and unresectable at the time of initial presentation. The tumor is nonencapsulated and often contains areas of necrosis which may result in a nondiagnostic FNA and require incisional biopsy to secure a diagnosis in addition to ruling out lymphoma. The cells are characteristically large and multinucleated with nuclear polymorphism and a high mitotic activity. At presentation, 25% of patients will have tracheal invasion, 90% will have regional metastases, and 50% will have distant spread, most commonly to the lung. Surgery rarely has a role in this disease; the most common procedures performed are isthmusectomy or debulking in order to palliate tracheal compression. The 1- and 5-year survival for a patient diagnosed with ATC is 25% and 5%, respectively, with 90% of patients dying of the disease within 6 months of diagnosis, usually secondary to local progression.

Lymphomas of the thyroid gland typically present in the seventh decade of life, affect women more commonly than men, and are often associated with a history of Hashimoto thyroiditis. They represent less than 2% of all thyroid malignancies and often present as a rapidly growing mass with symptoms of dysphagia and dysphonia, possibly confusing the diagnosis with ATC. The lymphoma may be primary or secondary with non-Hodgkin's B-cell lymphoma being the most common primary thyroid lymphoma although it has been reported that 23% to 77% of thyroid lymphomas are of mucosa-associated lymphoid tissue (MALT) origin. Histologically, the cells are monomorphic and stain positive for lymphocyte markers such as CD20. Tumors of MALT origin generally have a better prognosis and are often able to be treated with radiation therapy alone, instead of the multimodality therapy necessary to treat non-MALT lymphomas. Survival rates for lymphoma isolated to the thyroid gland (stage IE) are generally favorable, with a 5-year survival rate of 75% to 85%. However, patients with disease on both sides of the diaphragm (stage IIIE) or disseminated disease (stage IV) have a 5-year survival rate of less than 35%.

Diagnosis

Thyroid cancer is often discovered incidentally during neck imaging (computed tomography, positron emission tomography, magnetic resonance imaging, or ultrasonography) for unrelated complaints. Most patients with thyroid cancer have no specific symptoms and imaging modalities such as these will often trigger a diagnostic work-up. When patients do present to a physician with a specific symptom, it is often with the finding of a new thyroid mass/nodule, an enlargement of a previously detected nodule, pain secondary to hemorrhage into a nodule, or a palpable cervical lymph node. Symptoms of dysphagia, dysphonia, or dyspnea often portend a poor prognosis as these symptoms result from local invasion and usually are due to undifferentiated thyroid cancer since DTCs rarely invade surrounding structures.

Obtaining a thorough history and physical examination is a vital first step in the work-up of a patient suspected of having thyroid cancer. Particular attention should be paid to a past history of radiation exposure, family history of thyroid malignancy, or thyroid cancer syndrome (multiple endocrine neoplasia, Cowden's syndrome, familial adenomatous polyposis, Carney complex). In addition, inquiring about symptoms of dysphagia, dysphonia, or dyspnea may suggest an invasive component. The presence of diarrhea or flushing in association with nodular thyroid disease should raise the possibility of MTC. The physical examination should concentrate on findings suggestive of invasion or regional metastases which may include fixation to surrounding structures, presence of tracheal deviation, or vocal cord paralysis. In the absence of these findings, the presence of discrete 1 to 2 cm lymph nodes in conjunction with a thyroid nodule suggests regional metastases. Palpable lymphadenopathy is most commonly identified along the middle and lower portion of the jugular chain. Finally, prior to any operative intervention, the degree of neck extension should be assessed in anticipation of operative positioning. Condition of the larynx and vocal cords should also be evaluated, either indirectly with a mirror or directly with a flexible fiberoptic scope.

Once the history and physical examination have been completed, various diagnostic tests are available to help distinguish benign from malignant disease. The ultimate goal is to avoid unnecessary surgeries, and their possible complications, for benign lesions whenever possible. Most patients will present with a single thyroid nodule, either discovered incidentally on imaging, or by physical examination. The initial test of choice involves measurement of thyroid-stimulating hormone (TSH) in order to initiate the workup for a hyper-functioning nodule and subsequent treatment for hyperthyroidism if appropriate (Fig. 16.1). If the TSH is below normal limits, a thyroid radionucleotide scan (^{99}Tc or ^{125}I) should be performed to ascertain if the nodule is hyperfunctioning and if so, appropriate treatment for hyperthyroidism implemented. Because hyperfunctioning nodules rarely harbor malignancy, such a nodule seldom requires cytologic evaluation.

Thyroid ultrasound should be performed in all patients with a known or suspected thyroid nodule. The function of the ultrasound is to determine the size, character, and number of thyroid nodules, assess the status of the cervical lymph node basin, and allow for image-guided FNA of any suspicious or dominant nodules. FNA, either ultrasound-guided or performed by direct palpation of a nodule, has supplanted radionuclide scanning as the initial diagnostic test of choice in patients with thyroid nodules. The higher diagnostic yield, accessibility, and cost-effectiveness of FNA for thyroid nodules has reserved radionuclide scanning for those individuals with clinical or subclinical hyperthyroidism and a thyroid nodule. Ultrasound will detect clinically unsuspected nodules in 20% to 70% of patients and several ultrasound characteristics of the nodule(s) can help to assess the risk of malignancy and enable an ultrasound-guided FNA of any suspicious nodules and lymph nodes (Table 16.3). On the basis of the characteristics of the nodule, several independent risk factors for malignancy have been identified which include: presence of microcalcifications, increased vascularity within the nodule, and a blurred/irregular border. The exact role of ultrasound, however, in distinguishing benign from malignant nodules is still unresolved. Ultrasound can be used to perform surveillance on patients with benign nodules or in those who have been operated on for carcinoma. One of the most useful utilizations of the ultrasound is to guide the FNA of difficult to palpate lesions or to increase the yield from aspirations of small or complex lesions.

FNA of thyroid lesions is a safe and cost-effective means to diagnose a thyroid malignancy. It is the single most useful diagnostic tool as it provides direct diagnostic information on a lesion and has the greatest accuracy for lesions that are 1 to 4 cm. Lesions that are less than 1 cm are more difficult to sample, even with

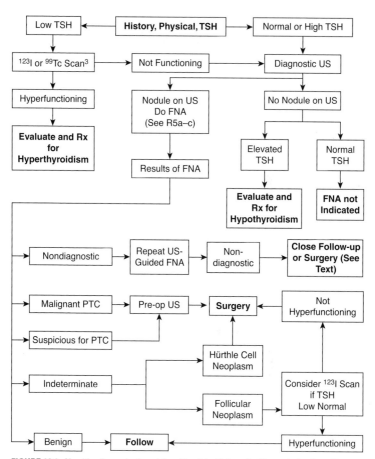

FIGURE 16.1 Algorithm for evaluation of thyroid nodule. (Adapted with permission from *Thyroid* 2009;19(11):1167–1214.)

ultrasound, while lesions that are greater than 4 cm have a greater chance for sampling error because of their larger size. The accuracy of FNA to diagnose a thyroid malignancy can be as high as 90% with a false-negative rate of less than 5% when an experienced physician performs the procedure and the collected cells are evaluated by an experienced cytopathologist. Lesions sampled by FNA are subsequently classified as benign, follicular lesion of undetermined significance, neoplasm (follicular or Hürthle cell variety), suspicious for malignancy, malignant, or nondiagnostic. The cytological diagnosis achieved by FNA plays a critical role in the subsequent treatment algorithm of patients with a thyroid nodule (Table 16.4). The risk of malignancy for a specimen categorized as "benign" on FNA is <1% while those labeled "malignant" have up to a 100% risk of malignancy. Clinical decision making and knowledge of malignancy plays the most important role for those lesions categorized as "follicular lesion of undetermined significance," "neoplasm," or "suspicious

| TABLE 16.3 | FNA Recommendations Based on Suspicious Characteristics of Thyroid Nodules and Lymph Nodes |

Thyroid Nodule
  Complex mass
  Solitary mass
  Calcification
  Vascular flow

Lymph Node
  Calcification
  Cystic component
  Disorganized vascular flow
  Rounded or full appearance
  Disruption or absence of normal echogenic hilum

for malignancy." Follicular lesions of undetermined significance have a 5% to 10% risk of malignancy and are a heterogeneous group of lesions that are not convincingly benign yet lack characteristics to label them as a follicular neoplasm or suspicious for malignancy. Often this is secondary to inferior quality of a specimen either from hypocellularity, poor fixation techniques, or presence of blood that obscures the sampled cells. In these cases, a repeat FNA can be very beneficial. FNA samples that are categorized as "follicular/Hürthle cell neoplasm" (also denoted as "suspicious for follicular/Hürthle cell neoplasm") have a 15% to 45% risk of malignancy

| TABLE 16.4 | The Bethesda System for Reporting Thyroid Cytopathology: Implied Risk of Malignancy and Usual Management |

Diagnostic Category	Risk of Malignancy (%)	Usual Management
Nondiagnostic	1–4	Repeat FNA with ultrasound guidance
Benign	<1%	Clinical follow-up
Atypical cells of undetermined significance (ACUS)	~5–10%	Clinical/imaging correlation, repeat FNA for most
Suspicious for a follicular neoplasm	15–30	Surgical lobectomy
Suspicious for a Hürthle cell neoplasm	15–45	Surgical lobectomy
Suspicious for malignancy • Suspicious for papillary carcinoma • Suspicious for medullary carcinoma • Suspicious for lymphoma • Suspicious for metastatic tumor • Other	60–75	Near-total thyroidectomy or surgical lobectomy
Malignant	97–99	Near-total thyroidectomy

Adapted with permission from *Am J Clin Pathol.* 2009;132(5):658–665.

and usual management involves surgical resection so that a definitive pathological diagnosis may be rendered. Finally, lesions that are read as "suspicious for malignancy" are malignant 60% to 75% of the time. When a lesion is suspicious for a papillary malignancy, these are most often follicular variants of PTC. Although PTC, MTC, and ATC can often be diagnosed by FNA, the distinction between FTC and a follicular adenoma cannot be made on the basis of solely on FNA because the presence of vascular or capsule invasion must be confirmed in order to diagnose FTC. This cannot be achieved with FNA alone and a tissue sample, usually in the form of a thyroid lobectomy, is needed in order to ascertain whether malignancy is present. Intraoperative frozen section evaluation of follicular neoplasms at the time of lobectomy is usually not definitive and we do not routinely recommend this practice. In cases where the FNA of a nodule is nondiagnostic, the patient should undergo a repeat FNA or surgery to obtain adequate tissue for diagnosis. The significant variability in the interpretation and reporting the results of FNA led to an effort to standardize the communication of FNA findings among physicians using the Bethesda system for reporting thyroid cytopathology (Table 16.4). In 15% to 25% of cases, the FNA will not yield enough material for diagnosis and a repeat FNA is necessary. Ultrasound, with its increased utilization and technological advancements, has increased the yield of FNA and reduced the need for repeat aspirations.

Treatment
In general, the goal of treatment for thyroid malignancies is multi-tiered and involves removal of the primary tumor with appropriate lymph node dissection while minimizing treatment-related morbidity. Surgical resection allows accurate staging to occur and guides postoperative treatment with radioactive iodine when appropriate. Finally, the treatment of thyroid malignancies should aim to reduce the risk of disease recurrence and permit accurate long-term surveillance to detect such recurrences.

Surgical Management
The primary management of thyroid cancer is surgical resection. The extent of thyroid gland resection for thyroid cancer was a highly debated topic in the 1980s and 1990s. The controversy revolved around the extent of resection with the proponents of thyroid lobectomy or near-total thyroidectomy arguing that the less extensive surgery decreases the risk of injury to the recurrent laryngeal nerves (RLNs) and parathyroid glands. In addition, it was debated that any remaining foci of differentiated cancer was rarely clinically significant and half of the clinically significant recurrences could be treated with reoperation. Finally, no survival benefit could be established for patients who underwent a total thyroidectomy versus lobectomy or near-total thyroidectomy. However, a recent evaluation of 52,173 patients from the National Cancer Database (NCDB) who underwent surgical treatment for PTC between 1985 and 1998 demonstrated a modest decrease in local recurrence and increase in survival benefit for patients with PTC >1 cm who underwent total thyroidectomy. This data coupled with the low incidence of RLN injury or permanent hypoparathyroidism (2%) by experienced surgeons makes total thyroidectomy the treatment of choice. In addition, foci of PTC are found bilaterally in 85% of thyroid specimens and 5% to 10% of recurrent disease occurs in the contralateral lobe when a thyroid lobectomy is performed. From a postoperative standpoint, the thyroid tissue that remains if a more conservative resection is undertaken makes radioactive iodine ablation of the remaining gland difficult and sometimes prohibitive. In addition, serum measurement of thyroglobulin as a marker of persistent or recurrent disease after thyroid lobectomy is more difficult to interpret given the remaining thyroid tissue. A total thyroidectomy avoids these pitfalls and minimizes reoperative surgery which is associated with increased complication rates.

On the basis of the data and advantages described above, our usual management is to perform a total thyroidectomy for all patients with PTC, FTC, and Hürthle cell carcinoma (refer to the Multiple Endocrine Neoplasia section of Chapter 14 for recommended surgical management of MTC). Unfortunately, the diagnosis of FTC or Hürthle cell carcinoma cannot be made utilizing FNA, for reasons explained earlier, and cannot be ascertained on the basis of frozen section pathology intraoperatively. Many times the diagnosis of FTC or Hürthle cell carcinoma is made postoperatively, in a patient who has already undergone a thyroid lobectomy. In these circumstances, a completion thyroidectomy is often performed in high-risk patients (age >45 years, prior neck radiation, lesion >1 cm, concerning pathologic features, or distant metastases) and in instances where radioactive iodine ablation is planned. Anaplastic carcinoma presents a unique challenge because it is rarely diagnosed in a timely fashion such that surgical management is more than a palliative option. In the rare instance where anaplastic carcinoma has been diagnosed either incidentally or early in its course, total thyroidectomy with central and ipsilateral modified radical lymphadenectomy offers the best opportunity for survival in the rare event that the tumor is intrathyroidal. Given the aggressive nature and limited survival for patients with anaplastic carcinoma, surgical intervention associated with excessive morbidity, such as resections of the larynx, pharynx, or esophagus, should be avoided. Resection of disease that extends beyond the thyroid gland may be appropriate in highly selected individuals as part of a multimodality treatment regimen along with radiation and chemotherapy.

In most cases of appropriately treated DTC, patients have a good prognosis with 10-year survival rates greater than 75% likely due to the indolent course of the disease. Where controversy once focused on the extent of surgical resection of the thyroid gland to achieve these high survival rates, the goals of treatment have changed and the controversy now focuses on the extent of the lymph node dissection in order to prevent local recurrence, provide more accurate staging, and increase survival. Given the low incidence of lymph node metastases with FTC, we do not routinely perform lymphadenectomy unless there is palpable lymphadenopathy at the time of surgery or preoperative ultrasonography demonstrates suspicious nodes. For PTC, however, prophylactic ipsilateral central lymphadenectomy is performed on most patients, especially in primary tumors >4 cm or when extrathyroidal extension is diagnosed at the time of surgery. Therapeutic bilateral central lymph node dissection (level VI) is appropriate if there is preoperative biopsy proven central or lateral compartment disease or central compartment nodal disease that is found intraoperatively. For patients with biopsy proven cervical lymph node metastases, a therapeutic lateral lymph node dissection is performed (levels IIa to IV with the addition of levels IIb, V, and VII based on the preoperative imaging or intraoperative findings). The distinction between a therapeutic versus elective (or prophylactic) central compartment dissection is that a therapeutic dissection implies that nodal disease has already occurred and been detected either clinically or by preoperative imaging (N1a disease). An elective or prophylactic central compartment dissection implies that there is no clinical or radiographic evidence for nodal metastases. This distinction is important because the impact of clinically detectable lymph node involvement on survival and local recurrence may differ from that observed with microscopic disease.

Surgical Technique
The neck is an anatomically complex site and removal of the thyroid gland requires precision and vigilance in identifying and preserving critical structures in this region. After the induction of general endotracheal anesthesia, the patient's arms are tucked and placed in semi-Fowler's position with the neck hyper-extended using a shoulder roll and appropriate support behind the head. Again, the patient's

ability to extend their neck should be ascertained preoperatively so as to not induce trauma during operative positioning. The field is then prepped and draped in the usual sterile fashion to include the chin, neck, and chest. A transverse incision, preferably utilizing a skin crease for cosmesis, is made approximately two finger-breadths above the suprasternal notch. Electrocautery is used to divide the platysma and flaps are created in the subplatysmal plane both superiorly and inferiorly to the level of the thyroid notch and suprasternal notch, respectively. A plane is then created between the strap muscles and the sternocleidomastoid muscles in order to facilitate exposure of the gland and allow inspection of the lower jugular lymph nodes. The strap muscles are then separated vertically along the median raphe. Strap muscles adherent to the gland or tumor should be resected en bloc with the specimen. In cases of reoperation, the thyroid compartment may be approached laterally along the anterior border of the sternocleidomastoid muscle.

Once proper exposure has been obtained, the sternothyroid muscle is freed from the underlying thyroid (unless precluded by tumor involvement in which case the muscle is resected en bloc with the thyroid) and the lobe of interest is retracted medially in order to identify and ligate the middle thyroid vein. This allows further medial mobilization of the lobe in order to enter the tracheoesophageal groove and identify and preserve the RLN as it runs caudally to cephalad. In approximately 1% of patients, a non-RLN is present on the right side and can be identified as it originates from the vagus nerve proximally. Blunt dissection is performed medial to the carotid artery to prevent injury to the recurrent laryngeal or superior laryngeal nerves. A Kittner dissector is useful for this maneuver as the dissection is carried superiorly to the superior pole vessels. At the superior pole, the external branch of the superior laryngeal nerve can be injured as it enters the cricothyroid muscle, resulting in difficulty with high-pitched tones. This nerve has a variable course and is intimately associated with the superior thyroid vessels in approximately 58% of the cases, either by traveling between branches of the superior thyroid artery, running in close proximately (<1 cm) superior to the vessels, or coursing posterior to the vessels and superior pole of the thyroid gland. The superior pole vessels must therefore be meticulously dissected close to the thyroid gland and divided in this manner, rather than placing a clamp across all superior pole structures blindly. At this point, the fascial attachments are carefully divided and dissection is continued medially and posterior to the gland, dividing the ligament of Berry and mobilizing the gland off the anterior surface of the trachea. If the RLN was unable to be identified earlier, it should become apparent now, lateral to the ligament of Berry, in the tracheoesophageal grove and dissected superiorly. The thyroid lobe is now attached only by the inferior thyroid artery which the RLN runs posterior to but may run between its branches as well. In 20% of cases, the nerve branches in this region and these branches should be preserved. The inferior thyroid artery branches, like the superior branches, must be individually ligated at the level of the thyroid gland in order to prevent injury to the RLN. Careful dissection of the inferior thyroid artery is not only meant to prevent RLN injury but to also maintain the blood supply to the parathyroid glands. The most common reason for postoperative hypoparathyroidism is compromise of the vascular supply during surgery. The superior parathyroid gland is usually located within the thyroid fascia and located within 1 cm of the intersection of the RLN and inferior thyroid artery in 80% of cases. The inferior parathyroid gland has a more variable location but is typically located posterior and medial to the RLN near the inferior pole of the thyroid gland in the thyrothymic tract. The parathyroid glands are carefully dissected free paying special attention to preserve the lateral vascular pedicle. On occasion, a small rim of thyroid tissue may need to be preserved in order to protect the vascular supply to the parathyroid glands. Should the vascular supply be compromised, the parathyroid gland should be carefully minced and autotransplanted into the ipsilateral sternocleidomastoid muscle after its identity has been confirmed on immediate pathologic evaluation. Resection of the contralateral thyroid lobe, when indicated, proceeds in the same manner as just described.

Depending on the pathology, a central compartment (level VI) lymph node dissection is performed to remove lymphatic tissue bordered superiorly by the hyoid bone, inferiorly by the level of the innominate vessel, and laterally by the carotid arteries with special attention to remove all lymphatic and areolar tissue posterior to the RLN. The goal is to clear all prelaryngeal, pretracheal, and paratracheal lymphatic tissue on the side of the tumor. Isolated removal of only grossly involved lymph nodes, referred to as "berry picking," violates the nodal compartment entered without adequately addressing its disease and may be associated with higher recurrence rates and morbidity from revision surgery. This technique should be discouraged in favor of the more oncologically sound anatomically based technique described above. Finally, when the removal of lateral lymph nodes is indicated for metastatic disease, a modified radical neck dissection is performed, removing all lymphatic tissue in levels II through V while sparing the sternocleidomastoid muscle, spinal accessory nerve, vagus nerve, phrenic nerve, and internal jugular vein (Fig. 16.2). The borders of such a dissection are defined posteriorly by the anterior border of the trapezius muscle (posterior aspect of level V), inferiorly by the clavicle (inferior aspect of levels IV and V), medially by the lateral limit of the

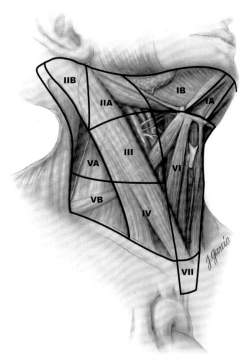

FIGURE 16.2 Anatomic compartments of the neck. (Adapted with permission from *Thyroid* 2009;19(11):1153–1158.)

sternohyoid muscle (medial aspect of levels III and IV), and superiorly by the lower border of the body of the mandible and skull base (superior aspect of level II). Although extrathyroidal extension is rare for most thyroid carcinomas, the surgeon must be prepared to resect any invaded structures including laryngeal or spinal accessory nerves, muscle, tracheal rings, or laryngeal cartilage.

Extent of Surgery

For PTC, therapeutic bilateral central neck lymph node dissection (level VI) is appropriate if there is biopsy proven central or lateral compartment disease prior to operation or central compartment nodal disease is found at the time of surgery. Prophylactic unilateral ipsilateral central lymph node dissection is appropriate for all other PTCs, especially primary tumors greater than 4 cm or when extrathyroidal extension is appreciated at the time of surgery. Extent of prophylactic lymph node dissection should be performed weighing the potential benefits for the individual patient with the associated risks of aparathyroidism and RLN injury. Therapeutic lateral lymph node dissection is appropriate for patients with biopsy proven metastatic lateral cervical lymphadenopathy. This dissection routinely includes levels IIA, III, and IV with the addition of levels IIB and V as warranted by preoperative imaging or intraoperative findings. For FTC and Hürthle cell cancer, no central or lateral neck dissection is indicated unless there is biopsy proven disease prior to surgery or palpable disease is found at the time of surgery. Regarding ATC, given the aggressive nature of this disease, surgical intervention associated with excessive morbidity should be avoided; resections of the larynx, pharynx, and esophagus are discouraged. Surgical resection offers the best opportunity for survival if the tumor is intrathyroidal (rare). Resection of disease that extends beyond the thyroid may be appropriate in highly selected patients as part of multimodal therapy along with radiation and chemotherapy.

Staging and Prognosis

Several staging classification systems have been proposed for thyroid carcinoma with the most commonly used systems being the AMES (age, metastasis, extent, size), MACIS (metastasis, age, completeness of resection, invasion, size), and American Joint Committee on Cancer (AJCC) TNM (tumor, node, metastasis) staging systems (Table 16.5). Research has demonstrated the superiority of the AJCC TNM staging system in predicting cancer related mortality and will be the focus of this section although the other staging systems are metioned for historical purposes. Unfortunately, none of the staging systems, including the AJCC system, has a high predictive value in forecasting recurrent disease, especially in individuals who develop thyroid cancer at a young age. Age at diagnosis is perhaps one of the most important predictive factors for patients with thyroid cancer as evident from its inclusion in each of the staging systems. Male gender has also been shown to be an independent predictor of survival, as thyroid cancer is more aggressive in men, although this variable is not specifically included in any staging system. In general, the prognosis of patients with well-differentiated thyroid carcinoma is based on their age, gender, extent of disease, and the size of their primary tumor. The issue of lymph node metastases and prognosis is still debated since lymph node involvement predicts local recurrence but does not contribute significantly to patient survival. Lymph node involvement affects staging classification only in those patients older than 45 years of age.

The AJCC staging for thyroid cancer stratifies patients into four stages based on the TNM classification except for ATCs, which are always considered stage IV. Staging is based on tumor histology and patient age, demonstrating the importance of these parameters in survival and prognosis. The seventh edition of the AJCC staging system for thyroid cancer has been updated from the sixth edition by the

| TABLE 16.5 | AJCC TNM Staging System for Thyroid Cancer |

Definition

Primary Tumor (T)[a]

Tx	Primary tumor cannot be assessed
T0	No evidence of primary tumor
T1	Tumor ≤2 cm and limited to the thyroid
T1a	Tumor ≤1 cm and limited to the thyroid
T1b	Tumor >1 cm but ≤2 cm and limited to the thyroid
T2	Tumor >2 cm but ≤4 cm and limited to the thyroid
T3	Tumor >4 cm and limited to the thyroid *or* any tumor with minimal extrathyroidal extension
T4	Tumor with advanced disease defined by extent of invasion
T4a	"Moderately advanced" with invasion of subcutaneous tissue, larynx, trachea, esophagus, or recurrent laryngeal nerve
T4b	"Very advanced" with invasion of prevertebral fascia, encasement of carotid artery, or mediastinal vessels

Anaplastic Carcinoma[b]

| T4a | Intra-thyroidal anaplastic carcinoma |
| T4b | Extra-thyroidal extension |

Regional Lymph Nodes (N)

Nx	Regional lymph nodes cannot be assessed
N0	No evidence of regional lymph node metastasis
N1	Regional lymph node metastasis present
N1a	Metastasis limited to level VI (pretracheal, paratracheal, and prelaryngeal lymph nodes)
N1b	Metastasis to unilateral, contralateral, or bilateral Levels I–V, VII, or retropharyngeal lymph nodes

Distant Metastasis (M)

| M0 | No distant metastasis |
| M1 | Distant metastasis |

Differentiated Thyroid Cancer (PTC, FTC, and Hürthle cell)

Under 45 years old

Stage I	Any T	Any N	M0
Stage II	Any T	Any N	M1

Over 45 years old

Stage I	T1	N0	M0
Stage II	T2	N0	M0
Stage III	T3	N0	M0
	T1	N1a	M0
	T2	N1a	M0
	T3	N1a	M0
Stage IVA	T1	N1b	M0
	T2	N1b	M0
	T3	N1b	M0
	T4a	Any N	M0

(*continued*)

TABLE 16.5 AJCC TNM Staging System for Thyroid Cancer (*continued*)

Definition			
Stage IVB	T4b	Any N	M0
Stage IVC	Any T	Any N	M1
Medullary Thyroid Cancer[c]			
Stage I	T1	N0	M0
Stage II	T2	N0	M0
Stage III	T3	N0	M0
	T1	N1a	M0
	T2	N1a	M0
	T3	N1a	M0
Stage IVA	T1	N1b	M0
	T2	N1b	M0
	T3	N1b	M0
	T4a	Any N	M0
Stage IVB	T4b	Any N	M0
Stage IVC	Any T	Any N	M1
Anaplastic Thyroid Cancer[d]			
Stage IVA	T4a	Any N	M0
Stage IVB	T4b	Any N	M0
Stage IVC	Any T	Any N	M1

[a]Primary tumor categories may be subdivided into solitary (s) tumor and multifocal (m) tumors.
[b]All anaplastic thyroid cancers are considered T4 tumors.
[c]Medullary thyroid cancer staging applies to all age groups.
[d]All anaplastic thyroid cancers are considered stage IV.
Adapted from the *AJCC Cancer Staging Manual,* 7th edition.

subdivision of T1 lesions into T1a (tumors ≤1 cm) and T1b (tumors >1 to 2 cm) that are limited to the thyroid. In addition, T category descriptors have been added to indicate solitary tumor (s) or multifocal tumor (m). Despite these modifications, none play a role in tumor staging or prognosis. N1 nodal disease is likewise subdivided on the basis of the location of the lymph node involvement. N1a represents nodal metastases to level VI lymph nodes (pretracheal, paratracheal, and prelaryngeal) while N1b represents nodal metastases to lymph nodes in levels I to V or level VII. This subdivision of lymph node status plays an important role in staging as it differentiates stage III patients from stage IV patients with DTC depending on tumor size. Survival rates for the various thyroid cancers are presented in Table 16.6. Although similar for stage I disease, survival for FTC is slightly worse than PTC and is likely due to the propensity for hematogenous spread and later age and stage at presentation. Anaplastic thyroid carcinoma has one of the worst survival rates of all malignancies with a 1-year survival of 17% and a 5-year survival of approximately 6%, demonstrating the aggressiveness of this disease. In general, the prognosis for patients diagnosed with thyroid cancer is good with survival rates >85% to 90% for most stages, likely as a result of the indolent nature of the disease.

Adjuvant Therapy
The goals of adjuvant treatment include prolonging survival and reducing the future recurrence of thyroid cancer. Retrospective studies of patient cohorts followed postoperatively for several decades suggest that multimodality adjuvant

TABLE 16.6	Stage-Specific Relative Survival for Thyroid Cancer			
	I	II	III	IV
Papillary				
1-Year	99.9	100	97.7	77.6
5-Year	99.8	100	93.3	50.7
Follicular				
1-Year	99.7	99.6	91.1	78.5
5-Year	99	99.7	71.1	50.4
Medullary				
1-Year	100	100	96	64.3
5-Year	100	97.9	81	27.7
Anaplastic				
1-Year	n/a	n/a	n/a	18
5-Year	n/a	n/a	n/a	6.9

Adapted from the *AJCC Cancer Staging Manual*, 7th edition.
Note: All anaplastic thyroid cancers are considered stage IV.

therapy can decrease local recurrence and may improve survival. The mainstay of adjuvant treatment for well-differentiated thyroid carcinoma is radioactive ^{131}I treatment and TSH suppression. The use of therapeutic radioactive ablation of remnant thyroid tissue after thyroidectomy is well established, but criteria for the use of this treatment vary among institutions.

The use of ^{131}I treatment after thyroidectomy improves clinical outcomes including recurrence and survival in selected patients with DTC. Such advantage has been observed in patients with advanced disease (stages III and IV), while patients with small primary tumors (<1 cm) confined to the thyroid may not benefit from radioactive iodine therapy. [131]I treatment is performed either through thyroid hormone withdrawal or using recombinant human TSH (rhTHS). Most DTC patients at MD Anderson Cancer Center (MDACC) undergo thyroid hormone withdrawal for 3 to 6 weeks along with 1 to 2 weeks of low iodine diet before ^{131}I therapy. rhTSH-assisted therapy has a role mainly in patients who are at significant risk for side effects from hypothyroidism (elderly patients, cardiac patients, patients with spine or brain metastases) or patients with central hypothyroidism who cannot produce enough TSH to allow therapy. While 2 to 3 weeks of thyroid hormone withdrawal is usually sufficient to achieve the desired TSH level to proceed with ^{131}I treatment (TSH > 25 to 30 µIU/mL), patients undergoing prolonged thyroid hormone withdrawal (4 to 6 weeks) can take short acting T3 (liothyronine) in the initial 2 weeks of withdrawal to ameliorate hypothyroid symptoms. While this practice is fairly common, the value of such an approach is unclear as most patients are asymptomatic in the initial few weeks of thyroid hormone withdrawal. Either ^{123}I or ^{131}I can be used to perform the initial diagnostic whole-body scan. At MDACC, ^{123}I is more commonly used due to factors related to imaging techniques and reducing the chance of theoretical tumor stunning effect. The initial diagnostic scan aids in disease staging and may assist with the dosing of ^{131}I therapy. [131]I therapy serves many goals including thyroid remnant ablation which simplifies future disease follow-up, as well as diagnosis and treatment of locoregional and distant metastatic disease. Radioactive iodine ablation in DTC is primarily used for patients who are 45 years of age or older, for patients whose primary tumor is greater than 1 cm in diameter or is multifocal, and for patients with extrathyroidal disease due to tissue invasion or metastases. Considering the risk:benefit ratio and the possibility of complications associated with ^{131}I therapy (including the small risk of secondary malignancies), lower doses are currently recommended compared to practices a decade ago. Most low-risk patients (primary tumor less than 1 cm with negative surgical margins without lymphovascular invasion or extrathyroidal extension) without uptake on initial postoperative thyroid scan do not receive [131]I. Patients with small volume disease (1 to 4 cm) limited to the thyroid and found to have radioiodine uptake in only the thyroid bed on initial postoperative thyroid scan often receive an empiric dose of 30 to 100 mCi of radioactive iodine. Patients who have evidence of extrathyroidal extension or lymph node metastases and have significant neck uptake on their initial postoperative thyroid scan receive higher doses of ^{131}I, in the range of 100 to 150 mCi. In patients with evidence of distant metastases preoperatively or on initial whole body iodine scan usually receive a dose between 150 and 200 mCi. Dosimetry is selectively used, aiming to reduce radiation exposure to certain body parts (mainly bone marrow and lungs), in elderly or very young patients or when attempting to administer a high ^{131}I dose.

After surgery and subsequent ^{131}I ablation therapy, patients receive hormonal replacement treatment (levothyroxine sodium) at a dose of 2 µg/kg/day. The dose may vary among patients and is adjusted to reach an appropriate level of TSH suppression for a patient as determined on the basis of the individual patient's disease status and the clinicopathological features of his or her tumor. TSH suppression and radioactive iodine are of no use in the management of medullary and anaplastic thyroid carcinomas because these tumors do not show consistent uptake of radioactive iodine and generally do not contain TSH receptors, making them insensitive to TSH suppression. The extent and duration of TSH suppression is influenced by disease stage, status of recurrence, as well as other comorbidities that may exist in DTC patients (cardiac arrhythmias, coronary artery disease, osteoporosis, or psychological disorders).

The role of external-beam radiation therapy (EBRT) as part of the initial adjuvant treatment regimen for DTC is also controversial. Several retrospective series have reported that local control can be improved with EBRT, specifically in patients with gross disease following surgical resection or in patients considered to be at high risk of relapse (>45 years of age, macroscopic residual disease, extensive extrathyroidal invasion); however, the potential side effects must be considered. Currently, EBRT is more often used to palliate metastatic or locally advanced disease, such as bone metastases or thyroid bed recurrences.

Overall, traditional cytotoxic chemotherapy has not been very effective in the treatment of thyroid carcinomas. Chemotherapy has limited use in the treatment of DTC, Hürthle cell carcinomas, and MTC. However, chemotherapy, in combination with EBRT and surgery, is more commonly used to treat ATC, for which there is a lack of effective therapies. Intravenous bisphosphonates can be given in patients with bony metastases. Arterial embolization has been used anecdotally to reduce pain in selected cases of metastatic follicular thyroid carcinoma where the lesions are highly vascular.

In the past decade, major advancement in treating metastatic DTC and MTC has occurred. Many phase 2 studies showed the benefit of targeted therapy to slow disease progression in as many as 60% to 70% of patients based on objective radiological criteria. These agents resulted in few complete responses, while the majority of patients had either partial response or disease stability after documented progression and failure of ^{131}I treatments. Agents commonly used and still under investigation are multitarget tyrosine kinase inhibitors. These agents primarily inhibit vascular endothelial growth factor receptor in addition to their effect on other tyrosine kinases. Pazopanib, sorafenib, and sunitinib are currently approved by the Food and Drug Administration (FDA) to treat various malignancies but none are

FDA approved for the treatment of metastatic DTC that is resistant to radioactive iodine therapy. Similarly, targeted therapy appears to be promising to treat progressive metastatic MTC using agents such as sorafenib, sunitinib, and vandetanib but none are currently FDA-approved to treat MTC.

Surveillance

Most recurrences of DTC occur within the first 5 years after initial treatment, but recurrences can also occur several decades later. Patients with PTC often recur in the neck, whereas patients with FTC more commonly recur at distant sites. The most common sites of distant metastases for thyroid cancers are the lungs, bone, soft tissues, brain, liver, and adrenal glands. Lung metastases are more common in young patients, whereas bone metastases occur more often in older patients.

A coordinated plan of follow-up for thyroid carcinomas must consider the varied presentations possible for recurrent disease. Most patients are seen every 6 months for 1 to 3 years postoperatively and yearly thereafter. Follow-up visits for DTC patients typically include clinical examination and blood tests measuring the serum thyroglobulin, TSH, and free T4 levels as well as cervical ultrasonography. A thorough physical examination and ultrasonography should be performed in order to detect locoregional recurrences in the surgical bed or neighboring lymph node basins. Thyroglobulin values normally drop after thyroidectomy and ablation and serve as a sensitive indicator of recurrent or persistent disease. However, it is important to keep in mind that thyroglobulin production is TSH dependent; therefore, TSH levels can affect the sensitivity of thyroglobulin measurements in detecting disease. As a result, stimulated serum thyroglobulin is often measured 1 year after initial treatment and is used to assess disease recurrence and plan future follow-up. In addition, 25% of patients with DTC have antithyroglobulin antibodies, which falsely lower measured thyroglobulin levels.

The surveillance for patients with MTC differs from FTC and PTC since it is not derived from follicular epithelium. Therefore, thyroid scanning and thyroglobulin measurement plays no role in the detection of recurrent disease in these patients. Instead, CEA and calcitonin levels are measured in addition to routine neck ultrasound. For patients diagnosed with MEN 2A or 2B, annual screening should be performed for pheochromocytoma and hyperparathyroidism as well. Patients with detectable serum markers (CEA or calcitonin) should undergo US of the neck and, depending on the level of calcitonin, CT or MRI of the chest, abdomen (with liver protocol) and axial skeleton to detect any recurrence. For those individuals who have elevated serum markers and repeat imaging fails to detect recurrent disease, conservative follow-up with repeat serum measurement of CEA and calcitonin every 6 months should be performed. Anaplastic carcinoma and lymphoma cannot be followed the same way as patients with DTC. Routine physical examinations, neck ultrasound, and measurement of CEA and LDH are therefore utilized.

Recurrent Disease

The risk of recurrence depends largely on tumor biology, extent of initial surgery, and other prognostic variables. Approximately 30% of patients with DTC will develop recurrent disease with 66% of patients recurring within the first decade after definitive treatment. Most recurrences (80%) will occur in the neck alone and involve the cervical lymph nodes in 74% of cases, thyroid remnant (20%), or tracheal and local muscle (6%). The remaining 20% of patients who recur develop distant metastatic disease, most commonly to the lungs, which is seen in approximately 60% of individuals. Half of the patients with distant metastatic disease will die of their disease.

The goal of a surveillance program is therefore to detect recurrent disease in a timely fashion so that appropriate medical and surgical intervention can be undertaken. The treatment of recurrent disease depends partly on the iodine avidity of the disease as well as the surgical resectability. In patients with recurrent well-differentiated disease (PTC, FTC, Hürthle cell carcinoma) in which stimulated thyroglobulin levels are 1 to 10 ng/mL but the disease is nonresectable and nonradioiodine responsive, TSH suppression should be undertaken with levothyroxine. If stimulated thyroglobulin levels are >10 ng/mL and all imaging is negative in detecting recurrence, radioiodine ablation should be considered, followed by a postablation radioactive thyroid scan to detect residual disease. In instances in which the recurrence is detected locoregionally by physical examination or imaging (usually ultrasound or CT), surgical resection is the preferred management option. Reoperation in the thyroid bed is associated with increased risk of RLN injury and potential avascularization of parathyroid glands; therefore, surgical intervention should be individualized. We most often recommend surgery in settings in which recurrent disease is greater than 1 cm, is in an anatomically worrisome location (concern for tracheal or nerve involvement) or continued growth is observed over time. Finally, treatment of distant metastatic disease depends on the site of metastases. Central nervous system (CNS) disease should be considered for neurosurgical resection in select patients followed by radioiodine ablation and/or image-guided radiation therapy. Bone and distant metastases other than the CNS should be treated surgically in the presence of enlarging lesions, for palliation in symptomatic patients, or for bone metastases involving weight-bearing extremities. External beam radiation is likewise an option for patients unable to tolerate surgery but with disease that is negative on radioiodine uptake scans. For iodine-avid disease, radioiodine ablation remains an option, but in non-iodine-avid disease which is progressive or symptomatic, referral for clinical trials should be considered.

PRIMARY HYPERPARATHYROIDISM AND PARATHYROID CARCINOMA

Primary Hyperparathyroidism

Epidemiology and Etiology

Although there are many causes for hypercalcemia (Table 16.7), primary hyperparathyroidism (PHPT) is defined as hypercalcemia resulting from the inappropriate or autogenous secretion of parathyroid hormone (PTH) by one or more parathyroid glands. PHPT is four times more common in females than males with approximately 100,000 new cases diagnosed annually in the United States. A solitary parathyroid adenoma is most commonly responsible for PHPT, present in 80% to 85% of patients, and less commonly it is caused by multigland parathyroid hyperplasia (15% to 20%).

Presentation

The presentation of patients with PHPT has changed over the last several decades with 80% to 85% of patients being asymptomatic and diagnosed on routine laboratory values obtained for other reasons. Patients with asymptomatic PHPT may not be truly asymptomatic as many symptoms of hypercalcemia go unrecognized or are thought to be related to medical conditions other than PHPT. Nonspecific symptoms of decreased energy, sleep disturbance, depression, muscle weakness, and bone/joint pain have all shown improvement when hypercalcemia secondary to PHPT is corrected demonstrating that these symptoms may be the initial, subtle presentation in patients with PHPT. Some patients present with more typical symptoms of hypercalcemia, triggering a workup for PHPT. Hypercalcemia may lead to symptoms of increased thirst and polyuria secondary to the inhibitory action of calcium on the antidiuretic hormone, resulting in a state similar to nephrogenic diabetes insipidus. Nephrolithiasis may occur secondary to the effect of PTH increasing renal tubular reabsorption of filtered calcium. Chronic PHPT may cause

TABLE 16.7 Differential Diagnosis of Hypercalcemia

- Primary hyperparathyroidism
  - Solitary adenoma
  - Multigland hyperplasia
  - Multiple gland adenoma
- Secondary/Tertiary hyperparathyroidism
- Familial hypocalciuric hypercalcemia
- Medication
  - Lithium
  - Hydrochlorothiazide
- Malignancy
  - Parathyroid carcinoma
  - Multiple myeloma
  - Tumors producing PTH-related peptide (ovarian, lung)
  - Acute or chronic leukemia
- Sarcoidosis
- Thyrotoxicosis
- Paget's disease
- Increased intake
  - Milk-alkali syndrome
  - Vitamin A toxicity
  - Vitamin D toxicity

severe bone demineralization leading to osteoporosis and fractures. Finally, severe hypercalcemia (>12 mg/dL) has cardiac implications such as shortened QT interval, hypertension (possibly from concomitant renal insufficiency or calcium-mediated vasoconstriction), and deposition of calcium leading to accelerated atherosclerosis as well as alterations in mental status. It is therefore imperative that patients undergo an expeditious workup when elevated or high-normal levels of calcium are discovered with or without the above symptoms.

Diagnosis

Primary hyperparathyroidism is defined as an elevated or high-normal calcium level with an inappropriately unsuppressed PTH levels. The diagnosis is contingent on the presence of normal renal function and normal to increased urinary calcium excretion. A classic, yet useful, test to distinguish cases of hypercalcemia caused by parathyroid versus nonparathyroid origin is the chloride/phosphate ratio. In cases of hypercalcemia secondary to PHPT, PTH inhibits resorption of bicarbonate from the proximal renal tubule resulting in a hyperchloremic renal tubular acidosis from the loss of bicarbonate. This slight increase in serum chloride, coupled with PTH reducing reabsorption of phosphate from the proximal renal tubule, results in a chloride/phosphorus >33 in approximately 94% of patients with PHPT. Thiazide diuretics have been shown to also produce a chloride/phosphorus ratio >33 so care must be taken in solely utilizing this test to diagnose PHPT. Perhaps the most sensitive and useful test to diagnose PHPT in patients with hypercalcemia is the measurement of serum intact parathyroid hormone (iPTH) levels. This test determines the active or "intact" form of PTH as older tests measured inactive forms of PTH or byproducts of PTH degradation that did not play a role in calcium homeostasis. In patients with mildly elevated calcium or iPTH, measurement of 24-hour urine calcium should be performed to rule out benign familial hypocalciuric hypercalcemia (FHH) which will typically be <100 mg/day with this condition. Finally, once the diagnosis of PHPT has been established by the serum measurement of calcium and iPTH, vitamin D deficiency should be ruled out and corrected if present. A deficiency in vitamin D (usually measured as 25-hydroxyvitamin D) will cause an increase in iPTH, mimicking PHPT. Once the vitamin D level has been corrected with supplementation, repeat calcium and iPTH should be measured to ensure the accurate diagnosis of PHPT. Once the diagnosis of PHPT has been established, the need for parathyroidectomy should then be established.

Indications for Surgery
Surgical removal of the parathyroid gland(s) responsible for autonomous production of PTH is the only effective treatment for patients with PHPT. All patients who have symptomatic PHPT should be referred for parathyroidectomy in order to relieve symptoms and prevent complications of chronic hypercalcemia. This category includes patients with overt nephrolithiasis, recent fractures, bone pain, osteitis fibrosa cystica, pancreatitis, mental status changes, or proximal muscle weakness. Many patients, as discussed earlier, present with asymptomatic disease and the criteria to operate on these individuals have changed over time as decided by an international consortium of experts in the field (Table 16.8). Twenty-four-hour measurement of urine calcium, while useful in ruling out FHH, is no longer considered an appropriate guideline to determine patients who are candidates for parathyroidectomy. This change was made because urinary calcium concentration is only one of many factors that determine calcium stone formation; calcium burden of the kidney is also related to serum calcium, renal blood flow, and glomerular filtration rate (GFR). The 24-hour measurement of urine calcium is a variable measurement and one of low precision to select candidates for parathyroidectomy. A GFR <60 mL/min is now used as a guideline for parathyroidectomy because based on the kidney disease outcome quality initiative (KDOQI), a GFR <60 mL/min is indicative of chronic renal insufficiency (stage III) that warrants evaluation and treatment of complications of chronic renal insufficiency. Below a GFR of 60 mL/min, serum iPTH and phosphorus exponentially increase with decreasing GFR and parathyroidectomy is thought to benefit such patients. Osteoporosis and/or history of fragility fractures, as well as age less than 50 years, are also indications to operate on patients with asymptomatic PHPT.

TABLE 16.8	Comparison of Guidelines for Surgical Management of Asymptomatic PHPT		
Measurement	**1990**	**2002**	**2008**
Serum Ca (>ULN)	1–1.6 mg/dL	1 mg/dL	1 mg/dL
24-hour urine calcium	>400 mg/dL	>400 mg/dL	Not indicated
Creatinine clearance (Calc)	Reduced by 30%	Reduced by 30%	Reduced to <60 mL/min
BMD	*Z*-score <−2 in forearm	*T*-score <−2.5 at any site	*T*-score <2.5 at any site and/or previous fracture/fragility
Age	<50	<50	<50

Adapted with permission from *J Clin Endocrinol Metab* 2009;94(2):335–339.
ULN, upper limit of normal; BMD, bone mineral density.

Preoperative Localization and Surgical Technique

While not recommended or necessary for the diagnosis of PHPT, preoperative imaging to help outline an operative strategy in patients with PHPT is necessary if a directed approach is planned. Imaging modalities commonly used in order to preoperatively localize parathyroid pathology include ultrasound, ^{99m}technetium-sestamibi radionuclide scan with or without single photon emission computed tomography (SPECT), and 4D-CT. A nomenclature system has been designed that takes into account the pathologic position of the parathyroid glands and helps radiologists communicate the location of abnormal parathyroid glands with the surgeon (Fig. 16.3).

Although ultrasonography is operator dependent, it is noninvasive, inexpensive, and can be used to evaluate concomitant thyroid pathology. Because of its reliance on the experience of the operator, the positive predictive value is low (50% to 70%) but when combined with sestamibi radionuclide scan can approach 90% and is a useful adjunct for equivocal sestamibi scans. The ^{99m}technetium-sestamibi scan relies on the fact that sestamibi is a lipophilic cation that concentrates in mitochondria. Since parathyroid adenomas and hyperplastic parathyroid glands are metabolically more active when compared to their normal counterparts, the mitochondrial concentration in these glands is higher and sestamibi therefore concentrates in these glands, allowing them to be imaged on radionuclide scan. When combined with SPECT imaging, sestamibi scan can more accurately detect smaller parathyroid glands and those that are more posteriorly located. The use of sestamibi radionuclide scan alone has a sensitivity of 65% to 90% in detecting parathyroid adenomas or hyperplastic glands.

The ability to localize parathyroid glands in the reoperative setting is decreased with the use of sestamibi scans. In this scenario, CT and MRI are useful to localize ectopic or "missed" glands as they provide accurate, and in many cases three-dimensional, imaging of the pertinent anatomy. They are costly however, and their ability to localize a parathyroid adenoma is sometimes limited. When MRI is utilized, parathyroid adenomas appear intense on T2-weighted imaging. Recently, 4D-CT has been utilized in the localization of parathyroid adenomas. This modality involves CT angiography of the neck using narrow slices with perfusion to the parathyroid glands calculated as perfusion over time. This perfusion is then extrapolated as an indicator of gland function since parathyroid adenomas as hyperplastic glands have higher metabolic activity and thus higher perfusion. The 4D-CT can therefore be used to gain information not only on the location of suspected glands but also their function.

Surgical Intervention

In the era of preoperative localization, minimally invasive parathyroidectomy has become the most common surgical treatment for PHPT. A standard cervical exploration involving four-gland evaluation as the primary procedure of choice is now often reserved for patients in whom multigland involvement is suspected prior to surgery (such as MEN1 or 2A) or in cases in which preoperative localization was not possible. The four-gland approach affords the ability to evaluate all four glands and resect as necessary based on the visualized pathology. In cases of parathyroid hyperplasia causing PHPT, a three and a half gland parathyroidectomy is performed with preservation of half of the most normal appearing parathyroid gland with its blood supply. Minimally invasive parathyroidectomy is becoming the most common surgical intervention for PHPT in part because of the high prevalence of a single adenoma as the cause for PHPT (80% to 85% of cases). The technique targets a specific gland and as such relies on accurate preoperative imaging and intraoperative PTH measurement in order to be successful. At the time of operation, a baseline PTH level is drawn and surgical dissection is then directed at the culprit

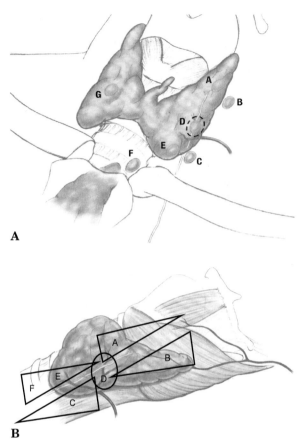

FIGURE 16.3 **A** and **B:** Nomenclature system for parathyroid location. In this classification scheme a *type A* gland is a "normal" superior gland in proximity to the posterior surface of the thyroid parenchyma. It may be compressed within the capsule of the thyroid. A *type B* gland is a superior parathyroid gland that has fallen posteriorly into the tracheoesophageal groove. There is minimal or no contact between the gland and the posterior surface of the thyroid tissue. A *type C* gland is a superior gland that has fallen posteriorly into the tracheoesophageal groove and lies at the level of or below the inferior pole of the thyroid. The *type D* gland lies in the mid region of the posterior surface of the thyroid parenchyma, near the junction of the RLN and the inferior thyroid artery. The *type D* gland may be either a superior or inferior gland, depending on its exact relationship to the nerve, which generally cannot be determined on imaging. The *type E* gland is an inferior gland in close proximity to the inferior pole of the thyroid parenchyma anterior to the trachea. The *type F* gland is an inferior gland that has descended into the thyrothymic ligament or superior thymus. It may appear to be "ectopic" or within the mediastinum. Finally, the *type G* gland is a rare intrathyroidal parathyroid gland. (Reprinted with permission from *Surgery* 2006;140(6):932–940.)

gland identified on preoperative imaging. Five and ten minutes after the gland is removed, a repeat PTH level is checked and a 50% decline in PTH level from baseline is predictive of cure in 96% of cases. Failure of the PTH to drop by 50%, a rebound of the PTH level, or a level that plateaus above the normal range indicates residual disease and a four-gland exploration should be performed.

Exploration of all four glands is the gold standard surgical approach for patients with PHPT and allows visualization of all glands prior to removal of any abnormal tissue. In experienced hands this approach has a low complication rate with a cure rate over 95%. After appropriate preoperative workup, the patient is brought to the operating room and general endotracheal anesthesia is induced. The patient's neck is extended, often facilitated by a shoulder roll, and placed in the semi-Fowler's position with arms tucked at the side for maximum exposure and surgeon access to the field. A transverse incision, utilizing a skin crease for cosmesis, is made approximately 2 cm superior to the sternal notch. Dissection is then carried through the subcutaneous tissue and platysma muscle and subplatysmal flaps are raised. The strap muscles are then divided along the median raphe and because statistically most parathyroid adenomas occur in the right inferior position, attention is directed here first. The strap muscles are then elevated off of the posteriorly positioned thyroid gland and the gland is retracted medially. With gentle retraction, the middle thyroid vein is encountered, ligated, and divided in order to allow additional elevation and medial retraction of the thyroid gland. This facilitates exposure of the carotid sheath and structures posterior to the thyroid which are then palpated, prior to any dissection, in order to discover any suspicious parathyroid glands. If no obvious pathology is identified, attention is turned to locating the right inferior gland first. With the thyroid gland rotated medially, the inferior thyroid artery is identified and preserved so as to not devascularize the parathyroid glands. The RLN is then identified and protected as it approaches the inferior thyroid artery. It is anterior to this position that the inferior parathyroid is often located, usually inferior to the thyroid gland in the thyrothymic tract but also possibly residing within the capsule of the lower thyroid pole. After the inferior gland is identified, the superior parathyroid gland is identified by tracing the RLN superiorly as it enters the cricothyroid membrane. The superior gland can usually be found within 1 cm of this location, posterior and lateral to the RLN and thyroid gland. Once both glands are discovered on one side, the contralateral side is explored where the glands are usually in mirror position to the previously identified parathyroid glands. Once all four glands have been discovered, the abnormal gland is gently teased from its position, paying special attention to preserving the RLN, and elevated on its vascular pedicle. The pedicle is then clipped or ligated and the parathyroid gland is removed. In cases where the glands are hyperplastic, attention should first be turned to partial resection of the most normal (smallest), clearly viable gland in order to preserve 50 to 80 mg of tissue. As resection of the other glands proceeds, the viability of the preserved gland should always be checked prior to resecting the next gland as this allows greater freedom in case the gland becomes nonviable. Less frequently, all four glands can be resected and the smallest one placed on ice in order to mince and reimplant approximately 50 to 80 mg of tissue in the sternocleidomastoid or nondominant brachioradialis muscle. The sternocleidomastoid is often chosen because it is already exposed during the procedure. However, some surgeons prefer to reimplant into the brachioradialis because if recurrent hyperparathyroidism occurs it would avoid a repeat operation in the neck. In any case, the fibers of the muscles are gently spread so as to retain the blood supply to the muscle and ultimately increase the likelihood of parathyroid gland neovascularization. Care should be taken to avoid a hematoma as this will severely compromise ability of the parathyroid glands to engraft. The minced parathyroid is then placed within this muscle pocket and the spread muscle is then gently reapproximated with either Prolene sutures or absorbable suture tagged with hemoclips. The hemoclips or Prolene sutures serve to identify the location of the gland in case reoperative surgery is necessary. Autotransplantation in this manner is successful in 80% of cases.

If preoperative imaging localizes a specific parathyroid gland as suspicious for a solitary adenoma, and intraoperative PTH levels can be measured, then a minimally invasive parathyroidectomy can be performed. Prior neck surgery is not necessarily a contraindication to a minimally invasive approach and may actually be preferred as it allows direct exposure to a solitary adenoma in an otherwise scarred operative field. This technique allows a solitary adenoma to be removed through a modest (2 cm) incision in an outpatient setting. At the time of surgery, the patient is placed into the semi-Fowler's position as previously described and a baseline PTH is drawn. The procedure can be performed under general or locoregional anesthesia which is desirable in older individuals or those for whom general anesthesia may be hazardous. A 2- to 3-cm incision is then made on the side of the localized adenoma medial to the sternocleidomastoid in line with a traditional Kocher incision. The adenoma is then resected as previously described and a repeat PTH level is drawn 5 and 10 minutes after removal of the gland to ensure a 50% or greater decrease in serum PTH. If the level does not drop, a traditional four-gland exploration should be performed.

Locating Parathyroid Glands

A thorough knowledge of parathyroid embryology is required in order to locate pathologic parathyroid glands. The superior parathyroid glands are derived from the fourth branchial pouch along with the thyroid gland. It is for this reason that the superior parathyroid glands do not descend significantly during development and remain closely associated with the posterior aspect of the thyroid gland during development. The inferior parathyroid glands, in contrast, are derived from the third branchial pouch, as is the thymus gland. As the inferior glands descend, they can be found anywhere along the thyrothymic tract (base of the skull to the anterior mediastinum), often in close association or embedded within the thymus gland.

The parathyroid location nomenclature system (Fig. 16.3) takes into account the embryologic migration of the glands and assists in locating glands. When a gland cannot be located, a systematic approach with knowledge of embryology must be utilized in order to locate the gland. If a superior gland cannot be located, attention should be turned to the cricothyroid membrane where the vast majority of superior parathyroids are located within 1 cm of this position. The posterior thyroid should be reinspected as the gland is often located under a fascial covering that once released will reveal the "missing" gland. The superior thyroid artery may be sacrificed in order to obtain better medial rotation of the thyroid gland and improved exposure of its posterior surface. If the gland cannot be located despite interrogating the posterior lateral aspect of the thyroid gland, the tracheoesophageal groove is then inspected, including posterior to the esophagus and subsequently following this into the upper mediastinum if necessary. Rarely are superior parathyroid glands located intrathyroidal and so hemithyroidectomy is seldom indicated. Finally, the carotid sheath should be opened and inspected for the presence of a missing gland. If an inferior parathyroid gland cannot be located, the posterior lateral border of the thyroid gland is inspected from the inferior border to above the junction where the RLN and inferior thyroid artery crosses each other. Because inferior parathyroid glands can be located in close association with the thyroid gland, the anterolateral surface of the thyroid is palpated to discover any suspicious areas and the overlying fascia divided to allow exposure to such a gland. It is in these situations that intraoperative ultrasound may be useful in order to identify a parathyroid gland that is situated deeper in the thyroid parenchyma.

In these cases a limited thyroidotomy can be performed to remove the gland. If these locations do not reveal the inferior parathyroid gland, a cervical thymectomy should be performed as upwards of 17% of inferior glands can be found in the thymus. This is a relatively simple maneuver that adds little time to the operative procedure. Finally, if the gland still cannot be located, a hemithyroidectomy or ligation of the inferior thyroid artery on the side of the missing gland can be performed although the better part of valor in many cases is to abort the procedure and re-image the patients. In the vast majority of instances, the "missing" gland is located in its normal anatomic position on re-exploration.

Parathyroid Carcinoma

Epidemiology

Although parathyroid carcinoma is a cause of PHPT, with calcium levels greater than 14 mg/dL (compared to 10 to 11 mg/dL in benign PHPT), it is a rare cause occurring in only 0.1% to 4% of cases. The incidence is equal among men and women with presentation usually occurring in the fifth decade. No true risk factors have been elucidated, likely due to the rarity of the disease. An association has been made between chronic renal failure and dialysis, thought to be due to malignant transformation of chronically hyperplastic glands. Associations have also been made with multiple endocrine neoplasia syndromes (1 and 2A) and external beam radiation but there is no definitive proof of this relationship. There is, however, an increased prevalence of parathyroid carcinoma in patients with hyperparathyroidism-jaw tumor syndrome. These patients most commonly have a germline mutation in the HRPT2/CDC73 gene whose product, parafibromin, is thought to regulate RNA polymerase-II mediated transcription and histone methylation for certain genes. The exact role of this gene product is not yet understood. Various inactivating mutations in the tumor suppressor gene, HRPT2/CDC73, have been found in the majority of patients with sporadic parathyroid carcinoma but much research is still needed in this particular field.

Presentation

The vast majority (95%) of parathyroid carcinomas are functional and as such, these patients present with severe signs and symptoms of hypercalcemia. In contrast to benign causes of PHPT, the PTH level of patients with parathyroid carcinoma is often five times the upper limit of normal with calcium levels greater than 14 mg/dL. In contrast to patients with benign PHPT in which 80% of cases are asymptomatic, only 20% of patients with parathyroid carcinoma are asymptomatic. It is the extreme levels of hypercalcemia that result in renal and skeletal symptoms in 60% and 50% of patients, respectively. These high levels more commonly cause symptoms of polyuria, polydipsia, nocturia, bone pain/fractures, nephrolithiasis, renal dysfunction, and pancreatitis when compared to benign PHPT where calcium levels are only mildly elevated. A significant number of patients (40%) with parathyroid carcinoma will present with a palpable neck mass and the diagnosis should therefore be entertained anytime a patient with PHPT presents with such a mass. Although hoarseness may be present, invasion of the RLN by a parathyroid cancer is actually infrequent, occurring 10% of the time.

Diagnosis and Treatment

Diagnosis of parathyroid carcinoma is suspected in patients diagnosed with PHPT as previously described but have significantly elevated calcium levels (>14 mg/dL) and/or a palpable neck mass. Preoperative FNA is contraindicated in these situations for risk of local tumor dissemination. It is extremely difficult to diagnose parathyroid cancer with an FNA biopsy and requires clinical examination of the gland intraoperatively or permanent pathologic sectioning to determine malignancy. Preoperative imaging can provide insight into the malignant potential as preoperative ultrasound will identify a gland with irregular margins or local invasion. Once the diagnosis of PHPT has been established and parathyroid carcinoma suspected, the patient is brought to the operating room and an en bloc resection of the parathyroid gland with ipsilateral thyroid lobe, ipsilateral central compartment lymph node dissection (level VI), and removal of the ipsilateral tracheoesophageal soft tissue and lymphatics. If the tumor is adherent to the strap muscles, RLN, or esophageal wall, they should be removed en bloc with the tumor. In cases where parathyroid cancer is not suspected preoperatively or preoperative imaging does not indicate signs of malignancy, parathyroid carcinoma should be suspected intraoperatively if the gland is adherent to surrounding structures, appears gray and firm in nature, or palpable lymph nodes are present. In these cases an en bloc resection should be performed as described. A modified radical neck dissection (levels II to VI) should be performed for clinically evident disease. Histologic criteria on final pathology that denote malignancy include capsular/vascular invasion, presence of mitotic figures, fibrous trabeculae, or rosette-like cellular architecture. Finally, if hypercalcemia recurs soon after treatment for PHPT, parathyroid carcinoma should be suspected with possible regional or distant metastatic disease.

Adjuvant Treatment and Treatment of Recurrence

Currently there is no staging system for parathyroid cancer as available data have not conclusively demonstrated tumor size or lymph node involvement as prognostic factors. The extent of surgery, with en bloc resection of the tumor, has been shown to correlate with improved overall and disease-free survival in multivariate analysis. Because of the rarity of this disease, accumulation of accurate survival data is difficult but suggests a 5-year survival of approximately 75% to 85% and 10-year survival of 50% to 75%. Local recurrence occurs in 25% to 80% of individuals at varying time periods from the initial surgery but typically occur 2 to 4 years after surgery. Distant metastases, most commonly to the lungs, bone, liver, or pancreas, occur in 25% of patients.

Originally thought to be ineffective for the treatment of parathyroid cancer, recent reports have demonstrated that adjuvant radiation may reduce local recurrence in these patients or be beneficial in patients with micrometastatic disease or tumor spillage at the time of surgery. In contrast, chemotherapy has not shown a survival benefit in patients with parathyroid carcinoma despite short-lived responses to single-agent dacarbazine or in combination with cyclophosphamide and fluorouracil for metastatic disease.

In patients with suspected recurrent disease, either locally or distant, imaging should be performed to identify the site and extent of disease with a sestamibi and CT scan. Recurrent hypercalcemia is often the first sign of tumor progression but reoperative surgery can be undertaken with the knowledge that a cure is unlikely but that symptoms of hypercalcemia can be improved in 70% to 85% of patients. The risk of reoperative neck surgery must be balanced with the ability to palliate the symptoms of hypercalcemia in a patient. A solitary focus of metastatic disease can be resected with the patient's understanding that this effort has not been shown to improve survival, only to improve symptoms. There is no benefit to partial resection of widely metastatic disease and these patients should be referred for medical treatment of their hypercalcemia which represents the main cause of morbidity and death in patients with recurrent parathyroid cancer.

The treatment of malignant hypercalcemia is particularly important in patients with disseminated disease or in patients with negative localization studies. In the acute setting, large volume intravenous fluid resuscitation is instituted with addition of a loop diuretic to increase renal calcium clearance. Agents such as mithramycin and calcitonin have proved to be effective but are limited by either toxicity or short duration of action. While not feasible in the chronic setting, intravenous infusion of bisphosphonates (pamidronate or zoledronic acid) have resulted in variable responses that may last for several weeks in some patients. Calcimimetic agents have proved to be the most effective agents for the long-term treatment of hypercalcemia secondary to parathyroid carcinoma. Cinacalcet is approved for the treatment of hypercalcemia secondary to inoperable parathyroid cancer based on a single-armed trial of the agent.

Recommended Readings

Ain KB. Anaplastic thyroid carcinoma: a therapeutic challenge. *Semin Surg Oncol.* 1999;16:64.

Anderson BJ, Samaan NA, Vassilopoulou-Sellin R, et al. Parathyroid carcinoma: features and difficulties in diagnosis and management. *Surgery.* 1983;94:906.

Austin JR, El-Naggar AK, Goepfert H. Thyroid cancers II: medullary, anaplastic, lymphoma, sarcoma, squamous cell. *Otolaryngol Clin North Am.* 1996;29:611.

Bilimoria KY, Bentrem DJ, Ko CY, et al. Extent of surgery affects survival for papillary thyroid cancer. *Ann Surg.* 2007;246:375–381 discussion. 381–384.

Bilimoria KY, Zanocco K, Sturgeon C. Impact of surgical treatment on outcomes for papillary thyroid cancer. *Adv Surg.* 2008; 42:1–12.

Brierley JD, Tsang RW. External beam radiation therapy in the treatment of differentiated thyroid cancer. *Semin Surg Oncol.* 1999;16:42.

Chen H, Udelsman R. Papillary thyroid carcinoma: justification for total thyroidectomy and management of lymph node metastases. *Surg Oncol Clin.* 1998;7:645.

Chow E, Tsang RW, Brierley JD, et al. Parathyroid carcinoma—the Princess Margaret Hospital experience. *Int J Radiat Oncol Biol Phys.* 1998;41:569.

Clayman GL, Gonzalez HE, El-Naggar A, et al. Parathyroid carcinoma: evaluation and interdisciplinary management. *Cancer.* 2004;5:900.

Devine RM, Edis AJ, Banks PM. Primary lymphoma of the thyroid: a review of the Mayo Clinic experience through 1978. *World J Surg.* 1981;5:33.

Duh QY, Sancho JJ, Greenspan FS, et al. Medullary thyroid carcinoma: the need for early diagnosis and total thyroidectomy. *Arch Surg.* 1989;124:1206.

Evans DB, Fleming JB, Lee JE, et al. The surgical treatment of medullary thyroid carcinoma. *Semin Surg Oncol.* 1999;16:50.

Gagel RF, Goepfert H, Callender DL. Changing concepts in the pathogenesis and management of thyroid carcinoma. *CA Cancer J Clin.* 1996;46:261.

Gimm O. Thyroid cancer. *Cancer Lett.* 2001; 2163:143.

Goldman ND, Coniglio JU. Thyroid cancers I: papillary, follicular, and Hürthle cell. *Otolaryngol Clin North Am.* 1996;29:593.

Hay ID, Grant CS, Taylor WF, et al. Ipsilateral lobectomy versus bilateral lobar resection in papillary thyroid carcinoma: a retrospective analysis of surgical outcome using a novel prognostic scoring system. *Surgery.* 1987;102:1089.

Hodgson NC, Button J, Solorzano CC. Thyroid cancer: is the incidence still increasing? *Ann Surg Oncol.* 2004;12:1093.

Hundahl SA, Fleming ID, Fremgen AM, et al. Two hundred eighty-six cases of parathyroid carcinoma treated in the U.S. between 1985–1995: a National Cancer Data Base Report. The American College of Surgeons Commission on Cancer and the American Cancer Society [see Comments]. *Cancer.* 1999;86:538.

Iacobone M, Lumachi F, Favia G. Up-to-date on parathyroid carcinoma: analysis of an experience of 19 cases. *J Surg Oncol.* 2004; 88:223.

Kebebew E, Clark OH. Differentiated thyroid cancer: complete rational approach. *World J Surg.* 2000;24:942.

Kenady DE, McGrath PC, Schwartz RW. Treatment of thyroid malignancies. *Curr Opin Oncol.* 1991;3:128.

Krubsack AJ, Wilson SD, Lawson TL, et al. Prospective comparison of radionucleotide, computed tomographic, sonographic, and magnetic resonance localization of parathyroid tumors. *Surgery.* 1989;106: 639.

Learoyd DL, Messina M, Zedenius J, et al. Molecular genetics of thyroid tumors and surgical decision making. *World J Surg.* 2000;24:922.

Maffioli L, Steens J, Pauwels E, et al. Applications of 99mTc-sestamibi in oncology. *Tumori.* 1996;82:12.

Mazzaferri EL, Jhiang SM. Long-term impact of initial surgical and medical therapy on papillary and follicular thyroid cancer. *Am J Med.* 1994;97:418.

Mazzaferri EL, Robyn J. Postsurgical management of differentiated thyroid carcinoma. *Otolaryngol Clin North Am.* 1996; 29:637.

McLeod MK, Thompson NW. Hürthle cell neoplasm of the thyroid. *Otolaryngol Clin North Am.* 1990;23:441.

Merino MJ, Boice JD, Ron E, et al. Thyroid cancer: a lethal endocrine neoplasm. *Ann Intern Med.* 1991;115:133.

Moley JF, Wells SA. Compartment mediated dissection for papillary thyroid cancer. *Langenbeck's Arch Surg.* 1999;384:9.

Nel CJC, van Heerden JA, Goellner JR, et al. Anaplastic carcinoma of the thyroid: a clinicopathological study of 82 cases. *Mayo Clin Proc.* 1985;60:51.

Niederle B, Roka R, Schemper M, et al. Surgical treatment of distant metastases in differentiated thyroid cancer: indication and results. *Surgery.* 1986;100:1088.

Norton JA. Reoperative parathyroid surgery: indication, intraoperative decision-making and results. *Prog Surg.* 1986;18:133.

Obara T, Fujimoto Y. Diagnosis and treatment of patients with parathyroid carcinoma: an update and review. *World J Surg.* 1991;15:738.

Obara T, Okamoto T, Kanbe M, et al. Functioning parathyroid carcinoma: clinicopathologic features and rational treatment. *Semin Surg Oncol.* 1997;13:134.

Pasieka JL. Anaplastic cancer, lymphoma, and metastases of the thyroid gland. *Surg Oncol Clin North Am.* 1998;7:707.

Ron E, Saftlas AF. Head and neck radiation carcinogenesis: epidemiologic evidence. *Head Neck Surg.* 1996;115:403.

Rosen IB, Sutcliffe SB, Gospodarowicz MK, et al. The role of surgery in the management of thyroid lymphoma. *Surgery.* 1988;104:1095.

Samaan NA, Schultz PN, Hickey RC, et al. The results of various modalities of treatment of well differentiated thyroid carcinoma: a retrospective review of 1599 patients. *J Clin Endocrinol Metab.* 1992;75:714.

Sandelin K, Auer G, Bondeson L, et al. Prognostic factor in parathyroid cancer: a review of 95 cases. *World J Surg.* 1992; 16:724.

Sandelin K, Thompson NW, Bondeson L. Metastatic parathyroid carcinoma: dilemmas in management. *Surgery.* 1991; 110:978.

Shaha AR. Management of the neck in thyroid cancer. *Otolaryngol Clin North Am.* 1998;31:823.

Sherman SI. Surgery for differentiated thyroid carcinoma. In: Rose B, ed. *Up To Date in Medicine* [CD-ROM]. Wellesley, MA: UpToDate; 1996.

Sherman SI. Clinicopathologic staging of differentiated thyroid carcinoma. In: Rose B, ed. *UpToDate in Medicine* [CD-ROM]. Wellesley, MA: UpToDate; 1997.

Sherman SI. Management of differentiated thyroid carcinoma: an overview. In: Rose B, ed. *UpToDate in Medicine* [CD-ROM]. Wellesley, MA: UpToDate; 1997.

Sherman SI. Radioiodide treatment of differentiated thyroid cancer. In: Rose B, ed. *UpToDate in Medicine* [CD-ROM]. Wellesley, MA: UpToDate; 1997.

Sherman SI. Adjuvant therapy and long-term management of differentiated thyroid carcinoma. *Semin Surg Oncol.* 1999;16:30

Sherman SI. Toward a standard clinicopathologic staging approach for differentiated thyroid carcinoma. *Semin Surg Oncol.* 1999;16:12.

Shortell CK, Andrus CH, Phillips CE, et al. Carcinoma of the parathyroid gland: a 30-year experience. *Surgery.* 1991;110:704.

Thomas CG. Role of thyroid stimulating hormone suppression in the management of thyroid cancer. *Semin Surg Oncol.* 1991; 7:115.

Vassilopoulou-Sellin R. Management of papillary thyroid cancer. *Oncology.* 1995; 9:145.

Woolam GL. Cancer statistics, 2000. *CA Cancer J Clin.* 2000;50:7.

Wynne AG, van Heerden JA, Carney JA, et al. Parathyroid carcinoma: clinical and pathological features in 43 patients. *Medicine.* 1992;71:197.

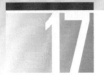

Hematologic Malignancies and Splenic Tumors

John D. Abad and Jorge A. Romaguera

Patients with hematologic malignancies represent an interesting and often challenging cancer population for the surgical oncologist. Whether to perform an excisional biopsy for a patient with suspicion of lymphoma or a therapeutic splenectomy in a patient with a hematologic malignancy, surgeons in cancer centers are frequently involved in the care of these individuals. Therefore, it is important for surgical oncologists to be familiar with these malignancies and the indications for appropriate interventions. The treatment plan almost always involves the participation of our medical oncology colleagues and a multidisciplinary approach.

Hematologic disorders are categorized based on the cell type of origin. This chapter will review hematologic malignancies and splenic tumors as they relate to the role of a clinical surgical oncologist and describe the therapeutic interventions necessary from a surgeon's perspective.

Leukemia and lymphoma represent 6% to 8% of adult cancers and 8% of all cancer deaths in the United States. For children younger than 15 years, leukemia is the most common malignancy. For patients less than 35 years, acute leukemia is the leading cause of cancer deaths. Non-Hodgkin lymphoma (NHL) is the fourth most common in children younger than 15 years.

THE LEUKEMIAS

Polycythemia Vera and Essential Thrombocythemia

Polycythemia vera is characterized by an autonomous expansion of red blood cell mass and volume with a variable effect on white blood cells and platelets. The etiologic mechanism is believed to involve a red blood cell clone highly sensitive to erythropoietin. Approximately three-fourths of patients with polycythemia vera develop palpable splenomegaly and half develop hepatomegaly. Essential thrombocythemia is associated with an increase in megakaryocytes and platelet count with a variable effect on erythrocytes and white blood cells. Increased risk of thrombosis and hemorrhage occur in both polycythemia vera and essential thrombocythemia.

The primary treatment for both diseases is phlebotomy, low-dose chemotherapy, or the combination of these approaches. The goal of treatment is to maintain a hematocrit less than 45%. Splenectomy has little to no role in the treatment of most patients with polycythemia vera or essential thrombocythemia. Although splenectomy has a minimal role in the treatment of these illnesses a condition similar to myelogenous metaplasia develops in a few patients who then require splenectomy. The operative risks are greater and the survival is poorer in this group than in patients with myelogenous metaplasia. Patients with polycythemia vera or essential thrombocythemia should be treated with aggressive nonoperative therapy and offered splenectomy only when pain or when anemia and thrombocytopenia are refractory to other treatments. Splenectomy does not increase the survival rate, but it may improve the quality of life.

Myelogenous Metaplasia

Myelogenous metaplasia is a chronic myeloproliferative disease where immature myeloid precursor cells settle in the reticuloendothelial organs, primarily the spleen, liver, and lymph nodes. It is characterized by fibrosis of the bone marrow and extramedullary hematopoiesis, resulting in massive splenomegaly in approximately 75% of patients. Some patients are asymptomatic; however, most present with fatigue, anorexia, or weight loss in addition to symptomatic splenomegaly. Either thrombocytopenia or thrombocytosis can occur. Active splenic destruction may be humorally or cell mediated. Bone marrow biopsy is necessary for diagnosis. Large platelets, nucleated red cells, anisocytosis, and immature myelogenous elements are often seen on peripheral blood smears.

Initial nonoperative management includes transfusions, steroids, androgens, cytotoxic chemotherapy, and splenic irradiation. Hypersplenism refractory to these primary treatments may warrant splenectomy. At M. D. Anderson Cancer Center, the indications for splenectomy in patients with myelogenous metaplasia with myelofibrosis are (a) severe anemia due to hypersplenism not responding to medical management; (b) chronically symptomatic splenomegaly; or (c) worsening congestive heart failure due to shunting through the spleen. Prior to splenectomy, adequate bone marrow activity must be documented by bone marrow biopsy and nuclear medicine bone marrow scan. If the major site of hematopoiesis is the spleen, a splenectomy may cause severe pancytopenia in these patients. Coagulation studies should also be performed preoperatively.

Postoperatively, these patients are at increased risk for portal vein thrombosis and thrombocytosis. The Mayo Clinic recently published a 30-year review of their splenectomy experience with myeloid metaplasia that suggested that postoperative thrombotic complications may be reduced with the use of platelet-lowering therapy. In this study, platelet-lowering therapy consisted of medical therapy with hydroxyurea, aspirin, or anagrelide, and platelet apheresis for platelet counts greater than one million. Postoperative portal vein thrombosis may present as a postoperative ileus, hepatic insufficiency, vague abdominal pain, or new-onset ascites. The treatment is 6 months of anticoagulation therapy while collateral circulation develops. To minimize the risk of portal vein thrombosis, the authors recommend ligating the splenic vein at its confluence with the superior mesenteric vein to maintain laminar blood flow.

Once again, splenectomy may improve the quality of life for these patients but does not provide a survival benefit. Following splenectomy, the response rates for anemia are 75% to 95%. For those patients that are poor candidates for surgery, low-dose radiation to the spleen may be used.

Chronic Myelogenous Leukemia

Also known as chronic granulocytic leukemia, chronic myelogenous leukemia (CML) involves the clonal proliferation of myelogenous stem cells. Ninety percent of CML patients have the Philadelphia chromosome, which is the characteristic translocation of chromosomes 9 and 22. Treatment response may be measured using PCR levels of the Philadelphia chromosome.

CML has a chronic benign phase and an acute blastic transformation. Most patients present with symptoms of the chronic phase, which include fatigue, weakness, night sweats, low-grade fever, and abdominal pain. On physical examination, splenomegaly may be an isolated finding. Anemia or thrombocytopenia may result from hypersplenism. The median duration of the chronic phase is about 45 months and patients should be followed every 3 to 6 months. Approximately 80% of patients with CML will progress from the chronic phase to the acute leukemic phase.

The acute blastic phase may present as progressive fatigue, high fevers, symptomatic splenomegaly, anemia, thrombocytopenia, basophilia, and bone or joint pain. Frequent infections and bleeding episodes may manifest with increased splenic destruction of blood components. Traditional treatments of CML included conventional chemotherapy with hydroxyurea or busulfan, interferon alpha, or bone marrow transplant with reported 5-year survival rates around 70%. However, with the FDA approval of imatinib mesylate (Gleevec) in 2001, 5-year survival for patients with CML reached 95%. Imatinib is a targeted therapy that inhibits tyrosine kinase and induces apoptosis of leukemic cells.

The indications for splenectomy in CML are to relieve the symptoms of splenomegaly or reduce the need for transfusions. Our experience with splenectomy for patients in accelerated or blastic phase CML at M. D. Anderson demonstrates that splenectomy can be performed safely during this phase and thrombocytopenia can be reliably reversed.

Chronic Lymphocytic Leukemia

Chronic lymphocytic leukemia (CLL) is characterized as a low-grade neoplastic disorder involving the accumulation of mature appearing but functionally incompetent B cells. It is the most common leukemia in the Western Hemisphere, and the median age of onset is in the seventh decade of life. Splenomegaly is common in the advanced stages of the disease. Common symptoms of hypersplenism include abdominal pressure, pain, gastric compression, anemia, or thrombocytopenia. Second malignancies develop in 20% of these patients, most commonly lung cancer, melanoma, or sarcoma. Overall survival is between 1 and 20 years, representing a wide range of indolent to aggressive disease courses. The most common cause of death in patients with CLL is infection from progressive immune system compromise.

At M. D. Anderson, chemotherapy is initiated in early-stage patients (Rai stage I or II) with poor prognostic signs and all patients with Rai stage III or IV disease (Table 17.1). The agent used is fludarabine combined with cyclophosphamide and rituximab. Splenectomy may be recommended for patients refractory to chemotherapy or with symptomatic splenomegaly. Splenectomy has been shown to improve thrombocytopenia in 70% to 80% and anemia in 60% to 70% of patients with CLL. Our experience at M. D. Anderson demonstrates that splenectomy provides an excellent hematologic response in patients with either isolated anemia or thrombocytopenia, but a poor response in patients with both. This suggests that hematopoietic reserve is necessary for a significant clinical response to splenectomy. In selected subgroups of patients with advanced-stage CLL, splenectomy demonstrates a significant survival advantage compared with conventional chemotherapy. This selected subgroup of CLL patients includes those with either hemoglobin levels $\leq$10 g/dL or platelet count $\leq$50 $\times$ 10^9 L.

TABLE 17.1	Rai Staging of Chronic Lymphocytic Leukemia

Stage	Criteria
0	Lymphocytosis (WBCs >15,000/mL with >40% lymphocytes in the bone marrow)
I	Lymphocytosis with lymphadenopathy
II	Lymphocytosis with enlarged liver or spleen (lymphadenopathy not necessarily present)
III	Lymphocytosis with anemia. Anemia may be due to hemolysis or due to decreased production (lymphadenopathy or hepatosplenomegaly need not be present)
IV	Lymphocytosis with thrombocytopenia (platelet count <100,000/μL), anemia, and lymphadenopathy

WBC, white blood cell.

Hairy Cell Leukemia

Hairy cell leukemia (HCL) is a monoclonal lymphoproliferative disorder of mature B cells characterized by the pathognomonic cytoplasmic projections that invade the bone marrow and spleen. It is considered a low-grade leukemic disorder that comprises only 2% to 5% of all leukemias with a 3:1 male predominance typically older than the age of 50 years.

Approximately 10% of HCL patients will have mild symptoms and not require treatment. Splenomegaly is almost universally present; other symptoms may include weakness and fatigue. Indications for treatment include neutropenia, splenomegaly, hypersplenism, or bone marrow failure. The most common cause of death is infection in the setting of neutropenia.

Prior to the development of effective chemotherapeutic agents, splenectomy was the traditional treatment of choice for HCL patients and was associated with an increased survival. However, since the discovery of more effective agents, splenectomy is no longer routinely performed in this setting. Pentostatin and cladribine result in complete response rates of 80% to 90% which are also more durable responses compared to splenectomy. Splenectomy may be considered in rare cases of the pure splenic form of disease or for palliation in HCL patients refractory to medical management.

Acute Lymphocytic Leukemia and Acute Myelogenous Leukemia

In general, there is no role for splenectomy in the treatment of acute lymphocytic leukemia or acute myelogenous leukemia during induction chemotherapy or relapse. Rare exceptions for splenectomy in these patients include cases of splenic rupture or persistent fungal granulomas of the spleen in patients in complete remission.

Splenic Rupture in Leukemia

Splenic rupture is a rare event in patients with leukemia and is almost exclusively the result of a traumatic injury. This is not due to the leukemia but rather the result of splenomegaly. The incidence of splenic rupture in leukemic patients is 0.2% and comprises 3.5% of all cases of spontaneous splenic rupture.

Patients most frequently present with abdominal tenderness, rigidity, and tachycardia. A chest radiograph may demonstrate an elevated hemidiaphragm or pleural effusion. An abdominal computed topography (CT) with intravenous contrast is the diagnostic imaging study of choice. Radiographic findings consist of perisplenic and free peritoneal fluid with possible active extravasation of contrast adjacent to a splenic capsular or hilar injury. For patients that are hemodynamically unstable in the setting of splenic rupture, emergent splenectomy is necessary. For those patients that are hemodynamically stable with evidence of active extravasation of intravenous contrast, emergent arterial embolization by interventional radiology frequently stops further hemorrhage and avoids operative intervention. In evaluating any patient with known splenomegaly and abdominal pain, a clinician must maintain a high index of suspicion for a splenic rupture. Leukemic patients that survive splenectomy after rupture maintain a similar life expectancy as other patients with the same type of leukemia.

THE LYMPHOMAS

Hodgkin Disease

Over the past 25 years, the overall survival of patients with Hodgkin disease (HD) has improved significantly. As our understanding of this tumor biology has improved, so has the use of multiple chemotherapy agents and radiation therapy to treat HD. The role of staging laparotomy has become of historical interest in these patients. The procedure involves liver biopsy, splenectomy, sampling from the periaortic, mesenteric, hepatoduodenal, splenic lymph nodes, as well as any enlarged or abnormal appearing lymph nodes. Adequate staging information is currently based on physical examination and cross-sectional imaging using chest, abdomen, and pelvis CT.

HD is characterized by the presence of multinucleated Reed–Sternberg cells or a variant of these cells. In contrast to NHL in which the predominant cells are malignant lymphocytes, the inflammatory cells outnumber the malignant cell population in HD. The initial symptoms of HD are typically nontender lymphadenopathy, most commonly in the cervical lymph node basins. The axillary, inguinal, mediastinal, and retroperitoneal lymph nodes are less frequently involved at presentation. The presence of B symptoms should also be identified. These include unexplained fever with temperature >38°C, night sweats, or weight loss of >10% body weight over 6 months.

The initial evaluation includes a comprehensive physical examination focusing on all lymph node basins and palpation for hepatomegaly and splenomegaly. Laboratory workup should include a complete blood count with differential and liver function tests. CT of the chest, abdomen, and pelvis and bone marrow biopsy are performed to determine the extent of disease. To confirm the suspected diagnosis of HD, core needle biopsy may be used. In cases where the diagnosis remains unclear, excisional biopsy of suspected lymph node involvement may be necessary. For a surgical oncologist, targeting an enlarged lymph node for excisional biopsy that is relatively accessible is the preferred strategy and lends itself to the lowest possible morbidity.

The prognosis of HD depends on the histologic subtype, stage of disease, and response to therapy. The World Health Organization classification of HD identifies four histologic subtypes divided into two main groups: nodular lymphocyte predominant and classical HD, which itself has four categories—nodular sclerosis, mixed cellularity, lymphocyte depleted, and lymphocyte-rich.

The Ann Arbor staging system (Table 17.2) was developed in 1971 and used to stage HD based on the extent of disease. Clinical staging includes data from the history, physical examination, and nonoperative diagnostic studies. Pathologic staging historically involves tissue analysis from staging laparotomy. The stages are subclassified to reflect lymphatic disease and extranodal involvement, E; and splenic involvement, S. The presence of systemic symptoms, B, further subclassifies patients with HD.

TABLE 17.2 Ann Arbor Staging System for Hodgkin Disease

Stage	Criteria
I	Involvement of a single lymph node region (I) or a single extralymphatic organ or site (IE)
II	Involvement of two or more lymph node regions on the same side of the diaphragm (II) or of an extralymphatic organ and its adjoining lymph node site (IIE)
III	Involvement of lymph node sites on both sides of the diaphragm (III) or localized involvement of an extra-lymphatic site (IIIE), spleen (IIIS), or both (IIISE)
IV	Diffuse or disseminated involvement of one or more extralymphatic organs with or without associated lymph node involvement
A	Asymptomatic
B	Fever, night sweats, or weight loss of more than 10%

Staging laparotomy was initially performed in the setting of all patients with HD to define the extent of disease. Over the years, laparotomy was used to determine early-stage disease, which could benefit from radiation vs. those with extensive disease requiring systemic chemotherapy. A combination of improved noninvasive imaging modalities and more aggressive use of early systemic treatment and radiation therapy have virtually eliminated the role for staging laparotomy for this disease process. At the M. D. Anderson Cancer Center, nonoperative staging and prognostic factors are used to guide therapy in these patients. This approach is supported by data failing to demonstrate a significant survival advantage between clinical and surgical staging. Performing an invasive staging laparotomy or laparoscopy therefore provides no benefit to HD patients and may delay the initiation of systemic chemotherapy.

The role for splenectomy, however, does occasionally exist in the HD population for two indications. The first is symptomatic splenomegaly. Second are hematologic disturbances such as thrombocytopenia and leucopenia that may result in chemotherapy delays.

Non-Hodgkin Lymphoma

NHL is the most common type of lymphoma and is characterized by the monoclonal proliferation of lymphocytes. Approximately 80% of NHL is derived from B-cell origin and the remainder 20% are from T cells. B-cell NHL is diagnosed and classified into subsets based on the identification of histopathologic markers using monoclonal antibodies and cellular morphology. These criteria for diagnosis depend on diffuse versus follicular (nodular) pattern of lymph node involvement, small versus large cell type, cell surface marker expression, and molecular/cytogenetic findings. Using these differences and others, patients with NHL may be placed into three categories that include mature B-cell, mature T and NK cell, and immunodeficiency-associated lymphomas.

Patients with NHL present with superficial nontender lymphadenopathy, most commonly in the cervical lymph nodes. The Ann Arbor Staging System initially developed for HD was adopted for the staging of NHL. It is generally less helpful for NHL because greater than half of NHL patients present with stage III or higher disease and 20% have B symptoms. Hematogenous spread versus lymphatic spread is more common in NHL compared to HD.

Surgical oncologists may be asked to evaluate patients with NHL for a variety of reasons. These include performing a diagnostic biopsy, providing vascular access for chemotherapy or rarely, splenectomy. Staging laparotomy is not indicated for NHL. Splenectomy is indicated for NHL patients with symptomatic splenomegaly or pancytopenia requiring frequent transfusion requirements as a result of hypersplenism. NHL patients with a persistent isolated splenic focus of disease may also benefit from splenectomy. The prognosis of these selected individuals is similar to other stage I patients.

Diagnostic Biopsy for Lymphoma

The pathologic diagnosis for a suspected lymphoma relies on the appropriate planning and communication between the medical oncologist, surgical oncologist, and pathologist. The targeted lymph node for excisional biopsy should be the largest node found on physical examination. Other radiographic signs can be used to select the lymph node to be biopsied, such as whether there is necrosis in the node or is there is high uptake of radioactive tracer as detected by the positron emission tomography (PET) testing. If multiple enlarged lymph nodes are present, the preferential biopsy sites are cervical lymph nodes, then axillary lymph nodes, then inguinal lymph nodes. For cases of matted lymph nodes or extranodal disease, a generous biopsy sample is helpful for diagnosis. The fundamental principle in making the pathologic diagnosis is preservation of architecture; therefore, sharp dissection is preferred over electrocautery. Once excised, the specimen should be sent directly to the pathologist as a fresh specimen in saline or a saline-soaked sponge. It should be clearly communicated to the pathologist that the biopsy is for a suspected lymphoma to further aid in the appropriate processing of the tissue. Needle biopsies may be helpful to rule out a carcinoma or sarcoma or to provide evidence for a suspected relapse of lymphoma; however, they tend not to be as helpful for the initial diagnosis of lymphoma since the histologic architecture is not preserved.

MISCELLANEOUS SPLENIC TUMORS

Splenic Cysts

Splenic cysts are typically classified as either primary (true) or secondary (false or pseudocysts) based on the presence of an epithelial lining. Primary cysts may be further classified as parasitic and nonparasitic. Nonparasitic cysts comprise 75% of splenic cysts in the United States and include both congenital and neoplastic cysts. Congenital cysts are characterized as epidermoid or dermoid cysts. These are usually diagnosed in children and young adults. Approximately 90% of nonparasitic true cysts are epidermoid cysts. Neoplastic cysts include lymphangiomas and cavernous hemangiomas. Parasitic cysts are very rare in the United States and most commonly the result of an echinococcal infection. Secondary cysts are more common than primary cysts and are generally believed to be the result of splenic injury and hematoma formation. Pseudocysts may also develop after acute pancreatitis, infections, or splenic infarcts. Patients with splenic cysts often present with vague symptoms of left upper quadrant pain and early satiety. Splenic cysts are often detected on physical examination as a palpable mass or on CT imaging. For nonparasitic splenic cysts <5 cm, conservative management with ultrasound follow-up is recommended. Indications for surgical management for patients with splenic cysts include size >5 cm, symptoms, hemorrhage, infection, or cyst perforation. The surgical options include complete or partial splenectomy, unroofing or marsupialization of the cyst, and fenestration. These can be performed through an open incision, hand-assisted or completely laparoscopic techniques. Percutaneous drainage of splenic cysts is generally avoided due to the high incidence of recurrence and difficulty with subsequent operations due to the resulting inflammatory response.

Inflammatory Pseudotumor

Inflammatory pseudotumor, also known as plasma cell granuloma, has features of inflammation and mesenchymal repair. These pseudotumors may be found throughout the body, including the respiratory and gastrointestinal tracts, orbit, and lymph nodes. Similar to pseudocysts, they are believed to result from prior trauma or infection. These lesions are often mistaken for lymphoma, therefore requiring tissue diagnosis with immunohistochemical stains and flow cytometry to differentiate them from lymphoproliferative diseases.

Nonlymphoid Tumors

Nonlymphoid tumors of the spleen may be either benign or malignant. The most common malignant nonlymphoid tumors of the spleen are angiosarcomas. These tumors tend to have an aggressive biology allowing them to grow quickly and metastasize early in their clinical course. Angiosarcomas are associated with exposure to thorium dioxide, vinyl chloride, and arsenic. Splenectomy is indicated in these patients but rarely curative. The overall prognosis is poor. Other rare malignant nonlymphoid splenic tumors include Kaposi sarcoma, malignant fibrous histiocytoma, fibrosarcoma, leiomyosarcoma, plasmacytomas, hemangiosarcomas, and lymphangiosarcomas.

Splenic Metastases

Splenic metastases are rare events given the large amount of total blood flow to the spleen. This may be related to the immunologic function of the spleen and its ability to clear microscopic metastatic disease. When they occur, they are usually associated with disseminated disease. The incidence of splenic metastases in autopsy studies ranges from 1.6% to 30%. The most frequently detected metastases originate from melanoma, breast, and lung cancer. Other primary sites include ovarian, endometrial, gastric, colonic, and prostate cancers. Splenectomy may be considered for solitary metastases with stable or treated primary disease such as melanoma or as part of a debulking procedure for ovarian, primary peritoneal, or appendiceal cancers. Other possible indications for splenectomy for metastatic disease include the treatment of complications of perforation of adjacent viscera, hemorrhage, or splenic vein thrombosis.

SPLENECTOMY

Splenectomy for Hypersplenism

Anemia, neutropenia, and thrombocytopenia may occur for a number of reasons in patients with hematologic malignancies. Because only patients with excessive destruction of a blood component will benefit from a splenectomy, a careful workup should be done to identify the etiology of the process. Patients with hypersplenism may present with a normal-sized spleen, and others may have massive splenomegaly without hypersplenism.

Infusion of the patient's or normal donor platelets tagged with ^{111}indium is helpful in determining whether the spleen is the site of destruction. Patients with an acquired hemolytic anemia generally have a positive Coombs test, and the detection of the warm antibody is a good indication that splenectomy will be beneficial. Although chromium-labeled red blood cell scans may be useful in demonstrating decreases in red blood cell survival, they are not as helpful in identifying the site of sequestration. In cases of suspected splenic sequestration, a bone marrow biopsy is important to determine whether adequate precursor cells are available or whether the patient depends on the hematopoietic activity of the spleen.

Splenectomy in patients with CML has been associated with severe bleeding problems. These may be related to impaired clot formation caused by proteases and serases produced by granulocytes. Patients with CML and severe leukocytosis should receive chemotherapy in an attempt to decrease the WBC count to approximately 20,000 cells/mL. Experience at M. D. Anderson suggests that splenectomy is best avoided in patients with CML in whom WBC counts cannot be controlled with chemotherapy. Splenectomy should also be avoided in patients with CML who have had splenic irradiation due to significant technical surgical difficulty from the radiation-induced scarring and fibrosis.

Bleeding and infection are the greatest perioperative risks after splenectomy for hypersplenism. Qualitative platelet function should be evaluated rather than relying on a platelet count. The template bleeding time is currently the most widely available laboratory value for identifying adequacy of platelet function. The patient's current and recent medications should be carefully reviewed to identify any drugs that may impair coagulation.

Although splenectomy may be performed through either a midline or a subcostal approach, the midline incision is preferred when coagulation defects, thrombocytopenia, or splenomegaly is present. After the splenic pedicle is clamped, thrombocytopenic patients are transfused with fresh platelets. Careful hemostasis at the conclusion of the procedure is mandatory. Postoperatively, patients should be monitored closely during the first 48 hours for signs of bleeding. A blood cell count with differential and platelet counts should be obtained every 6 hours for the first 24 hours after the operation. Decreasing platelet and blood counts, despite adequate replacement, suggest an ongoing bleeding process.

Splenectomy for the Massively Enlarged Spleen

Indications for splenectomy in patients with massively enlarged spleens include debilitating symptoms of splenomegaly, excessive destruction of blood components, and concerns of possible splenic rupture. These patients often complain of chronic severe upper abdominal and back pain, impaired respiration, and early satiety. Hypersplenism may be present. Depending on the size of the spleen and the body habitus, the patient may be judged to be at increased risk of splenic trauma.

Preoperatively, it is important to check quantitative and qualitative platelet function values and coagulation studies because hemorrhage is the major complication of splenectomy in this group. Portal venous contrast studies should be performed in patients with possible portal hypertension. If the splenic vein is thrombosed, splenectomy is appropriate, but otherwise it may deprive a patient with portal hypertension of the option of a splenorenal shunt.

Adequate blood products must be available preoperatively. The blood of these patients may be difficult to crossmatch because of numerous past transfusions, and fresh single-donor platelets may be required. Patients should undergo routine bowel preparation, and prophylactic antibiotics should be given.

A midline, rather than subcostal, incision is preferred because the rectus muscles are not severed, which limits bleeding. With increasing size, the spleen becomes more of a midline structure and lends itself to this approach. Before mobilization of the spleen, its vessels should be isolated. The gastrocolic omentum is divided, the lesser sac is entered, and the splenic artery is identified along the posterior-superior surface of the pancreas. The artery is ligated but left intact. The splenic vein is not disturbed yet. The spleen may decrease 20% to 30% in size at this point and allow platelet transfusion without consumption. The splenic flexure of the colon is mobilized, the splenic ligaments are divided, and the spleen is delivered from the splenic fossa. The normally avascular splenic ligaments often contain small vessels in the presence of hematologic malignancies. Dense adhesions between the spleen and the diaphragm may complicate mobilization, and when dissection is particularly difficult, it is better to resect part of the diaphragm with the spleen than to risk hypertrophy of splenic remnants. Such adhesions are formed in areas of splenic infarction and are the most frequent sites of postoperative bleeding in this group of patients.

After the spleen is mobilized, the artery and vein are suture ligated and divided. Liver biopsy may be indicated if involvement by lymphoma is suspected. If an injury to the pancreatic tail is recognized, it should be repaired and drained appropriately. Achieving hemostasis in the splenic bed is crucial and may require suture ligation, cautery, platelet transfusions, and thrombostatic agents. Drains do not reliably warn off postoperative hemorrhage or prevent infection, and except in cases of pancreatic injury, they are not routinely used. Postoperatively, patients should be closely monitored for signs of bleeding or infection.

Laparoscopic Splenectomy

Minimally invasive surgery techniques are utilized in several areas of surgical oncology including the use of laparoscopic splenectomy for hematologic and splenic malignancies. The laparoscopic approach has several traditional advantages, most obviously, less morbidity from smaller incisions. These generally translate to shorter hospitalizations post-op, less pain and need for narcotics, and fewer wound-related issues including subsequent incisional hernia development. The disadvantages historically have been longer operative time; however, this tends to be somewhat surgeon and experience dependent. Absolute contraindications for a laparoscopic approach include emergent conditions such as splenic rupture. Relative contraindications to laparoscopic splenectomy include massive splenomegaly (>25 cm in length), portal hypertension, and pregnancy; however, there have been successful reports in all of these conditions. The hand-assisted laparoscopic surgery approach is often used as a bridge between open and laparoscopic splenectomy for those surgeons learning minimally invasive techniques. This hybrid approach may also be helpful in manipulating a larger spleen without causing trauma.

There are two large recent meta-analyses published comparing the use of laparoscopic and open splenectomy, which include mostly patients with benign hematologic conditions. Overall, these reviews identify complication and mortality rates significantly lower with the laparoscopic compared with the open approach. These complications are generally related to pulmonary and infectious complications including wound infections. For benign hematologic disease and splenic tumors, laparoscopic splenectomy has become the standard approach. For malignant conditions without contraindications, its role has been generally accepted provided that fundamental oncologic surgical principles are observed.

Prophylaxis for Asplenic Sepsis

Patients with hematologic malignancies who undergo splenectomy are at greater risk for asplenic sepsis than are those who have the procedure for other indications. Some patients with hematologic malignancy, especially those with CML and CLL, are at increased risk for sepsis even before splenectomy. The risk of overwhelming postsplenectomy infection (OPSI) is greatest for children. The expected death rate from OPSI in children is one in every 300 to 350 patient-years, and in adults, one in every 800 to 1,000 patient-years. For all patients, the risk is greatest for the first few years following splenectomy, but deaths attributed to OPSI have occurred 30 or more years after splenectomy.

Following splenectomy, there is loss of the opsonins, tuftsin and properdin, a decrease in immunoglobulin M production, impaired phagocytosis, and altered cellular immunity. Poorly opsonized bacteria are best cleared by the spleen, and following the spleen's removal, patients are particularly susceptible to encapsulated bacteria.

Vaccination can decrease the risk of postsplenectomy pneumococcal infection. The 23-valent form of the pneumococcal vaccine should be used. The vaccine is most effective when given several weeks preoperatively. Nevertheless, despite the diminished immunity obtained if the vaccine is given after splenectomy, adequate protection is still achieved in most patients. In patients who are not immunized preoperatively there is no benefit from delaying the immunization for several weeks after surgery, so these patients should be vaccinated without delay. Leukemic patients may not be able to develop antibodies in response to pneumococcal vaccine, but it may still be worthwhile to vaccinate this group. Booster immunizations with the pneumococcal vaccine have no proven benefit, although reimmunization at 3 to 5 years may be required if a decrease in specific antibody levels is documented. Certain subsets of patients are at increased risk of infection with *Haemophilus influenzae* and *Neisseria meningitidis* and, therefore, patients should receive these vaccinations as well. Patients are also instructed to keep a supply of antibiotics such as amoxicillin and Augmentin (amoxicillin; clavulanate potassium) with them, which should be taken at the first sign of a febrile episode. This should also be followed by immediate contact with a physician.

Long-term use of prophylactic oral antibiotics is often recommended in the pediatric population or in patients who may have difficulty reaching a physician. Penicillin is commonly prescribed to these patients. Data have shown benefit of prophylactic penicillin in preventing pneumococcal infection in children with sickle cell disease, but the benefit of this practice has never been proved for other subsets of asplenic patients.

Recommended Readings

Berman RS, Yahanda AM, Mansfield PF, et al. Laparoscopic splenectomy in patients with hematologic malignancies. *Am J Surg.* 1999;178:530–536.

Bouroncle BA. Thirty-five years in the progress of hairy cell leukemia. *Leuk Lymphoma.* 1994;14:1.

Bouvet M, Babiera GV, Termuhlen PM, et al. Splenectomy in the accelerated or blastic phase of chronic myelogenous leukemia: a single institution, 25-year experience. *Surgery.* 1997;122:20.

Brenner B, Nagler A, Tatarsky I, et al. Splenectomy in agnogenic myelogenous metaplasia and postpolycythemic myelogenous metaplasia. *Arch Intern Med.* 1988;148:2501.

Burch M, Misra M, Phillips E. Splenic malignancy: a minimally invasive approach, *Cancer J.* 2005;1:36.

Canady MR, Welling RE, Strobel SL, et al. Splenic rupture in leukemia. *J Surg Oncol.* 1989;41:194.

Carde P, Hagenbeek A, Hayat M, et al. Clinical staging versus laparotomy and combined modality with MOPP versus ABVD in early-stage Hodgkin's disease: the H6 twin randomized trials from the European Organization for Research and Treatment of Cancer Lymphoma Cooperative group. *J Clin Oncol.* 1993;11:2258.

Coad JE, Matutes E, Catovsky D. Splenectomy in lymphoproliferative disorders: a report on 70 cases and review of the literature. *Leuk Lymphoma.* 1993;10:245.

Cortes J, Talpaz M, Kantarjian H. Chronic myelogenous leukemia: a review. *Am J Med.* 1996;100:555.

Cusack JC, Seymour JF, Lerner S, et al. The role of splenectomy in chronic lymphocytic leukemia. *J Am Coll Surg.* 1997;185:237.

Dawes LG, Malangoni MA. Cystic masses of the spleen. *Am Surg.* 1986;52:333.

Edwards MJ, Balch CM. Surgical aspects of lymphoma. *Adv Surg.* 1989;22:225.

Farrar WB, Kim JA. Biopsy techniques to establish diagnosis and type of malignant lymphoma. *Surg Oncol Clin North Am.* 1993;2:159.

Feldman EJ, Arlin ZA. Modern management of chronic myelogenous leukemia (CML). *Cancer Invest.* 1988;6:737.

Fielding AK. Prophylaxis against late infection following splenectomy and bone marrow transplant. *Blood Rev.* 1994;8:179.

Flexner JM, Stein RS, Greer JP. Outline of treatment of lymphoma based on hematologic and clinical stage with expected end results. *Surg Oncol Clin North Am.* 1993;2:283.

Hagemeister FB, Fuller LM, Martin RG. Staging laparotomy: findings and applications to treatment decisions. In: Fuller L, ed. *Hodgkin's Disease and Non-Hodgkin's Lymphoma in Adults and Children.* New York, NY: Raven; 1988.

Harris NL. The pathology of lymphomas: a practical approach to diagnosis and classification. *Surg Oncol Clin North Am.* 1993;2:167.

Hubbard SM, Longo DL. Treatment-related morbidity in patients with lymphoma. *Curr Opin Oncol.* 1991;3:852.

Johnson HA, Deterling RA. Massive splenomegaly. *Surg Gynecol Obstet.* 1989;168:131.

Kalhs P, Schwarzinger I, Anderson G, et al. A retrospective analysis of the long-term effect of splenectomy on late infections, graft-versus-host disease, relapse, and survival after allogenic marrow transplantation for chronic myelogenous leukemia. *Blood.* 1995;86:2028.

Kantarjian H, Sawyers C, Hochhaus A, et al. Hematologic and cytogenetic responses to imatinib mesylate in chronic myelogenous leukemia. *N Engl J Med.* 2002; 346(9):645.

Kantarjian HM, Smith TL, O'Brien S, et al. Prolonged survival in chronic myelogenous leukemia after cytogenetic response to interferon-a therapy. *Ann Intern Med.* 1995;122:254.

Klein B, Stein M, Kuten A, et al. Splenomegaly and solitary spleen metastasis in solid tumors. *Cancer.* 1987;60:100.

Kluin-Nelemans HC, Noordijk EM. Staging of patients with Hodgkin's disease: what should be done? *Leukemia.* 1991;4:132.

Kojouri K, Vesely SK, Terrell DR, et al. Splenectomy for adult patients with idiopathic thrombocytopenic purpura: a systematic review to assess long-term platelet count responses, prediction of response, and surgical complications. *Blood.* 2004;104:9.

Kraus MD, Fleming MD, Vonderhide RH. The spleen as a diagnostic specimen: a review of 10 years' experience at two tertiary care institutions. *Cancer.* 2001;91:11.

Kurzrock R, Talpaz M, Gutterman JU. Hairy cell leukaemia: review of treatment. *Br J Haematol.* 1991;79(suppl 1):17.

Mahon D, Rhodes M. Laparoscopic splenectomy: size matters. *Ann R Coll Surg Eng.* 2003;85:248.

McBride CM, Hester JP. Chronic myeloge-nous leukemia: management of splenec-tomy in a high-risk population. *Cancer.* 1977;39:653.

Morgenstern L, Rosenberg J, Geller SA. Tumors of the spleen. *World J Surg.* 1985; 9:468.

Mower WR, Hawkins JA, Nelson EW. Postsple-nectomy infection in patients with chronic leukemia. *Am J Surg.* 1986;152:583.

Noordijk EM, Carde P, Mandard AM, et al. Preliminary results of the EORTC-GPMC controlled clinical trial H7 in early stage Hodgkin's disease. *Ann Oncol.* 1994; 5(suppl 2):107.

Parker SL, Tong T, Bolden S, et al. Cancer sta-tistics 1997. *CA Cancer J Clin.* 1997;47:5.

Pittaluga S, Bijnens L, Teodorovic A, et al. Clinical analysis of 670 cases in two trials of the European Organization for the Research and Treatment of Cancer Lym-phoma Cooperative Group subtyped according to the Revised European-American Classification of lymphoid neoplasms: a comparison with the Work-ing Formulation. *Blood.* 1996;10:4358.

Pollock R, Hohn D. Splenectomy. In: Roh MS, Ames FC, eds. *Advanced Oncologic Sur-gery.* New York, NY: Mosby-Wolfe; 1994.

Schrenk P, Wayand W. Value of diagnostic laparoscopy in abdominal malignancies. *Int Surg.* 1995;80:353.

Shaw JHF, Print CG. Postsplenectomy sepsis. *Br J Surg.* 1989;76:1074.

Styrt B. Infection associated with asplenia: risks, mechanisms, and prevention. *Am J Med.* 1990;88:33N.

Tefferi A, Silverstein MN, Noel P. Agnogenic myelogenous metaplasia. *Semin Oncol.* 1995;22:327.

Wiernik PH, Rader M, Becker NH, et al. Inflammatory pseudotumor of spleen. *Cancer.* 1990;66:597.

Winslow ER, Brunt LM. Perioperative out-comes of laparoscopic versus open sple-nectomy: a meta-analysis with an emphasis on complications. *Surgery.* 2003; 134(4):647.

18 Genitourinary Cancer

Jose A. Karam and Christopher G. Wood

Global cancer statistics reveals that genitourinary cancers represented approximately 10.4% of new cancers diagnosed worldwide in 2005. These cancers occur in approximately 300,000 patients within the United States each year, and prostate cancer is now the most common malignancy and second leading cause of cancer death in U.S. men. Recognizing these facts, practicing physicians require an essential understanding of the diagnosis and treatment of these diseases. In this chapter, we review the current management of prostate, bladder, renal, and testicular neoplasms.

PROSTATE CANCER
Epidemiology and Etiology
In men, prostate cancer is the most common malignancy and the second leading cause of solid cancer mortality. In the United States, it is estimated that one of six men will be diagnosed with prostate cancer during their lifetime. Prostate cancer alone accounted for 25% of incident cases in 2009. Average mortality rates (2000 to 2005) are estimated to be 59.4 per 100,000 in African American males and 24.6 per 100,000 in white males. Prostate cancer screening was introduced in the United States in 1986. Since this introduction, the pattern of disease incidence has changed. From 1988 to 1992, the annual percent increase of prostate cancer incidence was estimated at 17.5% per year. From 1992 to 1995, the incidence decreased to 10.3% per year. This decrease has leveled off and from 1995 to 1997, the average annual decrease in incidence was 2.1%, and the average annual incidence was 149.7 cases per 100,000. These cancer trends are not equivalent between whites and African Americans. Prostate cancer incidence in white males is 156 per 100,000 compared to 248 per 100,000 in African Americans, while the resulting mortality is 24 per 100,000 versus 59 per 100,000, respectively (2001 to 2005). Furthermore, although the average annual mortality rates have decreased 4.4% per year (2001 to 2005) overall, African Americans have only experienced an average mortality rate decrease of 3.6% per year throughout 1993 to 2001. It is unclear whether the increased mortality rate of prostate cancer in African Americans is due to unique racial biological and genetic factors, rather than dietary influences, the existence of confounding medical comorbid conditions, lifestyle differences, and/or access to health care issues. Occupational exposure to cadmium has been associated with increased risk of prostate cancer, but this relationship is not yet proven to be causal.

Prostate cancer rarely occurs before the age of 50 years, and the incidence increases through the ninth decade of life; however, some of this increase may be attributable to an increase in prostate cancer screening in the later decades. It is estimated that 30% to 50% of men older than 50 years have histologic evidence of prostate cancer at autopsy, while at the age of 75 or older, it is estimated that this figure increases to 50% to 70%.

Many factors have been proposed to be associated with the development of prostate cancer. The presence of an intact hypothalamic–pituitary–gonadal axis and advanced age are the most universally accepted risk factors. Migration studies support a role for environmental influences on prostate cancer. Higher rates of prostate cancer have been found among populations with higher amounts of fat in the diet. Beneficial dietary associations include isoflavonoids and lycopenes. Until recently, selenium, and vitamin E were considered to exert a protective effect against prostate cancer. However, the Selenium and Vitamin E Cancer Prevention Trial (SELECT trial, 2009) showed no difference in prostate cancer incidence in subjects who received selenium and vitamin E. Two large prospective trials have recently shown that inhibiting 5-alpha reductase (which converts testosterone into dihydrotestosterone [DHT]) can prevent prostate cancer in a subset of patients. The Prostate Cancer Prevention Trial (PCPT trial, 2003) reported a 24.8% decrease in the incidence of prostate cancer in patients on finasteride; however, high-grade cancer rates was increased, which was later reported as an artifact resulting from shrinkage of the prostate and selective inhibition of low-grade cancers. The Reduction by Dutasteride of Prostate Cancer Events (REDUCE, unpublished) reported that dutasteride also decreased prostate cancer incidence by 23%, but with no associated increase in high-grade cancers.

Evidence has shown that a man with one, two, or three first-degree relatives affected with prostate cancer has a 2, 5, or 11 times greater risk, respectively, of the development of prostate cancer than the general population. A Mendelian pattern of autosomal dominant transmission of prostate cancer accounts for 43% of disease occurring before the age of 55 years and 9% of all prostate cancers occurring by the age of 85 years. Recent data have implicated the 8q24 chromosomal locus as a risk factor for prostate cancer.

Anatomy

The normal prostate gland weighs 15 to 20 g and is divided into three major glandular zones. The *peripheral zone* constitutes 70% of the prostate gland and is the area palpated during digital rectal examination (DRE). The area around the ejaculatory ducts is called the *central zone* and accounts for 25% of the gland. The *transitional zone* comprises 5% of the prostate gland around the urethra. In a pathological review of 104 prostate glands from patients who underwent radical prostatectomy, 68% of the cancers were located in the peripheral zone, 24% in the transitional zone, and only 8% in the central zone. Almost all stage T1 (nonpalpable) cancers in that study were found in the transitional zone, the area most susceptible to benign prostatic hyperplasia, which can be associated with urinary symptoms secondary to bladder neck obstruction.

Screening

Although good screening methods for prostate cancer are available, controversy surrounds the concept of screening for this disease. It is estimated that less than 10% of men with prostate cancer die because of the disease. This leads to a lack of consensus on the optimal management of early-stage disease and to questions regarding the cost-effectiveness of a national screening effort for all men older than 50 years. Two large randomized studies recently questioned the utility of screening for prostate cancer. The Prostate, Lung, Colorectal, and Ovarian Cancer Screening Trial (PLCO, 2009) compared one group of men that underwent prostate-specific antigen (PSA) screening with another group that did not undergo screening, and found no difference in mortality rates from prostate cancer. However, almost 44% of the patients in both arms of this trial underwent PSA testing prior to enrollment in the trial. On the other hand, the European Randomized Study of Screening for Prostate Cancer (ERSPC, 2009) reported that screening with PSA resulted in a 20% reduction in the rate of death from prostate cancer, but was associated with a high risk of overdiagnosis. Currently, the American Urological Association recommends that men with a life expectancy of at least 10 years undergo baseline PSA testing and DRE starting at the age of 40 years; and the American Cancer Society recommends discussing screening with patients and offering a DRE and measurement of

PSA starting at the age of 50 years for men with a life expectancy of at least 10 years. Screening should begin at age 45 for African American men or men with one first-degree relative with prostate cancer, and at age 40 for men with even higher risk, such as history of prostate cancer in many first-degree relatives, diagnosed at an early age.

Diagnosis
Patients with low-volume, clinically localized prostate cancer are typically asymptomatic; abnormalities are detected by DRE, increased serum PSA level, or both. Advanced prostate cancer can be asymptomatic; present as local symptoms of urinary hesitancy, frequency, and urgency; or present as systemic symptoms of weight loss, fatigue, and bone pain. Rarely, neurologic sequelae of impending spinal cord compression secondary to bone metastasis or uremia secondary to bilateral ureteral or urethral obstruction can be found in the presentation of advanced cases.

PSA is a serine protease produced by the epithelium of the prostate. PSA is not specific for prostate cancer and can be increased in benign conditions of the prostate such as prostatitis, prostatic infarction, and benign prostatic hyperplasia. Traditionally, a PSA threshold of 4 ng/mL was used as a trigger to perform biopsy. This PSA threshold has been lowered recently to 2.5 ng/mL, although the risk of cancer is also dependent on age, prostate volume, and PSA velocity. In fact, prostate cancer can be found in 6.6% of men with PSA <0.5 ng/mL, 10.1% of men with PSA 0.6 to 1.0 ng/mL, 17% of men with PSA 1.1 to 2.0 ng/mL, 23.9% of men with PSA 2.1 to 3.0 ng/mL, and 26.9% of men with PSA 3.1 to 4.0 ng/mL. It can also be increased as a consequence of recent ejaculation, and patients should be counseled to abstain from sexual activity for periods of up to 1 week prior to PSA screening. Transurethral resection of the prostate (TURP) and prostatic needle biopsy significantly increase the serum PSA level above baseline for up to 8 weeks. DRE (without prostate massage), cystoscopy, and transrectal ultrasound (TRUS) do not alter serum PSA to a clinically significant degree. The positive predictive value of a PSA level greater than 4 ng/mL for the detection of prostate cancer is 34.4%, while the positive predictive value for an abnormal DRE is 21.4%. Detection rates demonstrate that DRE and PSA together (5.8%) are superior to either DRE (3.2%) or PSA (4.6%) alone. Free PSA is a form of PSA not conjugated to protease inhibitors in the serum. Decreased percentage-free PSA (<25%) is associated with prostate cancer, and measurement of free PSA is performed to improve the specificity of PSA testing in the range of 4 to 10 ng/mL and thus eliminate unnecessary biopsies. The primary utility of free PSA is in the patients with a PSA in the 4 to 10 ng/mL range with a history of previously negative prostatic biopsies. In this clinical scenario, the free to total PSA ratio, or alternatively, complexed PSA, can be used to determine the need for repeat biopsies with continued elevation of the serum PSA. A low free to total PSA ratio (<20%) is an indication to repeat TRUS and biopsies of the prostate to rule out the presence of carcinoma.

TRUS is performed using real-time imaging with a 7-MHz transducer, which allows both transverse and sagittal imaging of the prostate gland. Prostate cancer can appear as a hypoechoic region within the prostate, although most experts agree that this is a nonspecific finding. TRUS can also be used to measure the dimensions of the prostate gland to calculate the glandular volume.

Pelvic lymphatic metastases can be detected by computed tomography (CT) or magnetic resonance imaging (MRI). The risk of pelvic nodal metastasis depends on tumor grade, clinical stage, and PSA level. Nomograms incorporating these three factors have been developed to predict the risk of nodal metastasis. However, the only definitive method for staging pelvic lymph nodes is a pelvic lymphadenectomy.

Radionuclide bone scan remains the most sensitive test to detect skeletal metastases. However, in 1993, Oesterling found the yield of a bone scan was 2% if a patient has a PSA level less than 20 ng/mL and evidence of skeletal metastasis, while no patients had a positive bone scan with a PSA less than 8 ng/mL. Therefore, based on this data, radionuclide bone scans are not necessary for staging prostate cancer patients who have a low serum PSA level (<10 ng/mL) and no skeletal symptoms, particularly in cases of low-grade cancers. When bone metastases are present, 80% are osteoblastic, 15% are mixed osteoblastic–osteolytic, and 5% are osteolytic. A chest radiograph is performed to detect the presence of pulmonary metastases, which are extremely rare.

The diagnosis of prostate cancer is made by the histologic finding of prostate cancer in a prostatic biopsy, in tissue obtained from prostatectomy for benign disease, or in the biopsy of a suspicious metastatic focus. In the past, sextant biopsies of the prostate were considered adequate in the patient with an elevated PSA, with site-specific biopsies directed at palpable or ultrasonographic abnormalities (hypoechoic regions). More recent data based on whole mount step sectioning of radical prostatectomy specimens suggest that sextant biopsies are inadequate, in favor of 12 core strategies that focus on the peripheral zone, but also include the anterior horns of the prostate and the transition zone bilaterally. Adenocarcinoma is the predominant cell type of prostate cancer and is the only type discussed in this chapter.

Grading and Staging

The Gleason grading system is the most widely used grading system. It recognizes five histologic patterns of prostate cancer, graded on a scale of 1 to 5, from most to least differentiated. The Gleason score is arrived at through the addition of the predominant and secondary grade patterns to yield a range of tumor Gleason scores from 2 to 10, with most prostate cancers falling in the Gleason 5 to 10 range. Prostate cancer is well known to be multifocal in nature, so not uncommonly, multiple biopsies from a prostate may be positive, each with a reported Gleason score. The biology of the cancer is frequently dictated by the most aggressive variant found in the prostate.

The biological behavior of the tumor can be further categorized by stage, which accounts for tumor volume and location. Prostate cancer typically spreads to the pelvic lymph nodes, bone, and lungs. The 2010 American Joint Committee on Cancer prostate cancer staging is shown in Table 18.1.

Management of Early Disease

In 1987, the National Cancer Institute published a consensus statement on the treatment of early-stage prostate cancer. The report concluded: "Radical prostatectomy and radiation therapy are clearly effective forms of treatment in the attempt to cure tumors limited to the prostate for appropriately selected patients. . . . What remains unclear is the relative merit of each in producing lifelong freedom from cancer recurrence. . . . Properly designed and completed randomized trials that evaluate both disease control and quality of life after modern radiation therapy compared with radical prostatectomy are essential." These criteria have yet to be fulfilled and probably never will; however, there appears to be little difference in clinical and biochemical outcomes between the two modalities when similar patient groups are compared.

Active Surveillance

As many prostate cancers are detected early, when PSA is still less than 10 ng/mL and Gleason scores are 6 or 7, active surveillance has emerged as a novel strategy for the management of this class of prostate cancers. In 2005, Bill-Axelson et al. prospectively compared surveillance with radical prostatectomy in patients with PSA <50 and clinical stage T2 or less, and found that patients who underwent radical prostatectomy were less likely to develop metastases (15% vs. 25%) and less

Staging Systems for Prostate Cancer

Primary Tumor Clinical (T)

TX	Primary tumor cannot be assessed
T0	No evidence of primary tumor
T1	Clinically inapparent tumor not palpable or visible by imaging
	T1a: Tumor incidental histologic finding in 5% or less of tissue resected
	T1b: Tumor incidental histologic finding in more than 5% of tissue resected
	T1c: Tumor identified by needle biopsy because of increased PSA
T2	Tumor confined within the prostate gland
	T2a: Tumor involves one-half of one lobe or less
	T2b: Tumor involves more than one-half of one lobe, but not both lobes
	T2c: Tumor involves both lobes
T3	Tumor extends through the prostate capsule
	T3a: Extracapsular extension (unilateral or bilateral)
	T3b: Seminal vesicle invasion
T4	Tumor is fixed or invades the bladder, rectum, external sphincter, levator muscles, or pelvic side wall

Regional Lymph Nodes (N)

NX	Regional lymph nodes cannot be assessed
N0	No regional lymph node metastasis
N1	Metastasis in regional lymph node or nodes

Distant Metastases (M)

MX	Distant metastasis cannot be assessed
M0	No distant metastasis
M1	Distant metastasis
	M1a: Nonregional lymph nodes
	M1b: Bone(s)
	M1c: Other site(s)

Prostate Cancer-Anatomic Stage/Prognostic Groups

Group	T	N	M	PSA	Gleason
I	T1a–T2a	N0	M0	<10	≤6
	T1a–T2a	N0	M0	X	X
IIA	T1	N0	M0	<20	7
	T1	N0	M0	≥10 <20	≤6
	T2a–T2b	N0	M0	<20	≤7
	T2b	N0	M0	X	X
IIB	T2c	N0	M0	Any	Any
	T1–T2	N0	M0	≥20	Any
	T1–T2	N0	M0	Any	≥8
III	T3a–T3b	N0	M0	Any	Any
IV	T4	N0	M0	Any	Any
	Any T	N1	M0	Any	Any
	Any T	Any N	M1	Any	Any

PSA, prostate-specific antigen.

likely to die of prostate cancer (10% vs. 15%). This reduction in prostate cancer deaths was most significant in patients younger than 65 years of age. Klotz et al. recently reported on 450 patients with low-risk prostate cancer that underwent active surveillance. During follow-up, 30% of patients were classified as high risk and 117 underwent radical therapy, of whom 50% experienced treatment failure. Patients with a fast PSA doubling time (less than 3 years) were at a higher risk of treatment failure. Overall survival was 78%, while 10-year actuarial prostate cancer-specific survival was 97%, indicating that most deaths resulted from causes other than prostate cancer. The PIVOT trial (Prostate Cancer Intervention Versus Observation Trial) is a more contemporary trial in progress comparing active surveillance with radical prostatectomy.

Cryotherapy
Prostate cryotherapy has been used since 1996. The current third-generation cryotherapy uses high-quality transrectal ultrasound guidance, argon-based freezing system, multisensor temperature probes, and urethral warming device. These features give urologists excellent control of ice ball formation during cryotherapy. Cryotherapy is typically reserved for early stage and low-grade disease. Large contemporary series have shown a 5-year disease-free survival rate of 77% for primary cryotherapy. The main side effect of whole-gland cryotherapy is that it results in 100% impotence rate. Focal cryotherapy has been investigated as an alternative, but is not widely accepted at present. The main use of cryotherapy though is in patients who have local prostate recurrence after radiation therapy (so called salvage cryotherapy for radiorecurrent prostate cancer). In this patient population, the 5-year disease-free survival rate decreases to 58.9%.

Surgery
The surgical excision of prostate cancer by complete removal of the prostate gland, seminal vesicles, and ampullae of the vasa deferentia was first performed in the early 1900s. This procedure, known as a *radical prostatectomy*, can be performed using a perineal or retropubic approach. Newer, minimally invasive surgical techniques such as laparoscopic radical prostatectomy and robot-assisted laparoscopic prostatectomy are now becoming more mainstream, with similar oncologic and functional outcomes (continence and erectile function), but less blood loss, narcotic and transfusion requirements, and shorter hospital stays compared to open techniques. Zincke et al. reported their experience with radical prostatectomy in 1,143 patients with 10- and 15-year cause-specific survival rates of 90% and 83% and metastasis-free survival of 83% and 77%, respectively. Complication rates are low. Mortality is less than 0.7% and the incidence of severe incontinence is 1.4%. In 1992, Leandri et al. reported on 620 patients and found a 6.9% early complication rate, 1.3% late complication rate, and 0.2% mortality rate. Sexual potency was maintained in 71% in whom a nerve-sparing technique was used, and 5% experienced stress incontinence after 1 year. Factors that predict for postoperative potency include preoperative erectile function, patient age, and number of cavernosal nerve fibers spared. Factors that influence continence results include nerve sparing, patient age, and obesity.

Radiation Therapy
Brachytherapy and external-beam radiation therapy are used for the definitive treatment of localized prostatic adenocarcinoma. Permanent brachytherapy typically uses Palladium-103 (doses of 125 Gy) or Iodine-125 (doses of 145 Gy) and is mainly reserved for patients with small prostates and low-risk prostate cancer (PSA <10, Gleason 6 or less, and clinical stage T2a or less). For patients with intermediate or high-risk prostate cancer, brachytherapy should not be given as single-modality

therapy, and needs to be combined with external beam radiotherapy. Intensity modulated radiation therapy (IMRT) is currently used to decrease adverse local side effects of radiation therapy and increase total dosage to the prostate, and is the external beam radiotherapeutic modality of choice due to improved prostate targeting and side effect profile compared to previous generation radiotherapy. For low-risk patients, IMRT is used alone at doses of up to 75 Gy, while for patients with intermediate or high-risk disease, doses up to 80 Gy are given, and are combined with androgen deprivation therapy. At the M. D. Anderson Cancer Center, we recommend radical prostatectomy for the treatment of early-stage prostate cancer in the patient with minimal comorbidities, less than 70 years of age. Primary radiation therapy is reserved for patients with significant comorbid medical illnesses or patients older than 70 years of age.

Management of Locally Advanced Prostate Cancer/Lymph Node Metastasis

Locally advanced prostate cancer involves areas outside the prostatic capsule, such as fat, seminal vesicles, levator muscles, or other adjacent structures. Locally advanced prostate cancer is associated with a 53% incidence of lymph node metastases and decreased overall survival rate compared with early-stage disease. Locally advanced disease with or without lymph node metastasis can be treated with primary radiation therapy and androgen ablation with a 6-year biochemical failure rate of 13%, but longer follow-up is still needed. These patients with locally advanced disease at high risk for relapse are frequently enrolled in clinical protocols that use neoadjuvant systemic therapy in combination with surgical extirpation of the prostate followed by adjuvant radiotherapy to improve patient outcome. Our experience at the M. D. Anderson Cancer Center with locally advanced disease treated with primary radiation therapy demonstrated 5-, 10-, and 15-year uncorrected actuarial survival rates of 72%, 47%, and 17%, respectively. The local control rate was 75% at 15 years of follow-up.

Treatment modalities other than radiation therapy used for locally advanced disease include radical prostatectomy, TURP, and hormonal therapy. Tumor grade, stage, bulk of tumor, and seminal vesicle involvement in locally advanced disease are associated with a decreased interval between radical prostatectomy and disease progression. The actuarial 5-year survival rate for patients with locally advanced disease who have undergone TURP is 64%, making TURP an option for patients with short life expectancies who have significant local symptoms associated with their prostate cancer such as urinary obstruction or intractable hematuria. This strategy may be ideal in the elderly and in those with serious coexisting medical problems.

Metastatic Prostate Cancer

Patients with metastatic prostate cancer have a median survival duration of 30 months, with an estimated 5-year survival rate of 20%. The first-line treatment of metastatic prostate cancer is androgen ablation therapy. Trials examining the role of chemotherapy in combination with androgen ablative therapy have not, as yet, demonstrated an additional benefit with regard to progression-free or overall survival when compared with androgen ablation alone. The hypothalamus produces luteinizing hormone-releasing hormone (LHRH) and corticotropin-releasing factor, which stimulate the anterior pituitary gland to release adrenocorticotropic hormone (ACTH) and luteinizing hormone (LH). LH stimulates testosterone production by the testes, and ACTH stimulates the adrenal glands to produce androstenedione and dehydroepiandrosterone, precursors of testosterone and DHT. Although the testes are the major source of testosterone, the adrenal glands can supply up to 20% of the DHT found in the prostate gland.

Androgen ablation therapy consists of either bilateral orchiectomy or LHRH agonists, which chronically stimulate the pituitary gland, resulting in a decrease in LH release. Direct LHRH antagonists are now also available, but they have not gained widespread acceptance over the agonists that have a more extensive clinical background. Decrease in LH leads to castrate levels of testosterone production by the testes, defined typically as less than 50 ng/mL. Several oral antiandrogens exist that work by blocking uptake or binding of androgen in target tissues. Combination of antiandrogens with either surgical or medical androgen ablation is termed combined androgen blockade.

Bilateral orchiectomy and LHRH agonists appear to have equal efficacy when used as monotherapy for metastatic prostate cancer. The Medical Research Council of the United Kingdom performed a randomized prospective trial with 934 patients and found that immediate androgen ablation delays disease progression and decreases pathological fractures. We recommend immediate androgen ablation for select patients. Combined androgen blockade with an LHRH agonist plus an antiandrogen is controversial. Many studies have shown no benefit to combined therapy with an antiandrogen versus LHRH agonist monotherapy. Intermittent androgen therapy has been demonstrated to improve quality of life, but its long-term effects on survival are unknown. Androgen ablation, although useful as first-line therapy in patients with metastatic prostate cancer, has been shown to increase the risk of osteoporosis, metabolic syndrome and cardiovascular disease. The median time to castration-resistant state for patients with metastatic prostate cancer treated with hormonal therapy is approximately 2 years. The median survival of patients with hormone refractory disease is on the order of 12 to 18 months. Chemotherapeutic regimens are the mainstay of therapy for hormone refractory prostate cancer with taxane-based regimens showing significant activity that includes decreases in PSA, improved quality of life, objective disease regression, and prolonged survival. Second-line chemotherapeutic regimens have recently emerged, such as satraplatin, a third-generation oral platinum compound that has been shown to delay progression of disease and pain without significantly improving overall survival; and sipuleucel, an intravenous immunotherapeutic agent that decreased overall mortality by 33% compared to placebo. In addition to antineoplastic therapy, patients with metastatic prostate cancer typically receive bone-protecting agents (such as the bisphosphonate zoledronic acid), especially when hormone ablation is instituted. Clinical trials continue to be the main and best treatment option for patients; however, some treatment options (primarily taxane-based chemotherapy regimens) now exist that demonstrate objective benefit where none existed previously. Clinical research is now focused on the efficacy of targeted therapies that act on specific molecular pathways involved in metastatic progression in the management of hormone refractory disease. Two promising therapies are currently under intense investigation: abiraterone acetate, a steroidal antiandrogen that inhibits CYP17A1 to reduce testosterone production; and MDV3100, an antiandrogen that blocks testosterone binding to the androgen receptor and interferes with its nuclear translocation and binding to DNA.

BLADDER CANCER

Epidemiology and Etiology

Bladder cancer is the second most common genitourinary malignancy in the United States. It is the fourth most common cancer in men and the tenth most common cancer in women. In 2009, almost 71,000 new cases were reported, and approximately 14,000 deaths were attributed to bladder cancer. The lifetime probability of developing bladder cancer is 1 in 27 in males and 1 in 84 in females, and is lower for African Americans compared to whites.

The etiology of bladder cancer, of which urothelial (or transitional cell) carcinoma is the most common, is well established. Cigarette smoking has been linked to 30% to 40% of all cases of bladder cancer. The chemicals 1-naphthylamine, 2-naphthylamine, benzidine, and 4-aminobiphenyl have been shown to promote urothelial carcinogenesis. Workers in the textile, leather, aluminum refining, rubber, and chemical industries who are exposed to high levels of these chemicals have an increased incidence of bladder cancer. Other chemicals that have been linked to urothelial cancer are MBUCCA (plastics industry), phenacetin, and the antineoplastic agent cyclophosphamide. In addition, recurrent bladder infections, as well as infections with the parasite *Schistosoma haematobium*, have been associated with squamous cell carcinoma of the bladder.

Pathology

The urinary bladder is a hollow viscus that functions in both the storage and the evacuation of urine. Histologically, the bladder is composed of mucosa, lamina propria, muscularis, and serosa (limited to the dome). Localized bladder cancer is classified as *nonmuscle invasive disease*, which is limited to the mucosa and lamina propria, or *muscle invasive disease*, which extends into the muscularis propria and beyond. Approximately 70% of newly diagnosed bladder cancers are superficial, whereas the remaining 30% are invasive. Once a bladder cancer extends through the basal layer of the mucosa, it may invade blood vessels and lymphatics, thereby providing a route of metastasis. Carcinoma in situ, an aggressive form of *nonmuscle invasive* disease, is composed of poorly differentiated cells limited to the mucosal layer.

The World Health Organization (WHO) classifies epithelial tumors of the bladder into four histologic types: urothelial carcinoma (91%), squamous cell carcinoma (7%), adenocarcinoma (2%), and undifferentiated carcinoma (<1%). However, up to 20% of urothelial carcinomas contain areas of squamous differentiation, and up to 7% contain areas of adenomatous differentiation. The remainder of this section discusses urothelial carcinomas.

Clinical Presentation

Eighty percent of all patients who present with bladder carcinoma have gross or microscopic hematuria, typically painless and intermittent. Approximately 20% of patients complain of symptoms of vesical irritability, including urinary frequency, urgency, dysuria, and stranguria. Other symptoms include pelvic pain, flank pain (from ureteral obstruction), and lower-extremity edema. Patients with systemic disease may present with anemia, weight loss, and bone pain.

Diagnosis

A patient who presents with hematuria or other symptoms of bladder cancer should undergo a thorough urologic evaluation consisting of a history, physical examination, urinalysis, cystoscopic examination of the urinary bladder, voided urine for cytologic examination, and intravenous contrast-enhanced CT scan of the abdomen and pelvis. The most useful of these steps is the direct visual examination of the bladder using a flexible cystoscope in the office. Papillary and sessile tumors are easily visualized through the cystoscope; carcinoma in situ, however, can appear as normal mucosa or as erythematous patches throughout the bladder. Fewer than 60% of bladder tumors can be seen on a CT scan, but this examination is obtained primarily to identify other abnormalities that may be present in the upper genitourinary tract (renal tumors, hydronephrosis, etc.) in addition to evaluating the primary bladder tumor, presence of local extension into soft tissues, and presence of regional lymphadenopathy. Urine cytology is reported as positive in ~30% of patients with low-grade tumors, and 65% to 100% of patients with high-grade tumors or carcinoma in situ (see the next section for definition of grades).

Grading and Staging

The WHO grading system, updated in 2002, is based on the cytologic features of the tumor. Low-grade tumors are well differentiated and high-grade tumors are poorly differentiated.

Once a bladder tumor is diagnosed, the urologist must accurately stage the tumor. The initial transurethral resection of the bladder tumor (TURBT), typically done in association with random biopsies of the bladder and prostatic urethra, will determine the histologic depth of invasion of the tumor and the presence or absence of dysplasia or carcinoma in situ. A bimanual examination should be performed at the time of resection to determine whether a mass is present and, if so, whether it is fixed or mobile.

Further workup for detecting metastasis consists of a CT scan, liver function tests, a chest radiograph, and a bone scan (if the alkaline phosphatase level is elevated or the patient's symptoms suggest systemic disease). American Joint Committee on Cancer International Union Against Cancer TNM staging systems are listed in Table 18.2.

Management

Nonmuscle Invasive Bladder Cancer

Approximately two-thirds of bladder cancers present as nonmuscle invasive disease (e.g., Ta, T1, or Tis). An estimated 60% of these cancers are Ta and 30% are T1. Ten percent of all bladder cancers present with Tis or carcinoma in situ (CIS). After the initial treatment of nonmuscle invasive bladder cancer, the cancer can be cured, can recur with the same stage and grade, or can recur with progression of stage or grade. Risk factors associated with both disease recurrence and progression include a high tumor grade, lamina propria invasion, dysplasia elsewhere in the bladder, positive urinary cytology findings, tumor diameter larger than 5 cm, vascular or lymphatic invasion, multicentricity, and expression of either epidermal growth factor or transforming growth factor-alpha. Mutations in the P53 gene may also be associated with a significant risk of disease progression.

Initial treatment of nonmuscle invasive bladder cancer focuses on eradication of the existing disease and prophylaxis against disease recurrence or progression. TURBT has been the standard treatment for existing stage Ta and T1 tumors and visible stage Tis tumors. Laser fulguration is another therapeutic option that results in fewer bleeding complications. The advantage of transurethral resection over laser fulguration is that it provides tissue for histologic examination. Patients with apparently nonmuscle invasive disease at the time of TURBT should receive a single dose of intravesical mitomycin C, if no bladder perforation is evident. This single dose has been shown to decrease the risk of bladder cancer recurrence by about 40%. Patients who have T1 disease should undergo a repeat TURBT 2 to 6 weeks after initial TURBT, as these patients have a 30% risk of being upstaged into T2 disease or higher.

Patients with Tis, high-grade Ta or T1 lesions, multiple tumors, recurrent tumors, tumors larger than 5 cm, or persistently positive cytology findings may be candidates for adjuvant intravesical therapy. Intravesical agents can be used as therapeutic, adjuvant, or prophylactic treatment for bladder cancer. Thiotepa, mitomycin C, and valrubicin are the chemotherapeutic agents used most frequently. Bacille Calmette–Guérin (BCG), a live attenuated tuberculosis organism, has become the most widely used intravesical agent in nonmuscle invasive bladder cancer, either alone or in combination with alpha-interferon. BCG enhances the

	Staging Systems for Bladder Cancer

Primary Tumor Clinical (T)

TX	Primary tumor cannot be assessed
T0	No evidence of primary tumor
Ta	Noninvasive papillary carcinoma
Tis	Carcinoma in situ
T1	Tumor invades subepithelial connective tissue
T2	Tumor invades muscle
	T2a: Tumor invades superficial muscularis propria
	T2b: Tumor invades deep muscularis propria
T3	Tumor invades perivesical tissue
	T3a: Microscopically
	T3b: Macroscopically (extravesical mass)
T4	Invasion of any of the following: prostate stroma, seminal vesicles, uterus, vagina, pelvic wall, or abdominal wall
	T4a: Tumor invades prostate stroma, uterus, or vagina
	T4b: Tumor invades pelvic or abdominal wall

Regional Lymph Nodes (N)

NX	Regional lymph nodes cannot be assessed
N0	No regional lymph node metastasis
N1	Metastasis in a single regional lymph node in the true pelvis
N2	Metastasis in multiple regional lymph nodes in the true pelvis
N3	Metastasis in a common iliac node

Distant Metastases (M)

MX	Distant metastasis cannot be assessed
M0	No distant metastasis
M1	Distant metastasis

Bladder Cancer-Anatomic Stage/Prognostic Groups

Group	T	N	M
0a	Ta	N0	M0
0is	Tis	N0	M0
I	T1	N0	M0
II	T2	N0	M0
III	T3–T4a	N0	M0
IV	T4b	N0	M0
	Any T	N1–N3	M0
	Any T	Any N	M1

patient's own immune response against the tumor, providing resistance to disease recurrence thereby potentially delaying progression. BCG is typically started 4 to 6 weeks after TURBT, as starting BCG too soon after TURBT (before urothelial healing occurs) may result in BCG sepsis. Although specific dose scheduling varies, most treatment regimens include intravesical treatment weekly for 6 weeks, followed by an optional series of maintenance treatments administered over many months. BCG has been shown to eliminate CIS in 80% of patients at a 5-year follow-up, reduce tumor recurrence rate for patients with T1 disease to 30% at 4 years, and eliminate residual tumor in up to 59% of patients. Maintenance therapy regimens with BCG appear to offer the best outcomes for patients. In 2000, Lamm et al.

randomized 384 patients with superficial bladder cancer to receive induction and maintenance BCG or just induction BCG therapy only. Median recurrence-free survival time was longer for those who received induction and maintenance therapy; however, at 5-year follow-up there was no difference in survival. In 2002, Sylvester et al. performed a meta-analysis of 24 clinical trials and found that only patients who received maintenance BCG after TURBT had a decreased risk of progression into muscle invasive disease.

There is good evidence that T1 high-grade cancer has a high rate of progression and therefore confers a high risk of death. Therefore, we recommend early radical cystectomy (before developing muscle invasion) for select patients with high-grade T1 bladder cancer. Furthermore, we also recommend cystectomy for patients who recur despite an adequate trial of BCG therapy because these patients have been shown to be at high risk for disease progression if their bladder remains in situ.

Invasive Bladder Cancer

Tumors that have penetrated the muscularis propria are considered invasive. Several options are available for treatment of patients with invasive tumors. A small subset of patients may be eligible for bladder-sparing therapy. In 2001, Herr demonstrated a 76% overall survival rate, with 57% of the patients preserving their bladders in 45 patients treated with aggressive transurethral re-resection of invasive bladder tumors (median follow-up: 61 months). Patients with a muscle-invasive tumor that is primary and solitary, does not have surrounding urothelial atypia, and allows for a 2-cm surgical margin may be candidates for partial cystectomy. At the M. D. Anderson Cancer Center, data have shown that approximately 5% of patients are actually suitable for bladder-sparing surgery; 5-year survival rates have been comparable to those achieved with radical cystectomy, when negative margins of resection can be achieved.

Primary external-beam radiation therapy has been used to treat invasive bladder cancer. Treatment protocols advocate doses of 65 to 70 Gy. Five-year survival rates range from 21% to 52% for stage B2 and from 18% to 30% for stage C. Local recurrence occurs in 50% to 70% of these patients. Stage T4 lesions fare worse, with 5-year survival rates consistently less than 10%. Our experience at the M. D. Anderson Cancer Center found a 26% 5-year survival rate with primary external-beam radiation. Thus, external-beam radiation therapy may be useful in patients who do not want to have surgery or for whom radical surgery is medically contraindicated; however, the results with radiation therapy, stage for stage, are significantly worse than those seen with radical surgery.

In an attempt to improve survival and bladder preservation rates, multimodality strategies have combined TURBT, chemotherapy, and radiation. In 1997, Kachnic et al. from Massachusetts General Hospital reported on 106 patients with stages T2 to T4 bladder cancers who were treated with TURBT, two cycles of methotrexate, cisplatin, vinblastine (MCV), and 40 Gy radiation therapy plus concurrent cisplatin. Overall 5-year survival was 52%, and overall 5-year survival rate with the bladder intact was 43%. These results are comparable to contemporary radical cystectomy series; however, this regimen involves significant morbidity and patient investment in complex treatment schedules. Moreover, patients are subjected to a considerable risk of eventual cystectomy and superficial bladder cancer recurrence.

Radical cystectomy with pelvic lymphadenectomy is performed with the intent of removing all localized and lymphatic disease. There is evidence that an extended pelvic lymphadenectomy (starting cranially from the inferior mesenteric artery takeoff) improves detection of nodal metastasis and could have a therapeutic benefit, especially in patients with minimal nodal disease. In 2001, Stein et al. reported on 1,054 patients who were treated with open radical cystectomy and pelvic lymphadenectomy at a single institution. Perioperative mortality was 2.5% and 28% experienced early complications postoperatively. Ten-year recurrence-free survival in node-negative patients was 86% for pT0, 89% for pTcis, 74% for pTa, 78% for pT1, 87% for pT2, 76% for pT3a, 61% for pT3b, and 45% for pT4. Twenty-four percent of all patients had positive lymph nodes, with a corresponding 10-year recurrence-free survival of 34%. Median time to recurrence in this patient cohort was 12 months (22% of patients had distant recurrence, and 7% had a local pelvic recurrence). In recent years, several centers have started using laparoscopic and robotic-assisted laparoscopic radical cystectomy with extracorporeal urinary diversion. However, long-term oncologic efficacy for these procedures cannot be evaluated yet due to short follow-up.

Once a patient undergoes cystectomy, the ureters must be diverted into an alternate drainage system. The most common urinary diversion used today is the orthotopic urinary diversion with an ileal segment used for bladder substitution. Patients who are unable to undergo an orthotopic diversion include patients with elevated serum creatinine, evidence of lymph node metastasis, prostatic urethral invasive urothelial carcinoma or CIS, or inflammatory bowel disease. Furthermore, these patients must be willing and able to undergo a vigorous voiding re-education program. Radiation therapy may render continence difficult; therefore, some patients may not benefit from this type of diversion. Catheterizable cutaneous reservoirs are also used as methods of urinary diversion in selected patients. In the end, if a patient is unable to meet these criteria, then a cutaneous ileal conduit is recommended.

Grossman et al. conducted a phase III randomized trial comparing radical cystectomy alone with neoadjuvant chemotherapy followed by radical cystectomy and reported a 33% decrease in the estimated risk of death for the latter approach. At the M. D. Anderson Cancer Center, adjuvant chemotherapy is used for select patients with unfavorable disease characteristics, which include resected nodal metastases, extravesical involvement, lymphovascular invasion, or involvement of pelvic viscera. Previously, treatment with adjuvant chemotherapy in select patients at the M. D. Anderson Cancer Center resulted in a 70% 5-year survival rate, which is comparable to patients without unfavorable features. Currently, several targeted therapies are being investigated in the neoadjuvant and metastatic setting.

Metastatic Disease
Cisplatin appears to be the agent with the greatest activity against urothelial carcinoma of the bladder; however, single-agent therapy response rates are only in the range of 10% to 30%. Traditionally, chemotherapy for bladder cancer included cisplatin, methotrexate, vinblastine, and doxorubicin (M-VAC). In the M. D. Anderson Cancer Center trial of M-VAC, a complete response rate of 35% and a partial response rate of 30% were observed. Other trials have documented similar response rates, with median a survival of approximately 1 year. Newer regimens using gemcitabine and cisplatin have demonstrated no significant difference in survival when compared with M-VAC, but adverse side effects and toxicity are decreased with the newer regimen, which is now used most commonly in this setting.

RENAL CANCER
Epidemiology and Etiology
Tumors of the renal and perirenal tissues comprise 3% of cancer incidence and mortality in the United States. Renal cell carcinoma (RCC) represents 85% of all renal parenchymal tumors and is the only renal tumor discussed in this chapter. In 2009, an estimated 57,000 people were diagnosed with malignancies of the kidney and renal pelvis, and close to 13,000 people died of this disease. From 1975 to 1995,

both the incidence and mortality rates of RCC have increased. The upward trend in mortality rates suggests that the increased incidental diagnosis of early-stage asymptomatic tumors does not fully account for the overall increase in incidence. This rise in incidence is seen more significantly in African Americans. Males are affected twice as often as females. RCC most frequently occurs in the fifth to sixth decades of life.

Several risk factors have been identified to be associated with RCC. Case–control studies have found strong correlations with smoking and obesity. Hypertension, diabetes mellitus, and diuretic use have also been found to be associated with RCC; however, it is unclear whether this is a causal relationship. RCC can occur either sporadically or genetically. Hereditary RCC tends to occur at an earlier age of onset and tends to be bilateral and multifocal. A well-described familial syndrome is von Hippel-Lindau (VHL) disease, which is characterized by cerebellar hemangioblastoma, retinal angiomata, bilateral clear cell RCC, and islet cell tumors of the pancreas. Both sporadic and VHL disease types have a common genetic mechanism that includes loss of a region of chromosome 3. Approximately 70% of clear cell renal cell carcinomas are believed to have loss of the VHL gene either through mutation, deletion, or silencing by methylation. Hereditary papillary RCC (papillary type 1) is an autosomal dominant syndrome associated with abnormalities of the *met* gene on chromosome 7. Other genetic RCC syndromes include Hereditary Leiomyomatosis and Renal Cell Cancer (papillary type 2) associated with mutations in the Krebs cycle enzyme fumarate hydratase, and Birt–Hogg–Dube syndrome, which manifests as bilateral multifocal tumors with both chromophobe RCC and oncocytoma histology. RCC is also associated with polycystic kidney disease, tuberous sclerosis, "horseshoe kidneys," and acquired renal cystic disease.

Pathology

Clear cell histology is the most common RCC subtype. Most RCCs originate in the proximal tubular cells of the kidney. The tumor is multifocal in 6.5% to 10% of cases, more commonly with papillary histology. The renal capsule and Gerota's fascia surrounding the kidney typically limit local extension of the tumor. The predominant cell type is clear cell, but granular and spindle-shaped cells also may be present. The tumor cells are typically rich in glycogen and lipid, giving the tumor a clear cell appearance microscopically and a characteristic yellow appearance grossly. Less common pathologies include papillary and chromophobe RCC. Unclassified RCC is a waste basket classification for tumors that do not fit the criteria of the classically described histologies. Sarcomatoid differentiation, once believed to be a separate histologic classification, is now recognized as a dedifferentiation pathway that can occur with any histology, including clear cell, papillary, and chromophobe. Oncocytoma is a benign tumor with no malignant potential that can be problematic to differentiate from chromophobe renal cell carcinoma on needle biopsy.

Clinical Presentation

RCC was traditionally called the "internist's tumor" because of its subtle presentation. Now more than 40% of clinically unsuspected tumors are found incidentally by abdominal imaging done for other reasons. Gross or microscopic hematuria, the most common presenting symptom, is present in more than half of patients with RCC. The classic "too late" triad of hematuria, abdominal mass, and flank pain occurs in approximately 19% of patients. Paraneoplastic syndromes occur in 10% to 40% of cases and consist of pyrexia, anemia, erythrocytosis, hypercalcemia, liver dysfunction (Stauffer syndrome), and hypertension. Other common symptoms include bone pain and central nervous system abnormalities, due to the fact that up to 30% of patients present with bone and brain metastases.

Diagnosis

The workup of a patient with the preceding symptoms should include a history, physical examination, complete blood cell count, serum chemistry panel (including alkaline phosphatase and liver function tests), urinalysis, urine culture, and a contrast-enhanced CT scan. In most cases, the CT scan will define the nature of the mass. If any of the studies obtained suggests involvement of the renal vein or vena cava, an MRI or CT scan with three-dimensional reconstruction should be obtained to assess the extent of the tumor thrombus. In contrast to the management of other renal tumors, RCC may be treated surgically without preoperative histologic diagnosis of the tumor. Biopsy of a renal mass is rarely indicated unless the radiographic characteristics of the mass suggest an etiology other than RCC, such as an abscess, lymphoma, urothelial carcinoma, or a metastasis from another malignant primary.

If a mass suggests RCC, a metastatic workup consisting of a chest radiograph, CT scan (if not already obtained), and liver function tests should be performed. The most common sites of metastases of RCC in decreasing order are the lung, bone, and regional lymph nodes. If the patient does not have an increased alkaline phosphatase level or skeletal pain, a bone scan is usually not required. A CT scan of the brain can be performed if there is any suspicion of brain metastases; however, this is not done routinely in the absence of symptoms referable to the CNS.

Grading and Staging

The most widely used grading system for RCC is the Fuhrman system, which is based on nuclear and nucleolar morphology, rated on a scale of 1 to 4.

The TNM system is the most commonly used for staging in the United States (see Table 18.3).

Management

Localized Renal Cell Carcinoma

To date, surgical excision remains the only proven effective treatment of localized RCC. In a radical nephrectomy, the kidney, ipsilateral adrenal gland, and surrounding Gerota's fascia are all resected en bloc. Although no randomized study has proved its benefit over simple nephrectomy, radical nephrectomy has the theoretical advantage of removing the lymphatics within the perinephric fat. Up to 20% of patients can have evidence of regional lymphatic metastases without distant disease, although the incidence of occult nodal involvement is in the range of 3% to 5%. The 5-year survival rates for patients with positive lymph nodes range from 8% to 35%; however, patients with papillary histology and node metastases that undergo aggressive surgical resection can enjoy an extended progression-free and overall survival, in contrast to those patients with nodal metastases from clear cell histology. Extended lymphadenectomy has never been proven to be of benefit in patients who undergo radical nephrectomy, except in the presence of clinically positive lymph nodes, and many surgeons prefer a limited node dissection, which has limited morbidity, for prognostic information. There is clear data that all evidence of gross disease should be removed, if feasible, at the time of nephrectomy.

The surgical approach to radical nephrectomy is determined by the size and location of the tumor and the surgeon's preference. A modified flank, midline, or subcostal (chevron) incision can be used. Large upper-pole tumors may be approached through a thoracoabdominal incision for greater exposure. Because the incidence of ipsilateral adrenal metastasis in lower-pole tumors is rare, not removing the adrenal gland at the time of nephrectomy for a lower-pole lesion is acceptable.

Approximately 15% to 20% of RCCs invade the renal vein, and 8% to 15% invade the vena cava. RCC invasion of the renal vein usually does not pose a

TABLE 18.3 Staging Systems for Renal Cell Cancer

Primary Tumor Clinical (T)

TX	Primary tumor cannot be assessed
T0	No evidence of primary tumor
T1	Tumor 7 cm or less in greatest dimension, limited to the kidney
	T1a: Tumor ≤4 cm, confined to kidney
	T1b: Tumor >4 cm, ≤7 cm, confined to kidney
T2	Tumor >7 cm in greatest dimension, confined to the kidney
	T2a: Tumor >7 cm, ≤10 cm, confined to kidney
	T2b: Tumor >10 cm, confined to kidney
T3	Tumor extends into major veins or perinephric tissues but not into the ipsilateral adrenal gland and not beyond Gerota's fascia
	T3a: Tumor grossly extends into the renal vein or its segmental (muscle containing) branches, or tumor invades perirenal and/or renal sinus fat but not beyond Gerota's fascia
	T3b: Tumor grossly extends into the vena cava below diaphragm
	T3c: Tumor grossly extends into the vena cava above diaphragm or invades the wall of the vena cava
T4	Tumor invades beyond Gerota's fascia (including contiguous extension into the ipsilateral adrenal gland)

Regional Lymph Nodes (N)

NX	Regional lymph nodes cannot be assessed
N0	No regional lymph node metastasis
N1	Metastasis in regional lymph node(s)

Distant Metastases (M)

MX	Distant metastasis cannot be assessed
M0	No distant metastasis
M1	Distant metastasis

Kidney Cancer-Anatomic Stage/Prognostic Groups

Group	T	N	M
I	T1	N0	M0
II	T2	N0	M0
III	T1–T2	N1	M0
	T3	N0–N1	M0
IV	T4	Any N	M0
	Any T	Any N	M1

significant surgical problem. Vena caval involvement, however, may require additional extensive procedures to completely excise the tumor. Vena caval thrombi have been divided by many authors into three groups. Type 1 thrombi (50%) are completely infrahepatic, type 2 (40%) are intrahepatic, and type 3 (10%) extend up into the right atrium of the heart. In cases with vena caval involvement, it is imperative that the surgeon be familiar with techniques of vascular surgery, and consideration should be given to consulting with a cardiothoracic surgeon, especially for type 3 thrombi. Cardiopulmonary bypass, deep hypothermic arrest, and venovenous bypass have been used in the resection of these locally advanced tumors that extend to the suprahepatic vena cava.

There are situations in which nephron-sparing surgery is indicated for patients with RCC. For example, in cases of tumors smaller than 4 cm, bilateral tumor involvement, renal insufficiency, solitary kidney, or VHL, a parenchyma-sparing procedure may be indicated. In this procedure, the renal artery is temporarily occluded, the kidney cooled down, and a partial nephrectomy or wedge resection performed. Frozen sections of the surgical margins are typically analyzed to ensure adequacy of resection. After restoration of arterial blood flow, the renal capsule is closed or, alternatively, perirenal fat or biodegradable hemostatic material is sutured to the defect to promote healing and hemostasis. Five-year survival rates after partial nephrectomy for patients with stage I or II disease are approximately 90% and 70%, respectively. Most urologic oncologists agree that partial nephrectomy has demonstrated oncologic equipoise with radical nephrectomy in patients with anatomically favorable tumors, even those greater than 4 cm.

Currently, partial nephrectomy constitutes the standard of care for patients with localized renal tumors less than 4 cm in size. Nephron-sparing surgery and radical nephrectomy provide equally effective curative treatments for single, small, well-localized tumors; partial nephrectomy yields 5-year cancer-specific survival rates of 92% to 97%. The incidence of tumor recurrence within the renal remnant is reported to be from 0% to 6%. Recent data also demonstrate that performing partial nephrectomy on anatomically favorable tumors between 4 and 7 cm is feasible, and when carefully performed in centers of excellence, cancer-specific survival is equivalent to those treated with radical nephrectomy. More importantly, several investigators have recently reported that radical nephrectomy is associated with a higher rate of cardiovascular complications, chronic kidney disease, noncancer mortality, and overall mortality when compared to partial nephrectomy, emphasizing the role of nephron preserving surgery whenever feasible.

More recent advances in the surgical therapy of localized RCC have focused on minimally invasive strategies. Laparoscopic radical nephrectomy, performed either through standard or hand-assisted approaches, is rapidly becoming the gold standard for the treatment of patients with localized RCC that is not amenable to nephron-sparing approaches. Laparoscopic partial nephrectomy has also been reported with some success, although hemostasis issues, warm renal ischemia times, and increased risk of urological complications have prevented this minimally invasive technique from being widely assimilated. Recently, robotic-assisted laparoscopic partial nephrectomy is gaining ground in treatment of small renal tumors, as it is less technically challenging than the pure laparoscopic counterpart. More recent clinical research has focused on energy ablative strategies such as cryotherapy and radiofrequency ablation, either through laparoscopic or percutaneous approaches, as strategies to treat the small (<4 cm) renal mass. These energy ablative strategies have recently reported encouraging intermediate term results, but long-term oncological efficacy is still lacking. These modalities remain investigational and should be used primarily in the setting of a clinical trial or for patients where surgical resection is contraindicated. Several centers are currently investigating active surveilance of renal masses less than 3 cm in elderly patients with severe medical comorbidities who cannot undergo surgery. A recent meta-analysis of 10 studies of active surveillance that included 331 patients with localized RCC demonstrated a metastatic progression rate of only 0.9%, which is encouraging. However, the long-term results of such approaches are still pending.

Advanced Renal Cell Carcinoma

Approximately 40% to 50% of patients either present with or develop metastases during the course of the natural history of their disease. The median survival for patients with metastatic RCC is 12 months. Two randomized phase III trials have demonstrated a significant survival benefit for patients who undergo cytoreductive nephrectomy prior to the administration of systemic immunotherapy in those that present with metastatic disease and their primary tumor in situ. The presence of nodal metastases, in the setting of distant metastatic disease, portends a worse prognosis and a decreased likelihood of responding to systemic therapy, which may be altered by aggressive surgical resection of the nodes at the time of cytoreductive surgery.

Distant metastatic disease can be categorized as a solitary metastasis or bulky metastatic disease. Several studies have shown higher 3-year survival rates, ranging from 20% to 60%, after radical nephrectomy with removal of a solitary metastasis. Solitary lung metastases appear to be associated with better survival rates than metastases to other organ sites. Multiple metastases or multiple sites of metastases portend a significantly worse prognosis and are usually approached with systemic therapy options, although the benefit of surgical consolidation following maximum response to systemic therapy has been demonstrated in selected patients with metastatic RCC.

Cytotoxic chemotherapy has been largely ineffective in RCC; the highest objective response rate for single-agent therapy is only 16%. More recently, regimens with gemcitabine and capecitabine have shown significant activity in selected patients. Interleukin-2 (IL-2) has yielded durable response rates of 15% to 19% in various trials, primarily with the use of high-dose bolus intravenous regimens. Subcutaneous IL-2, either alone or in combination with interferon, is believed to be inferior to intravenous IL-2 regimens, but associated with significantly less toxicity. Until recently, IL-2 was the gold standard of therapy for patients with metastatic disease, but recent inroads into the understanding of the molecular pathways associated with renal cell carcinogenesis and progression have resulted in the development of specific molecular targeted therapies that have rapidly replaced IL-2 in the armamentarium of the oncologist. Since 2005, five drugs (bevacizumab, sunitinib, sorafenib, temsirolimus, and everolimus) have been approved for the treatment of metastatic RCC. The usage of these drugs depends on histology, previous treatments received and failed, and patient risk stratification. So far, only temsirolimus has shown an improvement in overall survival in patients with poor-risk features. Unfortunately, these drugs, at best, only yield partial responses in a minority of patients, with no evidence of complete responses. A great deal of research is currently being conducted in the field of targeted therapy of renal cell carcinoma, with many new targeted agents in the pipeline.

TESTICULAR CANCER

Epidemiology and Etiology

Malignant tumors of the testis are rare. It is estimated that 8,400 cases of testicular cancer were diagnosed in 2009, but only 380 men will die of this disease. Ninety-five percent of these tumors are of germ cell origin. Although testicular tumors can occur at any age, specific tumor types tend to occur at different ages. Choriocarcinomas tend to occur between 24 and 28 years of age, embryonal carcinomas from 26 to 34 years of age, seminomas from 32 to 42 years of age, and lymphomas and spermatocytic seminomas after the age of 50 years.

The most well-known etiologic factor in the development of testicular cancer is cryptorchidism. Between 3% and 11% of all cases of testis cancer occur in cryptorchid testes. Although trauma to the testis has been linked to testis cancer, there is no evidence of a definite relationship. Genetic factors may also play a significant role.

Carcinoma in situ (otherwise known as intratubular germ cell neoplasia) is a precursor of testicular germ cell cancer. A total of 5% to 6% of men with a unilateral germ cell tumor have CIS in the contralateral testis, and a germ cell tumor will develop in 50% of these men. Other men with a high risk of CIS are individuals with intersex, cryptorchidism, infertility, or an extragonadal germ cell tumor.

Clinical Presentation

Testicular cancer typically presents as a painless testicular enlargement. Advanced disease can present as back pain, flank pain, or systemic symptoms. The differential diagnosis includes varicocele, hydrocele, hematoma, epididymitis, orchitis, and inguinal hernia.

Diagnosis

Although the diagnosis is usually evident at physical examination to an experienced clinician, scrotal ultrasound can be useful in establishing the diagnosis and evaluating local extension. Any solid testicular mass is considered a testicular tumor until proven otherwise. Patients with testicular enlargement that is believed to be inflammatory in nature (epididymo-orchitis) must be re-examined after the infection has been treated to rule out the presence of an occult testicular mass. Once a testicular tumor is suspected, the patient's levels of the tumor markers alpha-fetoprotein (AFP), human chorionic gonadotropin (hCG), and lactate dehydrogenase (LDH) should be tested. Following this, the patient should undergo a radical (inguinal) orchiectomy. There is no role for fine-needle aspiration or Tru-cut biopsy in the workup of this disease.

After radical orchiectomy, a CT scan of the chest, abdomen, and pelvis should be performed. If they were initially elevated, tumor markers should be reanalyzed following orchiectomy, after allowing the appropriate time for each marker to return to baseline. This would be approximately 1 week for hCG and 5 weeks for AFP.

Staging

The American Joint Committee on Cancer and International Union Against Cancer TNM testicular cancer staging system is outlined in Table 18.4. In terms of biological behavior and therapy, testicular tumors can be categorized as seminomatous or nonseminomatous germ cell tumors (NSGCTs). Seminomas are radiation-sensitive and chemosensitive tumors that undergo lymphatic spread in an orderly fashion. In contrast, NSGCTs are minimally radiation sensitive and have a higher metastatic potential than seminomas.

Management

Seminomatous Germ Cell Tumors

After radical orchiectomy, stage I seminomas are typically treated with radiation therapy to the retroperitoneal nodes up to the level of the diaphragm (doses of ~20 Gy) while stage IIA seminomas are treated with radiation therapy to the retroperitoneal nodes and ipsilateral pelvic nodes up to the level of the diaphragm (doses of 30 to 35 Gy). Using radiation therapy, the cure rate for stage I disease approaches 100%. Other treatment options include active surveillance (which requires a highly compliant patient) or the use of single agent carboplatin chemotherapy. Although 10% to 15% of patients with stage IIA disease have relapses, more than half of these respond successfully to salvage therapy, yielding a survival rate of 95% for patients with stage IIA disease.

Stage IIB or III disease is usually treated with cisplatin-based chemotherapy. Surgery is generally reserved for lymphatic disease that does not respond to chemotherapy or radiation therapy and is rarely performed in the setting of metastatic seminoma following radiation and/or chemotherapy. Using this approach, 5-year

American Joint Committee on Cancer/International Union Against Cancer Systems for Testicular Cancer

Primary Tumor Clinical (T)

pTX   Primary tumor cannot be assessed
pT0   No evidence of primary tumor (scar in testis)
pTis   Intratubular germ cell neoplasia (carcinoma in situ)
pT1   Tumor limited to the testis and epididymis and no vascular/lymphatic invasion
       Tumor may invade into the tunica albuginea but not the tunica vaginalis
pT2   Tumor limited to the testis and epididymis with vascular/lymphatic invasion or tumor
       invading into the tunica albuginea with involvement of the tunica vaginalis
pT3   Tumor invades the spermatic cord with or without vascular/lymphatic invasion
pT4   Tumor invades the scrotum with or without vascular/lymphatic invasion

Regional Lymph Nodes (N)

NX   Regional lymph nodes cannot be assessed
N0   No regional lymph node metastasis
N1   Lymph node mass 2 cm or less in greatest dimension; or multiple lymph nodes
       masses, none more than 2 cm in greatest dimension
N2   Lymph node mass, more than 2 cm but not more than 5 cm in greatest dimension; or
       multiple lymph node masses, any one mass greater than 2 cm but not more than
       5 cm in greatest dimension
N3   Lymph node mass more than 5 cm in greatest dimension

Distant Metastases (M)

MX   Distant metastasis cannot be assessed
M0   No distant metastases
M1   Presence of distant metastases
       M1a: Nonregional nodal or pulmonary metastases
       M1b: Distant metastases other than to nonregional lymph nodes and lungs

Serum Tumor Markers

Stage	LDH	hCG (mIU/mL)		AFP (ng/mL)
S0	≤Normal	≤N		≤N
S1	<1.5 × Normal	<5,000		<1,000
S2	1.5–10 × Normal	5,000–50,000		1,000–10,000
S3	>10 × Normal	>50,000		>10,000
Stage 0				
	pTis	N0	M0	S0
Stage I				
IA	T1	N0	M0	S0
IB	T2–T4	N0	M0	S0
IS	Any T	N0	M0	S1–S3 (postorchiectomy)
Stage II				
IIA	Any T	N1	M0	S0–S1
IIB	Any T	N2	M0	S0–S1
IIC	Any T	N3	M0	S0–S1
Stage III				
IIIA	Any T	Any N	M1a	S0–S1
IIIB	Any T	Any N	M0–M1a	S2
IIIC	Any T	Any N	M0–M1a	S3
	Any T	Any N	M1b	Any S

LDH, lactic dehydrogenase; hCG, human chorionic gonadotropin; AFP, alpha-fetoprotein.

disease-free survival rates of 86% and 92% have been obtained for patients with stages IIB and III disease, respectively.

Nonseminomatous Germ Cell Tumors

The optimal therapy for stage I disease is controversial; options include surveillance, retroperitoneal lymph node dissection (RPLND), and primary systemic chemotherapy. Overall, approximately 20% to 30% of patients with stage I disease who undergo surveillance experience relapse. Patients at high-risk of relapse include those with elevated AFP, lymphovascular invasion and >40% embryonal histology present in the primary tumor.

The recurrence rate after RPLND for low-volume stage II disease is less than 20%. Thus, both RPLND and primary systemic chemotherapy have been used to treat low-volume retroperitoneal disease. Survival rates of 97% or better have been associated with both forms of therapy. At the M. D. Anderson Cancer Center, patients with stage II disease are treated with primary chemotherapy, and RPLND is used to subsequently remove residual disease.

Because of the high recurrence rates associated with RPLND for stage IIB, IIC, and III NSGCTs, primary systemic chemotherapy is the treatment of choice for this disease. RPLND is used to remove any residual disease that may be present after primary chemotherapy and to determine the need for further therapy. Recent experience with chemotherapy for advanced NSGCT at the M. D. Anderson Cancer Center has shown 5-year survival rates of 96% and 76% for low- and high-volume stage III disease, respectively.

Despite the relatively early age of onset of testicular cancer, this disease remains one of the most curable cancers in humans. A majority of NSGCTs produce either AFP or β-hCG, rendering these markers helpful in monitoring the patient for treatment response and recurrent disease. RPLND can be performed in the primary setting (before chemotherapy, usually in stage I and IIA NSGCT) with excellent sparing of the sympathetic nerves, and resulting preservation of ejaculatory function. RPLND in this setting is performed using modified templates (and not just simply a mass excision). For residual masses after chemotherapy (in the setting of normal markers), postchemotherapy RPLND is performed with the goal of removing any residual viable tumor or teratoma. Teratomas can be life threatening, as it can grow very fast, invade adjacent vital organs, degenerate into a sarcoma or carcinoma, and is resistant to current chemotherapeutic regimens. Typically, with postchemotherapy RPLND, a full bilateral template is performed, aiming to remove all retroperitoneal lymph nodes. Postchemotherapy RPLND is a technically challenging procedure that should only be done in centers of excellence, as it is associated with higher complication rates, and could require resection of nearby involved organs (kidney, ureter, spleen, vena cava, colon) in as many as 25% of cases.

Recommended Readings

Prostate Cancer

Ahmed S, Lindsey B, Davies J. Emerging minimally invasive techniques for treating localized prostate cancer. *BJU Int.* 2005; 96:1230–1234.

Andriole GL, Crawford ED, Grubb RL III, et al. Mortality results from a randomized prostate-cancer screening trial. *N Engl J Med.* 2009;360:1310–1319.

Ash D. Advances in radiotherapy for prostate cancer. *Br J Radiol.* 2005;78(2):S112–S116.

Berthold DR, Sternberg CN, Tannock IF. Management of advanced prostate cancer after first-line chemotherapy. *J Clin Oncol.* 2005;23:8247–8252.

Beyer D, Nath R, Butler W, et al. American brachytherapy society recommendations for clinical implementation of NIST-1999 standards for (103) palladium brachytherapy. The clinical research committee of the American Brachytherapy Society. *Int J Radiat Oncol Biol Phys.* 2000;47:273–275.

Bill-Axelson A, Holmberg L, Ruutu M, et al. Radical prostatectomy versus watchful waiting in early prostate cancer. *N Engl J Med.* 2005;352:1977–1984.

Catalona WJ, Partin AW, Slawin KM, et al. Use of the percentage of free prostate-specific antigen to enhance differentiation of prostate cancer from benign prostatic disease: a prospective multicenter clinical trial. *JAMA.* 1998;279:1542–1547.

Catalona WJ, Richie JP, Ahmann FR, et al. Comparison of digital rectal examination and serum prostate specific antigen in the early detection of prostate cancer: results of a multicenter clinical trial of 6,630 men. *J Urol.* 1994;151:1283–1290.

Chen Y, Clegg NJ, Scher HI. Anti-androgens and androgen-depleting therapies in prostate cancer: new agents for an established target. *Lancet Oncol.* 2009;10: 981–991.

Chybowski FM, Keller JJ, Bergstralh EJ, et al. Predicting radionuclide bone scan findings in patients with newly diagnosed, untreated prostate cancer: prostate specific antigen is superior to all other clinical parameters. *J Urol.* 1991;145:313–318.

Cooner WH, Mosley BR, Rutherford CL Jr, et al. Prostate cancer detection in a clinical urological practice by ultrasonography, digital rectal examination and prostate specific antigen. *J Urol.* 1990;143:1146–1152; discussion 1152–1154.

D'Amico AV, Manola J, Loffredo M, et al. 6-month androgen suppression plus radiation therapy vs radiation therapy alone for patients with clinically localized prostate cancer: a randomized controlled trial. *JAMA.* 2004;292:821–827.

Higano CS, Schellhammer PF, Small EJ, et al. Integrated data from 2 randomized, double-blind, placebo-controlled, phase 3 trials of active cellular immunotherapy with sipuleucel-T in advanced prostate cancer. *Cancer.* 2009;115:3670–3679.

Jemal A, Siegel R, Ward E, et al. Cancer statistics, 2009. *CA Cancer J Clin.* 2009;59: 225–249.

Klotz L, Zhang L, Lam A, et al. Clinical results of long-term follow-up of a large, active surveillance cohort with localized prostate cancer. *J Clin Oncol.* 28:126–131.

Laufer M, Denmeade SR, Sinibaldi VJ, et al. Complete androgen blockade for prostate cancer: what went wrong? *J Urol.* 2000;164:3–9.

Leandri P, Rossignol G, Gautier JR, et al. Radical retropubic prostatectomy: morbidity and quality of life. Experience with 620 consecutive cases. *J Urol.* 1992;147: 883–887.

Lippman SM, Klein EA, Goodman PJ, et al. Effect of selenium and vitamin E on risk of prostate cancer and other cancers: the Selenium and Vitamin E Cancer Prevention Trial (SELECT). *JAMA.* 2009;301:39–51.

McNeal JE, Redwine EA, Freiha FS, et al. Zonal distribution of prostatic adenocarcinoma. Correlation with histologic pattern and direction of spread. *Am J Surg Pathol.* 1988;12:897–906.

Oesterling JE, Cooner WH, Jacobsen SJ, et al. Influence of patient age on the serum PSA concentration. An important clinical observation. *Urol Clin North Am.* 1993; 20:671–680.

Oesterling JE, Martin SK, Bergstralh EJ, et al. The use of prostate-specific antigen in staging patients with newly diagnosed prostate cancer. *JAMA.* 1993;269:57–60.

Petrylak D. Therapeutic options in androgen-independent prostate cancer: building on docetaxel. *BJU Int.* 2005;96(Suppl 2):41–46.

Saad F, Gleason DM, Murray R, et al. Long-term efficacy of zoledronic acid for the prevention of skeletal complications in patients with metastatic hormone-refractory prostate cancer. *J Natl Cancer Inst.* 2004;96:879–882.

Scardino PT, Frankel JM, Wheeler TM, et al. The prognostic significance of post-irradiation biopsy results in patients with prostatic cancer. *J Urol.* 1986;135:510–516.

Schroder FH, Hugosson J, Roobol MJ, et al. Screening and prostate-cancer mortality in a randomized European study. *N Engl J Med.* 2009;360:1320–1328.

Smith JA Jr, Herrell SD. Robotic-assisted laparoscopic prostatectomy: do minimally invasive approaches offer significant advantages? *J Clin Oncol.* 2005;23: 8170–8175.

Speight JL, Roach M III. Radiotherapy in the management of clinically localized prostate cancer: evolving standards, consensus, controversies and new directions. *J Clin Oncol.* 2005;23:8176–8185.

Sternberg CN, Petrylak DP, Sartor O, et al. Multinational, double-blind, phase III study of prednisone and either satraplatin or placebo in patients with castrate-refractory prostate cancer progressing after prior chemotherapy: the SPARC trial. *J Clin Oncol.* 2009;27:5431–5438.

The Medical Research Council Prostate Cancer Working Party Investigators Group. Immediate versus deferred treatment for advanced prostatic cancer: initial results of the Medical Research Council Trial. *Br J Urol.* 1997;79:235–246.

Thompson IM, Goodman PJ, Tangen CM, et al. The influence of finasteride on the development of prostate cancer. *N Engl J Med.* 2003;349:215–224.

Thompson IM Jr, Tangen CM, Paradelo J, et al. Adjuvant radiotherapy for pathologically advanced prostate cancer: a randomized clinical trial. *JAMA.* 2006;296: 2329–2335.

Thompson IM, Pauler DK, Goodman PJ, et al. Prevalence of prostate cancer among men with a prostate-specific antigen level < or = 4.0 ng per milliliter. *N Engl J Med.* 2004;350:2239–2246.

Zagars GK, Pollack A, von Eschenbach AC. Management of unfavorable locoregional prostate carcinoma with radiation and androgen ablation. *Cancer.* 1997;80:764–775.

Zincke H, Bergstralh EJ, Blute ML, et al. Radical prostatectomy for clinically localized prostate cancer: long-term results of 1,143 patients from a single institution. *J Clin Oncol.* 1994;12:2254–2263.

Bladder Cancer

Cummings KB, Barone JG, Ward WS. Diagnosis and staging of bladder cancer. *Urol Clin North Am.* 1992;19:455–465.

Grossman HB, Natale RB, Tangen CM, et al. Neoadjuvant chemotherapy plus cystectomy compared with cystectomy alone for locally advanced bladder cancer. *N Engl J Med.* 2003;349:859–866.

Heney NM, Ahmed S, Flanagan MJ, et al. Superficial bladder cancer: progression and recurrence. *J Urol.* 1983;130:1083–1086.

Herr HW. Tumour progression and survival in patients with T1G3 bladder tumours: 15-year outcome. *Br J Urol.* 1997;80:762–765.

Herr HW. Transurethral resection of muscle-invasive bladder cancer: 10-year outcome. *J Clin Oncol.* 2001;19:89–93.

Kachnic LA, Kaufman DS, Heney NM, et al. Bladder preservation by combined modality therapy for invasive bladder cancer. *J Clin Oncol.* 1997;15:1022–1029.

Kirkali Z, Chan T, Manoharan M, et al. Bladder cancer: epidemiology, staging and grading, and diagnosis. *Urology.* 2005; 66:4–34.

Lamm DL. Long-term results of intravesical therapy for superficial bladder cancer. *Urol Clin North Am.* 1992;19:573–580.

Lamm DL, Blumenstein BA, Crissman JD, et al. Maintenance bacillus Calmette-Guerin immunotherapy for recurrent TA,

T1 and carcinoma in situ transitional cell carcinoma of the bladder: a randomized Southwest Oncology Group Study. *J Urol.* 2000;163:1124–1129.

Logothetis C, Swanson D, Amato R, et al. Optimal delivery of perioperative chemotherapy: preliminary results of a randomized, prospective, comparative trial of preoperative and postoperative chemotherapy for invasive bladder carcinoma. *J Urol.* 1996;155:1241–1245.

Logothetis CJ, Dexeus FH, Finn L, et al. A prospective randomized trial comparing MVAC and CISCA chemotherapy for patients with metastatic urothelial tumors. *J Clin Oncol.* 1990;8:1050–1055.

Logothetis CJ, Johnson DE, Chong C, et al. Adjuvant cyclophosphamide, doxorubicin, and cisplatin chemotherapy for bladder cancer: an update. *J Clin Oncol.* 1988;6:1590–1596.

Pollack A, Zagars GK, Swanson DA. Muscle-invasive bladder cancer treated with external beam radiotherapy: prognostic factors. *Int J Radiat Oncol Biol Phys.* 1994;30:267–277.

Shipley WU, Kaufman DS, Zehr E, et al. Selective bladder preservation by combined modality protocol treatment: long-term outcomes of 190 patients with invasive bladder cancer. *Urology.* 2002;60:62–67; discussion 67–68.

Stein JP, Lieskovsky G, Cote R, et al. Radical cystectomy in the treatment of invasive bladder cancer: long-term results in 1,054 patients. *J Clin Oncol.* 2001;19:666–675.

Stockle M, Wellek S, Meyenburg W, et al. Radical cystectomy with or without adjuvant polychemotherapy for non-organ-confined transitional cell carcinoma of the urinary bladder: prognostic impact of lymph node involvement. *Urology.* 1996;48:868–875.

Sylvester RJ, Oosterlinck W, van der Meijden AP. A single immediate postoperative instillation of chemotherapy decreases the risk of recurrence in patients with stage Ta T1 bladder cancer: a meta-analysis of published results of randomized clinical trials. *J Urol.* 2004;171:2186–2190, quiz 2435.

Sylvester RJ, van der MA, Lamm DL. Intravesical bacillus Calmette-Guerin reduces the risk of progression in patients with superficial bladder cancer: a meta-analysis of the published results of randomized clinical trials. *J Urol.* 2002; 168: 1964–1970.

Vogeli TA. The management of superficial transitional cell carcinoma of the bladder:

a critical assessment of contemporary concepts and future perspectives. *BJU Int.* 2005;96:1171–1176.

Renal Cancer

Blom JH, van Poppel H, Marechal JM, et al. Radical nephrectomy with and without lymph-node dissection: final results of European Organization for Research and Treatment of Cancer (EORTC) randomized phase 3 trial 30881. *Eur Urol.* 2009; 55:28–34.

Cohen HT, McGovern FJ. Renal-cell carcinoma. *N Engl J Med.* 2005;353:2477–2490.

Couillard DR, deVere White RW. Surgery of renal cell carcinoma. *Urol Clin North Am.* 1993;20:263–275.

Escudier B, Eisen T, Stadler WM, et al. Sorafenib in advanced clear-cell renal-cell carcinoma. *N Engl J Med.* 2007;356: 125–134.

Escudier B, Pluzanska A, Koralewski P, et al. Bevacizumab plus interferon alfa-2a for treatment of metastatic renal cell carcinoma: a randomised, double-blind phase III trial. *Lancet.* 2007;370:2103–2111.

Flanigan RC, Salmon SE, Blumenstein BA, et al. Nephrectomy followed by interferon alfa-2b compared with interferon alfa-2b alone for metastatic renal-cell cancer. *N Engl J Med.* 2001;345:1655–1659.

Hudes G, Carducci M, Tomczak P, et al. Temsirolimus, interferon alfa, or both for advanced renal-cell carcinoma. *N Engl J Med.* 2007;356:2271–2281.

Kletscher BA, Qian J, Bostwick DG, et al. Prospective analysis of multifocality in renal cell carcinoma: influence of histological pattern, grade, number, size, volume and deoxyribonucleic acid ploidy. *J Urol.* 1995; 153:904–906.

Lam JS, Belldegrun AS, Pantuck AJ. Long-term outcomes of the surgical management of renal cell carcinoma. *World J Urol.* 2006;24:255–266.

Mickisch GH, Garin A, van Poppel H, et al. Radical nephrectomy plus interferon-alfa-based immunotherapy compared with interferon alfa alone in metastatic renal-cell carcinoma: a randomised trial. *Lancet.* 2001;358:966–970.

Motzer RJ, Escudier B, Oudard S, et al. Efficacy of everolimus in advanced renal cell carcinoma: a double-blind, randomised, placebo-controlled phase III trial. *Lancet.* 2008;372:449–456.

Motzer RJ, Hutson TE, Tomczak P, et al. Sunitinib versus interferon alfa in metastatic renal-cell carcinoma. *N Engl J Med.* 2007; 356:115–124.

Wirth MP. Immunotherapy for metastatic renal cell carcinoma. *Urol Clin North Am.* 1993;20:283–295.

Testis Cancer

Albers P, Albrecht W, Algaba F, et al. Guidelines on testicular cancer. *Eur Urol.* 2005; 48:885–894.

Carver BS, Serio AM, Bajorin D, et al. Improved clinical outcome in recent years for men with metastatic nonseminomatous germ cell tumors. *J Clin Oncol.* 2007;25: 5603–5608.

Carver BS, Sheinfeld J. Germ cell tumors of the testis. *Ann Surg Oncol.* 2005;12:871–880.

Carver BS, Sheinfeld J. Management of postchemotherapy extra-retroperitoneal residual masses. *World J Urol.* 2009;27: 489–492.

Feldman DR, Bosl GJ, Sheinfeld J, et al. Medical treatment of advanced testicular cancer. *JAMA.* 2008;299:672–684.

Logothetis CJ. The case for relevant staging of germ cell tumors. *Cancer.* 1990;65: 709–717.

Spiess PE, Brown GA, Liu P, et al. Predictors of outcome in patients undergoing postchemotherapy retroperitoneal lymph node dissection for testicular cancer. *Cancer.* 2006;107:1483–1490.

Spiess PE, Kassouf W, Brown GA, et al. Surgical management of growing teratoma syndrome: the M. D. Anderson cancer center experience. *J Urol.* 2007;177: 1330–1334; discussion 1334.

Svatek RS, Spiess PE, Sundi D, et al. Long-term outcome for men with teratoma found at postchemotherapy retroperitoneal lymph node dissection. *Cancer.* 2009;115:1310–1317.

Wishnow KI, Johnson DE, Swanson DA, et al. Identifying patients with low-risk clinical stage I nonseminomatous testicular tumors who should be treated by surveillance. *Urology.* 1989;34:339–343.

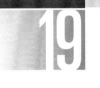

Gynecologic Cancers

Liz Y. Han, Brian M. Slomovitz,
Pamela T. Soliman, and Judith K. Wolf

Surgical oncologists are often consulted by general obstetrician/gynecologists to assist in the management of patients with primary gynecologic malignancies. It is therefore important to understand the surgical staging procedures involved with each disease process (i.e., ovarian, fallopian tube, uterine, cervical, vulvar, and vaginal). This chapter discusses the basic principles of gynecologic oncology so appropriate management can occur when these neoplasms are unexpectedly encountered. Emphasis is placed on diagnosis, staging, and surgical management.

OVARIAN CANCER

Ovarian cancer is the deadliest of gynecologic malignancies. Every year in the United States, approximately 21,000 new cases are diagnosed, and 14,000 women die from this disease. Ovarian cancers are heterogeneous, and subtypes are defined by histology. The most common, and "typical," is epithelial ovarian cancer. Other less common subtypes are germ cell tumors and sex cord stromal tumors.

Epithelial Ovarian Cancer

Incidence and Risk Factors
Epithelial ovarian cancer occurs in 1 in 70 women and constitutes 90% of all ovarian cancers. The median age at diagnosis is 61 years. Approximately 10% of these cases are hereditary, and these are transmitted in an autosomal dominant fashion. Hereditary breast ovarian cancer syndrome (BRCA-1 and BRCA-2 mutations) and Lynch syndrome/hereditary nonpolyposis colorectal cancer (in which colon, endometrial, ovarian, and other cancers cluster in first- and second-degree relatives) are known hereditary forms of ovarian cancer; other genetic mutations likely remain to be identified.

Factors believed to increase the risk of a woman developing epithelial ovarian cancer are increased age (peak age is 70 years), nulliparity, early menarche, late menopause, delayed childbearing, and Ashkenazi Jewish descent. Early studies suggested an association with fertility drugs (i.e., clomiphene and gonadotropin), but more recent studies have not confirmed this link. The use of oral contraceptives for more than 5 years appears to protect against the development of epithelial ovarian cancer.

Pathology
Tumor subtypes are listed in Table 19.1. The incidence of concomitant endometrial carcinoma is 15% to 30% in cases of endometrioid ovarian carcinoma. Cases of synchronous appendiceal and ovarian mucinous tumors have also been reported, but because it is not unusual for appendiceal cancer to spread to the ovaries, it can be difficult to determine the true site of the primary disease.

Routes of Spread and Sites of Metastasis
Because exfoliated cells tend to assume the circulatory path of the peritoneal fluid and implant along this path, the most common route of metastasis is by seeding.

TABLE 19.1	Percentage Distribution of Epithelial Ovarian Carcinomas and Percentage that are Bilateral, by Histologic Subtype	
Histologic Subtype	**Percentage Distribution**	**Bilaterality (%)**
Serous	46	73
Mucinous	36	47
Endometrioid	8	33
Clear cell	3	13
Transitional	2	—
Mixed	3	—
Undifferentiated	<2	53
Unclassified	<1	—

Epithelial ovarian cancer may also metastasize to the lymph nodes. Hematogenous spread is uncommon.

Clinical Features

Symptoms. The interval from onset of disease to diagnosis is often prolonged because of lack of specific symptoms, with the significant complaint being persistent urinary and abdominal problems. The diagnosis is often not made until patients have disseminated disease, with approximately 65% of cases presenting at stage III or IV. Patients with stage IV disease and malignant pleural effusions may present with a cough or shortness of breath. It is uncommon for ovarian cancer to be diagnosed by abnormal Papanicolaou (Pap) smear results.

Physical Findings. An adnexal mass noted on routine pelvic examination and a palpable fluid wave are often found in patients with advanced-stage epithelial ovarian cancer. Five percent of patients with presumed ovarian cancer have another primary tumor that has metastasized to the ovary. The most common primary cancers that metastasize to the ovary are breast, gastrointestinal tract, and other gynecologic cancers.

Pretreatment Workup

Careful physical examination, including pelvic examination with rectovaginal examination, is required. Pretreatment workup also includes clinical tests (e.g., complete blood cell count, serum glucose, blood urea nitrogen, creatinine, liver function, serum albumin, and CA-125 [which is elevated in approximately 80% of cases]), chest radiography, and mammography. Computed tomography (CT) analysis may help determine the extent of disease. Barium enema is useful in examining the colon and can be particularly helpful in distinguishing between a primary ovarian and primary colon cancer, which may present in the same way.

Staging

The surgical staging schema for epithelial ovarian cancer is outlined in Table 19.2.

Treatment

The initial step in treatment is surgical cytoreduction with appropriate intraoperative staging procedures, including abdominal and pelvic cytologic analysis (or collection of ascites), careful exploration of all abdominal and pelvic structures and surfaces, total abdominal hysterectomy and bilateral salpingo-oophorectomy

TABLE 19.2	Surgical Staging of Epithelial Ovarian Cancer

Tumor Stage	Description
I	Growth limited to the ovaries
IA	Growth limited to one ovary, no ascites, no tumor on the external surfaces, intact capsules
IB	Growth in both ovaries, no ascites, no tumor on the external surfaces, intact capsules
IC	Stage IA or IB characteristics but with tumor on the surface of one or both ovaries, ruptured capsules, or malignant ascites with positive peritoneal cytologic results
II	Growth involving one or both ovaries with pelvic extension
IIA	Extension and/or metastases to the uterus and/or tubes
IIB	Extension to other pelvic tissues
IIC	Stage IIA or IIB characteristics but with tumor on the surface of one or both ovaries, ruptured capsules, or malignant ascites with positive peritoneal cytologic results
III	Growth involving one or both ovaries with peritoneal implants outside the pelvis and/or positive retroperitoneal or inguinal nodes; superficial liver metastasis equal to stage III; tumor limited to the true pelvis but with histologically proven malignant extension to the small bowel or omentum
IIIA	Tumor grossly limited to the true pelvis with negative nodes but histologically confirmed microscopic seeding of abdominal peritoneal surfaces
IIIB	Tumor involving one or both ovaries with histologically confirmed implants of abdominal peritoneal surfaces ≤2 cm in diameter; negative nodes
IIIC	Abdominal implants >2 cm in diameter and/or positive retroperitoneal or inguinal nodes
IV	Growth involving one or both ovaries with distant metastases; positive cytologic results from pleural effusion or pathological confirmation of parenchymal liver metastases

(except in cases of concern about fertility or of early-stage disease), omentectomy, and selective pelvic and para-aortic lymph node sampling. In patients with a mucinous tumor or an involved appendix, appendectomy should be performed. Primary cytoreduction is a key component in advanced cases because survival is inversely correlated to the amount of residual tumor remaining. Optimal tumor reductive surgery is loosely defined as the diameter of the largest residual tumor implant being less than 1 cm. If the residual mass is larger than 1 cm, then cytoreduction is deemed suboptimal. Recently, there has been a movement to update the definition of optimal tumor reductive surgery as no visible residual disease.

Although "second-look" laparotomy or laparoscopy was routinely performed in the past, it is no longer performed unless required as part of an investigational trial.

After surgical cytoreduction, patients should be treated with combination platinum- and taxane-based chemotherapy. After six to eight courses of chemotherapy, treatment decisions are based on the presence of persistent disease or the disease-free interval.

In select cases, there may be a role for neoadjuvant ("up-front") chemotherapy followed by an interval cytoreduction procedure. In patients with advanced cancer, neoadjuvant chemotherapy may be warranted for those with multiple medical comorbidities that preclude aggressive surgical debulking or extensive disease that cannot be optimally reduced (as determined by CT scan or diagnostic laparotomy or laparoscopy). A European collaborative trial showed noninferiority when comparing neoadjuvant to adjuvant chemotherapy with debulking in patients with stage IIIC and IV disease. Furthermore, the strongest independent predictor of prolonged survival is the absence of residual tumor after surgery.

Prognostic Factors

Prognostic pathological factors include tumor grade (Table 19.3), histologic subtype, and DNA ploidy. Clinical factors of prognostic significance include surgicopathologic stage, extent of residual disease remaining after primary cytoreduction (Table 19.3), volume of ascites, patient age, and patient performance status. Patients with poor performance status before treatment (Karnofsky score <70%) have significantly shorter survival than do patients with good performance status.

TABLE 19.3 Five-Year Survival Rates for Patients with Epithelial Ovarian Cancer, by Tumor Stage and Grade, Amount of Residual Disease, and Disease Status

Tumor Stage	All Grades	Survival Rate (%)		
		Grade 1	Grade 2	Grade 3
I				
IA	85	92.5	86	63
IB	69	85	90	79
IC	59	78	49	51
II				
IIA	62	64	65	39
IIB	51	79	43	42
IIC	43	68	46	20
III				
IIIA	31	58	38	20
IIIB	38	73	42	21
IIIC	18	46	22	14
IV	8	14	8	6

	Survival Rate (%)
Amount of residual disease after primary cytoreductive surgery	
Microscopic (residual disease)	40–75
Macroscopic (optimal debulking)	30
Macroscopic (suboptimal debulking)	5
Disease status at second look	
No evidence of disease	50
Microscopic disease	35
Macroscopic disease	5

Recommended Surveillance
Patients should be followed up every 2 to 4 months for the first 2 years, then every 3 to 6 months for the next 3 years, and then annually after 5 years. A physical examination with pelvic examination as well as specific labs (e.g., CA-125) should be checked at each visit. As clinically indicated, a CT of the chest, abdomen and pelvis, +/− a PET component can be performed.

Ovarian Tumors of Low Malignant Potential

Incidence and Risk Factors
Sometimes referred to as borderline tumors, ovarian tumors of low malignant potential (LMP) constitute as many as 5% to 15% of epithelial ovarian malignancies. The highest incidence is among white women, and the mean age at diagnosis is 39 to 45 years (approximately 10 to 15 years younger than that for epithelial ovarian cancer). No risk factors have been identified, and pregnancy and exogenous hormones do not appear to be protective. There is no apparent association with family history.

Pathology
The most common histologic subtypes of ovarian tumors of LMP are serous and mucinous (Table 19.4). Diagnosis requires the absence of frank stromal invasion. Distinct pathological features that may be associated with a more aggressive disease course include micropapillary architecture, microinvasion, and invasive implants.

Clinical Features
Patients with ovarian tumors of LMP, as well as those with epithelial ovarian cancers, present similarly. The most common symptoms are lower abdominal pain or discomfort, early satiety, dyspepsia, and a sense of abdominal enlargement. Ovarian tumors of LMP can also be identified as an adnexal mass on routine pelvic examination. The CA-125 levels may be elevated in serous tumors.

Treatment
Compared with patients with invasive epithelial ovarian cancer, it is more common for patients with ovarian tumors of LMP to be diagnosed with early-stage disease. Recommended treatment for all patients is primary surgery; fertility-sparing procedures should be performed in patients with stage I disease who desire children in the future. There has been no proven benefit to adjuvant therapy in treating this cancer, even in patients with advanced-stage disease. Typically, these tumors have an indolent clinical course and may recur after a long disease-free interval. Tumor

TABLE 19.4	Distribution of Ovarian Tumors of Low Malignant Potential, by Tumor Stage and Histologic Type	
	Histologic Type (%)	
Tumor Stage	**Serous**	**Mucinous**
I	65	89.5
II	14	1
III	20	9
IV	1	0.5

	Five-Year Survival Rates for Patients with Ovarian Tumors of Low Malignant Potential, by Tumor Stage

Tumor Stage	Survival Rate (%)
I	95
II	75–80
III	65–70

stage is the most important predictor of survival (Table 19.5). Secondary cytoreduction can be considered in select patients with recurrent disease.

Ovarian Germ Cell Tumors

Incidence and Risk Factors
Germ cell tumors are the second most common type of ovarian tumor. Among persons 20 years of age or younger, 70% of ovarian tumors are of germ cell origin, and one-third of these are malignant. The mean age at diagnosis is 19 years; germ cell tumors rarely occur after the third decade of life. Sixty to 75% of cases are stage I at diagnosis.

Pathology
The histologic subtypes of germ cell tumors and their incidences are listed in Table 19.6.

Routes of Spread and Sites of Metastasis
Germ cell tumors have the same potential as epithelial ovarian tumors to metastasize.

Clinical Features
Germ cell malignancies grow rapidly and are often characterized by pain secondary to torsion, hemorrhage, or necrosis. They may also cause bladder, rectal, or

	Clinical Features of Ovarian Germ Cell Tumors, by Histologic Subtype

			Tumor Markers		
Histologic Subtype	Incidence (%)	Bilaterality	AFP	β-hCG	LDH
Dysgerminoma	40	10%–15% of cases	−	−	±
Endodermal sinus tumor	22	Rare; dermoids common in contralateral ovary	±	−	−
Immature teratoma	20	Rare; dermoids common in contralateral ovary	−	−	−
Embryonal carcinoma	1–3	Rare	±	±	−
Choriocarcinoma	1–3	Rare	−	±	−
Polyembryonal	1–3	Rare	−	−	−
Mixed tumor	10–15	Varies	−	−	−

AFP, α-fetoprotein; β-hCG, beta subunit of human chorionic gonadotropin; LDH, lactic dehydrogenase; +, negative result; −, positive/negative result; ±, positive result.

menstrual abnormalities. Dysgerminomas account for 20% to 30% of malignant ovarian tumors diagnosed during pregnancy. Embryonal carcinomas may produce estrogen and cause precocious puberty.

Pretreatment Workup
Careful physical examination, including pelvic examination, is required. Other components of the pretreatment workup include clinical tests (e.g., complete blood cell count, serum glucose, blood urea nitrogen, creatinine, liver function, serum albumin) and chest radiography. Serum markers, including α-fetoprotein, β-human chorionic gonadotropin (β-hCG), and lactic dehydrogenase, should be measured (Table 19.6). Premenstrual women with an ovarian mass should undergo karyotyping because the incidence of dysgenic gonads is increased in patients with these tumors.

Staging
The surgical staging criteria are the same as those for epithelial ovarian cancer (Table 19.2).

Treatment
In general, surgical staging includes unilateral salpingo-oophorectomy (if there is a desire to preserve fertility), peritoneal cytology, omentectomy, and selective biopsies of retroperitoneal lymph nodes and abdominal structures. For patients whose disease is inadequately staged, there are two options: surgical re-exploration and appropriate staging, and initiation of chemotherapy without re-exploration. In most cases, it is imprudent to delay chemotherapy by re-exploration and staging because these tumors are highly chemosensitive.

Chemotherapy is recommended for all patients with germ cell tumors, except for those with stage I tumors. Chemotherapy should begin 7 to 10 days after surgical exploration because of rapid tumor growth. The first-line regimen is bleomycin, etoposide, and cisplatin administered for three or four cycles in 21-day intervals. Radiotherapy may have a limited role in treatment of dysgerminomas.

Prognostic Factors
The survival rates for individual ovarian germ cell tumor subtypes are listed in Table 19.7. Dysgerminomas larger than 10–15 cm in diameter or with a high mitotic index and anaplasia are more likely to recur. Prognostic factors for immature teratomas include tumor grade, extent of disease at diagnosis, and amount of residual tumor. The tumor grade of immature teratomas is determined by the presence of immature neural elements. Tumor stage is also an important prognostic factor for all ovarian germ cell tumors (Table 19.8).

Recommended Surveillance
Surveillance is similar to that for epithelial ovarian tumors. Patients should be followed up every 2 to 4 months for the first 2 years, then every 3 to 6 months for the next 3 years, and then annually after 5 years. A physical examination with pelvic examination should be performed at each visit. Labs (e.g., CA-125, α-fetoprotein, β-hCG, and lactic dehydrogenase) should be checked at each visit if they were initially elevated. As clinically indicated, a CT of the chest, abdomen and pelvis, +/– a PET component can be performed.

Sex Cord Stromal Tumors

Incidence and Risk Factors
Sex cord stromal tumors account for 5% to 8% of ovarian malignancies and up to 5% of childhood malignancies. Occurrence before menarche is often associated with precocious puberty.

TABLE 19.7	Survival Rates for Patients with Ovarian Germ Cell Tumors, by Histologic Subtype, Tumor Stage or Grade, and Time Interval	

Histologic Subtype and Tumor Stage or Grade	Interval (y)	Survival Rate
Dysgerminoma	5	
Stage I		90%–95%
All stages		60%–90%
Endodermal sinus tumor	2	
Stages I and II		90%
Stages III and IV		50%
Immature teratoma	5	
Stage I		90%–95%
All stages		70%–80%
Grade 1		82%
Grade 2		62%
Grade 3		30%
Embryonal carcinoma	5	39%
Choriocarcinoma		Low
Polyembryonal		Low
Mixed tumor		Variable; depends on tumor composition

Pathology

As their name suggests, these tumors are derived from sex cords or stroma. Derivatives include granulosa cells, theca cells, stromal cells, Sertoli cells, Leydig cells, and cells resembling embryonic precursors of these cell types (Table 19.9).

Routes of Spread and Sites of Metastasis

The pattern and sites of metastatic spread are analogous to that of epithelial ovarian cancers.

Clinical Features

Fibromas and Fibrosarcomas. Fibromas and fibrosarcomas are the most common sex cord stromal tumors and constitute 4% of ovarian neoplasms. The mean age at diagnosis is 46 years. Ten percent of these lesions are bilateral. Symptoms include

TABLE 19.8	Five-Year Survival Rates for Patients with Ovarian Germ Cell Tumors, by Tumor Stage

Tumor Stage	Survival Rate (%)
I	72
II	38
III	18
IV	0

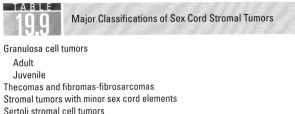

TABLE 19.9 Major Classifications of Sex Cord Stromal Tumors

Granulosa cell tumors
   Adult
   Juvenile
Thecomas and fibromas-fibrosarcomas
Stromal tumors with minor sex cord elements
Sertoli stromal cell tumors
   Sertoli cell
   Leydig cell
   Sertoli–Leydig cell
Gynandroblastomas
Sex cord tumors with annular tubules
Unclassified tumors

ascites in 50% of patients with tumors larger than 6 cm in diameter, increased abdominal girth, Meigs syndrome (right pleural effusion and ascites), and Gorlin syndrome with basal nevi. These tumors are primarily inert but may secrete small amounts of estrogen.

Granulosa Cell Tumors. Granulosa cell tumors comprise 1% to 2% of ovarian tumors. Adult-type tumors (90% to 95% of granulosa cell tumors) are characterized by secretion of excess estrogen. Patients may experience menstrual irregularities or postmenopausal bleeding. Five percent of patients present with an acute abdomen caused by tumor hemorrhage. Patients with juvenile-type granulosa cell tumors (5% to 10% of granulosa cell tumors) can also present with menstrual abnormalities, abdominal pain, and (rarely) postmenopausal bleeding. Because granulosa cell tumors produce estrogen, coexisting endometrial pathological processes occur in up to 30% of patients. In rare cases, these tumors may produce testosterone and cause some virilizing features.

Thecomas. Thecomas are one-third as common as granulosa cell tumors. The mean age at diagnosis is 53 years, and 2% to 3% of these tumors are bilateral. Menstrual abnormalities and postmenopausal bleeding are the most common presenting symptoms. Thecomas also produce estrogen.

Sertoli Cell Tumors. The average age at diagnosis of Sertoli cell tumors is 27 years, but these tumors can occur at any age. Sertoli cell tumors are unilateral. Seventy percent of patients have symptoms related to excess estrogen, whereas 20% exhibit signs of virilization. Rarely, hyperaldosteronemia manifested as hypertension and hyperkalemia may develop. Seventy percent of these tumors produce both estrogen and androgens, whereas 20% produce androgens alone.

Leydig Cell Tumors. Leydig cell tumors occur at an average age of 50 to 70 years but can occur at any age. These tumors are often unilateral. Eighty percent produce androgens and 10% produce estrogen, which often results in hormonally related side effects. Leydig cell tumors are often associated with thyroid disease and may be hereditary.

Sertoli–Leydig Cell Tumors. Sertoli–Leydig cell tumors occur at an average age of 25 to 40 years but can occur at any age. These tumors are rarely bilateral. Symptoms include amenorrhea, and virilization may occur in up to 50% of patients. Most of these tumors produce testosterone, and some may produce α-fetoprotein.

Gynandroblastomas. Gynandroblastoma are unilateral tumors that can occur at any age. Patients may experience estrogenic effects or virilization secondary to the hormone products of these tumors. Histologically, both granulosa cell and Sertoli–Leydig cell components may be present in these tumors. These tumors may produce androgens or estrogen, or they may be inert.

Sex Cord Tumors with Annular Tubules. The average age of patients with sex cord tumors with annular tubules is 25 to 35 years. These tumors may be associated with Peutz–Jeghers syndrome, and in these cases, 66% are bilateral and most produce estrogen. Among those that occur in women without Peutz–Jeghers syndrome, only 40% produce excess estrogen. These tumors are also associated with endocervical adenocarcinomas.

Pretreatment Workup
Careful physical examination, including pelvic examination, is required. Other components of the pretreatment workup include clinical tests (e.g., complete blood cell count, serum glucose, blood urea nitrogen, creatinine, liver function, serum albumin, CA-125), chest radiography, and mammography. Evaluation of serum concentrations of estradiol, dehydroepiandrosterone, testosterone, 17-OH-progesterone, and hydrocortisone may be helpful in diagnosis. CT and ultrasonography should be performed to evaluate the adrenal glands and ovaries. Although imaging studies may be helpful, they do not often change the planned staging procedure.

Staging
The surgical staging criteria are the same as those for epithelial ovarian cancer (Table 19.2).

Treatment
In general, surgical staging of sex cord stromal tumors can be accomplished by unilateral salpingo-oophorectomy (if there is a desire to maintain fertility), peritoneal cytology, infracolic omentectomy, selective biopsies of nodes and abdominal structures, and appropriately targeted biopsies. If a hysterectomy is not performed at the time of surgery, dilatation and curettage and endocervical curettage should be performed to evaluate any coexistent pathological processes. These tumors are surgically staged according to the criteria used for epithelial ovarian cancer (Table 19.2).

Tumors of stromal origin (i.e., thecomas and fibromas) and Leydig cell tumors generally follow a benign course; surgery is the only treatment. Sertoli cell or granulosa cell tumors are generally of LMP, tend to recur late, and rarely metastasize. Chemotherapy should be considered for advanced disease. Postoperative adjunctive therapy with bleomycin, etoposide, and cisplatin or other platinum-based chemotherapy should be considered in patients with Sertoli cell or Leydig cell tumors with poor differentiation and heterologous components and in patients with advanced or recurrent stromal tumors; pelvic radiation therapy can also play a role in treatment of these patients.

Prognostic Factors
Survival rates are described in Table 19.10.

TABLE 19.10	Five-Year Survival Rates for Patients with Sex Cord Stromal Tumors, by Histologic Subtype	

Histologic Subtype	Survival Rate
Granulosa cell tumor	
Tumors confined to the ovary	85%–90%
Tumors with extraovarian extension	55%–60%
Sertoli or Leydig cell tumor with poor differentiation	Low
Other tumors of sex cord stromal origin	Consistent with benign processes and low-grade malignancies

Recommended Surveillance

Surveillance is similar to that for epithelial ovarian tumors. Patients should be followed up every 2 to 4 months for the first 2 years, then every 3 to 6 months for the next 3 years, and then annually after 5 years. A physical examination with pelvic examination should be performed at each visit. Labs (e.g., CA-125, inhibin A and B for granulose cell tumors, and testosterone for Sertoli–Leydig cell tumors) should be checked at each visit if they were initially elevated. As clinically indicated, a CT of the chest, abdomen and pelvis, +/– a PET component can be performed.

Management of Incidental Cancers Found at Laparotomy

The finding of an unsuspected ovarian mass at the time of exploratory laparotomy or at laparotomy for an unrelated condition can pose a therapeutic dilemma to the surgeon. Appropriate treatment depends on several factors, including the patient's age, the size and consistency of the mass, possible bilaterality, and gross involvement of other structures. Informed consent is a key component to the decision making. Unless there is a life-threatening situation, a hysterectomy and bilateral salpingo-oophorectomy should be performed only with proper informed consent, especially in women of childbearing age.

Ovarian Mass in Premenopausal Women: Functional Cysts. An unsuspected mass in a young patient is most likely benign. The most frequently found benign masses involving the adnexa are functional cysts, which are related to the process of ovulation. These cysts are significant because they cannot be easily distinguished from true neoplasms on clinical grounds alone. If ovulation does not occur, a clear, fluid-filled follicular cyst up to 10 cm in diameter may develop. This follicular cyst usually resolves spontaneously within several days to 2 weeks. Ovulating women can also present with functional ovarian cysts. These are usually asymptomatic but can cause lower abdominal or pelvic pain; signs of an acute abdomen are rare. The corpus luteum, which is formed during ovulation, may become abnormally large if there is hemorrhage within it. A patient with a hemorrhagic corpus luteum may present with an acute abdomen, which necessitates laparotomy. Often the bleeding area may be oversewn without the need for removal of the cyst, fallopian tube, or ovary.

    Simple cysts up to 5 cm in diameter may be found incidentally at the time of surgery. These can often be observed safely in women who are in their reproductive years. If it is a functional cyst, it should resolve after the patient's next menstrual period. Resolution can be evaluated with physical examination alone or in conjunction with pelvic ultrasonography. Functional cysts are more common in patients who have anovulatory cycles, such as women who are obese or those who have polycystic ovarian syndrome.

Dermoid Cysts. Dermoid cysts, or benign cystic teratomas, are the most common ovarian tumors in women in the second and third decades of life. These cystic masses may be of any size, and up to 15% are bilateral. Torsion is the most frequent complication and commonly occurs in children, young women, and pregnant women. Severe acute abdominal pain is usually the initial symptom, and this condition constitutes an emergency. Treatment is cystectomy and close inspection of the other ovary.

Cystadenomas. Other common benign neoplasms that occur in young patients are serous and mucinous cystadenomas. These are treated with unilateral salpingo-oophorectomy if the other ovary appears normal.

Endometriomas. Endometriomas, which are also called chocolate cysts of endometriosis, can also occur in young women. These patients may have a history of endometriosis or chronic pelvic pain. Often, other endometriosis implants may be seen in the pelvis or abdominal cavity; this finding may be helpful in establishing a diagnosis. The treatment of endometriomas may be cystectomy or unilateral oophorectomy and depends on the degree of the remaining normal-appearing ovarian tissue. Every effort should be made to salvage the normal-appearing portion of ovary.

Treatment

If ascites is present on opening of the abdomen, it should be evacuated and submitted for cytologic analysis. After careful inspection and palpation, if the ovarian mass appears to be confined to one ovary and malignancy is suspected, unilateral salpingo-oophorectomy is appropriate in most circumstances. If the mass is believed to be benign, ovarian cystectomy may be preferable. The ovarian capsule should be inspected for any evidence of rupture, adherence, or excrescence. Once removed, the ovarian specimen should be sent for frozen-section examination. If malignancy is diagnosed, surgical staging should be performed. This should include biopsies of the omentum, peritoneal surfaces of the pelvis and upper abdomen, and retroperitoneal lymph nodes (including both the para-aortic and the bilateral pelvic regions).

If the contralateral ovary appears normal, random biopsy or wedge resection is probably not indicated because it may interfere with future fertility due to peritoneal adhesions or ovarian failure. If the histologic diagnosis is questionable based on frozen-section results, it is always preferable to wait for permanent section results before proceeding with a hysterectomy and bilateral salpingo-oophorectomy in a young patient. General criteria for conservative management include young patients desirous of future childbearing; patient and family consent and agreement to close follow-up; no evidence of dysgenetic gonads; any unilateral malignant germ cell, stromal, or borderline tumor; and stage IA invasive epithelial tumor.

Advances in assisted reproduction have greatly influenced intraoperative management decisions. Traditionally, if a bilateral salpingo-oophorectomy is indicated, a hysterectomy has also been performed. Current technology for donor oocyte transfer and hormonal support, however, allows a woman without ovaries to sustain a normal intrauterine pregnancy. Similarly, if the uterus and one tube and ovary are removed because of tumor involvement, current techniques allow for retrieval of oocytes from the patient's remaining ovary, in vitro fertilization with sperm from her partner, and implantation of the embryo into a surrogate's uterus.

Ovarian Mass in Postmenopausal Women. The risk of an ovarian mass being malignant begins to increase at 40 years of age and rises steadily thereafter. Therefore, the finding of an unsuspected ovarian mass in a postmenopausal woman is more ominous. The most common malignant neoplasms in this age group are malignant epithelial tumors; germ cell and stromal cell tumors rarely occur. Benign lesions, such as epithelial cystadenomas and dermoid cysts, can still occur in this population, although they do so much less frequently than in younger patients. Treatment of an unanticipated ovarian mass in a postmenopausal patient includes salpingo-oophorectomy and further staging if the frozen section reveals a diagnosis of cancer. Appropriate staging biopsies should also be performed. A gynecologic oncologist should be consulted.

Laparoscopy for the Management of Ovarian Cancer

Laparoscopy has been widely used as the standard surgical approach for benign and suspicious adnexal masses. The role of laparoscopy in the treatment of ovarian cancer is less clear, but some studies have suggested that it can be used safely at the time of second-look surgery or to stage and treat patients with early ovarian cancer. The role of laparoscopy in treating ovarian cancer still needs to be defined, although laparoscopic surgery is associated with significantly less morbidity than laparotomy.

FALLOPIAN TUBE CANCER

Incidence and Risk Factors

Fallopian tube cancer accounts for 0.1% to 0.5% of gynecologic malignancies. The average age at diagnosis is 55 years. No known risk factors exist for the development of this disease.

Pathology

The most common histologic subtype is adenocarcinoma, and the most common tumors of the fallopian tube are metastatic lesions from other sites. To establish a diagnosis of primary fallopian tube cancer, Hu's criteria must be met: The main tumor must be in the fallopian tube, the mucosa should be involved microscopically and exhibit a papillary pattern, and the transition between benign and malignant tubal epithelium should be demonstrated if the tubal wall is significantly involved with the tumor.

Routes of Spread and Sites of Metastasis

Fallopian tube cancer metastasizes in a manner similar to that of epithelial ovarian cancer. Lymphatic spread tends to play more of a role in fallopian tube cancer. Because of the presence of extensive lymphatics, one-third of patients exhibit evidence of nodal metastases.

Clinical Features

The classic triad of primary fallopian tube cancer is watery vaginal discharge, pelvic pain, and a pelvic mass. However, this triad is present in less than 15% of patients. Watery discharge and vaginal bleeding are the most commonly reported symptoms.

Pretreatment Workup
Careful physical examination, including pelvic examination, is required. Other components of the pretreatment workup include clinical tests (e.g., complete blood cell count, serum glucose, blood urea nitrogen, creatinine, liver function, serum albumin, and CA-125), chest radiography, and mammography. Imaging studies may be helpful but usually do not change the planned staging procedure. CT may help determine the extent of disease. Barium enema is useful in examining the colon. It can also be particularly helpful in distinguishing a colonic primary in older patients from either fallopian tube or ovarian cancer, which may present with similar symptoms. Intravenous pyelography is also helpful in certain clinical situations.

Staging
There is no official International Federation of Gynecology and Obstetrics (FIGO) staging system for fallopian tube cancer. By convention, the surgical staging criteria used for epithelial ovarian cancer is used (Table 19.2).

Treatment
Treatment of fallopian tube cancer is analogous to that of epithelial ovarian cancer.

Prognostic Factors
It is difficult to determine the prognostic factors specific to fallopian tube cancer because this disease is rare, but they are likely similar to those of epithelial ovarian cancer. The overall 5-year survival rate is estimated to be 40%, which is higher than the 5-year survival rate for patients with epithelial ovarian cancer. This difference in survival is likely related to diagnosis at an earlier stage in fallopian tube cancer than in ovarian cancer.

Recommended Surveillance
Recommended surveillance is the same as for epithelial ovarian cancer.

UTERINE CANCER

Cancers of the uterus are divided into three main categories: those arising from the endometrium (endometrial cancer), those arising from the myometrium or muscle layer (uterine sarcomas), and those associated with pregnancy (gestational trophoblastic disease).

Endometrial Cancer

Incidence and Risk Factors
Endometrial cancer is the most common malignancy of the female genital tract and the fourth most common cancer among women in the United States (following breast, lung, and colon cancers). Approximately 40,000 new cases are diagnosed annually, and approximately 7,000 women die yearly from this disease. The median age at onset is 63 years, although up to 25% of patients are premenopausal at the time of diagnosis. Up to 10% of cases of endometrial cancer are hereditary. Lynch syndrome/hereditary nonpolyposis colorectal cancer is a hereditary cancer predisposition syndrome characterized by the development of multiple cancers, including endometrial, colorectal, and ovarian cancer. Risk factors for endometrial cancer include nulliparity, early menarche, late menopause, obesity, unopposed estrogen therapy, and chronic diseases such as diabetes mellitus and hypertension.

Pathology
Ninety percent of endometrial cancers are endometrioid adenocarcinomas (70% grade 1, 15% grade 2, and 15% grade 3), 5% to 7% are papillary serous carcinomas, and

the remaining 3% to 5% are clear cell carcinomas. The latter two histologic subtypes are more aggressive, accounting for more than 50% of the recurrences and deaths due to endometrial cancer.

Routes of Spread and Sites of Metastasis
Endometrial cancer metastasizes primarily by myometrial invasion and direct extension to adjacent structures, including the cervix, vagina, and adnexa. Lymphatic embolization and hematogenous dissemination can also occur.

Clinical Features
Patients commonly present complaining of abnormal uterine bleeding or postmenopausal bleeding; approximately 15% of patients with postmenopausal bleeding have uterine cancer. Patients may also experience pelvic pressure and pelvic pain. Other associated findings include pyometra, hematometra, heavy menses, intermenstrual bleeding, and, in some cases, an abnormal Pap smear result. The presence of atypical glandular cells on a Pap smear requires that an endometrial biopsy be performed to rule out malignancy.

Pretreatment Workup
Careful physical examination, including pelvic examination, is required. Pathological confirmation of the disease by endometrial biopsy or dilatation and curettage is essential. Other components of the pretreatment workup include clinical tests (e.g., complete blood cell count, serum glucose, blood urea nitrogen, creatinine, and CA-125), chest radiography, and mammography. Diagnostic tests, including CT, barium enema, proctosigmoidoscopy, cystoscopy, and, in some cases, magnetic resonance imaging (MRI) should be performed as indicated by symptoms or examination findings.

Staging
The surgical staging schema for endometrial cancer is described in Table 19.11. The FIGO grading schema is based on the prevalence of a nonsquamous or nonmorular solid growth pattern (grade 1, 5% or less; grade 2, more than 5% and less than 50%; and grade 3, 50% or higher) (Table 19.12).

TABLE 19.11	Surgical Staging of Endometrial Cancer

Tumor Stage	Description
I	Carcinoma confined to the uterine corpus
IA	Tumor confined to the uterus, no or $<\frac{1}{2}$ myometrial invasion
IB	Tumor confined to the uterus, $>\frac{1}{2}$ myometrial invasion
II	Cervical stromal invasion, but not beyond uterus
III	Extension of the tumor outside the uterus but confined to the true pelvis or para-aortic area
IIIA	Tumor invades serosa or adnexa
IIIB	Vaginal and/or parametrial involvement
IIIC1	Pelvic node involvement
IIIC2	Para-aortic involvement
IV	Distant metastases or involvement of adjacent pelvic organs
IVA	Tumor invasion of the bowel or bladder mucosa
IVB	Distant metastases, including intra-abdominal and/or inguinal lymph nodes

| TABLE 19.12 | International Federation of Gynecology and Obstetrics Grading of Endometrial Cancer |

Tumor Grade	Description
1	≤5%, a nonsquamous or nonmorular solid growth pattern
2	>5%–50%, a nonsquamous or nonmorular solid growth pattern
3	>50%, a nonsquamous or nonmorular solid growth pattern

Treatment

Unless a patient has comorbidities that do not allow for surgical intervention, exploratory laparotomy, hysterectomy, and possibly bilateral salpingo-oophorectomy are required for patients with endometrial cancer. Additional surgical staging biopsies, omentectomy, and lymph node dissection are also recommended in certain cases. Low-risk patients with grade 1 or 2 endometrioid adenocarcinoma with myometrial invasion of 50% or less and a primary tumor diameter of 2 cm or less do not benefit from lymphadenectomy. Furthermore, if lymphadenectomy is performed in high-risk patients (i.e., those with high grade tumors), a systematic clearance of lymph nodes up to the renal vessels is advised.

Up to 20% of patients with endometrial cancer have a synchronous or metastatic ovarian malignancy, so in young patients who want to preserve their ovarian function, the ovaries should be carefully inspected at the time of exploration. After surgical staging, adjuvant chemotherapy, radiation, or both may be indicated. For patients at risk for pelvic or vaginal cancer recurrence, whole pelvic radiotherapy with vaginal brachytherapy has been shown to decrease local recurrence. However, radiation has not been shown to improve overall survival.

Estrogen antagonists and aromatase inhibitors, with a more tolerate side effect profile when compared to conventional chemotherapy, may have a role in the treatment of recurrent and advanced disease.

Prognostic Factors

Tumor stage is the most important prognostic variable for endometrial cancer (Table 19.13). Other prognostic factors are myometrial invasion, lymphovascular space invasion, nuclear grade, histologic subtype, tumor size, patient age, positive peritoneal cytologic findings, hormone receptor status, and type of primary treatment used (surgery vs. radiation therapy).

Recommended Surveillance

Physical and pelvic examinations should be performed every 3 months in the first year after diagnosis, every 4 months in years 2 and 3, every 6 months in years 4 and

| TABLE 19.13 | Five-Year Survival Rates for Patients with Endometrial Cancer, by Tumor Stage |

Tumor Stage	Survival Rate (%)
I	90
II	75
III	40
IV	10

5, and annually thereafter. A Pap smear and chest radiograph should also be obtained annually.

Uterine Sarcomas

Incidence and Risk Factors

Uterine sarcomas account for approximately 3% to 5% of uterine cancers. Most patients have no known risk factors. A small number of patients have a history of pelvic irradiation.

Pathology

Uterine sarcomas arise from mesodermal derivatives that include uterine smooth muscle, endometrial stroma, and blood and lymphatic vessel walls. The number of mitoses per 10 high-power fields, the degree of cytologic atypia, and the presence of coagulative necrosis are the most reliable predictors of biological behavior. This disease is classified according to the types of elements involved (pure, only mesodermal elements present and mixed, both mesodermal and epithelial elements present) and whether malignant mesodermal elements are normally present in the uterus (homologous, only smooth muscle and stroma present and heterologous, striated muscle and cartilage present) (Table 19.14). Half of endometrial sarcomas are carcinosarcomas (formally known as malignant mixed Müllerian tumors). Other common histologic subtypes are leiomyosarcomas (40%) and endometrial stromal sarcomas (8%). Less common subtypes are adenosarcomas, pure heterologous sarcomas, and other variants, which together comprise 1% to 2% of uterine sarcomas.

Routes of Spread and Sites of Metastasis

Sarcomas demonstrate a propensity for early hematogenous dissemination and lymphatic spread. Metastasis is exhibited in one-third of patients.

Pretreatment Workup

Careful physical examination, including pelvic examination, is required. Clinical features of uterine sarcomas are listed in Table 19.15. Endometrial biopsy, dilatation and curettage, or both are essential to providing pathological confirmation of disease. Other components of the pretreatment workup include clinical tests (e.g., complete blood cell count, serum glucose, blood urea nitrogen, creatinine, and liver function), chest radiography, mammography, and cystoscopy or

TABLE 19.14	Classification of Uterine Sarcomas	
Tumor Type	**Homologous**	**Heterologous**
Pure	Leiomyosarcoma Endometrial stromal sarcoma	Rhabdomyosarcoma Chondrosarcoma Osteosarcoma Liposarcoma
Mixed	Carcinosarcoma Previously known as mixed mesodermal (müllerian) sarcoma or malignant mixed mesodermal (müllerian) tumor with homologous components	Mixed mesodermal (müllerian) sarcoma or malignant mixed mesodermal (müllerian) tumor with heterologous components

TABLE 19.15 Clinical Features of Uterine Sarcomas and Basis for Pathological Confirmation of the Disease, by Histologic Subtype

Histologic Subtype	Patient's Age	Signs and Symptoms	Pathological Basis for Confirmation of Disease
Endometrial stromal sarcoma	42–53 y	Vaginal bleeding Uterine enlargement Lower abdominal pain or pressure	EMB or D&C
Leiomyosarcoma	45–55 y	Vaginal bleeding Rapid uterine enlargement Lower abdominal pain or pressure	Preoperative diagnosis is difficult: only 15% diagnosed by EMB or D&C
Carcinosarcoma	65–75 y	Several factors in common with endometrial cancer (e.g., nulliparity, obesity, and diabetes) Vaginal bleeding Uterine enlargement	EMB or D&C; in up to 50% of cases, the tumor protrudes through the cervix
Adenosarcoma	Any age, but most common in the fifth decade of life	Vaginal bleeding Uterine enlargement	EMB or D&C; in up to 50% of cases, the tumor protrudes through the cervix

EMB, endometrial biopsy; D&C, dilatation and curettage.

proctoscopy, depending on the site and extent of the lesion. Preoperative medical clearance is necessary for patients with chronic disease or other appropriate indications.

Staging
In 2009, FIGO defined surgical staging criteria specifically for uterine sarcomas in order to better reflect its clinical behavior (Table 19.16).

Treatment
Surgical excision is the only treatment of curative value. Pelvic radiation therapy has a role in local control of the tumor, but because of the propensity of uterine

TABLE 19.16 Surgical Staging of Uterine Sarcomas (Leiomyosarcoma, Endometrial Stromal Sarcoma, and Adenosarcoma

Tumor Stage	Description
IA	Tumor limited to uterus <5 cm
IB	Tumor limited to uterus >5 cm
IIA	Tumor extends to the pelvis, adnexal involvement
IIB	Tumor extends to extra-uterine pelvic tissue
IIIA	Tumor invades abdominal tissues, one site
IIIB	Tumor invades abdominal tissues, more than one site
IIIC	Metastasis to pelvic and/or para-aortic lymph nodes
IVA	Tumor invades bladder and/or rectum
IVB	Distant metastasis
Adenosarcoma Stage I Differs from the Other Uterine Sarcomas	
IA	Tumor limited to endometrium/endocervix
IB	Tumor limited to the uterus, invasion to <½ myometrium
IC	Tumor limited to the uterus, invasion to >½ myometrium

sarcomas for early hematogenous spread, this treatment does not affect outcome. Leiomyosarcomas generally do not respond to radiation therapy. Cisplatin, doxorubicin, and ifosfamide have shown some activity against uterine sarcomas; leiomyosarcomas are more sensitive to doxorubicin. However, there is emerging evidence to support the use of gemcitabine and docetaxel in the treatment of leiomyosarcoma. There may be some benefit to hormonal therapy with megestrol acetate; tamoxifen is recommended in cases where hormone receptors have been identified. Hormonal therapy is the treatment of choice for low-grade endometrial stromal sarcomas.

Prognostic Factors
The most important prognostic factor for uterine sarcomas is tumor stage: Diagnosis at stage I has a 5-year survival rate of 50%, whereas diagnosis at any other stage has a 5-year survival rate of 15% or less (Table 19.17). Sarcomatous overgrowth and deep myometrial invasion must be considered in cases of adenosarcoma because they adversely affect prognosis.

Recommended Surveillance
Physical and pelvic examinations should be performed every 3 months for 2 years after diagnosis, then every 6 months in years 3 through 5, and annually thereafter. A chest radiograph should also be obtained annually.

TABLE 19.17 Five-Year Survival Rates for Uterine Sarcomas, by Tumor Stage

Tumor Stage	Survival Rate (%)
I	50
II–IV	≤15

Gestational Trophoblastic Disease

Incidence and Risk Factors

Gestational trophoblastic disease is characterized by an abnormal proliferation of trophoblastic tissue; all forms develop in association with pregnancy. Because this disease is associated with a gestational event, the age of occurrence spans the entire reproductive spectrum. In the United States, hydatidiform moles occur in 1 in 600 therapeutic abortions and 1 in 1,000 to 2,000 pregnancies; of these, approximately 20% develop malignant sequelae, including invasive moles, placental site trophoblastic tumors, and gestational choriocarcinoma. Choriocarcinoma is estimated to occur in 1 in 20,000 to 40,000 pregnancies. One-half of these cases follow term gestations, one-fourth follow molar gestations, and one-fourth follow other gestational events.

A number of well-established risk factors are positively associated with hydatidiform mole. These include age younger than 20 years or older than 40 years, previous molar pregnancy (women who have had one molar pregnancy have a 0.5% to 2.5% risk of a second occurrence, and women who have had two molar pregnancies have a 33% risk of a third occurrence), previous spontaneous abortion (the risk increases with each subsequent spontaneous abortion), and Asian race. Black race is negatively associated with hydatidiform mole.

Pathology

Gestational trophoblastic disease is categorized as hydatidiform mole, invasive mole, placental site trophoblastic tumor, and choriocarcinoma. Nonmetastatic disease after molar evacuation may be hydatidiform (invasive) mole or choriocarcinoma. Gestational trophoblastic disease persisting after a nonmolar pregnancy is predominantly choriocarcinoma or, rarely, placental site trophoblastic tumor. Metastatic gestational trophoblastic disease diagnosed in the early months after molar evacuation may be hydatidiform mole or choriocarcinoma. When gestational trophoblastic disease is found remote from a gestational event, it is characteristically choriocarcinoma.

Routes of Spread and Sites of Metastasis

Malignant gestational trophoblastic disease spreads primarily by hematogenous route. The most frequent site of metastasis is in the lung (80%). Other common sites are the vagina (30%), pelvis (20%), brain (10%), liver (10%), and bowel, kidney, and spleen (less than 5% each).

Clinical Features

Hydatidiform Mole. Vaginal bleeding, uterus size larger than expected for gestational age, and the presence of prominent theca lutein ovarian cysts are characteristic clinical features of hydatidiform mole. Features of partial and complete hydatidiform moles are listed in Table 19.18. Other associated findings include toxemia, hyperemesis, hyperthyroidism, and respiratory symptoms such as dyspnea and respiratory distress. Patients with partial moles may present in the same manner as those with missed or incomplete abortions: vaginal bleeding and the passage of tissue through the vagina.

Malignant Gestational Trophoblastic Disease. Malignant gestational trophoblastic disease can be categorized as nonmetastatic or locally invasive, or as metastatic. The clinical features of molar pregnancy and the associated incidences of malignant gestational trophoblastic disease are shown in Table 19.19.

Pretreatment Workup for Molar Pregnancy

Careful physical examination, including pelvic examination, is required. Other components of the pretreatment workup include clinical tests (e.g., complete

Classification of Hydatidiform Moles

Feature	Complete Mole	Partial Mole
Hydatidiform swelling of villi	Diffuse	Focal
Trophoblast	Cytotrophoblastic and syncytial hyperplasia	Syncytial hyperplasia
Embryo	Absent	Present
Villous capillaries	No fetal red blood cells	Many fetal red blood cells
Gestational age at diagnosis	8–16 wk	10–22 wk
β-hCG concentration	Usually >50,000 mIU/mL	Usually >50,000 mIU/mL
Proportion that progress to choriocarcinoma	15%–25%	5%–10%
Karyotype	46XX (95%), 46XY (5%)	Triploid (80%)
Uterine size for gestational dates		
Small	33%	65%
Large	33%	10%

β-hCG, beta subunit of human chorionic gonadotropin.

blood cell count, serum glucose, blood urea nitrogen, creatinine, liver function, serum albumin, thyroid function tests, serum β-hCG [in less than 5% of cases, the β-hCG antigen titer may be elevated without clinical or radiographic evidence of disease]) and chest radiography.

Metastatic Workup for Malignant or Persistent Gestational Trophoblastic Disease

Metastatic workup for malignant or persistent gestational trophoblastic disease consists of the tests described for molar pregnancy plus pelvic sonography; CT scan of the abdomen, pelvis, brain, and chest; and MRI of the brain. Metastatic lesions

Clinical Features of Molar Pregnancy and Associated Incidences of Malignant Gestational Trophoblastic Disease

Clinical Feature	Incidence of Malignant Gestational Trophoblastic Disease (%)
Delayed postmolar evacuation hemorrhage	75
Theca lutein cyst >5 cm	60
Acute pulmonary insufficiency after mole evacuation	58
Uterus large for gestational dates	45
Serum β-hCG concentration >100,000 mIU/mL	45
Second molar gestation	40
Maternal age >40 y	25

β-hCG, beta subunit of human chorionic gonadotropin.

International Federation of Gynecology and Obstetrics Staging of Gestational Trophoblastic Disease	
Tumor Stage	**Description**
I	Confined to the uterine corpus
II	Metastasis to the pelvis and vagina
III	Metastasis to the lung
IV	Distant metastasis to the brain, liver, kidneys, or gastrointestinal tract

(e.g., a vaginal nodule) should not be biopsied because these lesions are very vascular and patients have exsanguinated from such biopsies.

Staging

The FIGO staging schema of gestational trophoblastic disease is outlined in Table 19.20.

Treatment

Molar Pregnancy. Dilation and curettage is the standard treatment for molar pregnancy and is followed by close monitoring of the β-hCG antigen titer. Hysterectomy may be performed if fertility is not an issue.

Nonmetastatic Gestational Trophoblastic Disease (Figo Stage I). If preserving fertility is not a consideration, a total hysterectomy can be offered. If preserving fertility is desirable, adjuvant single-agent chemotherapy with methotrexate is the most common treatment choice. Chemotherapy should be continued until at least one menstrual cycle beyond normalization of the β-hCG antigen titer. If there is disease resistance (i.e., the β-hCG antigen titer increases or plateaus), the patient should be treated with an alternate single agent, most commonly dactinomycin. If resistance persists, combination chemotherapy with EMA-CO (etoposide, methotrexate, dactinomycin, cyclophosphamide, and vincristine) or MAC (methotrexate, actinomycin, and cyclophosphamide) should be administered.

Metastatic Gestational Trophoblastic Disease (Figo Stages II to IV): Low-Risk Disease (World Health Organization Risk Score 0 to 6). For initial treatment, patients generally receive single-agent therapy with methotrexate. If there is disease resistance, the patient should be treated with an alternate single agent, typically dactinomycin. If resistance persists, combination chemotherapy with EMA-CO or MAC should be administered. If there is resistance to EMA-CO and MAC, salvage therapy includes the combination of cisplatin, bleomycin, and vinblastine. Ifosfamide may have a role in refractory cases.

High-Risk Disease (World Health Organization Risk Score 7 or Higher). Combination chemotherapy is the treatment of choice. EMA-CO is the initial chemotherapeutic regimen, and cisplatin, bleomycin, and vinblastine are used as salvage treatment.

Special Considerations. Patients with brain metastases may be treated with radiotherapy for local control and prophylaxis against hemorrhage. Patients with residual solitary liver or lung lesions may be candidates for surgical resection.

TABLE 19.21 Prognostic Indicators for Patients with Gestational Trophoblastic Disease, by World Health Organization Prognostic Index Score

Prognostic Indicator	World Health Organization Prognostic Index Score			
	0	1	2	4
Age (y)	<39	>39		
Type of antecedent pregnancy	Hydatidiform mole	Abortion	Term	—
Interval between antecedent pregnancy and start of chemotherapy (mo)	<4	4–6	7–12	>12
β-hCG concentration (mIU/mL)	<10^3	10^3–10^4	10^4–10^5	>10^5
Diameter of largest tumor (cm)		3–5	>5	—
Site of metastasis	Lung, vagina, pelvis	Spleen, kidney	Gastrointestinal tract, liver	Brain
Number of metastases identified	0	1–4	4–8	>8
Prior chemotherapy			1 drug	≥2 drugs

β-hCG, beta subunit of human chorionic gonadotropin.
Low risk 0–6, high risk >6.

Prognostic Factors

Factors that may affect a patient's prognosis and response to treatment are outlined in Table 19.21. The cure rate for stage I, II, and III disease is greater than 80%, whereas the cure rate for stage IV disease is approximately 50%.

Recommended Surveillance

Surveillance is essentially the same for all cases of gestational trophoblastic disease, except for patients with stage IV disease, who require a longer period of surveillance. β-hCG antigen titers are measured weekly until the level is normal for 3 consecutive weeks and then measured monthly until the level is normal for 12 consecutive months. Patients with stage IV disease are typically followed for 24 months after normalization of β-hCG antigen titer values. Contraception is mandatory throughout the follow-up period.

Management of Incidental Uterine Masses Found at Laparotomy

The finding of an enlarged or abnormal uterus at the time of exploratory laparotomy or surgery for an unrelated condition can pose a therapeutic dilemma to the surgeon. Uterine fibroids, which are benign tumors of the uterus, are the most common cause of uterine enlargement. In most cases, immediate surgical intervention is unnecessary. Unless the situation is life threatening, hysterectomy and bilateral salpingo-oophorectomy should be performed only after proper informed consent has been obtained, especially in women of childbearing age.

Laparoscopy for the Management of Endometrial Cancer

The use of laparoscopy in the staging of endometrial cancers has gained popularity, and at many institutions it is now the preferred surgical approach. With this approach, a thorough inspection of the peritoneal cavity, peritoneal washings (only if required by study protocols), and appropriate staging biopsies are still important. Laparoscopy has been compared with laparotomy for comprehensive surgical staging of endometrial cancer in a multicenter collaborative trial (GOG LAP2). This study established that the laparoscopic approach is not only feasible and safe but also results in fewer complications and shorter hospital stays.

CERVICAL CANCER

Incidence and Risk Factors

Approximately 500,000 women worldwide develop cervical cancer each year. It is the most common cause of cancer-related death among women in underdeveloped countries. In the United States, an estimated 10,000 new cases of cervical cancer and 4,000 deaths due to this disease occur annually.

Cervical cancer is a sexually transmitted disease. It was the first solid tumor to be linked to a virus: infection with human papillomavirus, specifically types 16 and 18, is associated with the development of this disease. Other risk factors include early age at first intercourse, multiple sexual partners, multiparity, smoking, and other behaviors associated with exposure to the human papillomavirus. Half of women with newly diagnosed invasive cervical cancer have never had a Pap smear, and another 10% have not had a Pap smear in the previous 5 years.

Pathology

Eighty-five percent of cervical cancers are squamous cell carcinomas, and 10% to 15% are adenocarcinomas, including the less common adenosquamous subtype. Rare histologic subtypes include small cell tumors, sarcomas, lymphomas, and melanomas.

Routes of Spread and Sites of Metastasis

Cervical cancer spreads through various mechanisms. It can directly invade surrounding structures, including the parametria, the corpus, and the vagina. Lymphatic spread commonly occurs in an orderly and predictable sequence involving the parametrial, pelvic, iliac, and finally para-aortic lymph nodes. Hematogenous metastases and intraperitoneal implantation can also occur.

Clinical Features

Symptoms. Discharge and abnormal bleeding, including postcoital, intermenstrual, menorrhagia, and postmenopausal bleeding, are often the first signs of cervical cancer. Frequent voiding and pain on urination can also occur and may indicate advanced disease.

Physical Findings. Findings on examination vary depending on the site of the lesion (endocervix or ectocervix). Careful inspection and palpation, including bimanual and rectovaginal examinations, are required to determine the size and extent of the lesion.

Pretreatment Workup

Careful physical examination must be performed, including pelvic examination and biopsy of the lesion. Other components of the pretreatment workup include clinical tests (e.g., complete blood cell count, serum glucose, blood urea nitrogen, creatinine, liver function), chest radiography, and mammography.

Cervical cancer is staged by the results of the clinical examination. Therefore, unlike endometrial and ovarian cancer, staging is performed before treatment planning and not at the time of diagnosis. The following studies should be performed for patients with stage IB2 to stage IV cervical cancer: cystoscopy, proctoscopy, intravenous pyelography (or CT of the abdomen or pelvis), and chest X-ray or CT. MRI may be useful, especially in distinguishing endometrial and endocervical lesions.

Staging
The clinical staging scheme for cervical cancer is outlined in Table 19.22. The term microinvasive cervical cancer is sometimes used interchangeably with stage IA lesions. This diagnosis must be made from a cone biopsy or hysterectomy specimen.

Treatment

Stage IA1. Lesions that qualify as microinvasive disease may be treated conservatively with simple hysterectomy, cervical conization in cases where maintenance of

TABLE 19.22 Clinical Staging of Cervical Cancer

Tumor Stage	Description
I	Lesions generally confined to the cervix; uterine involvement is disregarded
IA	Preclinical cervical cancers diagnosed by microscopic analysis alone
IA1	Stromal invasion ≤3 mm deep and ≤7 mm wide
IA2	Stromal invasion >3 mm but ≤5 mm deep and ≤7 mm wide
IB	Lesions larger than stage IA lesions, regardless of whether seen clinically
IB1	Clinical lesions ≤4 cm
IB2	Clinical lesions >4 cm
II	Extension beyond the cervix but not to the pelvic sidewall or the lower third of the vagina
IIA1	Involvement of the upper two-third of the vagina, without parametrial invasion, <4 cm in greatest dimension
IIA2	Involvement of the upper two-third of the vagina, without parametrial invasion, >4 cm in greatest dimension
IIB	With parametrial involvement
III	Extension to the pelvic wall with no cancer-free space between the tumor and the pelvic wall; tumor involving the lower third of the vagina; hydronephrosis or nonfunctioning kidney unless secondary to an unrelated cause
IIIA	Involvement of the lower third of the vagina; no extension to the pelvic sidewall
IIIB	Extension to the pelvic wall, hydronephrosis, or nonfunctioning kidney
IV	Extension beyond the true pelvis or clinical involvement of the mucosa of the bladder or rectum
IVA	Spread to adjacent organs
IVB	Spread to distant organs

fertility is an issue, or intracavitary radiation therapy for patients who do not qualify for surgery.

Stage IA2. Lesions that have >3 mm of invasion are significantly more likely to recur when treated conservatively; therefore, radical hysterectomy and lymph node dissection or radiation therapy should be performed.

Stages IB and IIA. Surgery or chemosensitizing radiation therapy results in similar cure rates when patients are carefully selected; patients with squamous lesions 4 to 5 cm in diameter and adenocarcinomas smaller than 3 cm in diameter are potential surgical candidates. The standard surgical option is radical hysterectomy with pelvic lymph node dissection. Nonsurgical management may include sensitizing radiation therapy with weekly chemotherapy and 40 to 45 Gy external-beam irradiation followed by two intracavitary brachytherapy. Among patients who undergo surgery, chemoradiation is used postoperatively in those believed to be at high risk for disease recurrence. Simple hysterectomy after pelvic radiation therapy is indicated primarily for patients whose tumors respond slowly to radiation therapy or when pelvic anatomy precludes optimal intracavitary placement.

Stages IIB to IVA. Radiation therapy is the treatment of choice for locally advanced disease. Surgery may be used as adjuvant therapy for stage IVA disease without parametrial involvement and in cases of central disease persisting after radiation therapy.

Stage IVB. Stage IVB disease is treated primarily with chemotherapy because the disease is disseminated. Platinum-based chemotherapy regimen remains the treatment cornerstone for advanced cervix cancer. In investigational settings, biologic therapy, particularly anti-angiogenic agents such as bevacizumab, is being used in combination with a cytotoxic agent for treatment. Radiation therapy may be used in certain cases for local control and palliation of symptoms.

Recurrent Disease

Treatment of recurrent cervical cancer depends on the location of the disease and the type of primary treatment the patient received. Central recurrence may be managed with pelvic exenteration if there are no contraindications. Patients who have had prior radiation therapy and extensive pelvic recurrence or distant metastatic disease are treated with systemic chemotherapy.

Prognostic Factors

The most important prognostic factors for stage I disease include lymphovascular space involvement, tumor size, depth of invasion, and presence of lymph node metastases (Table 19.23). For patients with stage II to IV disease, tumor stage, presence of lymph node metastases, tumor volume, age, and the patient's performance status are key prognostic factors. The survival rates for patients with cervical cancer are shown in Table 19.24. Among patients who have recurrent cervical cancer, more than 50% are diagnosed with the recurrence within 1 year after primary treatment is completed. Seventy-five percent of patients are diagnosed with their recurrent disease within 2 years, and 95% within 5 years.

Recommended Surveillance

Physical and pelvic examinations should be performed every 3 months in the first year after diagnosis, every 4 months in years 2 and 3, every 6 months in years 4 and 5,

TABLE 19.23 Incidence of Cervical Cancer Lymph Node Metastasis, by Tumor Stage

Tumor Stage	Incidence (%) as Indicated by Lymph Node Metastasis	
	Pelvic	Para-Aortic
I		
IA1	0	
IA2 (lesion 1–3 mm in diameter)	0.6	0
IA2 (lesion 3–5 mm in diameter)	4.8	<1
IB	15.9	2.2
II		
IIA	24.5	11
IIB	31.4	19
III	44.8	30
IVA	55	40

and annually thereafter. A Pap smear and chest radiograph should also be obtained annually.

VULVAR CANCER

Incidence and Risk Factors

Vulvar cancer accounts for 3% to 5% of gynecologic malignancies and 1% of malignancies in women. Between 2,000 and 3,000 new cases are diagnosed annually in the United States. The incidence of vulvar cancer tends to be bimodally distributed. Most cases are solitary lesions that occur in postmenopausal women, and the tumors are often associated with chronic vulvar dystrophy. Recently, a subset of tumors has been identified in a younger population; these tumors tend to be multifocal and are associated with human papillomavirus infection.

The cause of vulvar cancer appears to be multifactorial. Risk factors include human papillomavirus infection (although the association is not as strong as that

TABLE 19.24 Five-Year Survival Rates for Patients with Cervical Cancer, by Tumor Stage and Histologic Subtype

Tumor Stage and Histologic Subtype	Survival Rate (%)
Stage I	
Squamous	65–90
Adenocarcinoma	70–75
Stage II	
Squamous	45–80
Adenocarcinoma	30–40
Stage III	
Squamous	≤60
Adenocarcinoma	20–30
Stage IV (both types)	<15

TABLE 19.25	Surgical Staging of Vulvar Cancer

Tumor Stage	Description
IA	Lesion ≤2 cm in size and stromal invasion ≤1 mm; negative nodes
IB	Lesion >2 cm in size and stromal invasion >1 mm; negative nodes
II	Tumor of any size with adjacent spread (1/3 lower urethra, 1/3 lower vagina, anus); negative nodes
IIIA1	1 lymph node metastasis ≥5 mm
IIIA2	1–2 lymph node metastasis(es) <5 mm
IIIB1	2 or more lymph nodes metastases ≥5 mm
IIIB2	3 or more lymph node metastases <5 mm
IIIC	Positive node(s) with extracapsular spread
IVA1	Tumor invades other regional structures (2/3 upper urethra, 2/3 upper vagina), bladder mucosa, rectal mucosa, or fixed to pelvic bone
IVA2	Fixed or ulcerated inguinofemoral lymph nodes
IVB	Any distant metastasis, including to the pelvic nodes

with cervical cancer), advanced age, low socioeconomic status, hypertension, diabetes mellitus, prior lower genital tract malignancy (e.g., cervical cancer), and immunosuppression (Table 19.25).

Pathology
Eighty-five percent of vulvar malignancies are squamous cell carcinomas, and 8% are malignant melanomas. Less common histologic subtypes include basal cell carcinomas, Bartholin gland carcinomas, Paget disease, and adenocarcinomas arising from sweat glands.

Routes of Spread and Sites of Metastasis
Vulvar cancer spreads by direct extension to the vagina, urethra, and rectum. Embolization to regional lymphatics (e.g., the groin) and hematogenous spread to distant sites can also occur.

Clinical Features

Symptoms. Chronic pruritus, ulceration, and nodules on the vulva are the most common presenting symptoms of this disease.

Physical Findings. Lesions may arise from the labia majora (40%), labia minora (20%), periclitoral area (10%), and perineum or posterior fourchette (15%). Lesions may appear as a dominant mass, warty area, ulcerated area, or thickened white epithelium.

Diagnosis
Five percent of cases are multifocal. Any suspicious area must undergo biopsy, using a Keyes punch biopsy and lidocaine without epinephrine for anesthesia.

Pretreatment Workup
Careful physical examination, including pelvic examination and measurement of the lesion, is required. Other components of the pretreatment workup include

clinical tests (e.g., complete blood cell count, serum glucose, blood urea nitrogen, creatinine, liver function), chest radiography, mammography, and cystoscopy or proctoscopy, depending on the site and extent of the lesion. Barium enema, CT, and MRI should be performed if indicated. Preoperative medical clearance is necessary for patients with chronic disease or other appropriate indications.

Staging
In 2009, FIGO updated vulvar staging criteria to better reflect the clinical and prognostic factors related to this disease.

Treatment
Stage I. Wide local excision should be performed if the lesion has less than 1 mm of invasion into the underlying tissue. Wide radical excision with a traditional 2-cm gross margin (measured with a ruler) and superficial dissection of the ipsilateral groin are appropriate for all other stage I lesions. Bilateral superficial groin dissection should be performed if the lesion is within 2 cm of the midline.

Stage II. Radical vulvectomy with dissection of bilateral nodes, including superficial and deep inguinal nodes, is the standard approach to stage II disease. The local recurrence rate is similar when the more conservative approach of radical wide excision is used instead of radical vulvectomy. Adjuvant radiation therapy may be indicated if the tumor-free margin of resection is less than 8 mm, the tumor is thicker than 5 mm, or the lymphovascular space invasion is present.

Stage III. Treatment must be individualized for each patient with stage III disease. Options include surgery, radiation, and a combination of treatment modalities. A modified radical vulvectomy (or a radical wide local excision) with inguinal and femoral node dissection can be performed; pelvic and groin radiation therapy should be administered if positive groin nodes are found. Preoperative radiation therapy (with or without radiation-sensitizing chemotherapy) can be given to increase the operability of the lesion and decrease the extent of resection and is followed by radical excision with bilateral superficial and deep groin node dissection. Radiation therapy alone is an option if the patient is ineligible for radical surgery or the lesion appears to be inoperable.

Stage IV. Treatment of stage IV disease must also be individualized. Options include radical vulvectomy and pelvic exenteration, radical vulvectomy followed by radiation therapy, preoperative radiation therapy (with or without radiation-sensitizing chemotherapy) followed by radical surgical excision, and radiation therapy (with or without radiation-sensitizing chemotherapy) if the patient is ineligible for surgery or the lesion is deemed inoperable.

Recurrent Disease
Treatment of recurrent disease depends on the site and extent of the recurrence. Options include radical wide excision with or without radiation therapy (depending on prior treatment and extent of recurrence), groin node debulking followed by radiation therapy (depending on prior treatment), and pelvic exenteration. Regional or distant metastasis is difficult to treat, and palliative therapy is often the only option.

Prognostic Factors
The prognostic factors for vulvar carcinoma are various. Inguinal node metastasis appears to be the single most important prognostic variable. Other factors

TABLE 19.26	Five-Year Survival Rates for Patients with Vulvar Cancer, by Tumor Stage	
Tumor Stage	**Survival Rate (%)**	
I	95	
II	75–85	
III	5	
IV		
IVA	20	
IVB	5	

include lymphovascular space invasion, tumor stage (Table 19.26), lesion size, lesion site, histologic grade, and depth of invasion.

Recommended Surveillance
Physical and pelvic examinations should be performed every 3 months the first year, every 4 months in years 2 and 3, every 6 months in years 4 and 5, and annually thereafter. A Pap smear should be performed annually.

VAGINAL CANCER

Incidence and Risk Factors
Primary vaginal cancer represents 1% to 2% of malignancies of the female genital tract. The average age at diagnosis is 60 years. Most vaginal neoplasms represent metastases from another primary source.

Risk factors associated with vaginal cancer include low socioeconomic status, history of human papillomavirus infection, chronic vaginal irritation, prior abnormal Pap smear result with cervical intraepithelial neoplasia, prior hysterectomy (59% of patients with primary vaginal cancer), prior treatment for cervical cancer, and in utero exposure to diethylstilbestrol during the first half of pregnancy. Diethylstilbestrol was used from 1940 to 1971 to prevent pregnancy complications such as threatened abortion and prematurity. Clear cell carcinoma of the vagina developed in approximately 1 in 1,000 women exposed to diethylstilbestrol in utero. Since this agent is no longer available, the incidence of this disease has dramatically declined.

Pathology
Eighty-five percent of vaginal cancers are squamous cell neoplasms. Other histologic subtypes include adenocarcinoma (9%), sarcoma (6%), melanoma (<1%), and clear cell carcinoma (<1%).

Routes of Spread and Sites of Metastasis
Vaginal cancer metastasizes via direct extension to adjacent structures. It can also spread through a well-established lymphatic drainage distribution. Lesions of the upper two-thirds of the vagina metastasize directly to pelvic lymph nodes, and lesions of the lower third of the vagina metastasize primarily to the inguinofemoral nodes and secondarily to pelvic nodes. Hematogenous spread is likely a late occurrence because, in most cases, the disease is confined primarily to the pelvis.

Clinical Features

Symptoms. Painless vaginal bleeding and vaginal discharge are the primary symptoms associated with vaginal cancer. Bladder symptoms, tenesmus, and pelvic pain, which are usually indicative of locally advanced disease, are less commonly seen.

Physical Findings. Lesions are located primarily in the upper third of the vagina, usually on the posterior wall. The appearance of lesions varies. Surface ulceration is usually not present, except in advanced cases. Visualization of lesions identified by Pap smear may require colposcopy.

Pretreatment Workup
Careful physical examination, including pelvic examination with colposcopy, is required unless the lesion is visible. Other components of the pretreatment workup include clinical tests (e.g., complete blood cell count, serum glucose, blood urea nitrogen, creatinine, and liver function), chest radiography, mammography, and cystoscopy or proctoscopy, depending on the site and extent of the lesion. Barium enema, CT, and MRI should be performed if indicated. Preoperative medical clearance is necessary for patients with chronic disease or other appropriate indications.

Staging
The clinical staging scheme for vaginal cancers is outlined in Table 19.27.

Treatment

Stage 0. Stage 0 disease may be treated by surgical excision, laser ablation, and, in some cases, topical 5-fluorouracil.

Stage I. Lesions of the upper vaginal fornices may be treated with radical hysterectomy and lymphadenectomy or with radiation therapy alone. All stage I lesions (including lesions of the upper vaginal fornices) may be treated with radiation therapy, usually in the form of an intracavitary cylinder.

Stages II to IV. External-beam radiation therapy and intracavitary or interstitial radiation therapy are used for stage II to stage IV disease. If the tumor involves the

TABLE 19.27 Clinical Staging of Vaginal Cancer

Tumor Stage	Description
0	Carcinoma in situ, intraepithelial carcinoma
I	Carcinoma limited to the vaginal wall
II	Carcinoma involving subvaginal tissue but not extending to the pelvic wall
III	Extension to the pelvic wall
IV	Extension beyond the true pelvis, or involvement of the bladder or rectal mucosa
IVA	Spread to adjacent organs and/or direct extension beyond the pelvis
IVB	Spread to distant organs

TABLE 19.28	Five-Year Survival Rates for Patients with Vaginal Cancer, by Tumor Stage

Tumor Stage	Survival Rate (%)
I	80
II	45
III	35
IV	10

lower third of the vagina, radiation to the groin nodes should be included in the treatment plan.

Recurrent Disease
Treatment of recurrent vaginal cancer depends on the extent of recurrence. Options include wide local excision, partial vaginectomy, and exenteration. Chemotherapy may be given for distant metastatic disease; however, the efficacy of chemotherapy is not well known because of the rarity of the disease.

Prognostic Factors
The most important prognostic factor for vaginal cancer is the tumor stage (Table 19.28).

Recommended Surveillance
Physical and pelvic examinations should be performed every 3 months the first year, every 4 months in years 2 and 3, every 6 months in years 4 and 5, and annually thereafter. A Pap smear should be performed annually.

Recommended Readings

Epithelial Ovarian Cancer

Berek JS, Hacker NF. *Practical Gynecologic Oncology*. 3rd ed. Baltimore, MD: Williams & Wilkins; 2000.

Cannistra SA. Cancer of the ovary. *N Engl J Med*. 1993;329:1550.

Dembo AJ, Davy M, Stenwig AE. Prognostic factors in patients with stage I epithelial ovarian cancer. *Obstet Gynecol*. 1990;75:263.

Einzig AI, Wiernik PH, Sasloff J, et al. Phase II study and long-term follow-up of patients treated with taxol for advanced ovarian adenocarcinoma. *J Clin Oncol*. 1992;10:1748.

Eisenhauer EA, ten Bokkel Huinink WW, Swenerton KD, et al. European-Canadian randomized trial of paclitaxel in relapsed ovarian cancer: high-dose versus low-dose and long versus short infusion. *J Clin Oncol*. 1994;12:2654.

Flam F, Einhorn N, Sjovall K. Symptomatology of ovarian cancer. *Eur J Obstet Gynecol Reprod Biol*. 1988;27:53.

Gershenson DM, Mitchell MF, Atkinson N, et al. The effect of prolonged cisplatin-based chemotherapy on progression-free survival in patients with optimal epithelial ovarian cancer: "maintenance" therapy reconsidered. *Gynecol Oncol*. 1992; 47:7.

Goff BA, Mandel LS, Melancon CH, et al. Frequency of symptoms of ovarian cancer in women presenting to primary care clinics. *JAMA*. 2004;291:2705.

Goodman HM, Harlow BL, Sheets EE, et al. The role of cytoreductive surgery in the management of stage IV epithelial ovarian carcinoma. *Gynecol Oncol*. 1992;46: 367.

Han LY, Kipps E, Kaye SB. Current treatment and clinical trials in ovarian cancer. *Expert Opin Investig Drug* 2010;10:521.

Hakes TB, Chalas E, Hoskins WJ, et al. Randomized prospective trial of 5 versus 10 cycles of cyclophosphamide, doxorubicin, and cisplatin in advanced ovarian carcinoma. *Gynecol Oncol.* 1992;45:284.

Heintz APM, Hacker NF, Lagasse LD. Epidemiology and etiology of ovarian cancer: a review. *Obstet Gynecol.* 1985;66:127.

Hogberg T, Kagedal B. Long-term follow-up of ovarian cancer with monthly determinations of serum CA 125. *Gynecol Oncol.* 1992;46:191.

Hoskins WJ. Surgical staging and cytoreductive surgery of epithelial ovarian cancer. *Cancer.* 1993;71(4, suppl):1534.

Hoskins WJ, Bundy BN, Thigpen JT, et al. The influence of cytoreductive surgery on recurrence-free interval and survival in small-volume stage III epithelial ovarian cancer: a Gynecologic Oncology Group study. *Gynecol Oncol.* 1992; 47:159.

Hoskins WJ, McGuire WP, Brady MF, et al. The effect of diameter of largest residual disease on survival after primary cytoreductive surgery in patients with suboptimal residual epithelial ovarian carcinoma. *Am J Obstet Gynecol.* 1994; 170:974.

Kohn EC, Sarosy G, Bicher A, et al. Dose-intense taxol: high response rate in patients with platinum-resistant recurrent ovarian cancer. *J Natl Cancer Inst.* 1994;86:18.

Krag KJ, Canellos GP, Griffiths CT, et al. Predictive factors for long term survival in patients with advanced ovarian cancer. *Gynecol Oncol.* 1989;34:88.

Landen CN, Birrer MJ, Sood, AK. Early events in the pathogenesis of epithelial ovarian cancer. *J Clin Oncol.* 2008;26:495.

Lynch HT, Watson P, Lynch JF, et al. Hereditary ovarian cancer: heterogeneity in age at onset. *Cancer* 1993;71(2 suppl):573.

Martinez A, Schray MF, Howes AE, et al. Postoperative radiation therapy for epithelial ovarian cancer: the curative role based on a 24-year experience. *J Clin Oncol.* 1985;3:901.

McGuire WP, Hoskins WJ, Brady MF, et al. Cyclophosphamide and cisplatin compared with paclitaxel and cisplatin in patients with stage III and stage IV ovarian cancer. *N Engl J Med.* 1996;334:1.

Morris M, Gershenson DM, Wharton JT, et al. Secondary cytoreductive surgery for recurrent epithelial ovarian cancer. *Gynecol Oncol.* 1989;34:334.

NIH Consensus Conference. Ovarian cancer: screening treatment, and follow-up. *JAMA.* 1995;273:491.

Omura GA, Brady MF, Homesley HD, et al. Long-term follow-up and prognostic factor analysis in advanced ovarian carcinoma: the Gynecologic Oncology Group experience. *J Clin Oncol.* 1991;9:1138.

Omura GA, Bundy BN, Berek JS, et al. Randomized trial of cyclophosphamide plus cisplatin with or without doxorubicin in ovarian carcinoma: a Gynecologic Oncology Group study. *J Clin Oncol.* 1989;7:457.

Pecorelli S, Bolis G, Colombo N, et al. Adjuvant therapy in early ovarian cancer: results of two randomized trials. *Gynecol Oncol.* 1994;52:102.

Pettersson F. *Annual Report of the Results of Treatment in Gynecologic Cancer. International Federation of Gynecology and Obstetrics,* vol. 20. Stockholm: Panoramic Press; 1988.

Piver MS, Baker TR, Jishi MF, et al. Familial ovarian cancer: a report of 658 families from the Gilda Radner Familial Ovarian Cancer Registry 1981–1991. *Cancer.* 1993; 71(2 suppl):582.

Piver MS, Malfetano J, Baker TR, et al. Five-year survival for stage IC or stage I, grade 3 epithelial ovarian cancer treated with cisplatin-based chemotherapy. *Gynecol Oncol.* 1992;46:357.

Potter ME, Partridge EE, Hatch KD, et al. Primary surgical therapy of ovarian cancer: how much and when? *Gynecol Oncol.* 1991;40:195.

Sigurdsson K, Alm P, Gullberg B. Prognostic factors in malignant ovarian tumors. *Gynecol Oncol.* 1983;15:370.

Trimble EL, Arbuck SG, McGuire WP. Options for primary chemotherapy of epithelial ovarian cancer: taxanes. *Gynecol Oncol.* 1994;55:S114.

van der Burg ME, van Lent M, Buyse M, et al. The effect of debulking surgery after induction chemotherapy on the prognosis in advanced epithelial ovarian cancer. *N Engl J Med.* 1995;332:629.

Vergote I, Trope CG, Amant F, et al. Neoadjuvant chemotherapy or primary surgery in stage IIIC or IV ovarian cancer. *N Engl J Med.* 2010;363:943.

Williams L. The role of secondary cytoreductive surgery in epithelial ovarian malignancies. *Oncology.* 1992;6:25.

Young RC, Gynecologic Oncology Group. Phase III randomized study of CBDCA/TAX administered for 3 vs 6 courses for selected stages IA–C and stages IIA–C ovarian epithelial cancer (summary last modified 10/95), GOG-157, clinical trial, active, March 20, 1995.

Young RC, Walton LA, Ellenberg SS, et al. Adjuvant therapy in stage I and stage II epithelial ovarian cancer: results of two prospective randomized trials. *N Engl J Med.* 1990;322:1021.

Zaino RJ, Unger ER, Whitney C. Synchronous carcinomas of the uterine corpus and ovary. *Gynecol Oncol.* 1984;19:329.

Ovarian Tumors of Low Malignant Potential

Bell DA, Scully RE. Serous borderline tumors of the peritoneum. *Am J Surg Pathol.* 1990;14:230.

Casey AC, Bell DA, Lage JM, et al. Epithelial ovarian tumors of borderline malignancy: long-term follow-up. *Gynecol Oncol.* 1993;50:316.

de Nictolis M, Montironi R, Tommasoni S, et al. Serous borderline tumors of the ovary. *Cancer.* 1992;70:152.

Fort MG, Pierce VK, Saigo PE, et al. Evidence for the efficacy of adjuvant therapy in epithelial ovarian tumors of low malignant potential. *Gynecol Oncol.* 1989; 32:269.

Gershenson DM, Silva EG. Serous ovarian tumors of low malignant potential with peritoneal implants. *Cancer.* 1990;65:578.

Hopkins MP, Kumar NB, Morley GW. An assessment of pathologic features and treatment modalities in ovarian tumors of low malignant potential. *Obstet Gynecol.* 1987;70:293.

Koern J, Trope CG, Abeler VM. A retrospective study of 370 borderline tumors of the ovary treated at the Norwegian Radium Hospital from 1970 to 1982. *Cancer.* 1993;71:1810.

Kurman RJ, Trimble CL. The behavior of serous tumors of low malignant potential: are they ever malignant? *Int J Gynecol Pathol.* 1993;12:120.

Leake JF, Currie JL, Rosenshein NB, et al. Long-term follow-up of serous ovarian tumors of low malignant potential. *Gynecol Oncol.* 1992;47:150.

Michael H, Roth LM. Invasive and noninvasive implants in ovarian serous tumors of low malignant potential. *Cancer.* 1986; 57:1240.

Rice LW, Berkowitz RS, Mark SD, et al. Epithelial ovarian tumors of borderline malignancy. *Gynecol Oncol.* 1990;39:195.

Slomovitz BM, Caputo TA, Gretz HF, et al. A comparative analysis of 57 serous borderline tumors with and without a noninvasive micropapillary component. *Am J Surg Pathol.* 2002;26:592.

Sutton GP, Bundy BN, Omura GA, et al. Stage III ovarian tumors of low malignant potential treated with cisplatin combination therapy (a Gynecologic Oncology Group study). *Gynecol Oncol.* 1991;41:230.

Trimble EL, Trimble CL. Epithelial ovarian tumors of low malignant potential. In: Markman M, Hoskins WJ, eds. *Cancer of the Ovary.* New York, NY: Raven Press; 1993.

Trope C, Kaern J, Vergote IB, et al. Are borderline tumors of the ovary overtreated both surgically and systematically? A review of four prospective randomized trials including 253 patients with borderline tumors. *Gynecol Oncol.* 1993;51:236.

Yazigi R, Sandstad J, Munoz AK. Primary staging in ovarian tumors of low malignant potential. *Gynecol Oncol.* 1988;31:402.

Ovarian Germ Cell Tumors

Gershenson DM. Update on malignant ovarian germ cell tumors. *Cancer.* 1993;71 (4 suppl):1581.

Gershenson DM, Morris M, Cangir A, et al. Treatment of malignant germ cell tumors of the ovary with bleomycin, etoposide, and cisplatin. *J Clin Oncol.* 1990;8:715.

Kurman RJ, Norris HJ. Malignant germ cell tumors of the ovary. *Hum Pathol.* 1977; 8:551.

Morrow CP, Curtin JP, Townsend DE. *Synopsis of Gynecologic Oncology.* 4th ed. New York, NY: Churchill Livingstone; 1993.

Munshi NC, Loehrer PJ, Roth BJ, et al. Vinblastine, ifosfamide and cisplatin (VeIP) as second line chemotherapy in metastatic germ cell tumors (GCT). *Proc Am Soc Clin Oncol.* 1990;9:134.

Romero R, Schwartz PE. Alpha-fetoprotein determinations in the management of endodermal sinus tumors and mixed germ cell tumors of the ovary. *Am J Obstet Gynecol.* 1981;141:126.

Schwartz PE, Morris JM. Serum lactic dehydrogenase: a tumor marker for dysgerminoma. *Obstet Gynecol.* 1988;72:511.

Serov SF, Scully RE, Robin IH. *International Histologic Classification of Tumours, No. 9. Histological Typing of Ovarian Tumours.* Geneva: World Health Organization; 1973.

Slayton RE, Park RC, Silverberg SG, et al. Vincristine, dactinomycin, and cyclophosphamide in the treatment of malignant germ cell tumors of the ovary. *Cancer.* 1985;56:243.

Williams S, Blessing JA, Liao SY, et al. Adjuvant therapy of ovarian germ cell tumors with cisplatin, etoposide, and bleomycin: a trial of the Gynecologic Oncology Group. *J Clin Oncol.* 1994;12:701.

Williams SD, Birch R, Einhorn LH, et al. Treatment of disseminated germ-cell tumors with cisplatin, bleomycin, and either vinblastine or etoposide. *N Engl J Med.* 1987;316:1435.

Williams SD, Blessing JA, Hatch KD, et al. Chemotherapy of advanced dysgerminoma: trials of the Gynecologic Oncology Group. *J Clin Oncol.* 1991;9:1950.

Williams SD, Blessing JA, Moore DH, et al. Cisplatin, vinblastine, and bleomycin in advanced and recurrent ovarian germcell tumors: a trial of the Gynecologic Oncology Group. *Ann Intern Med.* 1989; 111:22.

Williams SD, Gershenson DM. Management of germ cell tumors of the ovary. In: Markman M, Hoskins WJ, eds. *Cancer of the Ovary.* New York, NY: Raven Press; 1993.

Williams SD, Gynecologic Oncology Group. Phase II combination chemotherapy with BEP (CDDP/VP-16/BLEO) as induction followed by VAC (VCR/DACT/CTX) as consolidation in patients with incompletely resected malignant ovarian germ cell tumors (summary last modified 10/95), GOG-90, clinical trial, active, September 15, 1986.

Sex Cord Stromal Tumors

Berek JS, Hacker NF. *Practical Gynecologic Oncology.* 3rd ed. Baltimore, MD: Williams & Wilkins; 2000.

Bjorkholm E, Silversward C. Theca cell tumors. Clinical features and prognosis. *Acta Radiol.* 1980;19:241.

Bjorkholm E, Silversward C. Prognostic factors in granulosa-cell tumors. *Gynecol Oncol.* 1981;11:261.

Evans AT III, Gaffey TA, Malkasian GD Jr. Clinicopathologic review of 118 granulosa and 82 theca cell tumors. *Obstet Gynecol.* 1980;55:231.

Fox H, Agarical K, Langley FA. A clinicopathologic study of 92 cases of granulosa cell tumors of the ovary with special reference to the factors influencing prognosis. *Cancer.* 1975;35:231.

Gershenson DM. Management of early ovarian cancer: germ cell and sex cord-stromal tumors. *Gynecol Oncol.* 1994;55:S62.

Lappohn RE, Burger HG, Bouma J, et al. Inhibin as a marker for granulosa-cell tumors. *N Engl J Med.* 1989;321:790.

Meigs JV, Armstrong SH, Hamilton HH. A further contribution to the syndrome of fibroma of the ovary with fluid in the abdomen and chest, Meig's syndrome. *Am J Obstet Gynecol.* 1943;46:19.

Norris HJ, Taylor HB. Prognosis of granulosatheca tumors of the ovary. *Cancer.* 1968; 21:255.

Roth LM, Anderson MC, Govan AD, et al. Sertoli-Leydig cell tumors: a clinicopathologic study of 34 cases. *Cancer.* 1981; 48:187.

Scully RE. Ovarian tumors: a review. *Am J Pathol.* 1977;87:686.

Young RH, Scully RE. Ovarian sex cord-stromal tumors: recent progress. *Int J Gynecol Pathol.* 1982;1:101.

Young RH, Scully RE. Ovarian sex cord stromal and steroid cell tumors. In: Roth LM, Czernobilsky B, eds. *Tumors and Tumor-Like Conditions of the Ovary.* New York, NY: Churchill Livingstone; 1985.

Young RH, Welch WR, Dickersin GR, et al. Ovarian sex cord tumor with annular tubules. Review of 74 cases including 27 with Peutz-Jeghers syndrome and four with adenoma malignum of the cervix. *Cancer.* 1982;50:1384.

Fallopian Tube Cancer

Eddy GL, Copeland LJ, Gershenson DM, et al. Fallopian tube carcinoma. *Obstet Gynecol.* 1984;64:156.

Hu CY, Taymor ML, Hertig AT. Primary carcinoma of the fallopian tube. *Am J Obstet Gynecol.* 1950;59:58.

Morris M, Gershenson DM, Burke TW, et al. Treatment of fallopian tube carcinoma with cisplatin, doxorubicin and cyclophosphamide. *Obstet Gynecol.* 1990;76: 1020.

Rose PG, Piver MS, Tsukada Y. Fallopian tube cancer. *Cancer.* 1990;66:2661.

Sedlis A. Carcinoma of the fallopian tube. *Surg Clin North Am.* 1978;58:121.

Endometrial Cancer

American Cancer Society. *Cancer Facts and Figures.* Atlanta, GA: American Cancer Society; 1995.

Axelrod JH, Gynecologic Oncology Group. Phase II study of whole-abdominal radiotherapy in patients with papillary serous carcinoma and clear cell carcinoma of the endometrium or with maximally debulked advanced endometrial carcinoma (summary last modified 05/91), GOG-94, clinical trial, closed, February 24, 1992.

Boring CC, Squires TS, Tong T. Cancer statistics, 1991. *Cancer.* 1991;41:19.

Burke TW, Munkarah A, Kavanagh JJ, et al. Treatment of advanced or recurrent endometrial carcinoma with single-agent carboplatin. *Gynecol Oncol.* 1993;51:397.

Burke TW, Stringer CL, Morris M, et al. Prospective treatment of advanced or recurrent endometrial carcinoma with cisplatin, doxorubicin, and cyclophosphamide. *Gynecol Oncol.* 1991;40:264.

Creasman WT. New gynecologic cancer staging. *Obstet Gynecol.* 1990;75:287.

Creasman WT, Morrow CP, Bundy BN, et al. Surgical pathologic spread patterns of endometrial cancer: a Gynecologic Oncology Group study. *Cancer.* 1987;60:2035.

Gusberg SB. Virulence factors in endometrial cancer. *Cancer.* 1993;71(4 suppl):1464.

Hancock KC, Freedman RS, Edwards CL, et al. Use of cisplatin, doxorubicin, and cyclophosphamide to treat advanced and recurrent adenocarcinoma of the endometrium. *Cancer Treat Rep.* 1986;70:789.

Homesley HD, Zaino R. Endometrial cancer: prognostic factors. *Semin Oncol.* 1994;21:71.

Lanciano RM, Corn BW, Schultz DJ, et al. The justification for a surgical staging system in endometrial carcinoma. *Radiother Oncol.* 1993;28:189.

Lentz SS. Advanced and recurrent endometrial carcinoma: hormonal therapy. *Semin Oncol.* 1994;21:100.

Marchetti DL, Caglar H, Driscoll DL, et al. Pelvic radiation in stage I endometrial adenocarcinoma with high-risk attributes. *Gynecol Oncol.* 1990;37:51.

Mariani A, Dowdy SC, Cliby WA, et al. Prospective assessment of lymphatic dissemination in endometrial cancer: a paradigm shift in surgical staging. *Gynecol Oncol.* 2008;109:11.

Morrow CP, Bundy BN, Kurman RJ, et al. Relationship between surgical-pathological risk factors and outcome in clinical stage I and II carcinoma of the endometrium: a Gynecologic Oncology Group study. *Gynecol Oncol.* 1991;40:55.

Morrow CP, Curtin JP, Townsend DE. *Synopsis of Gynecologic Oncology.* 4th ed. New York, NY: Churchill Livingstone; 1993.

Nori D, Hilaris BS, Tome M, et al. Combined surgery and radiation in endometrial carcinoma: an analysis of prognostic factors. *Int J Radiat Oncol Biol Phys.* 1987;13:489.

Piver MS, Hempling RE. A prospective trial of postoperative vaginal radium/cesium for grade 1–2 less than 50% myometrial invasion and pelvic radiation therapy for grade 3 or deep myometrial invasion in surgical stage I endometrial adenocarcinoma. *Cancer.* 1990;66:1133.

Potish RA, Twiggs LB, Adcock LL, et al. Role of whole abdominal radiation therapy in the management of endometrial cancer: prognostic importance of factors indicating peritoneal metastases. *Gynecol Oncol.* 1985;21:80.

Quinn MA, Campbell JJ. Tamoxifen therapy in advanced/recurrent endometrial carcinoma. *Gynecol Oncol.* 1989;32:1.

Roberts JA, Gynecologic Oncology Group. Phase III randomized evaluation of adjuvant postoperative pelvic radiotherapy vs no adjuvant therapy for surgical stage I and occult stage II intermediate-risk endometrial carcinoma (summary last modified 08/95), GOG-99, clinical trial, closed, July 3, 1995.

Rutledge F. The role of radical hysterectomy in adenocarcinoma of the endometrium. *Gynecol Oncol.* 1974;2:331.

Seski JC, Edwards CL, Herson J, et al. Cisplatin chemotherapy for disseminated endometrial cancer. *Obstet Gynecol.* 1982;59:225.

Slomovitz BM, Burke TW, Eifel PJ, et al. Uterine papillary serous carcinoma (UPSC): a single institution review of 129 cases. *Gynecol Oncol.* 2003;91:463.

Walker JL, Piedmont MR, Spirtos NM, et al. Laparoscopy compared with laparotomy for comprehensive surgical staging of uterine cancer: Gynecologic Oncology Group study LAP2. *J Clin Oncol.* 2009;27:5331.

Uterine Sarcomas

Berek JS, Hacker NF. *Practical Gynecologic Oncology.* 3rd ed. Baltimore, MD: Williams & Wilkins; 2000.

Gershenson DM, Kavanagh JJ, Copeland LJ, et al. Cisplatin therapy for disseminated mixed mesodermal sarcoma of the uterus. *J Clin Oncol.* 1987;5:618.

Harlow BL, Weiss NS, Lofton S. The epidemiology of sarcomas of the uterus. *J Natl Cancer Inst.* 1986;76:399.

Hornback NB, Omura G, Major FJ. Observations on the use of adjuvant radiation therapy in patients with stage I and II uterine sarcoma. *Int J Radiat Oncol Biol Phys.* 1986;12:2127.

Major FJ, Blessing JA, Silverberg SG, et al. Prognostic factors in early-stage uterine sarcoma: a Gynecologic Oncology Group study. *Cancer.* 1993;71(4 suppl):1702.

Morrow CP, Curtin JP, Townsend DE. *Synopsis of Gynecologic Oncology.* 4th ed. New York, NY: Churchill Livingstone; 1993.

Norris HJ, Taylor HB. Postirradiation sarcomas of the uterus. *Obstet Gynecol.* 1965;26:689.

Olah KS, Dunn JA, Gee H. Leiomyosarcomas have a poorer prognosis than mixed mesodermal tumours when adjusting for known prognostic factors: the result of a retrospective study of 423 cases of uterine sarcoma. *Br J Obstet Gynaecol.* 1992; 99:590.

Omura GA, Blessing JA, Lifshitz S, et al. A randomized clinical trial of adjuvant Adriamycin in uterine sarcomas: a Gynecologic Oncology Group study. *J Clin Oncol.* 1985;3:1240.

Omura GA, Blessing JA, Major F, et al. A randomized clinical trial of adjuvant Adriamycin in uterine sarcomas: a Gynecologic Oncology Group study. *J Clin Oncol.* 1985;3:1240.

Silverberg SG, Major FJ, Blessing JA, et al. Carcinosarcoma (malignant mixed mesodermal tumor) of the uterus: a Gynecologic Oncology Group pathologic study of 203 cases. *Int J Gynecol Pathol.* 1990;9:1.

Sutton GP, Blessing JA, Barrett RJ, et al. Phase II trial of ifosfamide and mesna in leiomyosarcoma of the uterus: a Gynecologic Oncology Group study. *Am J Obstet Gynecol.* 1992;166:556.

Sutton GP, Gynecologic Oncology Group. Phase III study of IFF and the uroprotector mesna administered alone or with CDDP in patients with advanced or recurrent mixed mesodermal tumors of the uterus (summary last modified 08/95), GOG-108, clinical trial, active, February 15, 1989.

Sutton GP, Gynecologic Oncology Group. Phase II master protocol study of chemotherapeutic agents in the treatment of recurrent or advanced uterine sarcomas—IFF plus mesna (summary last modified 04/93), GOG-87B, clinical trial, completed, December 28, 1994.

Wheelock JB, Krebs H-B, Schneider V, et al. Uterine sarcoma: analysis of prognostic variables in 71 cases. *Am J Obstet Gynecol.* 1985;151:1016.

Gestational Trophoblastic Disease

Azab M, Droz JP, Theodore C, et al. Cisplatin, vinblastine, and bleomycin combination in the treatment of resistant high-risk gestational trophoblastic tumors. *Cancer.* 1989;64:1829.

Bagshawe KD. High-risk metastatic trophoblastic disease. *Obstet Gynecol Clin North Am.* 1988;15:531.

Berek JS, Hacker NF. *Practical Gynecologic Oncology.* 3rd ed. Baltimore, MD: Williams & Wilkins; 2000.

Lurain JR. Gestational trophoblastic tumors. *Semin Surg Oncol.* 1990;6:347.

Morrow CP, Curtin JP, Townsend DE. *Synopsis of Gynecologic Oncology.* 4th ed. New York, NY: Churchill Livingstone; 1993.

Mutch DG, Soper JT, Babcock CJ, et al. Recurrent gestational trophoblastic disease: experience of the Southeastern Regional Trophoblastic Disease Center. *Cancer.* 1990;66:978.

Newlands ES, Bagshawe KD, Begent RH, et al. Results with the EMA/CO (etoposide, methotrexate, actinomycin D, cyclophosphamide, vincristine) regimen in high risk gestational trophoblastic tumours, 1979 to 1989. *Br J Obstet Gynaecol.* 1991;98:550.

Surwit EA. Management of high-risk gestational trophoblastic disease. *J Reprod Med.* 1987;32:657.

World Health Organization Scientific Group. Gestational trophoblastic diseases. *WHO Tech Rep Ser.* 1983;692:1.

Cervical Cancer

Alberts DS, Kronmal R, Baker LH, et al. Phase II randomized trial of cisplatin chemotherapy regimens in the treatment of recurrent or metastatic squamous cell cancer of the cervix: a Southwest Oncology Group study. *J Clin Oncol.* 1987;5:1791.

American Cancer Society. *Cancer Facts and Figures.* Atlanta, GA: American Cancer Society; 2003.

Artman LE, Hoskins WJ, Bibro MC, et al. Radical hysterectomy and pelvic lymphadenectomy for stage IB carcinoma of the cervix: 21 years' experience. *Gynecol Oncol.* 1987;28:8.

Coia L, Won M, Lanciano R, et al. The patterns of care outcome study for cancer of the uterine cervix: results of the Second National Practice Survey. *Cancer.* 1990; 66:2451.

Coleman RE, Harper PG, Gallagher C, et al. A phase II study of ifosfamide in advanced and relapsed carcinoma of the cervix. *Cancer Chemother Pharmacol.* 1986;18: 280.

Creasman WF, Fetter BF, Clarke-Pearson DL, et al. Management of stage IA carcinoma of the cervix. *Am J Obstet Gynecol.* 1985; 153:164.

Creasman WT. New gynecologic cancer staging. *Gynecol Oncol.* 1995;58:157.

Dembo AJ, Balogh JM. Advances in radiotherapy in the gynecologic malignancies. *Semin Surg Oncol.* 1990;6:323.

Eifel PJ, Burke TW, Delclos L, et al. Early stage I adenocarcinoma of the uterine cervix: treatment results in patients with tumors ≤4 cm in diameter. *Gynecol Oncol.* 1991;41:199.

Fletcher GH, Rutledge FN. Overall results in radiotherapy for carcinoma of the cervix. *Clin Obstet Gynecol.* 1967;10:958.

Grigsby PW, Perez CA. Radiotherapy alone for medically inoperable carcinoma of the cervix: stage IA and carcinoma in situ. *Int J Radiat Oncol Biol Phys.* 1991; 21:375.

Hopkins MP, Morley GW. Squamous cell cancer of the cervix: prognostic factors related to survival. *Int J Gynecol Cancer.* 1991;1:173.

Morrow CP, Curtin JP, Townsend DE. *Synopsis of Gynecologic Oncology.* 4th ed. New York, NY: Churchill Livingstone; 1993.

Perez CA, Grigsby PW, Nene SM, et al. Effect of tumor size on the prognosis of carcinoma of the uterine cervix treated with irradiation alone. *Cancer.* 1992; 69:2796.

Rutledge FN, Smith JP, Wharton JT, et al. Pelvic exenteration: analysis of 296 patients. *Am J Obstet Gynecol.* 1977;129:881.

Sevin BU, Nadji M, Averette HE, et al. Microinvasive carcinoma of the cervix. *Cancer.* 1992;70:2121.

Stehman FB, Bundy BN, DiSaia PJ, et al. Carcinoma of the cervix treated with radiation therapy: a multivariate analysis of prognostic variables in the Gynecologic Oncology Group. *Cancer.* 1991;67: 2776.

Thomas G, Dembo A, Fyles A, et al. Concurrent chemoradiation in advanced cervical cancer. *Gynecol Oncol.* 1990;38:446.

Vermorken JB. The role of chemotherapy in squamous cell carcinoma of the uterine cervix: a review. *Int J Gynecol Cancer.* 1993;3:129.

Vulvar Cancer

Anderson JM, Cassady JR, Shimm DS, et al. Vulvar carcinoma. *Int J Radiat Oncol Biol Phys.* 1995;32:1351.

Berek JS, Heaps JM, Fu YS, et al. Concurrent cisplatin and 5-fluorouracil chemotherapy and radiation therapy for advanced-stage squamous carcinoma of the vulva. *Gynecol Oncol.* 1991;2:197.

Binder SW, Huang I, Fu YS, et al. Risk factors for the development of lymph node metastasis in vulvar squamous cell carcinoma. *Gynecol Oncol.* 1990;37:9.

Boyce J, Fruchter RG, Kasambilides E, et al. Prognostic factors in carcinoma of the vulva. *Gynecol Oncol.* 1985;20:364.

Burke TW, Stringer CA, Gershenson DM, et al. Radical wide excision and selective inguinal node dissection for squamous cell carcinoma of the vulva. *Gynecol Oncol.* 1990;38:328.

Chung AF, Woodruff JW, Lewis JL Jr. Malignant melanoma of the vulva: a report of 44 cases. *Obstet Gynecol.* 1975;45:638.

Creasman WT. New gynecologic cancer staging. *Gynecol Oncol.* 1995;58:157.

Hacker NF, Van der Velden J. Conservative management of early vulvar cancer. *Cancer.* 1993;71(4 suppl):1673.

Heaps JM, Fu YS, Montz FJ, et al. Surgical-pathologic variables predictive of local recurrence in squamous cell carcinoma of the vulva. *Gynecol Oncol.* 1990; 38:309.

Homesley HD, Bundy BN, Sedlis A, et al. Assessment of current International Federation of Gynecology and Obstetrics staging of vulvar carcinoma relative to prognostic factors for survival (a Gynecologic Oncology Group study). *Am J Obstet Gynecol.* 1991;164:997.

Homesley HD, Bundy BN, Sedlis A, et al. Prognostic factors for groin node metastasis in squamous cell carcinoma of the vulva (a Gynecologic Oncology Group study). *Gynecol Oncol.* 1993;49:279.

Hopkins MP, Reid GC, Morley GW. The surgical management of recurrent squamous cell carcinoma of the vulva. *Obstet Gynecol.* 1990;75:1001.

Keys H. Gynecologic Oncology Group randomized trials of combined technique therapy for vulvar cancer. *Cancer.* 1993; 71(4 suppl):1691.

Malfetano JH, Piver MS, Tsukada Y, et al. Univariate and multivariate analyses of 5-year survival, recurrence, and inguinal node metastases in stage I and II vulvar carcinoma. *J Surg Oncol.* 1985;30:124.

Perez CA, Grigsby PW, Galakatos A, et al. Radiation therapy in management of carcinoma of the vulva with emphasis on conservation therapy. *Cancer.* 1993;71:3707.

Podratz KC, Symmonds RE, Taylor WF, et al. Carcinoma of the vulva: analysis of treatment and survival. *Obstet Gynecol.* 1983;61:63.

Russell AH, Mesic JB, Scudder SA, et al. Synchronous radiation and cytotoxic chemotherapy for locally advanced or recurrent squamous cancer of the vulva. *Gynecol Oncol.* 1992;47:14.

Sedlis A, Homesley H, Bundy BN, et al. Positive groin lymph nodes in superficial squamous cell vulvar cancer: a Gynecologic Oncology Group study. *Am J Obstet Gynecol.* 1987;156:1159.

Shimm DS, Fuller AF, Orlow EL, et al. Prognostic variables in the treatment of squamous cell carcinoma of the vulva. *Gynecol Oncol.* 1986;24:343.

Stehman FB, Bundy BN, Dvoretsky PM, et al. Early stage I carcinoma of the vulva treated with ipsilateral superficial inguinal lymphadenectomy and modified radical hemivulvectomy: a prospective study of the Gynecologic Oncology Group. *Obstet Gynecol.* 1992;79:490.

Thomas GM, Dembo AJ, Bryson SC, et al. Changing concepts in the management of vulvar cancer. *Gynecol Oncol.* 1991;42:9.

Vaginal Cancer

Berek JS, Hacker NF. *Practical Gynecologic Oncology.* 3rd ed. Baltimore, MD: Williams & Wilkins; 2000.

Delclos L, Wharton JT, Rutledge FN. Tumors of the vagina and female urethra. In: Fletcher GH, ed. *Textbook of Radiotherapy.* 3rd ed. Philadelphia, PA: Lea & Febiger; 1980.

Herbst AL, Robboy SJ, Scully RE, et al. Clear cell adenocarcinoma of the vagina and cervix in girls: analysis of 170 registry cases. *Am J Obstet Gynecol.* 1974;119:713.

Kucera H, Vavra N. Radiation management of primary carcinoma of the vagina: clinical and histopathological variables associated with survival. *Gynecol Oncol.* 1991;40:12.

Morrow CP, Curtin JP, Townsend DE. *Synopsis of Gynecologic Oncology.* 4th ed. New York, NY: Churchill Livingstone; 1993.

Perez CA, Camel HM, Galakatos AE, et al. Definitive irradiation in carcinoma of the vagina: long-term evaluation of results. *Int J Radiat Oncol Biol Phys.* 1988;15:1283.

Stock RG, Chen AS, Seski J. A 30-year experience in the management of primary carcinoma of the vagina: analysis of prognostic factors and treatment modalities. *Gynecol Oncol.* 1995;56:45.

Neurosurgical Malignancies: Treating Tumors of Brain, Spine, and Peripheral Nerve and Their Effects on the Nervous System

Ian E. McCutcheon

The interplay of neurosurgery with other disciplines in the broader field of surgical oncology leads to frequent instances of neurosurgical treatment in patients whose tumors originated outside the central nervous system. Tumors also originate within the brain or spine and require neurosurgical care. To many oncologists the nervous system remains an arcane, poorly understood area yet it is one with profound implications on patient outcome. Neurosurgical oncologists aim to cure or palliate tumors when possible, but even more so to preserve function at the highest possible level and for the longest period of time. It is a technically demanding discipline very much concerned with maintaining the functions that make life worthwhile. This chapter will provide an overview of fundamental clinical scenarios and basic tumor types relevant to the practice of neurosurgical oncology in a cancer center.

CLINICAL EVALUATION

Neurological Examination

All encounters with patients suspected of harboring some form of neurological disease must perforce begin with an interview and neurological examination. All too often this portion of the physical examination is skipped, notated scantily, or not at all in the chart, or receives lip service of the most superficial type, yet a good history and intelligently focused neurological examination will yield 90% of the elements needed to make clinical decisions for a tumor affecting the neuraxis. Ultimately the interpretation of such information depends on a sound working knowledge of the anatomy of the nervous system. Each of the 10 subsystems (cerebral cortex, pyramidal tracts, basal ganglia, brainstem, cranial nerves, cerebellum, spinal cord, nerve roots, peripheral nerve, and muscle) cause different changes on neurological examination that allow accuracy in anatomical localization. Details of correlative clinical neuroanatomy are beyond the scope of this chapter, but it is possible to winnow out a number of key features of the neurological examination that should be tested even by those uninitiated in its mysteries.

Questions to Ask

First, *is the patient conscious?* The classic way of measuring consciousness is by grading eye movements, verbalization, and motor function on the Glasgow Coma Scale (GCS), in which perfect wakefulness and function result in a score of 15 and complete coma without even reflex movements yields a score of 3 (Table 20.1). Note that even a dead person has a score of 3, and prognosis is very poor in a living patient with this low GCS. The scale measures whether such responses occur spontaneously or only after varying degrees of stimulation. Even patients in deep coma will preserve flexor or (in the worst case) extensor motor responses to such deep painful stimuli as a sternal rub. In the relatively awake patient, speech function can be assessed by noting speech patterns during conversation, but subtle patterns of dysphasia may elude the observer unless he or she addresses pointed questions to

TABLE 20.1	Glasgow Coma Scale	
		Score
Eye opening	Spontaneously	4
	To speech	3
	To pain	2
	None	1
Verbal response	Oriented	5
	Confused	4
	Inappropriate	3
	Incomprehensible	2
	None	1
Motor response	Obeys commands	6
	Localizes to pain	5
	Withdraws from pain	4
	Flexion to pain	3
	Extension to pain	2
	None	1

the patient. In most patients the speech areas reside in the brain's left hemisphere. However, because speech function arises in the *right* hemisphere in 15% of left-handed subjects, this generalization is not absolute. Depending on which part of the speech network is affected by a lesion, patients can show difficulties with expressing words (Broca's area), with naming objects (uncinate fasciculus), with reading (posterior parasylvian), or with understanding spoken phrases (Wernicke area). In addition speech may be impaired from a motor perspective if the cranial nerves subserving coordination of tongue, throat muscles, and vocal cords are impaired.

Is the patient weakened or paralyzed in one or more limbs? Even in a comatose patient, differential degrees of withdrawal to painful stimuli can uncover a weakness. In the awake patient, a simple request to pull or push against resistance provided by the examiner, and made for each of the four limbs, can uncover various patterns of weakness. These include a hemiparesis (weakness of one side of the body), quadriparesis (weakness in all four limbs and implying a lesion of the cervical spinal cord or brain), or paraparesis (weakness of both legs, implying a spinal lesion above the lumbosacral junction). The list of causes of weakness is long, but in an oncology patient the possibility of tumor affecting neural elements at the appropriate location in the nervous system must be considered before other diagnoses common in the non-oncologic population (e.g., stroke, trauma).

Does the patient have a myelopathy? This term implies a disorder of the spinal cord as opposed to the brain, and ruling myelopathy in or out is done in any patient who complains of sensory or motor symptoms that could have arisen from such a spinal lesion. The delicacy of the spinal cord in the face of extrinsic (or for that matter, intrinsic) compression means that such compression cannot be allowed to persist for long before permanent deficits ensue. Thus, knowing whether myelopathy is present allows the surgeon to make timely decisions critical to the maintenance of neurological function. This is tested by examining (a) reflexes at the knees and elbow (quadriceps and biceps reflexes, respectively), (b) muscle tone, and (c) response of the toes to plantar stimulation, that is, the Babinski response. When myelopathy is present, reflexes and tone are increased and the plantar response is extensor. Subtle forms of myelopathy may not encompass all three of these categories but some portion of this description should apply in any patient with a clinically significant spinal cord lesion.

Can the patient see? Four of the 12 cranial nerves are used for seeing (optic nerve, cranial nerve II), eye movement (cranial nerves III, IV, and VI), or eyelid opening (cranial nerve III). Eye movements should be checked because they give an indicator of the function of the brainstem, where the nuclei of these cranial nerves reside, and because increases in intracranial pressure can affect ocular motility most commonly by causing a sixth nerve palsy in which lateral movement (abduction) of one or both eyes is impaired. In addition, increases in intracranial pressure (ICP) can cause papilledema visible on fundoscopy. Perfect vision requires maintenance of the integrity of a system that extends from the retina through the optic nerves, chiasm, and tracts back through the geniculate body of the thalamus, and thence through the optic radiations to the calcarine cortex in the occipital lobes at the posterior-most portion of the brain. If the patient passes a good visual examination then malfunction of a significant portion of the brain has been excluded.

Can the patient swallow? This aspect of the neurological examination is often overlooked, but the ability to swallow is critically important to good outcome for any patient undergoing surgery for tumor. Patients with impairment of the gag reflex or with pharyngeal dysmotility are harder to wean safely off ventilatory assistance, are more prone to aspiration and its consequences, and often cannot achieve oral intake sufficient to maintain the good nutrition needed for post-surgical healing. Decisions about gastrostomy or about transnasal tube feeding should be made early in patients in whom such issues have been discovered.

Finally, *can the patient walk?* Walking is a complex function that needs inputs from sensory systems, proprioceptive processing systems, and motor systems if falls are to be avoided. Thus, tumors in the cerebellum, which acts as a computer processing and modulating proprioceptive inputs and motor outputs, cause ataxia. Intrinsic disease within nerves in diabetic neuropathy can reduce sensory input and cause a patient to stumble more easily. When the surgical oncologist is confronted with a patient with a recent history of stumbling or falling, it is particularly important to examine for signs of incipient myelopathy indicating an impending spinal cord compression. Patients are frequently brought to the hospital only after they have been bed-bound for 5 or more days, at a time when surgical intervention for their spinal metastasis will no longer allow restoration of function. As the window of opportunity in such cases is small (24 hours from loss of ambulation), a decline in the ability to walk can be a vitally important clue, and demands prompt investigation.

INCREASED INTRACRANIAL PRESSURE

Basic Principles

In humans the cranium is a rigid structure. Its contents include the brain, blood (arterial and venous), and cerebrospinal fluid (CSF). Because the intracranial volume is constant, when an intracranial mass is introduced compensation first occurs through a reciprocal decrease in the volume of venous blood and CSF. This concept, known as the Monro–Kellie doctrine, is most applicable in adults as children younger than the age at which skull suture close will show cranial expansion if the rise in pressure is chronic. CSF volume increases with age due to brain atrophy.

When compensatory mechanisms have been exhausted, minute changes in volume produce precipitous increases in pressure. The pressure–volume curve reflects very small increases in pressure when an expanding mass is introduced into the intracranial compartment. Such pressure begins to rise more precipitously as compensation allowed by egress of CSF and venous blood disappears. When ICP overcomes arterial pressure, perfusion ceases and brain death occurs.

The blood–brain barrier is formed by linked astrocytic foot processes along the adventitial surfaces of cerebral endothelial cells. It prevents many substances carried in the blood from reaching the brain and thus protects neural tissue from potentially toxic materials. It also regulates the flow of biologically active molecules into the brain. Lipid-soluble substances can usually penetrate more effectively than amino acids and sugars, which are transported across the endothelium by specific carrier-mediated mechanisms. When the barrier is disrupted, plasma components can cross it into the brain and cause vasogenic edema. The relevance of the blood–brain barrier in neurosurgical oncology rests in its relative disruption by intracranial tumors which results in local edema around the tumor leading to neurological malfunction in the edematous zone. In addition, the blood–brain barrier prevents most chemotherapy agents from penetrating into the brain and has stymied the development of effective medical treatments for brain tumors. In the past 35 years only two drugs have been approved by the FDA for brain tumor therapy: *bis*-chloronitrosourea (BCNU) which is now little used in its native form, but which has the advantage of being lipid-soluble; and temozolomide which has an oral route of administration, relatively good penetrance through the barrier, and a relatively low side effect profile. Polycarbonate wafer impregnated with BCNU (Gliadel®) has been separately approved for treatment of glioblastoma and is placed during surgery along the walls of the surgical resection cavity. However, it provides only a modest increase in survival through its mechanism of slow diffusion of the drug out of the wafer and into the sites of microscopic invasion in edematous peritumoral brain.

Cerebral edema is treated with steroids (usually dexamethasone) and in more refractory cases with osmotic agents such as mannitol, urea, or hypertonic saline. Use of steroids is routine after resection of intracranial or spinal tumors as a way of reducing the flare-up of edema commonly seen after intraoperative tumor manipulation. Patients are pre-treated with steroids before surgery if neurological dysfunction predates the operation. Vasogenic edema can be quite extensive with some tumor types more likely to provoke it than others. Tumors that produce copious amounts of vascular endothelial growth factor give the most extensive edema, with the emblematic tumor in this category being metastasis from renal cell carcinoma.

Mean cerebral blood flow is 55 to 60 mL/100 g/min. It is 20% higher in the more metabolically active cortex (grey matter) and 20% less in the white matter. Cerebral blood flow is determined most significantly by the cerebral perfusion pressure (CPP), defined as the difference between the incoming mean arterial pressure (MAP) and the opposing ICP. The formula is:

$$CPP = MAP - ICP = [diastolic\ pressure + [1/3\ (pulse\ pressure)]] - ICP$$

As ICP rises, CPP decreases. Under physiological conditions several factors regulate cerebral blood flow: systemic blood pressure, pCO_2 and pH in the arterial blood, and pO_2. Autoregulation maintains blood flow to the brain at a constant level over a wide range of MAP. When MAP is low, cerebral arterioles dilate to allow adequate flow at decreased pressure. By contrast, increased systemic blood pressure causes arterioles to constrict and thereby maintain flow. However, at MAP < 50 mm Hg perfusion is inadequate; with MAP > 150 the autoregulatory system fails and cerebral blood flow increases with resulting increase in vasogenic edema leading to a hypertensive encephalopathy.

Arterial pCO_2 is the most potent stimulus for dilation of cerebral arterioles. As pCO_2 decreases from 80 to 15 mm Hg, cerebral blood flow decreases, thus hyperventilation can be used as a treatment for increased ICP by diminishing cerebral blood flow and blood volume. A patient with decreased level of consciousness (GCS ≤9)

TABLE 20.2	Common Causes of Increased Intracranial Pressure (ICP)
Pathological Process	**Examples**
Localized masses	Hematomas: epidural, subdural, intracerebral
	Neoplasms: gliomas, meningiomas, metastases
	Abscesses
	Focal edema: from trauma, infarction, tumor
Obstruction of CSF pathway	Obstructive hydrocephalus
	Communicating hydrocephalus
Obstruction of major venous sinus	Depressed skull fracture over sinus
	Thrombosis from dehydration or oral contraceptive use
Diffuse brain edema	Encephalitis, meningitis
	Diffuse head injury
	Subarachnoid hemorrhage
	Water intoxication
	Lead poisoning causing encephalopathy
Idiopathic	Pseudotumor cerebri

from increased ICP is typically intubated for airway protection and prevention of aspiration, but also for hyperventilation to a pCO_2 of 28 mm Hg. Such patients are maintained normoxic or slightly hyperoxic. Hypoxia causes cerebral arteriolar dilation and thus maintaining good oxygenation also prevents further contribution to increases in ICP.

The normal ICP is 10 to 15 mm Hg (13 to 20 cm H_2O) in an awake patient. Causes of raised ICP are given in Table 20.2. Increased ICP harms the brain in two ways. First, ischemia can occur when CPP reaches critically low levels and can lead to stroke. Second, focal masses (e.g., tumors) cause distortion of the brain which if profound enough causes compression of brainstem structures vital to life. Herniation of the cerebellar tonsils through the foramen magnum or of the midbrain and aqueduct of Sylvius through the tentorial incisura further elevates ICP by blocking CSF pathways. Increases in ICP are better tolerated when shift of brain structures is absent. When pressure in increased slowly and chronically by generalized syndromes such as pseudotumor cerebri (a little-understood condition labeled variously as a disorder of CSF absorption or a structural defect in venous sinuses), neurological dysfunction may be absent or limited to specific cranial neuropathies.

Herniation occurs when the brain moves within the cranial cavity relative to the edge of dural folds intended to prevent its movement. The four main types of brain herniation are as follows:

1. *Cingulate herniation,* in which pressure is greater in one hemisphere than the other, leading to shift of the cingulate gyrus beneath the falx and accompanying shift of the nearby ventricular system.
2. *Uncal herniation,* which is the most clinically dramatic and most common herniation syndrome. It occurs when a lesion in the middle cranial fossa (temporal lobe) such as tumor or hematoma expands the uncus, the most inferomedial structure of the temporal lobe, and displaces it against the peduncle of the midbrain. Uncal herniation gives a clinical syndrome of progressively impaired consciousness, dilation of the ipsilateral pupil

("blown pupil"), and contralateral hemiplegia. Disturbance of consciousness comes from disturbance of the reticular activating system in the midbrain, pupillary dilation from compression of the oculomotor nerve and its parasympathetic pupillary constrictors, and hemiplegia from the compression of the corticospinal tract above its decussation.

3. *Central transtentorial herniation,* which is caused by hemispheric lesions in the frontal or parietal areas of the brain. Here the diencephalon and midbrain shift down through the tentorial incisura. The clinical syndrome is more difficult to recognize than that of uncal herniation and may include small reactive pupils, obtundation, loss of vertical gaze, and Cheyne–Stokes respiration.

4. *Tonsillar herniation* is caused by expansion of posterior fossa masses. The cerebellar tonsils move through the foramen magnum into the upper spinal canal and compress the dorsolateral medulla and upper cervical cord. This leads to hypertension, cardiorespiratory impairment, neurogenic hyperventilation, and impaired swallowing and consciousness. Ultimately death occurs due to cardiac and respiratory instability.

Symptoms of increased ICP include headache, worse in the early morning due to a rise of pCO_2 from hypoventilation during sleep and increased venous pressure from the recumbent position. However, headache is not a specific symptom and it is perfectly possible to have increased ICP without headache. The combination of headache and vomiting is suggestive and accompanying neurological signs like papilledema and cranial neuropathies are further confirmatory. The speed of onset of the increase in ICP influences symptoms as well. More chronic or slowly progressive rises in pressure are less likely to cause obtundation or pronounced neurological decline.

Monitoring ICP

Continuous monitoring of ICP is important in patients whose neurological and radiological examinations support the suspicion of increased pressure. Controlling such pressure rises significantly reduces morbidity and mortality in neurosurgical patients. Although the most common indicators for such monitoring are closed head injury and subarachnoid hemorrhage, patients in the oncology setting may require it in a number of circumstances including after posterior fossa surgery (to determine whether pre-existing hydrocephalus has cleared); when brain injury has led to coma and thus abrogated use of the neurological examination as an index of brain function; or when an intracranial hemorrhage caused by chemotherapy-induced thrombocytopenia leaves the patient at risk for hydrocephalus or further bleeding, with decisions about shunting or clot evacuation assisted by ICP measurement over time.

The most effective method of measuring ICP is through placement of a ventriculostomy drainage catheter. This is usually inserted through a burr hole made either at the bedside or in the operating room and located at or just anterior to the coronal suture at the mid-pupillary line. The catheter is tunneled a short distance to prevent infection and exits the scalp through a separate stab incision. It is connected to a pressure transducer and a drainage system. The major advantage of this method is that the catheter can be used to measure the pressure but also to treat ICP increases by allowing continuous drainage of CSF when the pressure exceeds a pre-specified limit. This limit is set by raising or lowering the loop of the drain, which provides resistance to CSF egress. For example, when the loop is set at 10 cm above the external auditory meatus (the typical "zero" point) no drainage occurs unless CSF pressure exceeds 10 cm of H_2O.

In some centers a fiberoptic transducer (Camino catheter) is implanted through a burr hole into the ventricle, brain parenchyma, or subdural space depending on the clinical situation. Such systems give pressure readings but do not allow drainage of fluid. Their advantages are that the zero position need not be reset when head position changes, and they are not susceptible to blockage by air or debris as are fluid-coupled systems. However, they cannot be tunneled and thus carry a higher risk of infection, and they provide a regional reading rather than a global one and so may not reflect ICP as truly as the intraventricular catheter does.

Treatment of Increased ICP

The first order of business in ICP treatment is always to address the cause directly. If the increased pressure results from the presence of an intracranial mass such as a tumor or clot, it should be promptly removed. Such surgery will restore ICP to normal more effectively than any other measure. However, the clinical situation is often complex with other causes of increased ICP at play such as hydrocephalus or cerebral edema. The main methods for ICP control (other than direct surgery) are as follows:

1. *Ventricular drainage.* This can be maintained for 10 to 14 days before catheter change is recommended to reduce the risk of ventriculitis or meningitis. Antibiotic-coated catheters are now standard and help keep the rate of infection low.

2. *Mannitol.* The usual dose is 0.25 gm/kg i.v. q4–6 hours. It is given in small boluses rather than continuously and an increase in serum osmolality of as little as 10 mosm/mL can be enough to reduce cerebral edema significantly. Mannitol also improves perfusion by reducing blood viscosity. It is effective for 48 to 72 hours, but its use is not recommended beyond that time frame.

3. *Hypertonic saline.* This has been used increasingly in the past 10 years, and studies have shown that it is as effective as mannitol.

4. *Hyperventilation.* This requires intubation and in a patient above the level of coma may also require paralysis and sedation. Hyperventilation should be moderate with end-tidal pCO_2 lowered to 28 to 32 mm Hg. Reducing pCO_2 below that level will compromise cerebral blood flow and compound the ischemia already produced by increased ICP.

5. *Loop diuretics* (furosemide; Lasix®). This is sometimes used as an adjunct to mannitol, although it is not dependable when used alone for the reduction of ICP.

6. *Steroids.* Dexamethasone is given at a loading dose of 10 mg i.v. followed by 4 to 8 mg q6h. Dexamethasone should be tapered once its therapeutic effect has been achieved, with the taper extending over 7 to 10 days. Other steroids (hydrocortisone or methylprednisolone) are not used, as they are either insufficiently potent or have inconsistent metabolism that impairs their effectiveness.

7. *Barbiturate coma.* The use of short-acting barbiturates to induce coma is a measure of last resort in managing increased ICP. These agents reduce cerebral metabolism and reduce cerebral blood flow; the most commonly used drug is thiopental given as a loading dose of 3 to 10 mg/kg i.v. over 10 min with a maintenance dose of 1 to 2 mg/kg/hour. Serum levels are checked and should be maintained at 3 to 4 mg/L. Patients in barbiturate coma need intensive monitoring and may require vasopressors to counteract arterial hypotension. Spectral electroencephalogram (EEG) monitoring confirms burst suppression.

SEIZURES

Seizures in the tumor patient are caused by cortical irritation provoked by brain tumor (either primary or metastatic), intracranial bleeding (usually subdural), electrolyte abnormality (in sodium, calcium, or magnesium), infections like meningitis or encephalitis, or head trauma after a fall. As they are most easily corrected, metabolic causes should always be eliminated, but radiological investigation is usually needed as well. Seizures should be controlled because they are distressing to the patient and his or her family, but also because the hypermetabolic effects of active epilepsy can impair function in already compromised brain around a tumor or in a zone of cerebral edema. Seizures can be focal or general, simple or complex, and occur with or without loss of contact with surroundings. A patient with a chronic seizure disorder need not be scanned every time a new seizure is noted. However, a patient without a history of seizures should undergo scanning by computed tomography (CT) or magnetic resonance imaging (MRI) to examine the brain for bleeding, edema, or increased ICP needing intervention. The seizure itself can usually be suppressed by use of levetiracetam (Keppra) or the older drugs, phenytoin (Dilantin) or valproic acid (Depakote). Occasionally seizures will be refractory and will require more than one drug or in cases of status epilepticus, intubation and intravenous barbiturates. The most common cause of new-onset seizure in a previously healthy adult is not tumor but stroke. Nevertheless, brain tumors are associated with seizures as a presenting symptom in 20% to 30% of cases. After surgery, the seizure tendency does not decrease for at least 2 weeks after an offending mass lesion has been resected, likely due to the persistence of edema and the presence of blood products in the resection cavity during that time. If a patient has had seizures prior to surgery and is on anticonvulsants to control them, we continue the drug therapy for 3 to 6 months after surgery before attempting a taper in those who have been seizure-free. For those who have had an uncomplicated craniotomy without a prior history of seizure, we do not routinely use anticonvulsants after surgery. For those with complicated cases involving significant brain trauma in epileptogenic zones, like the temporal lobe or motor cortex, anticonvulsant prophylaxis after surgery is used by surgeon preference.

MYELOPATHY

Myelopathy refers to the clinical syndrome caused by dysfunction of the spinal cord, but does not specify where in the spinal cord such dysfunction has arisen. Syndromes differ depending on the spinal level, as lesions in the cervical cord can produce weakness and sensory loss in all four limbs, whereas lumbar lesions produce such loss only in the legs because of their location well below the exit point of the nerves supplying the arms. The spinal cord also influences bladder and bowel function and in the neck gives rise to the phrenic nerve (C3–5) controlling diaphragmatic excursion. The most common reason for myelopathy in an oncology practice is extrinsic compression of the spinal cord by a metastatic tumor within a vertebral body or pedicle immediately adjacent to the cord. Such patients commonly present with an ascending sensory loss that begins in the feet and can ascend no higher than the level of the lesion itself. In addition, they often show weakness more likely affecting the legs and impairing the ability to walk. They also can complain of bladder and sometimes bowel incontinence. The key to successful treatment of a compressive myelopathy is early intervention before loss of the ability to walk. A patient who has been bed-bound for more than 24 hours is unlikely to benefit from a decompressive operation. Indeed, the first symptom is often not a neurological dysfunction at all but back pain caused by compression of nerve roots or by local instability due to bony collapse or ligamentous disruption. Any patient with a history of cancer who presents with back pain should have an MRI of the affected spinal region to rule out spinal involvement by tumor. Certainly an aging population can contain patients with cancer who also have coincident degenerative disease of the spine with spondylosis, disc protrusion, and osteophyte formation causing a typical degenerative pain syndrome. However, it is never wise to assume the absence of neoplasm in a patient with a history of systemic cancer, and MRI will also help in diagnosing non-tumor pathologies.

RADIOLOGICAL ASSESSMENT

Imaging for tumors of the brain and spine has evolved significantly during the past 20 years and now depends heavily on computerized scans of various types to diagnose lesions, select which are appropriate for surgery, and provide data helpful in planning operative strategies.

Computed Tomography

CT is a vital component of oncological diagnosis for sites in the chest, abdomen, and pelvis. However, its utility in diagnosing brain lesions has diminished somewhat with the advent of the more anatomically detailed images provided by MRI. When oncologists suspect intracranial tumor they often order CT almost by reflex, but MRI will generally be needed whether the CT finding is positive or negative. As the cost differential is not great, the exposure to ionizing radiation is eliminated, and the sensitivity is greater, we recommend using MRI rather than CT as the first-line scanning modality for patients being screened for intracranial or spinal tumor. The advantages of MRI include the anatomical detail that it provides, the multiplanar capacity that permits three-dimensional visualization, the sensitive depiction of the extent of edema, and the ability of MRI to show subtle lesions through the hypersensitive FLAIR sequence usually included in such scans.

CT remains useful in certain limited areas. First, it is much quicker to obtain than an MRI, thus should be used for any patient in whom urgent imaging is needed. In a post-operative patient in whom concern has arisen over the possibility of a clot in the resection cavity, CT is typically requested. Second, the scanner is more open and allows easier access to an unstable patient than the closed tube of an MRI, so CT is favored for very sick patients in the ICU for whom constant nursing access is necessary. Third, the depiction of bone is better on CT than MRI, thus a tumor of the skull vault or skull base usually requires a CT as part of the radiological workup. It can also be used to detect calcification in tumor as a way of narrowing the differential diagnosis. Examples of this include meningiomas and craniopharyngiomas, both benign tumors that often calcify. Showing calcification by CT may allow the diagnosis to be established. Fourth, CT angiography has supplanted digital subtraction angiography as a mode of screening for intracranial aneurysm or other vascular malformations. Formal angiography is still required for patients with vascular lesions who require surgical or endovascular intervention, but CT angiography is an excellent way of deciding whether a patient with an intracerebral hematoma of the temporal lobe and a history of cancer has an aneurysm or a metastatic tumor as the inciting cause of the bleed. Finally, patients with pacemakers may not be able to undergo MRI safely and thus a CT may be required for them.

In the spine, depiction of bony anatomy can be done with great precision by CT using reconstructed sagittal and coronal, as well as axial views. 3-D reconstruction of the spine in patients with complex bony defects, particularly those who have had prior surgery, can be a very valuable tool in planning further surgery.

Magnetic Resonance Imaging

MRI is the most useful radiographic modality in neurosurgical oncology. Frequently used sequences for imaging tumors of the brain include T1-weighted spin-echo before and after injection of gadolinium contrast agent; T2-weighted spin-echo or fast-spin echo sequences; and FLAIR images. Fat suppression can be used as needed to enhance image clarity. Standard depiction of tumors occurs on T1 pre- and post-contrast sequences, with T2 sequences useful for showing edema, cyst, or tumor water content. FLAIR sequences bring out subtle abnormalities than can be missed on other less sensitive images. In addition, diffusion-weighted images show areas of diminished perfusion indicative of stroke, and diffusion tensor imaging can be used for mapping fiber tracts such as the corticospinal tract or uncinate fasciculus, the localization of which can enhance safety during surgery. Functional MRI is now commonly used for patients in whom preoperative mapping of speech areas is desirable. Such patients include those with a tumor near Broca's or Wernicke's area or the left-handed patient in whom localization of speech to the left hemisphere is not guaranteed. Motor mapping can also be done on functional imaging but is less often requested because intraoperative methods of motor mapping are easy to apply and highly accurate.

MRI spectroscopy has been advocated as a method of distinguishing one tumor type from another by virtue of the varied metabolic spectra produced by tumors in vivo. This is a controversial area, and spectroscopy is not a modality that we would apply routinely for that purpose. Its main utility is in distinguishing tumor from post-treatment effect in patients who have undergone prior radiotherapy or chemotherapy. Even in that group, however, the sensitivity and specificity are somewhat imperfect and biopsy may ultimately be needed to make that distinction. The classic tumor signature is an increase in the choline/creatinine ratio over that of normal brain.

In the larger world of oncology, combining CT with positron emission tomography is commonly done now for metastatic surveys. This is not particularly helpful for brain imaging because of the diffuse hypermetabolism exhibited by the brain on such images. However, they can be helpful in detecting metastatic deposits in the spine and pinpointing areas that should undergo MRI for anatomic delineation. In addition, such imaging is quite useful in assessing tumors of peripheral nerve as it can depict formerly benign tumors undergoing dedifferentiation to neurofibrosarcoma, an absolute indication for surgical resection.

PRIMARY TUMORS OF CENTRAL NERVOUS SYSTEM

Brain

Primary brain tumors arise in most cases from neuroglial cells and fall into an umbrella category, the gliomas. These make up 50% to 65% of intracranial tumors in most series. Their pathology, locations, and prognosis are diverse. Annually in the United States approximately 17,000 new cases of malignant primary brain tumors are detected, and gliomas form >90% of these. The median age at diagnosis is the mid- to late 50s, but such tumors can occur in childhood and there is an increase in the incidence of the most malignant form (glioblastoma) in the elderly. Rare familial syndromes, e.g. the Li–Fraumeni syndrome, which link gliomas with other non-neural cancers, but most are sporadic and lack specific risk factors. Basic types are listed in Table 20.3.

Histological Classification

Since the initial attempts at histological classification of gliomas by Cushing and others in the 1920s and 1930s, the multiplicity of definitions has muddied the literature tremendously. Such inconsistency in labeling tumor types and grades has made it difficult to compare the utility of new glioma therapies, and neuropathologists have made strenuous recent efforts to codify their systems. Both three- and four-tiered systems have been suggested, but the current WHO classification contains four grades for astrocytomas. Grade I lesions, which include the subependymal giant cell astrocytomas and pilocytic astrocytomas, are uncommonly seen and grade II are the classical "low-grade" astrocytomas. The uniformly invasive group of anaplastic astrocytomas (grade III) represents the first level of malignancy, and glioblastomas and gliosarcomas are classified in grade IV. Neuropathology has traditionally been as much an art as a science and disagreements among its practitioners are relatively frequent over the subtleties of such grading. With the current and

	Patchell et al. (1990)	**Vecht et al. (1993)**	**Mintz et al. (1996)**
TABLE 20.3 Randomized Trials Comparing [Surgery + Postop Radiotherapy] Versus [Radiotherapy Alone]			
No. of patients	48	63	84
Inclusion criteria	>17 years old	>17 years old	<80 years old
	Single lesion	Single lesion	Single lesion
	KPS >60	Functional level at least 2	KPS >40
	Lesion surgically accessible	Life expectancy >6 months	Lesion surgically accessible
	No LMD	No LMD	No LMD
	Very radiosensitive tumor excluded	No SCLC or lymphoma	No SCLC, lymphoma, or nonmelanoma skin cancer
Disseminated cancer	38%	32%	45%
Imaging	MRI	CT	CT
Histological proof in radiotherapy group	Yes	No	Occasional
Radiotherapy regimen	36 Gy/12 fractions	40 Gy/20 fractions (b.i.d.)	30 Gy/10 fractions
Outcome (weeks)	Surgery better	Surgery better	No difference
Surgery	40	40	24
Radiotherapy	15	24	24

LMD, leptomeningeal disease; SCLC, small cell carcinoma of lung; CT, computed tomography; MRI, magnetic resonance imaging; KPS, Karnofsky performance scale.

growing emphasis on genomic analysis, several molecular alterations can be used as distinguishing characteristics beyond the traditional grading schemes that rely on histology alone.

Astrocytic Tumors

Pilocytic Astrocytomas
These WHO grade I tumors commonly affect patients in the second decade of life and do not invade adjacent brain tissue, nor do they usually undergo malignant degeneration. The majority (two-thirds) occur in the cerebellum; 30% in the optic nerves, chiasm, and hypothalamus; and the rest in the cerebral hemispheres. The treatment for these is surgery which if complete is generally curative. Although some have advocated using radiotherapy and chemotherapy at recurrence, this methodology is controversial and reoperation is often advocated in that circumstance. Such tumors in the cerebellum or cerebral hemisphere are typically resectable with minor or no morbidity. However, those termed "optic gliomas," typically seen in patients with neurofibromatosis type 1 (NF1), are much less amenable to surgery without compromise of vision. Typically such patients are observed and followed conservatively with the therapeutic intervention being radiotherapy should they progress. Surgery is reserved for patients unresponsive to irradiation who have already lost all visual function and in whom the resection is done on a palliative basis.

Astrocytomas

The low-grade (grade II) astrocytomas make up 10% to 25% of gliomas in most series and are usually detected in the fourth or fifth decade. Such tumors grow slowly and often present with seizures or are incidentally found. They do not show well on CT in many cases, and MRI is a more reliable modality for comparative imaging over time. Traditionally these tumors have been managed conservatively, but in the past decade a growing consensus has arisen in the literature over the desirability of resection prior to malignant transformation. The mean time from detection to such transformation is 8 years at which point they become much more aggressive and have a significant likelihood of killing the patient. Because mitosis is so sparse in such tumors, chemotherapy and radiotherapy have not been particularly effective in controlling them long term. In one large study by Karim et al. (2002), the 5-year survival rate was 80% in those with gross total resection, 50% for those with partial resection, and 45% for those who underwent stereotactic biopsy only. Early postoperative radiotherapy lengthens time to progression but not overall survival, and the 5-year median survival rate is 63% to 72% in the studies of Karim et al. and Shaw et al. (2002). Patients with such tumors may be reluctant to undergo surgical resection because of their lack of symptoms, but we do advocate early removal to as complete a degree as possible given local functional anatomy. Enhancing completeness of resection in these relatively subtle lesions is facilitated greatly by the use of an intraoperative MRI (Fig. 20.1). These units are not widely available due to their cost but will become more accessible in the future. Our studies show a significant improvement in radiographically complete resection with such technology relative to historical controls, but the effect on survival is not yet proven.

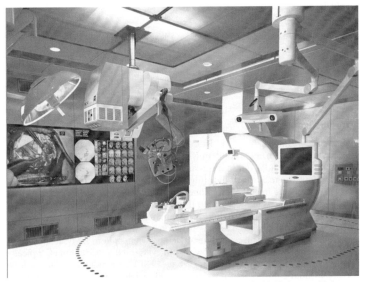

FIGURE 20.1 The intraoperative MRI is located within a magnetically shielded room with integrated components allowing efficiency of workflow. The patient lies on a bed outside the 5-Gauss line for surgery, then is covered to maintain sterility and rotated into the MRI scanner for imaging at intervals during the operation.

Anaplastic Astrocytoma

These tumors occur in a slightly older age group (fifth or sixth decades of life) either de novo or as a result of malignant degeneration within a low-grade astrocytoma. They form 10% to 15% of the gliomas and commonly present in the cerebral hemi-spheres with seizures and focal neurological deficits. These tumors, unlike the low-grade tumors, frequently show contrast enhancement on MRI and have more surrounding edema, mass effect, and rapidity of growth. Age and preoperative functional status are prognostic, but the goal of treatment is not to cure but to extend life and maintain function. Current standard treatment consists of surgical resection followed by radiotherapy and then chemotherapy with temozolomide. A variety of chemotherapy regimens have been tried in the past, but most have been unsuccessful in prolonging life by more than a few months. Most of these tumors will recur eventually as glioblastomas. The median survival is 3 years with about 20% surviving 5 years.

Glioblastoma

This is the most common intrinsic brain tumor and forms half of gliomas in most series. It usually occurs in the sixth or seventh decade, but it can arise at any age. The common location is the cerebral hemisphere with occasional tumors in the corpus callosum giving rise to the classic "butterfly glioma" pattern that extends into both hemispheres from its central point of origin. Inception in the basal ganglia leads quickly to hemiparesis and hemiplegia. Personality change and headache are common, but seizures are seen sometimes only. Glioblastoma is much less common in the posterior fossa and very rare in the spinal cord.

Such tumors have a heterogeneous pattern of enhancement with typically a centrally necrotic area that is relatively hypointense on MRI (Fig. 20.2). The edges are indistinct and such tumors may cross the midline. They have significant perilesional edema in many instances. The histology is characterized by vascular proliferation, frequent mitotic figures, hypercellularity, and necrosis, which is the hallmark of these tumors.

Glioblastomas are the most aggressive brain tumors. Their treatment should be aggressive as well and include a meaningful attempt at radical surgical resection followed by whole-brain radiotherapy and chemotherapy in patients able to tolerate it. Lacroix et al. (2001) have shown at MDACC that the greatest positive influence on survival occurs after resection of ≥98% of the contrast-enhancing portion of the lesion. However, increasing benefit was seen at all percentages of resection above 90%. Thus, if resection is to be done, it makes little sense to remove less than 90% of these tumors, and the ideal approach is complete radiographic removal. Since these tumors have an infiltrating edge and have been shown through biopsy of theoretically unaffected brain to have infiltrating cells as far as 4 cm from the radiographic edge of the tumor, the "gross total" resection is by no means total. For this reason, adjunctive therapies must be used and must be developed further in the future to make a more meaningful impact on this disease. In the realm of chemotherapy, the most studied drugs are the nitrosoureas (BCNU and its analogue CCNU), which give a 10% increase in 18-month survival and little change in median survival. With temozolomide and newer multi-drug combinations, the median survival in our institution is 21 months. This is significantly better than the 9 to 12 months of survival quoted in most textbooks, but still far too short for the patient struck by this tumor in the peak of life, as many are.

Innovative approaches include biologically based therapies such as immunotherapy and gene therapy. Trials are currently underway at MDACC using each of these approaches. In immunotherapy, tumors that are positive for the endothelial growth factor receptor variant III (35% to 40% of glioblastomas) showed significant prolongation of survival to 30 months after which all recurred through the growth

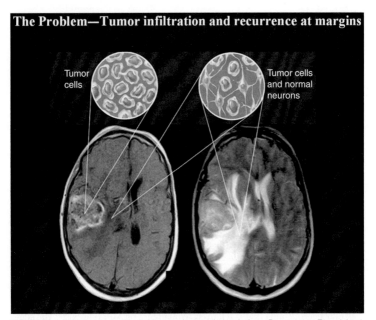

FIGURE 20.2 MRI of patient with glioblastoma in the right hemisphere. Post-contrast T1-weighted image is on the left side of the panel, and T2-weighted image shows edema on the right. Even when gross total removal of contrast-enhancing portions is achieved, the margins remain with infiltrating tumor cells that cannot be controlled by surgery.

of clones not positive for that epitope. A study using the delta 24 oncolytic virus given through intraparenchymal injection of the tumor or the edges of its resection cavity is underway at MDACC. Kunwar et al. (2010) have used convection-enhanced delivery to infuse IL-13-PE38QQR (IL-13 linked to pseudomonas exotoxin) into the brain's interstitial space in patients with glioblastoma, but without significant added benefit. Given that this approach combines a new mode of delivery with a new therapeutic agent, it is hard to tell whether the agent would be effective if delivered by other means.

The 5-year survival for glioblastoma is <5% and recurrence occurs within 2 to 3 cm of the original resection margin in 80% of patients. The remaining patients also show recurrence, but farther afield within the brain, and even in the opposite hemisphere. Metastasis to extraneural sites is vanishingly rare. Occasional patients are seen with gliomatosis, that is, a multifocal involvement of more than one lobe of the brain. Because many patients with systemic cancer are elderly and glioblastoma tends to be a disease of older patients, it is not infrequent to find glioblastoma arising in a patient being treated for a second cancer, so it is important for general oncologists to recognize its manifestations, implications, and modes of therapy.

Oligodendrogliomas

These tumors form 10% to 15% of gliomas and typically involve the cerebral hemispheres, with involvement of the thalamus and brainstem much less likely. They present in the fifth or sixth decade, frequently with seizures although headache and focal deficit may also occur. They are more likely to be calcified than are the astrocytomas, indicative of their slower pace of growth. The majority present as grade II lesions, but the occasional anaplastic tumor arises de novo as a grade III lesion. The classic histological finding is a perinuclear halo known as a "fried egg" appearance which is caused by shrinkage of the cellular components during exposure to formalin. Mixed oligo-astrocytomas are possible and are defined by staining with glial fibrillary acid protein, an astrocytic marker not present in oligodendroglioma.

Cairncross et al. (1998) have shown that chromosomal analysis further differentiates a subgroup of oligodendrogliomas forming 60% to 70% of the whole, with deletions of chromosome 1p, 19q, or both. Those tumors with such deletions are more sensitive to chemotherapy (prototypically, procarbazine, CCNU, and vincristine), radiotherapy, or both. Thus, the median survival is affected by the presence or absence of these chromosomal alterations. It is 3 to 5 years for patients with tumors without loss of heterozygosity and 10 to 12 years for those with loss of heterozygosity. Therapy for oligodendrogliomas mirrors that for astrocytomas, with surgery followed by radiotherapy and chemotherapy used in most cases. Chemotherapy is overall more effective in oligodendrogliomas than astrocytomas. However, recent work shows a survival difference within the glioblastoma population based on patients' mutational status in the *IDH1* gene. Such molecular analyses will be increasingly important in personalizing therapeutic choices of drugs most likely to work in tumors most likely to respond.

Ependymomas

These tumors arise from the ependymal lining of the ventricles and most commonly produce tumors in the fourth ventricle or its recesses. They arise more often in children, but do occur occasionally in adults in whom the supratentorial location is more typical. A related tumor is the subependymoma, which is less common and more indolent. Classic ependymomas can be low grade or anaplastic, and CSF seeding occurs more often in the latter category (8%) than in the low-grade tumors (4%). Because of the possibility of such seeding, imaging should include the entire craniospinal axis and CSF should be obtained for cytological analysis. Treatment is surgery followed by either whole-brain irradiation or craniospinal axis irradiation, then chemotherapy. The extent of radiotherapy depends on the tumor's location, grade, and whether cytology is positive. When drop metastases are present, low-dose irradiation of the spinal axis should be performed with a boost to the specific area involved. The 5-year survival rate is 40% to 60% with local recurrence within 2 years in half of patients overall.

NEURONAL TUMORS

This unusual category includes gangliogliomas and central neurocytomas, both of which arise from presumptive neuronal rather than glial elements. As their name implies, gangliogliomas include glial fibrillary acid protein-positive cells, although the neoplastic component is believed to be the ganglion cell portion of the tumor. Gangliogliomas are most commonly found in the temporal lobes and present classically with seizures, although they can also be found in other intracranial locations. Neurocytomas arise along the edge of the lateral ventricles where they can grow to a large size due to their slow rate of expansion and their filling of the ventricle before they achieve meaningful neurological compression and compromise. Gangliogliomas are usually eminently resectable and can be cured by surgery alone. About 10% are malignant and that category requires radiotherapy and chemotherapy. The central neurocytomas are typically treated with surgery alone although focused radiotherapy may be useful for unresectable portions of a large tumor. Because of the intraventricular location of most central neurocytomas, shunting may be required after their resection to control communicating hydrocephalus.

METASTATIC BRAIN TUMORS

Between 20% and 40% of patients with systemic cancer develop brain metastasis. Such tumors can be extra-axial (involving the dura and subdural space, or lepto-meninges and subarachnoid space) but usually occur within the brain parenchyma. MRI confirms that two-third of such patients have more than one metastasis in the brain and that the classic solitary metastasis is uncommon. As with other tumor types, available methods for treating brain metastases include surgery, focused or diffuse irradiation, or chemotherapy.

The true incidence of brain metastasis is unknown. CT under-represents the number of metastases in many patients and is insufficiently sensitive to use as a proper screening study. MRI is the imaging modality of choice as it can show not only subtle lesions but also leptomeningeal disease, the presence of which greatly impacts prognosis and mode of treatment. Brain metastases are the most common intracranial tumors in adults. Their incidence has risen because of increased detection by MRI and because of longer survival from more effective systemic therapies. The biology and thus the nuances of surgical treatment differ among the various histologies, so brain metastasis cannot be considered as a single disease. About 1% to 2% of ovarian and prostate cancers spread to the brain, but at least half of melanomas do so when other systemic metastases are present. These tumors are supratentorial in 80%. The most common histological type of brain metastasis is carcinoma of the lung which makes up 40% to 60%, followed by those derived from breast cancers (15% to 20%) and melanoma (10% to 20%) with the data differing between clinical and autopsy series. Colorectal and renal cell carcinomas account for 5% to 10% each. These five sources yield most cerebral metastases. Melanoma has the highest propensity to spread to the brain but is less represented than lung cancer because of the much greater incidence of the latter in the general population. In children with systemic cancer, the incidence of intracerebral metastasis is <5% and arises mainly from neuroblastoma, Wilms tumor, and sarcoma (especially rhabdomyosarcoma).

Two-third of patients with brain metastasis present with neurological decline, usually focal deficits or impairment of cognitive function. Many asymptomatic patients actually have disordered cognition unrecognized by external observers. Increase in ICP through edema or blockage of CSF pathways can combine with local ischemia to give localized cerebral dysfunction. In 20% to 30% of patients seizures occur, more often in those with multiple metastases. Two histologies are particularly prone to intratumoral bleeding: melanoma and choriocarcinoma in which the bleeding rates are 45% and 95%, respectively. On MRI a large amount of edema around a recent hematoma (<6 hours old) suggests but does not confirm a tumor beneath the hematoma. Metastases can produce cysts, especially carcinomas of the breast and adenocarcinomas of the lung, but other histologies can also provoke them.

Radiology

MRI is the most sensitive test and thus should be used for surveillance unless it is contraindicated. Most metastases are hypo- to isointense on T1-weighted images and hyperintense on T2-weighted images. Hemorrhage may be suggested by the presence of a hemosiderin ring hypointense on T2 along the tumor margin or by hyperintensity on pre-contrast T1-weighted images. Some small tumors may fail to enhance due to relative preservation of the blood–brain barrier but can still be detected on FLAIR sequences.

These tumors are classically located at the junction between grey and white matter. However, they can grow anywhere in the brain. Radiological diagnosis is sometimes inexact, but presumed metastases meeting the above criteria may turn out to be other tumor types when resected. Patchell et al. (1990) reported that 11% of patients thought to have a single brain metastasis actually had other pathology.

Multiple brain lesions in patients without a history of cancer represent metastasis in only 15% of cases. Spinal tap is the only other diagnostic test sometimes helpful in workup of such patients. If cytological analysis is positive for malignant cells in CSF, the patient by definition has leptomeningeal dissemination of tumor and may benefit from intrathecal instillation of chemotherapy. This is usually done through an Ommaya reservoir, which is a silastic chamber placed beneath the scalp in the frontal area with a ventriculostomy tube leading into the frontal horn of the lateral ventricle. As the ventricles are the site of origin for CSF, this places the drug at the beginning point of the pathways of CSF flow, which are thus able to carry it widely through the subarachnoid space.

Life expectancy of patients with brain metastasis depends more on the status of their systemic disease than the status of their brain metastasis (which can usually be controlled); however, patients with leptomeningeal dissemination of tumor have the worst prognosis with a median survival of 3 months. They are at risk for hydrocephalus and survival can be prolonged by shunting, but their prognosis remains poor even with aggressive multimodality therapy including intrathecal chemotherapy and radiotherapy.

Unknown Primary Tumors

One-third of patients with symptomatic brain metastases have no systemic cancer previously diagnosed. Such patients should undergo metastatic workup to screen the most likely primary sites (lung, breast, kidney, colon, and skin). Lung cancer is the culprit in 70% of these patients. Thus, chest x-ray, mammography (in women), and a skin survey should be obtained. CT of the chest, abdomen, and pelvis, or positron emission tomography–CT, should also be done. In the absence of any accessible extracranial tumor, stereotactic biopsy or (more often) open resection of the cerebral tumor should be done to confirm diagnosis prior to treatment. The source of an unknown primary brain metastasis remains occult in 15% of patients despite extensive investigation.

Treatment

The management of brain metastasis is both complex and controversial. It includes surgery, stereotactic radiotherapy, whole-brain radiotherapy, and chemotherapy. Patients with edema on MRI receive steroids to suppress it. Clinical improvement is generally noted within 12 hours of beginning steroid therapy in 70% to 80% of cases, but the peak effect may be delayed for up to a week. After surgery a steroid taper is instituted over 1 to 2 weeks. We reserve anticonvulsants for patients with a known seizure history.

Single Brain Metastasis

The median survival for patients without treatment is 6 weeks. Adding steroids improves this to 3 months, and external beam (whole-brain) radiotherapy improves survival to 4 to 6 months. Randomized clinical trials comparing surgery + radiotherapy with radiotherapy alone suggest a significant benefit from surgery on overall survival and quality of life. If systemic disease is not controlled, however, the benefits of controlling brain metastasis are eroded.

The variables to be considered when selecting patients with a single metastasis for surgery are (a) the overall clinical status, (b) the surgical accessibility of the tumor, and (c) its radiosensitivity. Only patients with absent or controlled systemic disease and no leptomeningeal dissemination of tumor derive significant benefit from the removal of brain metastasis. Obviously distinguishing "controlled" from "uncontrolled" systemic disease can be somewhat arbitrary. We usually look for expected survival of ≥4 months in patients being considered for surgery, while advanced age, poor medical condition, and KPS <70 argue against surgery.

Ultimately brain metastasis is a multifocal or even a diffuse process. Focal treatments like surgery or radiosurgery can suppress the disease, but eliminating it may require whole-brain irradiation to treat microscopic foci unseen on MRI as well as small tumor fragments left at sites of resection. However, standard radiotherapy is less effective than radiosurgery for radiographically evident tumors because the dose must be lowered to prevent toxicity to normal brain. Standard whole-brain radiotherapy uses 10 fractions of 3 Gy each for a total dose of 30 Gy.

Surgery Versus Radiosurgery: The Conundrum

The basic dilemma for most patients with brain metastasis is whether to treat with surgery or use focused methods of stereotactic irradiation to target the lesion(s) (Fig. 20.3). Attempts at randomized trials have not been wholly successful due to the difficulty of convincing patients to enroll. Many patients have a bias favoring

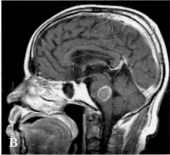

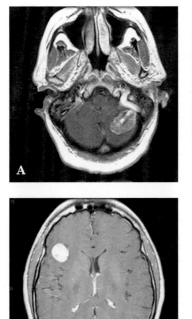

FIGURE 20.3 A: MRI showing metastasis from carcinoma of colon in left cerebellar hemisphere. This patient should have surgery, because the lesion's size puts it slightly above the 3-cm limit for stereotactic radiosurgery, and its location in the posterior fossa means that brainstem should be protected from the possibility of edema post-irradiation. **B:** This metastatic carcinoma of unknown primary sits within the brainstem, a site that is unsafe for surgery. It should be treated with stereotactic radiosurgery. **C:** This small metastasis from renal cell carcinoma sits in the right frontal lobe. This area is safe for both surgery and radiosurgery, and this patient can be assigned either treatment, with little advantage to be gained from choosing one over the other.

| | Advantages Versus Disadvantages of Surgery |

Advantages
No incision
Treats surgically inaccessible lesions
More easily tolerated by physiologically compromised patient
Short hospital stay (usually 1 day)

Disadvantages
Poor targeting for tumors >3 cm in diameter
Tumor persists on scans, so must be followed to prove success
No tissue diagnosis
Persistent edema or radionecrosis may require surgical removal of tumor
Cannot be used on targets within 5 mm of optic nerve/chiasm/tract without significant dose modification

stereotactic radiosurgery as it has the benefit of avoiding a surgical incision, anesthesia, and a hospital stay of several days with recovery over several weeks. Radiosurgery procedures are done in a single day and require little to no post-treatment recovery. They do require placement of a head frame with resulting moderate discomfort, but most patients tolerate this well. Retrospective comparison implies a similar outcome between surgery and stereotactic irradiation but is unreliable because of selection bias. Advantages and disadvantages of radiosurgery are shown in Table 20.4. At MDACC we now treat four patients with radiosurgery for each one treated surgically.

Drawbacks to radiosurgery remain. Even when local control of a tumor is achieved, patients with significant peritumoral edema may remain steroid-dependent for 3 months or even longer. Many tumors show temporary mild enlargement and intensification of enhancement during the first 1 to 2 months after radiosurgery. Persistence of edema, development of necrosis exerting mass effect, or frank tumor growth after radiosurgery imply treatment failure and are all indications for resection. With both surgery and radiosurgery, local rates of control of 85% to 95% are achieved, which are similar for various histologies, and median survivals range between 8 and 13 months depending on histology. The so-called radio-resistant tumors such as melanoma, renal cell carcinoma, and soft-tissue sarcomas do respond to radiosurgery because of the high dose used, but local rates of control are still lower than in carcinomas of the lung and breast.

Recent comparisons of patients operated by en bloc resection versus piecemeal removal have shown that en bloc resection yields better local control and also a lower rate of subsequent leptomeningeal dissemination. Clearly surgical technique is important in metastasis removal. Tumors that are soft and friable, necrotic, cystic, or hemorrhagic are particularly difficult to remove cleanly, and in such cases strong consideration should be given to subsequent adjuvant radiotherapy either as a stereotactic boost to the operative cavity or by whole-brain mode.

The morbidity after radiosurgery is comparable to that seen after surgery. In each the local recurrence rate is 5% to 15%. Hemorrhage and seizures can occur after either. Worsening of cerebral edema is unusual, however, after resection of a metastasis and most post-surgical patients improve neurologically and can stop steroids within 1 to 2 weeks. The 30-day post-operative mortality is 2% to 3% in major centers with an overall morbidity of 10% to 15%.

We recommend surgery to patients with a single metastasis who present with marked mass effect and neurological decline. When systemic disease is controlled the brain metastasis can usually be removed without inciting or worsening neurological deficits, and surgery is a good option. However, locations in deep portions of the brain or in/near eloquent areas may shift the balance in favor of radiosurgery. Very large tumors respond best to surgery. Radiosurgery is the preferred treatment for tumors <3 cm in diameter in patients whose age or medical condition renders them imperfect candidates for surgery or whose tumors are located in areas of relative surgical inaccessibility.

Patient preference is a major driving factor in making the choice between surgery and radiosurgery. The perception of radiosurgery as non-invasive often trumps the therapeutic benefits of surgery in the minds of patients and physicians alike.

Radiotherapy After Surgery

Whole-brain irradiation is often given after surgical resection of brain metastases to reduce local recurrence and eliminate any occult micrometastases. The conventional dosing scheme is 30 Gy/10 fractions. Larger fraction sizes give increased risk of neurotoxicity, but this regimen does not eliminate altogether the long-term cognitive effects of irradiating the entire brain. Given the longer survivals now achieved by multimodality or personalized treatment regimens for various cancers with a propensity for brain metastasis, such delayed toxicity (which usually takes ≥2 years to develop) has been seen more often recently and is very difficult to treat.

Patchell et al. (1998) described a randomized trial assigning surgical patients to postoperative observation versus radiotherapy. The study was limited to patients with a single, completely resected brain metastasis, and the radiotherapy consisted of 50.4 Gy in 28 fractions, a significantly longer course of treatment than is given in most centers. This regimen lowered the local rate of recurrence from 46% to 10% and the appearance of brain metastasis at new sites from 37% to 14%. Differences in overall survival and functionally independent survival were not statistically significant. This study is flawed in that a local recurrence rate of 46% is three times higher than expected with surgery alone, thus conclusions about the efficacy of whole-brain irradiation in controlling local recurrence are dubious at best. It does appear to reduce formation of new brain metastases, which suggests that micrometastases are indeed present in many patients.

Whole-brain radiotherapy for single lesions after surgical removal (or after radiosurgery) is thus a valid treatment option. It is equally valid to withhold radiotherapy and monitor closely for recurrence, at which point focal therapy can be repeated as needed. The decision to give such radiotherapy should be based on the number of tumors visible in the brain and on their size and radiosensitivity. Although we have traditionally favored whole-brain radiotherapy for patients with multiple tumors, we now often treat these with stereotactic radiotherapy focused on multiple separate targets to reduce the risk of provoking cognitive deficits. When used, it works best on small tumors (<2 cm) and on those with radiosensitive histology.

Multiple Metastases

A nihilistic attitude is maintained by many neurosurgeons toward patients with multiple brain metastases. However, studies from our institution have shown through retrospective and case-control analysis that multiple surgical resections via one or more simultaneous craniotomies are both safe and effective. In the case-control study by Bindal et al. (1993) survival of patients undergoing complete resection of up to three metastases was significantly better than that of patients in whom one or more tumors was left unresected and was similar to survival after removal of a single metastasis, without increase in morbidity or mortality. Surgery should definitely be considered for a single, dominant, surgically accessible metastatic tumor causing mass effect and neurological compromise, regardless of the presence of smaller and less dangerous tumors elsewhere in the brain. When a cluster of tumors can be removed through a single craniotomy, this too may be beneficial in preserving neurological function. In many large centers (including ours), local therapy (with or without subsequent whole-brain irradiation) is offered for multiple metastases in patients with controlled systemic disease, KPS >70, and life expectancy >3 to 4 months. Argument continues over the ideal cut-off number for brain metastases above which focal therapy should not be offered. In one typical clinical scenario, lesions >2 to 3 cm in diameter are resected and the remainder, especially those that are surgically inaccessible, are treated with radiosurgery. When all tumors are <3 cm in diameter, focal therapy should be offered for all tumors as treating some but not others yields little benefit.

Chemotherapy

Chemotherapy has not been very successful in controlling cerebral metastases. The blood–brain barrier provides a pharmacological sanctuary for metastatic lesions. Occasional responses by chemosensitive solid tumors such as breast cancer or non-seminomatous germ cell tumors of the testis belie the sturdiness of the barrier, and 10% of melanoma brain metastases will respond to temozolomide given systemically. In general, however, chemotherapy gives little improvement in survival or quality for brain metastasis and is usually a last resort after other therapies have failed.

Small Cell Carcinoma: A Special Case

Randomized prospective trials have shown that prophylactic whole-brain radiotherapy reduces the incidence of brain metastasis in patients with small cell carcinoma of the lung, a histology exquisitely sensitive to irradiation. Enthusiasm for this technique is tempered by concern over its effects on cognitive function in patients who survive longer than a year. In addition, radiation necrosis can occur idiosyncratically beyond 9 months from radiation delivery. Neurological toxicity can be limited by keeping fractions small and by withholding concurrent chemotherapy. The current consensus holds that prophylactic whole-brain irradiation confers a survival advantage of 5% at 3 years and a reduction in the incidence of brain metastasis by 25% and is thus considered standard treatment for patients with this disease who are in complete remission after initial treatment. The situation for patients who have not achieved complete remission is less clear.

Surgical Technique for Brain Metastasis

Ideally resection is done en bloc when removal of a circumferential 5-mm margin of brain is not limited by nearby functional areas. When it is so limited, or when tumors are friable or cystic, a careful piecemeal technique must often be used. When intratumoral hemorrhage eliminates the en bloc option, the blood should be carefully drained from the tumor pocket and not allowed to spill and produce seeding that leads to early recurrence. In addition, the wall of any associated cyst should be excised along with the tumor. The most friable tumors (melanoma, non-seminomatous germ cell tumors, and some lung cancers) should be isolated with cottonoids prior to resection to avoid tumor escape into the subdural space.

General Principles of Intracranial Surgery

In the majority of cases the goal of surgery is resection, either to the maximum possible degree or to a more limited degree for the purposes of decompression and open biopsy. Occasional patients will present with tumors in locations preventing safe resection or in whom the use of prior therapy has raised the possibility of the lesion's representing treatment effect rather than tumor. In those circumstances, stereotactic biopsy may be chosen over open resection.

Stereotactic biopsy involves the placement of a biopsy needle under image guidance at a radiologically specified target within a brain lesion. This can be done using a frame-based system or with frameless technology. When a frame is used, it is placed around the patient's head to provide a physical array of known linear and angular dimensions that serves as a Cartesian coordinate grid and thus a reference framework against which the location of the target can be plotted. A scan is done after frame placement and shows the lesion as well as the frame structure. Coordinates are acquired using specialized computer software and the fiducial bars are then removed from the frame. They are replaced with an adjustable superstructure through which the biopsy needle is passed. The coordinates are used to position the superstructure to direct the needle to the target at the appropriate angle and depth. A suction–aspiration method is used that pulls small portions of the lesion into the side window at the needle tip, where they are trapped in an inner sleeve that is removed to extract the specimen. Such biopsy is therefore not useful for achieving meaningful resection; if resection is the goal, a craniotomy should be done instead.

In frameless systems, small round fiducial markers are placed on the surface of the patient's scalp at multiple points. A scan (usually an MRI) is then performed and the patient brought to the operating room with the markers still in place. The patient is registered to the system by localizing each of the external markers with a wand whose position is determined by the workstation through an infrared detector. This process registers the patient's head into the three-dimensional space predicted by the scan and then similar infrared detection is used on the needle itself, which effectively becomes the localizing probe. Frameless systems are subject to slightly more error than frame-based systems and thus should not be chosen for brainstem biopsies, but their accuracy is quite sufficient for biopsy in supratentorial locations.

It is important to recognize that the heterogeneity of gliomas may lead to sampling error if biopsy is not taken from several points within the lesion. The main risk of stereotactic biopsy is the induction of bleeding at the biopsy site. Most such hematomas are clinically insignificant but in 1% a craniotomy must be done to relieve pressure from an expanding clot.

The advantage of surgical resection is that it is more likely to overcome the intratumoral heterogeneity (and thus give a more accurate pathological diagnosis), and of course, it does achieve physical removal of tumor with elimination of mass effect, reduction of ICP, and improvement in neurological impairment. Intraoperative mapping of cortical function allows the resection of tumors even when located in or near the so-called eloquent areas, that is, those containing important functions like speech or motor control. It is our routine practice to perform cortical mapping in any patient whose tumor is suspected by radiographic criteria of being within 2 cm of the motor strip, Broca's area, or Wernicke's area.

In patients in whom tumor is intimately involved with speech areas, we perform craniotomy awake with anesthesia induced through a laryngeal mask airway during the opening and close phases of the operation. The anesthesiologist removes the airway (and fully awakens the patient) for the core portion of the procedure when speech mapping and then tumor resection are performed. This is made possible by an extensive scalp block placed after the patient is asleep and lasting for a number of hours beyond completion of the procedure. Speech mapping is done in areas near tumor and suggested by preoperative functional MRI as containing speech function. Mapping proceeds by the surgeon applying a low-voltage electrical stimulus to the cortical surface at sites being tested while the patient carries on a conversation or names objects shown on cards. Interruption of speech by the electrical stimulus denotes active function at the site touched. It is possible to integrate within a navigational workstation not only standard anatomical information for tumor localization but also functional MRI information as an overlay, together with fiber tract localization obtained from diffusion tensor imaging acquired prior to surgery. In this way, the completeness of resection can be enhanced while reducing the risk of neurological injury to maximal degree.

The mortality rate from craniotomy in large series is 1% to 2%. Surgical morbidity includes increased neurological deficit (8% to 11%), hemorrhage at the operative site (4% to 5%, although no more than 1% require reopening and evacuation), and wound infection (1% to 2%). Medical complications such as deep vein thrombosis, myocardial infarction, and pneumonia occur in 3% to 9%. It is worth noting that venous Doppler studies of patients with glioblastoma before surgery have shown deep venous thrombosis in the legs of 30% to 40% of patients. Thus, the postoperative finding of such thrombosis may simply imply an ongoing hypercoagulable state that predated the surgery. In glioma surgery and in particular when resecting malignant gliomas, the added risk of an aggressive resection is less than the risk of leaving tumor behind and thereby provoking an ongoing edematous reaction within the residual tumor. Such edema causes worsening of pre-existing deficits and responds only slowly to osmotic dieresis and steroids. In accessible brain tumors, the main constraint on resection is the presence of nearby eloquent brain that cannot be breached without causing a functional decline in the patient.

CRANIAL SURGICAL APPROACHES

In planning resection for intracranial glioma or metastasis, four basic styles of craniotomy are applied.

1. The *pterional approach* gives access to frontal and temporal lobe tumors near the Sylvian fissure or skull base. This can be modified by creating a more posterior curve or greater extension to the vertex when necessary. Such patients are placed supine with the shoulder bumped up and the head tilted away from the affected side. The incision has the appearance of a reverse question-mark and starts just anterior to the tragus at the zygomatic process, then ends at its superior aspect behind the hairline between the mid-pupillary line and the midline.

2. A *bicoronal incision* can be used to approach the frontal lobe more anteriorly or medially than one can achieve through a pterional approach. This allows access to medial frontal lobe lesions and also permits a subfrontal approach to the anterior fossa floor or suprasellar space. Patients are placed supine with the head neutral or slightly angled to either side. The incision may extend from one zygomatic process to the other and again is kept behind the hairline. When a unilateral craniotomy is performed, the incision extends only to the contralateral superior temporal line. Care should be taken when a low craniotomy opening is done to avoid opening the frontal sinus (when possible), or if it is opened to occlude it with fat and then cover it with a pericranial flap harvested from the undersurface of the reflected scalp. This prevents communication between the contaminated frontal sinus cavity and the sterile intradural space, with subsequent onset of infection.

3. A *V-shaped or horseshoe-shaped incision* may be placed with a medial limb along the midline or near it and parallel to it. Such an approach gives good access to tumors in the medial half of the hemisphere. This also gives access to the interhemispheric fissure and thus to the corpus callosum and intraventricular space. These patients are placed neutral with the head flexed slightly forward. The incision can be shifted posteriorly for tumors in the parietal or occipital lobes, and for surgery in those locations the patient can be placed in lateral or prone position.

4. A *suboccipital craniotomy* is used for resection of infratentorial lesions. It can be located at the midline (our preferred location) or in a paramedian

position. If paramedian, it should be more than two finger-breadths lateral to the midline to avoid damaging the greater occipital nerve, which supplies sensation to a significant portion of the posterior scalp. The patient is generally placed prone or in a lateral position, and the patient's head may be rotated toward the floor and flexed for better access when the tentorial angle is steep. The incision goes from the inion to the spinous process of C2, and the muscles are reflected laterally with care taken to preserve the vertebral arteries as they loop over the lateral aspect of C1. We prefer to perform this operation as a craniotomy rather than the more traditional craniectomy, as retaining the bone plate permits less postoperative pain due to muscle adhesion to the pain-sensitive dura, which is left exposed in the craniectomy site. The dura in such cases is opened in a Y-fashion, and the cisterna magna opened to release CSF.

The use of computer-assisted navigational techniques is optional for most brain tumor cases but can be quite helpful in minimizing the size of the craniotomy opening and in identifying the extent of the lesion (Fig. 20.4). When such stereotactic navigation is used, four stages are followed: image acquisition, registration,

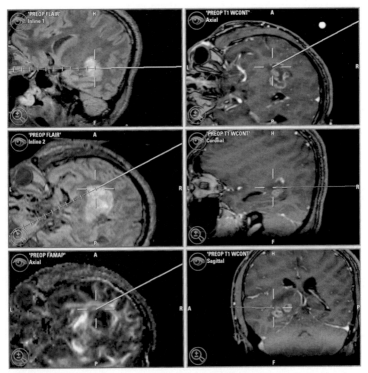

FIGURE 20.4 MRI acquired before surgery and imported into BrainLab neuronavigational workstation. It shows a glioblastoma in the deep posterior right temporal area, localized by wand guidance that will allow optimal creation of the craniotomy opening and of the transcerebral corridor needed to expose the tumor.

planning, and intraoperative navigation. Typically the images are acquired before the operation after fiducial markers have been placed on the skin of the anterior half of the head. The images acquired are transferred to the intraoperative computer workstation and can be overlaid on imaging data from functional MRI or tractography as mentioned above. When the patient is placed into final position in the operating room, registration is done to synchronize the patient's fiducial array with the array depicted in the previously acquired images. From that point on the surgeon can check the position of any point within the head in three dimensions relative to the tumor or to anatomical landmarks with accuracy of 1 to 2 mm. This accuracy diminishes, however, as the operation proceeds due to brain shift caused by hyperventilation, CSF loss, and tumor removal. Thus, we generally use intraoperative ultrasound for real-time imaging, as it is cheaper, provides immediate feedback, and is not subject to the vicissitudes of brain shift.

INTRACRANIAL BLEEDING

Hematomas occur within the head in the epidural, subdural, subarachnoid, and intracerebral spaces. The general differential diagnosis for such bleeding includes head trauma (the most common cause), arterial hypertension, vascular anomalies such as aneurysms and arteriovenous malformations, recent prior surgery, and coagulopathy.

In the setting of cancer with its predilection for the elderly, hypertensive intracerebral hematomas or spontaneous intracerebral hematomas caused by amyloid angiopathy are occasionally seen. These are only treated with craniotomy for evacuation of hematoma when mass effect has been produced leading to a decreased level of consciousness or when the clot expands on serial imaging. Most such cases are treated conservatively with control of blood pressure, anticonvulsant prophylaxis, and correction of coagulopathy.

Epidural hematomas are almost always traumatic in origin. Subdural hematomas can be traumatic or spontaneous from tumor abutting the subdural space. The trauma required to provoke a chronic subdural hematoma may be so minimal as not to be remembered by the patient. The elderly are especially prone to subdural hematomas because the cerebral atrophy that occurs with age causes stretching of the veins traversing the subdural space, rendering them more susceptible to disruption by a blow to the head, even a minor one.

Bleeding from a metastatic tumor can produce an intracerebral hematoma that can be difficult to distinguish from hypertensive or spontaneous bleeding. Edema around the clot suggests tumor but can be absent, and review of all MRI sequences sometimes shows subtle traces of a tumor inside the blood. If other brain metastases are present, the bleed is probably tumor-induced. If a clot is suspected of hiding a tumor, the need for operation is much greater. Otherwise, rebleeding can occur and tumor growth is inevitable over time.

The other common presentation of intracranial hematoma in a cancer center is an intracerebral, subarachnoid, or subdural hematoma caused by chemotherapy-induced coagulopathy. Patients with hematological malignancies (leukemia or lymphoma) routinely show very low platelet counts induced by either their disease or the treatment given for it. Even profound thrombocytopenia can be well tolerated in the absence of trauma. Low counts (<50,000) put patients at much higher risk for bleeding compared to a platelet count >100,000. As the quality of the platelets can also be compromised by chemotherapy, low counts can actually underestimate the risk of such bleeding. Minor bleeding seen on imaging but unaccompanied by any neurological decline can be followed conservatively with correction of coagulopathy, which may require platelet transfusions as well as infusion of clotting factors and exogenous vitamin K. When a patient with a subdural or other hematoma is coagulopathic and needs surgical evacuation of the blood due to neurological decline, surgery cannot be done safely and effectively unless the coagulopathy is first corrected. Different surgeons have different criteria for correction; we generally accept patients for surgery who have had correction of the platelet count to ≥75,000 and INR to ≤1.2. This permits control of intraoperative bleeding and gets the patient safely off the operating table. It is vital that such correction continues during the postoperative phase to prevent re-accumulation of the clot. Our policy is to offer surgery in the circumstance outlined above, but not to re-operate repeatedly when platelet counts cannot be maintained sufficiently high to prevent rebleeding. This policy also prevents patients who are fundamentally refractory to platelet transfusion from receiving surgery should they suffer an intra-cranial bleed.

HYDROCEPHALUS

Hydrocephalus is an accumulation of CSF within the head (generally, the ventricles) leading to a rise in ICP that when high enough will compromise brain function. It can be "non-communicating" when the CSF pathways are blocked somewhere along their course or "communicating" when the blockage is at the final point of the pathway, the arachnoid granulations near the superior sagittal sinus, where CSF is absorbed into the venous system. Patients with cancer develop hydrocephalus for any of several reasons:

1. Tumor may be located in the brain near the ventricular system, against which it produces mass effect sufficient to trap the upstream portion and cause it to balloon.

2. Leptomeningeal disease, defined as tumor cells in the subarachnoid space where CSF flow occurs, can clog the absorptive pathways or cause radiographically occult blockage at points of narrowing along the CSF pathways, for example, the aqueduct of Sylvius.

3. The effects of treatment may cause hydrocephalus. The likeliest scenario occurs after whole-brain radiotherapy with formation of scarring either in the ventricles or on the arachnoid granulations that interfere with CSF absorption or flow. Radiotherapy may additionally alter brain compliance and thereby magnify the effects of pathway blockage by shifting the pressure–volume curve.

Treatment

Medical therapies for hydrocephalus reduce CSF production to mitigate rises in pressure. The drugs generally used are Diamox (a carbonic anhydrase inhibitor) and dexamethasone. Both reduce the rate of CSF production but do not increase its absorption, and are temporizing measures useful while preparing a more definitive plan of action. The most direct way of treating hydrocephalus is to remove any mass that causes obstruction. In many patients, however, no such mass exists and placement of a shunt is the appropriate treatment.

A ventriculostomy is in effect a temporary shunt that diverts CSF out of the ventricle into an external collecting system. This may be placed to record CSF pressures to show whether a shunt is needed and if so, to help in selecting its valve strength. Indwelling shunts offer a more permanent solution, usually in the form of a ventriculoperitoneal system that runs from the lateral ventricle up through a burr hole into the subgaleal space over the cranium, and thence behind the ear and through the subcutaneous space of the neck, anterior chest, and abdominal wall to a point where it penetrates the peritoneum to deposit CSF into the peritoneal cavity. There the large surface area facilitates efficient CSF absorption. Shunts contain a valve usually located either at the burr hole where the shunt emerges or further downstream above or behind the ear. The valve allows the shunt to provide a set resistance to flow. This mechanism shuts off flow through the shunt when the ICP falls to the desired level and opens the shunt when the ICP rises above it.

Patients sometimes require instillation of intraventricular chemotherapy for leptomeningeal carcinomatosis with concomitant hydrocephalus. Such treatment would be ineffective in the presence of a standard shunt, which would immediately flush it from the ventricles. In such cases, we place a shunt with an "on-off" valve that allows the shunt to be closed or opened by external pressure on the valve. Just before chemotherapy is instilled into the ventricular system through an in-line Ommaya reservoir, the shunt is closed. It is reopened after a suitable interval (usually 3 to 5 hours later) to relieve built-up CSF pressure and carry the patient safely until the next treatment. As these patients are usually quite shunt-dependent, longer periods of occlusion are unsafe.

Once an indwelling shunt has been placed, it is expected to function for the remainder of the patient's life. However, later problems do arise including shunt blockage, infection, or shift in the dynamics of the hydrocephalus that require valve renewal at a different level of resistance. When a shunt is blocked or infected, reoperation is needed to unblock it or remove it. Shunt infection is particularly troublesome as the ongoing hydrocephalus requires "externalization" of the shunt, meaning it is replaced by a ventriculostomy catheter alone that must then be reinstalled as an indwelling system in a third procedure done only after the infection has cleared. To avoid the necessity for repeat operations done to change out the valve, systems have been developed with adjustable valves in which the setting can be changed by application of a magnetic wand external to the skin overlying the valve. The wand can increase or decrease the valve's resistance depending on the clinical need. The problem with their use in the cancer setting is that patients with tumor require frequent MRIs, and such systems are affected by the magnetic field of the scanner. They must be reset after any MRI scan. Each company's system uses a different wand device, and the lack of a universal wand makes it hard for patients to transfer care to hospitals that use a system other than the one originally placed. We try to avoid such systems for these reasons.

In some patients endoscopic third ventriculostomy serves as a substitute for an indwelling shunt. In this procedure an endoscope is inserted through a frontal burr hole and advanced under stereotactic guidance through the lateral ventricle, foramen of Munro, and into the third ventricle. There the surgeon can see the ventricular floor and create an opening that allows egress of CSF into the subarachnoid space, whence it can be absorbed. This technique is not universally applicable but can help patients with hydrocephalus due to aqueductal stenosis or other compressive etiologies within the posterior fossa. It is not useful in patients with non-communicating hydrocephalus as the success of the procedure depends on patency of absorptive pathways that are nonfunctional in this scenario.

SPINAL TUMORS

Tumors in the spine form a significant part of neurosurgical oncology and are subcategorized by their anatomic localization. They are either intradural or extradural, with extradural implying an intraosseous location within one or more vertebrae. Intradural tumors are further subdivided into those within the spinal cord, denoted as intramedullary, and those within the space between dura and spinal cord denoted as intradural/extramedullary. The latter tend to arise from nerve roots or from the dura itself and are usually schwannomas or meningiomas.

INTRADURAL TUMORS

Intramedullary Tumors

These form 4% to 10% of all CNS tumors. They grow within the spinal cord and thus can affect neurological function in a variety of ways depending on their precise site of origin and pattern of growth within that very small space. As always, the rate of growth has relevance to the way symptoms develop. Tumors of the cord create symptoms by direct compression of adjacent neural pathways. Because sensory and motor tracts are packed tightly together, either or both can be affected by such compression. In addition, when highly vascular a tumor in the cord can create neurological dysfunction by a steal phenomenon and tumors of any vascularity may provoke formation of a syrinx, that is, a cyst that extends within the cord above or below the tumor, sometimes for great distances. Almost all spinal cord tumors (about 99%) fall within one of three categories, to which we will confine this discussion.

Ependymomas

Ependymomas are the most common intramedullary tumor in adults and make up 60% to 65% of such lesions. They are generally discrete with a distinct interface with the cord and little tendency to invade. A cyst is commonly seen adjacent to the tumor and can be extensive. If the cyst is big enough, it can be used as part of the avenue of approach to the tumor. Although the histological appearance of ependymomas of the cord is similar to that of cerebral ependymomas, their behavior is quite different. Cord ependymomas are much less likely to produce metastases by CSF spread and rarely convert to malignant forms. A subtype, the myxopapillary ependymoma, is actually not an intramedullary tumor but an intradural/extramedullary one, which occurs at the origin of the filum terminale just below the conus medullaris and thus is classically found at the level of L2 among the roots of the cauda equina. Ependymomas of the cord tend to enhance on MRI and grow slowly with an insidious clinical onset (Fig. 20.5A). The exception to this comes when they hemorrhage (6% to 8%), in which case a sudden worsening occurs, often associated with neuropathic pain. They can occur anywhere along the cord although they are somewhat more common in the cervical region.

The primary mode of therapy for ependymomas of the cord is surgical removal via laminectomy, dural opening, and myelotomy. Complete resection is achieved in our hands in 90% of these tumors. Even with use of such intraoperative neurophysiological monitoring techniques as somatosensory-evoked potentials and motor-evoked potentials, about half of patients develop new deficits immediately after surgery, but these deficits are transient in all but 10% of those operated on. As the most important influence on the postoperative neurological status is the preoperative status, patients should ideally be operated before they show neurological decline. Those with longstanding deficits rarely improve after resection, even when tumor removal is complete. A recurrence rate of 5% to 10% over 5 years is typical and radiotherapy should not be used in ependymomas of the cord unless (a) gross total resection cannot be achieved despite valiant efforts to do so or (b) a remnant shows signs of growth while under surveillance by MRI. There is no role for chemotherapy in the treatment of these tumors.

Astrocytomas

Unlike astrocytomas in the brain, those in the cord are more likely to be well differentiated. Indeed, 90% of them fall into this category as either pilocytic astrocytomas or diffusely infiltrating (but benign) lesions. The infiltrating variety have pure tumor at the heart of the mass but tend to mingle with normal cord at their periphery and thus are difficult to remove in a truly complete fashion. Pilocytic astrocytomas, similar to those in the brain, are quite discrete and can be removed completely.

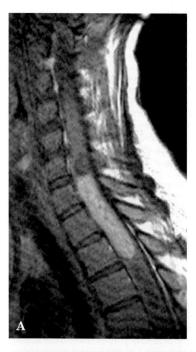

FIGURE 20.5 A: MRI (sagittal, post-contrast) of the cervical spine showing a well-defined enhancing tumor within the cord, consistent with ependymoma. Note the syrinx both rostral and caudal to the tumor. This patient presented with quadriparesis and recovered significantly after total removal of the tumor. **B:** MRI (T1-weighted) of thoracic spine of patient with metastatic renal cell carcinoma. The images show (left) an axial view at the site of maximum epidural compression. The vertebral body, pedicle, and lamina are involved and the cord is severely effaced. (Right) Sagittal view shows tumor in two contiguous vertebral segments (T2 and T3) with the epidural compression caused at T2. Both segments must be resected for long-term local control. This patient requires an operation done by transpedicular approach with reconstruction and posterior instrumentation by a rod-and-screw construct.

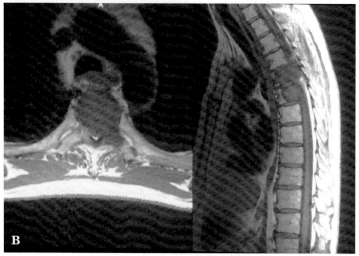

The main difficulty is identifying the interface with an accuracy sufficient to prevent resection of slivers of normal cord along with the tumor. Pilocytic astrocytomas can have associated cysts. Only 10% of the intramedullary astrocytomas are malignant and those are overwhelmingly anaplastic in grade. True glioblastomas of the cord occur, but at the minute incidence of 1/20 million people/year.

As with the ependymomas, neurological deficits come on quite slowly in patients with spinal astrocytoma. Such tumors are more common in children than are ependymomas (the reverse is true for adults), and 5-year survival varies between 60% and 85% with a 10-year survival of 55%. The mortality may reflect the fallout of profound neurological deficits imposed by the tumor or transformation to more malignant forms. Malignant astrocytomas have traditionally been quoted as having a mean postoperative survival of 6 to 12 months, although this is likely an underestimate for patients who have undergone aggressive resection, radiotherapy, and chemotherapy, as many now do.

The distinction between the infiltrating and the pilocytic varieties can sometimes be made on MRI. Infiltrating astrocytomas tend not to enhance, while pilocytic tumors enhance quite brightly after gadolinium infusion. However, the distinction is somewhat academic as both are treated with surgery, and radiotherapy is reserved (as is chemotherapy) for those showing malignant histology or a tendency to recur.

Hemangioblastoma

The third most common category of spinal cord tumor is the hemangioblastoma. These tumors grow slowly and form 5% to 8% of intramedullary tumors. They are highly vascular and often provoke syrinx formation that can be quite extensive (even occupying the entire cord) in some cases. The tumors have a characteristic orange or reddish color due to their extreme vascularity and their content of lipid-laden cells. When a cyst is present, it is the dominant portion of the mass and the source of compression on the cord. However, even a small hemangioblastoma can provoke a significant expansion of the coronal venous plexus through arteriovenous shunting causing venous hypertension that can itself affect cord function.

These tumors can be solitary or multiple, with multiple tumors always forming a component of von Hippel–Lindau disease (VHL), a genetic tumor syndrome in which renal cell carcinoma, pheochromocytoma, and hemangioblastomas of the brain are also seen. Thus, patients with one hemangioblastoma should undergo MRI of the entire craniospinal axis to search for others. Half of patients with spinal hemangioblastoma have VHL, while the other half represent sporadic cases without a germ-line mutation. Surgical resection of a sporadic versus a VHL-associated tumor is entirely similar, with the exception that in VHL multiple resections may be needed in one patient. In some, a cluster of tumors occurs within a single field and allows one laminectomy site to encompass all tumors planned for removal; in others the tumors sit in divergent locations and several incisions may be needed.

When the hemangioblastoma is removed, care should be taken to interrupt the arterial supply before the dominant draining vein. It can be difficult to sort out which vessel belongs in which category, and so a preoperative spinal angiogram may be useful. However, we have found that the discomfort and risk to the patient with angiography outweigh the benefits and that we can usually tell by direct inspection which vessels are arterial. The tumor is removed by entering its interface with the cord, preferably within the associated syrinx. If no syrinx is present, the surgeon adheres intimately to the tumor capsule and carefully dissects and incises the tumor's attachments to the cord at the pial surface. Once the tumor is freed from the pia it will tend to extrude slightly from the cord, and the remaining attachments can be divided without difficulty. If the draining vein is taken prematurely, the tumor will swell and the potential for damage to the cord is significant.

Patients who have extensive syrinx show excellent resolution of the cystic changes in the cord if tumor removal is complete. The cord generally continues to show some minor gliotic changes, but the syrinx will resolve during the 3 months after surgery.

We have found that resection of multiple hemangioblastomas is quite feasible and safe, although tumors located along the anterior edge of the cord or in its anterolateral quadrant pose more risk as the manipulation required to extract them is greater unless a truly lateral approach is taken. However, this is rarely done in intradural surgery to avoid spinal destabilization.

Metastatic Tumors

Metastasis confined within the spinal cord is unusual. Such tumors make up no more than 2% of all cord tumors and are most commonly seen in patients with carcinomas of the breast or lung. Renal cell carcinoma and melanoma also metastasize to the spinal cord with some regularity. The majority of such patients do not undergo surgery because the cord metastasis generally appears during the late stages of the disease when the patient is already somewhat debilitated. As patients with systemic metastasis live longer, metastasis to the spinal cord is becoming more common, but we still rarely perform surgery on these patients. At MDACC we have operated on only 10 patients with intramedullary metastasis in the past 17 years, usually because of diagnostic uncertainty or because the patient was in a relatively good medical and neurological condition and preservation of function was sought through surgical decompression. Such tumors usually have an incompletely defined plane with the cord and can therefore be debulked, but not cured, by surgery. Postoperative radiotherapy is typically used, but leptomeningeal dissemination nonetheless occurred in 30% of our patient cohort after surgery. No patient with already-diagnosed leptomeningeal metastasis underwent surgery, as we consider this a contraindication due to the relatively short survival of patients with that form of tumor spread. In our group, the median survival after surgery was 5 months and the two longest survivors lived for 7 and 15 months.

Intradural/Extramedullary Tumors

These are tumors that occur inside the dura but outside the spinal cord and thus usually arise from nerve roots or from the dura/arachnoid interface. The tumors are mainly meningiomas of dural origin or schwannomas arising from nerve roots, usually sensory. Each of these tumor types shows excellent delineation from the cord and can be resected completely. The tendency of the schwannoma to arise from a sensory root generally means that the root can be cut with minimal loss of function, as transfer of that function may already have occurred to adjacent sensory roots or enough anatomic overlap already exists to prevent the patient from noticing a deficit. Some schwannomas extend transdurally into the intervertebral foramen and can be chased there, while others form a "dumbbell" tumor which necessitates resection outside the spine as well as within the spinal canal. Schwannomas have a globular appearance on MRI with a sharp border and moderate enhancement. The presence of a dumbbell picture confirms the diagnosis of schwannoma when it is present. Meningiomas have a different appearance in that they tend to show a tapering, sloping defect with gradual narrowing of the subarachnoid space up to the point of contact between cord and tumor at both its rostral and caudal ends. They tend to be low grade and often calcify. The presence of calcification in a tumor in this compartment is pathognomonic for meningioma. The meningiomas are intimately apposed to the dura to which they may adhere or even invade; thus a complete resection may entail dural removal as well. If the durotomy is relatively anterior on the circumference of the spinal dura, no CSF leak will ensue. If it is posteriorly located a dural patch may be needed to prevent such leak.

Patients with multiple spinal meningiomas usually have NF2, and in such cases debulking the tumor achieves the goal of decompression as complete removal is generally not possible. In patients with NF1, nerve sheath tumors also arise in this space to a point that the cord may be crowded and compressed by tumor bilaterally at multiple levels, particularly in the cervical spine. The removal of such tumors, which tend to be neurofibromas rather than schwannomas, is something of an art form as it requires debulking of the tumors with maintenance of quite ill-defined nerve roots and removal of tumors from motor roots as well. These motor roots may be fully functional yet heavily overlain by tumor; they are very important as they provide motor function to the arms and hands, and their interruption is much noticed by the patient.

The general surgical approach for intradural/extramedullary tumors is similar to that used for the intramedullary tumors (laminectomy and durotomy), but no myelotomy is necessary. Intraoperative ultrasound localizes tumors nicely in both these categories. In patients who are at risk for swan neck deformity due to tumor impairment of nerves to the paraspinal muscles or because of multiple levels of root involvement, a laminoplasty may be more desirable than a laminectomy to allow better maintenance of spinal stability.

Metastasis can also be found within the intradural/extramedullary space, usually as drop metastasis from a tumor in the posterior fossa. Almost all patients with this rare phenomenon have known systemic metastasis to other sites, and the diagnosis is not difficult by MRI as the tumor will have an ill-defined and fuzzy border quite different from the typical meningioma or schwannoma. Even so, some patients may need to undergo surgery due to diagnostic confusion; meningiomas and schwannomas are quite curable, so if there is any room for belief that they belong in the differential diagnosis, an operation is indicated. As with intramedullary metastases, metastasis within the intradural/extramedullary space is not curable but can be debulked. Although this is best regarded as a focal form of leptomeningeal dissemination, the life expectancy of these patients may exceed that of patients with true leptomeningeal spread, so surgery may actually provide benefit in carefully selected cases.

TUMORS OF THE OSSEOUS (EXTRADURAL) SPINE

Patients with tumors within the vertebra present with pain or neurological deficit, patterns that depend on the level of spine involvement, the degree of root compression, and the degree of mechanical spinal instability. Surgery is more intended to help with diagnosis, palliation, and restoration of spinal stability rather than to achieve oncologic cure, although for primary tumors of the spine cure is a desirable objective. Just as with brain tumors, the multidisciplinary approach is crucial for optimal management of extradural spinal tumors.

Diagnostic Tests

Testing begins with plain x-rays which are inexpensive and easy to obtain, and the results may be diagnostic of tumor. Anteroposterior and lateral x-rays of the entire spine are also useful in assessing spinal alignment and stability and can be used to predict the quality of bone strength to be encountered during surgery. The classic findings on x-ray of a spinal bony tumor are loss of pedicle definition (metastases have a heavy predilection for the vertebral pedicle), compression fracture, or destruction of one or more vertebrae with disc preservation; all these features suggest a malignant lesion. However, plain films show an abnormality in only 60% to 80% of patients who have neurological deficits due to spinal cord compression and thus merely begin a radiological investigation of this problem.

Much more useful are MRI and CT in delineating the extent of tumor and the degree of spinal stability. Although MRI has optimal visualization of epidural compression and paraspinal soft tissue involvement, CT gives better insight into the degree of bony destruction. When metastasis is suspected the entire spine should be imaged to determine the presence of multiple coincident lesions. When MRI is contraindicated (e.g., by presence of a pacemaker) or images are obscured by artifact (e.g., by prior rod and screw placement) CT myelography can give good imaging of bony anatomy and neural constituents. CT-guided needle biopsy is performed when no prior malignancy exists and pathological diagnosis is needed. 3-D reconstruction of the CT is quite useful for surgical planning, particularly in those patients who have undergone prior operation in the same region. In those with potential need for spinal instrumentation and pedicle placement, CT is superior to MRI for providing accurate measurement of pedicle dimensions.

MRI is the key to studying spinal tumors completely and accurately. The degree of spinal cord compression is readily disclosed on T2-weighted images, and fat suppression techniques are quite useful in eliminating overshadowing from epidural or paraspinal fat. MRI is also the most sensitive and specific modality for distinguishing spinal metastases from osteoporotic compression fractures, common among patients with cancer. Osteoporotic fractures are most often seen in the thoracic spine, do not involve the pedicle, and on T1-weighted images lack signal change. Pathological fractures tend to have a homogeneous signal on T1-weighted images and often involve the pedicle. Radionuclide bone scanning is sensitive but not very specific in detecting metastatic spinal disease. It relies on osteoblastic bone deposition to detect tumor, so rapidly progressive tumors may not be well seen by this technique. It is also relatively insensitive to myelomas limited to the bone marrow. Furthermore, osteomyelitis, hemangiomas, fractures, and even degenerative spondylosis can show as increased uptake on bone scan.

PRIMARY BONE TUMORS

Such tumors are not common, as fewer than 10% of all primary tumors of bone involve the spine. They present with symptoms that include night pain, pain at rest (either in the back or as a radicular component), or neurological deficit. The course can be insidious with relatively nonspecific complaints. Once a lesion is suspected, CT or MRI will typically identify its location and offer clues to its cell type of origin.

Hemangioma

These are vascular lesions found more commonly in females than males and are solitary two-thirds of the time. They tend to be located in the lower thoracic or upper lumbar spine and have a characteristic honeycomb appearance on plain films due to linear reactive calcification around the radiolucent vascular tissue. Most are confined to their vertebral body and pose no particular clinical issue. Only occasionally do they cause compression of the cord due to extension of the vascular tissue into the epidural space. Pain alone is not an indication for surgery and only those patients in whom neurological symptoms have occurred are operated on. Asymptomatic lesions can generally be ignored until pain or neurological deficits develop. Complete resection is possible and surgery is the mainstay of treatment.

Aneurysmal Bone Cyst

These lesions occur most often in children and are not common in patients over 30 years of age. They tend to involve the posterior vertebral elements more than the anterior elements and the lumbar vertebrae more than other levels. These are benign lesions but can be proliferative and lytic and occasionally expand rapidly. When they spill into the canal they can cause neurological compromise. Surgical resection is the favored treatment, sometimes after preoperative embolization. Incomplete resection leads to a high rate of recurrence, but complete resection generally gives long-term cure. Radiotherapy is relatively ineffective.

Osteoblastic Lesions

These benign tumors of the spine occur more often in males and are categorized either as osteoid osteomas or as osteoblastomas. The distinction is purely made on the basis of size, with osteoid osteomas being <1.5 cm in diameter. Any young patient with back or neck pain, scoliosis, or radicular pain should be considered for such a lesion. X-rays show a dense sclerotic rim of reactive bone around a small central nidus. They have intense radionuclide uptake on bone scan. The pain secondary to these lesions can be treated with non-steroidal anti-inflammatory agents and occasionally the osteoid osteomas will spontaneously resolve. If pain is an ongoing issue and no resolution has occurred, surgical excision can be performed and if complete, will successfully eliminate the lesion. Osteoblastomas are more likely to come to surgery because of their larger size. Complete tumor removal by en bloc resection is curative. Intralesional debulking is more likely to lead to incomplete resection and thus carries a higher risk of recurrence.

Osteochondroma

These tumors are the most frequently encountered benign lesions of bone. They consist of cartilage-covered cortical bone with underlying medullary bone. The osteochondroma is formed when the cartilaginous cap undergoes calcification. These are most commonly seen in males in the third decade of life. They also tend to affect the posterior elements including the pedicle. They have a predilection for the cervical spine. The best diagnostic test for them is a CT scan as they show less radionuclide uptake on bone scan than do other lesions like osteoid osteoma. They tend to increase in size during adolescence and sometimes into adulthood. Malignant transformation is rare and surgical removal is the treatment of choice.

Giant Cell Tumor

These tumors are uncommon, locally aggressive, and occur more often in females. The most frequent spinal location is the sacrum but they can occur anywhere in the spine and usually involve a single vertebra in which an expansile mass has formed. They transform to a malignant state in 10% of cases and then can metastasize. Interestingly, the "giant cells" are not the neoplastic element of the tumor; rather this is usually the other cell component, traditionally believed to be the stromal cells. Thus this tumor is misnamed. The best resection of such lesions is done en bloc as recurrence is more common after intralesional curettage. When found in the sacrum, a sacrectomy with sacrifice of neural elements may be necessary to achieve cure. These tumors are quite vascular and preoperative embolization is useful. They may benefit as well from radiotherapy after a subtotal resection.

Plasmacytoma

These are the most common malignant lesions of the adult spine. Malignant proliferation of the plasma cells occurs in the bone marrow, spleen, and lymphoid tissues. A few patients have a solitary plasmacytoma but multiple plasmacytomas (called "multiple myeloma") are far more common. Such patients have infiltration of bone marrow by plasma cells with resulting reduction in immunoglobulin levels. However, with solitary plasmacytomas serum protein electrophoresis is normal because the bone marrow is largely functional. Bone in patients with multiple myeloma generally has a poor quality and thus aggressive resections necessitating vertebral reconstruction and instrumentation affixed to adjacent segments are not ideal. The treatment of choice is thus vertebroplasty for pain control and possibly radiotherapy thereafter for tumor control. Half of patients with solitary plasmacytoma progress to multiple myeloma within 5 years (and usually within 3 years), so patients with solitary disease should be followed closely to detect distant recurrence. Chemotherapy is often used for multiple myeloma and sometimes stem cell transplant, especially if progression is apparent.

Chordoma

These tumors arise from remnants of the embryonic notochord and tend to be indolent but locally progressive. They can metastasize when advanced. About 50% of chordomas occur in the sacrum, 40% in the clivus, and the rest in mobile regions of the spine. The 5-year survival rate ranges from 50% to 75% and the 10-year survival rate is about 50%. The consensus now is that en bloc resection is the ideal intervention for chordoma. For tumors of the sacrococcygeal spine, ventral, dorsal, or combined surgical approaches may be needed together with nerve sacrifice and sometimes resection of adjacent bowel leading to colostomy. Such cases are always done in conjunction with both neurosurgeon and colorectal surgeon and often with a plastic surgeon as well. There are no current indications for using chemotherapy to manage chordomas, but radiotherapy may have a role. It has been suggested that proton beam irradiation may be especially useful in treating clival chordomas in which an incomplete resection has been done due to the inability to perform en bloc resection in this difficult anatomical area. Resection of clival chordomas requires special skull base techniques, a subject beyond the scope of this chapter but often involving an anterior approach through the mid-face, with good results when this is followed by proton beam radiotherapy.

Ewing Sarcoma

These tumors are most common in the first two decades of life and occur more often in males. More than half of these involve the sacrum. Plain x-ray shows a lytic lesion with a sclerotic rim. Treatment often starts with chemotherapy with surgery reserved for those patients with an incomplete response or if decompression of the spinal canal is desirable. Radical resection may be necessary here, just as with chordoma.

Osteosarcoma

These are seen occasionally in the spine either as primary tumors or as metastases from sites of origin in the appendicular skeleton. Osteosarcomas can be primary in young adults or in older patients may be secondary lesions arising as a result of radiotherapy to bone. En bloc resection is now advocated followed by radiotherapy and aggressive chemotherapy. Occasional long-term survival is seen, but patients generally die of this disease through widespread metastasis.

Chondrosarcoma

Such tumors are typically indolent and show multiple local recurrences over long periods of time before switching to a metastatic mode. They are more common in men and have a poor prognosis despite their slow pace of growth. They are quite resistant to radiotherapy and chemotherapy, and thus complete (en bloc) resection is the ideal goal of an operation done for this tumor type.

SPINAL METASTASIS

About 5% to 10% of patient with all types of cancer combined develop symptomatic spinal metastasis at some point during the course of their disease. In one-fifth of patients with involvement of the vertebral column by metastasis, frank spinal cord compression ultimately occurs (Fig. 20.5B). The thoracic spine is the most common location for spinal metastasis, with the lumbar spine yielding 20% of cases and the cervical spine 10%. Over half of cases arise from carcinomas of breast, lung, and prostate, due to the fact that these cancers are relatively common and (in the case of breast and prostate cancer) because of their tendency to metastasize to other bones as well. Since pain is the most common symptom, back pain in a patient with known cancer should be assumed to be caused by metastasis until proven otherwise. The pain can be mechanical due to spinal instability from bony destruction or radicular due to nerve root irritation. Pain that worsens with movement and improves when the patient lies down suggests a component of mechanical instability and that stabilizing instrumentation should be part of any operation done. Although it is possible and indeed likely for spinal metastasis to present without myelopathy, a complete neurological examination is important in any patient suspected of having this condition.

The oncologist's weapons for treating metastatic spinal disease include chemotherapy, radiotherapy, and surgery. The most important factor affecting prognosis is the patient's ability to walk when treatment starts. Surgery is palliative in patients with metastatic disease to the spine. The clinical emphasis should focus on reduction of pain, preservation of neurological function, and restoration of mobility while maintaining sphincter control. Loss of such control predicts a poor outcome. The debate over the relative efficacy of radiotherapy versus surgery is complex and continues today. However, a patient in relatively good shape from the medical and oncological perspective with a reasonable life expectancy overall (>6 months) should be considered for surgery if spinal metastasis endangers neurological function but has not yet eroded it. In addition, pain of instability (axial loading pain) will be helped more by resection and stabilization than by radiotherapy, which controls the tumor but leaves the mechanical instability in place. The goal of surgery is to provide decompression of the spinal cord and nerve roots and to stabilize the spinal column. Radiotherapy is a good modality, however, for treating radiosensitive spinal tumors or those causing minimal or no neurological deficits. We have found that stereotactic radiosurgery for spinal metastases can be quite effective in suppressing focal deposits of disease with good safety to the nearby cord and that it shortens the time of treatment significantly without compromising effectiveness. Radiosurgical delivery requires five or fewer sessions, while standard external beam irradiation is given in 10 fractions to a total dose of 30 to 40 Gy.

Metastatic breast cancer is typically radiosensitive and also can respond to hormonal therapy, cytotoxic chemotherapy, or both. Thus, in breast cancer cases (and in particular those with multiple spinal lesions) surgical intervention is limited. Spinal involvement from a lung cancer can result from direct extension of a tumor from the chest wall to the nearby spine or may develop from hematogenous routes. Superior sulcus tumors in particular can involve the spine and require intricate cooperation between thoracic surgeon and neurosurgeon for ideal resection of the lung, chest wall, spinal, and occasionally neural components, with reconstruction of the chest wall needed in many cases. Because of its high degree of radiosensitivity, small cell carcinoma rarely needs surgery. Prostate cancer also responds more often than not to palliative efforts without surgery and is sensitive to radiotherapy at least for a time. Its spinal involvement tends to be multifocal, and thus surgical cases must be carefully chosen. The role of surgery in prostate cancer tends to focus on correction of spinal instability, control of intractable pain caused by a focal lesion, or prevention of neurological decline.

The non-small cell carcinomas of the lung (squamous cell carcinoma and adenocarcinoma) can metastasize to the spine and are resistant to radiotherapy. Although surgery can be considered for such patients, they often have poor pulmonary function in which case a transthoracic approach is less desirable. Transpedicular approaches through a midline posterior incision are preferred for them or indeed for any patient with a significant burden of lung metastasis compromising pulmonary mechanics. Renal cell carcinomas also resist radiotherapy and the systemic disease varies significantly in its clinical behavior. In many patients the pace of the disease is relatively indolent even when lung or other metastases are present. Renal cell carcinoma thus lends itself to surgery, but it is quite vascular and preoperative embolization is often helpful in staunching intraoperative hemorrhage. The key to resection of a renal cell carcinoma from the spine is a quick removal after a careful and comprehensive isolation of the tumor and as much devascularization as possible prior to tumor entry. Such tumors must usually be removed in piecemeal fashion and bleed significantly during that removal. When the tumor has been removed completely or almost so, the bleeding slows and stops or at least becomes much more responsive to the usual control measures of Gelfoam in thrombin, Avitene, and sometimes recombinant factor VII.

INDICATIONS FOR SPINAL SURGERY

Because patients with vertebral column tumors usually have a life expectancy limited to 1 to 2 years and may have multiple sites of disease when the tumor is metastatic, oncological cure is not the usual goal of an operation. The benefits must be balanced against the risks of a major procedure and the time needed for recuperation, usually 4 to 8 weeks. Thus, a patient with 3 to 4 months of predicted survival would not be a good candidate for such an operation as it would consume half his remaining life span in recovery time. The goals of surgery are dictated by the patient's life expectancy, functional (including neurological) status, tumor type, chance for oncological cure, degree and type of pain, degree and duration of compression of spinal cord or nerve roots, and the need to restore spinal stability.

The classic indication for surgery is rapid neurological decline due to epidural compression of spinal cord caused by a radioresistant tumor. Spinal instability is a commonly cited reason as well, but there is no uniformly accepted definition of that phrase. Commonly used definitions include disruption of two of the three bony columns of the thoracolumbar spine (although this does not apply to the cervical spine, whose structure is different); kyphotic deformity >20 degrees; or loss of >50% of vertebral body height in any portion of the spine. If patients meet one or more of these criteria and have a well-defined syndrome of axial loading pain, then surgery is a reasonable consideration as vertebral resection and reconstruction with appropriate anterior and/or posterior instrumentation may give excellent pain relief long term.

Overall the aims of spinal surgery are three in number. These include (a) decompression of the spinal cord to improve or maintain neurological status, (b) decompression of nerve roots to reduce radicular pain, (c) stabilization of the spine to reduce the pain of instability, and (d) correction, if possible, of kyphotic or scoliotic deformities or loss of vertebral height that add to the patient's pain burden.

Surgical Adjuncts

Embolization done prior to surgery (within 24 hours) can reduce blood loss during operations and may be useful for hypervascular metastases like renal cell carcinoma and thyroid carcinoma. Bleeding from thyroid carcinoma is the most profound and difficult to stop of any metastasis, and such tumors should be approached surgically with great caution and with an adequate supply of blood readily available. Embolization requires spinal angiography which carries risk and some discomfort to the patient. The embolization itself can cause spinal cord infarction and complete paralysis should the injection be done too proximally within the vascular tree. This procedure should only be performed by interventional neuroradiologist experts in its application.

Blood loss during resection of spinal metastases ranges from minimal to extreme. If large blood loss is expected, transfusion should begin as soon as tumor resection starts to avoid having to play "catch-up" and to prevent hemodynamic instability. Patients who have received multiple transfusions will take longer to recover and may be in the hospital for several weeks after the surgery. We do not advocate the use of cell savers out of concern that they may re-circulate malignant cells into the bloodstream. Cryocoagulation of the tumor in situ can be very effective in stopping intractable bleeding, but the cord must be excluded from the zone of freezing.

We routinely perform intraoperative monitoring of somatosensory evoked potentials and motor evoked potentials, which give immediate feedback on the integrity of neural pathways in the dorsal and ventral portions of the spinal cord, respectively. When motor-evoked potentials are used, anesthesia techniques must be modified to exclude paralytic agents.

Fluoroscopy is useful for localizing vertebral levels early in surgery. It also helps to ensure good screw placement during spinal fixation, with avoidance of pedicle breach or penetration of the vertebral endplate or cortex by a misdirected or overly long screw.

Surgical Techniques

Extradural spinal metastases can be approached from an anterior, posterior, or combined direction. The choice of approach is determined by tumor location (vertebral body vs. posterior elements), the spinal level, the extent of the tumor, and the degree of patient debility. When tumors involve only the posterior spine and laminae, decompression is done through a posterior laminectomy approach. However, it is more common to see the compression along the anterior aspect of the thecal sac, in which case effective decompression can be achieved either via an anterior/anterolateral or a posterolateral (transpedicular or costotransversectomy) approach. When the dural sac is surrounded by tumor from all directions, resection proceeds either by the posterolateral transpedicular method or by combined anterior and posterior approaches.

The anterior approach is awkward at the highest cervical and thoracic levels (C1, C2, and T1-T3) and the lowest lumbar and sacral segments (L5 and below). Access to the upper cervical spine can be done through a transoral or mandibular splitting approach but these are technically difficult procedures and in the context of malignant disease may be unrealistic for palliation. The high thoracic segments can be reached by performing a sternal split with reflection of the first and second ribs laterally. The heart and great vessels limit caudal exposure as does the natural spinal curve. We have preferred to approach tumors in these locations purely from a posterior transpedicular direction. The lumbosacral junction can be reached from the front without great difficulty, but stabilization at this level is difficult and requires complex posteriorly placed lumbo-pelvic rod constructs; thus such operations are always done as combined anterior-posterior cases. Sacral reconstruction is essentially impossible although replacement of the L5 vertebral body can be performed.

Spinal stabilization is needed after any anterior corpectomy and after most (but not all) posterolateral decompressions. When two or more vertebral body segments have been removed, anterior fixation alone is usually insufficient for long-term stability, and supplementation with posterior rods and screws is helpful. The current posterior instrumentation systems are highly developed and allow stabilization anywhere from the occipitocervical area to the lumbar spine. Lumbo-pelvic fixation remains a difficult area in which the perfect construct has not yet been achieved.

Patient debility plays an important role in selecting surgical approaches. Many patients have undergone previous radiotherapy, and surgery performed through an irradiated field carries a higher risk of wound complications. Thus, plastic surgical assistance can be quite helpful for wound closure in such patients.

Vertebral replacement can be done with autologous or allograft bone cut to appropriate size, methylmethacrylate, or an expandable titanium alloy cage.

We use expandable cages for the majority of our vertebrectomy patients as they permit adjustment in situ which can restore lost vertebral body height without drilling into the adjacent vertebral bodies, as must be done to anchor a methylmethacrylate strut graft. However, a number of patients still receive methylmethacrylate grafts when expandable cages will not fit the bony defect or when the corridor of access to the vertebrectomy site is offset and prevents placement of the tools necessary for cage expansion. We are least likely to use bone graft because long-term fusion is not generally necessary in a patient population whose life expectancy rarely extends beyond 2 to 3 years, and in which strenuous physical activity is not common.

Multidisciplinary cooperation between surgical services is frequently necessary in performing these operations. It is routine to engage the services of a thoracic surgeon for anterolateral approaches to the thoracic spine needing thoracotomy or a thoracoabdominal approach for spinal tumors near the diaphragm. Retroperitoneal or transabdominal approaches require the services of a general surgeon, and complex neck approaches from an anterolateral or posterolateral angle may benefit greatly from help by a head and neck surgeon. Although brain operations are exclusively the province of the neurosurgeon, spinal procedures can involve any of these named services as well as plastic surgery when significant tissue loss has occurred that compromises wound closure, or when the effects of prior treatment make wound healing tenuous.

Cervical Spine

High cervical (C1 and C2) vertebral tumors can be approached transorally with or without transmandibular modification, depending on the degree of rostral extension of the tumor. This approach is destabilizing and mandates posterior occipitocervical fixation as part of the procedure. Tumors in the anterior portion of the subaxial cervical spine can be approached through the anterolateral neck along the edge of the sternocleidomastoid muscle. This provides excellent exposure but puts the function of the recurrent laryngeal nerve at risk through potential stretch injury. To avoid postoperative hoarseness, retractors should be relaxed at 30-min intervals throughout the case. En bloc resection in the cervical spine is challenging and usually not possible due to the anatomic constraints imposed by the vertebral artery, nerve roots, and spinal dura.

Thoracic Spine

Tumors in the T1 vertebral body that do not extend laterally can be approached through an incision in the low anterolateral neck, but many cannot be well exposed without sternal split (trapdoor approach). Thoracic vertebral tumors with a lateral paraspinal extension require posterolateral thoracotomy from the side of greatest tumor bulk. Transpedicular vertebrectomy is useful for tumors in this region but will usually not clear disease as effectively as the transthoracic approach. Because the transpedicular method is facilitated by bilateral transection of nerve roots it is usually not used at T1, where the roots may be important for hand function.

Thoracolumbar Spine

Direct exposure of a thoracolumbar (T10-L1) vertebral tumor requires a thoracoabdominal approach in which a portion of the diaphragmatic crus is divided to uncover the spine not only over the tumor site but also over adjacent levels needed for fixation of an anterior plate-and-screw construct. The side of the approach is decided by the location of the tumor within the vertebral body; those extending equally to both sides are approached from the left to avoid the liver. En bloc resection of tumors in the thoracic, thoracoabdominal, and lumbar spine is challenging but is being used more as surgeons become familiar with this special technique.

Lumbar Spine
For vertebral tumors below L1, a retroperitoneal approach is favored. Transpedicular vertebrectomy in this region is difficult because of the larger size of the vertebral body and the obstruction by nerve roots that cannot be transected as they control leg strength and sensation. L4 and L5 are often best approached from an anterior direction because of obstruction of direct lateral access by the ilium that varies from patient to patient.

Sacrum
Tumors in the distal sacrum (S3 and below) can be approached solely from the back, usually without need for reconstruction, stabilization, or sacrifice of bowel or bladder function. Maintenance of such function requires that both S2 nerve roots be kept intact as well as one S3 nerve root. High sacral tumors (S1 and S2) require complete sacrectomy. This is a technically challenging and usually staged procedure with a total surgical time exceeding 24 hours and using the talents of multiple surgical services. Rehabilitation after total sacrectomy takes at least 3 months and the hospital stay is lengthy.

Postoperative Radiotherapy
Although en bloc resections are now being done in selected cases, most patients undergoing removal of spinal metastasis have an intralesional debulking. Although removal may appear complete both at the time of surgery and on postoperative imaging, microscopic disease almost invariably remains. Therefore, postoperative radiotherapy is given in most patients who have not previously undergone irradiation of the site. When used before surgery, radiotherapy is associated with infection and other problems of wound healing in one-third of patients. However, newer intensity-modulated methods and stereotactic radiosurgical techniques may allow tumor control without imposing such regional tissue compromise.

TUMORS OF PERIPHERAL NERVE

Tumors may arise on peripheral nerves anywhere that peripheral nerves go. Thus such tumors can be found anywhere in the extremities, trunk, soft tissues of neck and scalp, or on the skin surface. Most are benign and are identified either as neurofibromas or schwannomas. Solitary tumors often found in the paraspinal region are typically schwannomas. When tumors are multiple, neurofibroma is the more likely diagnosis.

Neurofibromas can be either solitary (intraneural), diffuse (cutaneous), or plexiform (involving several nerve branches). Solitary neurofibromas are the most commonly encountered benign tumors of peripheral nerve. They are slow growing and relative circumscribed lesions that cause pain and less often sensory loss or weakness when they grow to large size. Solitary neurofibromas are not linked to a genetic disorder, but multiple neurofibromas indicate the presence of NF1, caused by loss of function of the *NF1* tumor suppressor gene from chromosome 17. Diffuse neurofibromas occur on the skin and in subcutaneous tissue of children and adolescents and often are associated with NF1. Plexiform neurofibromas are pathognomonic for NF1 and appear as a fusiform and often quite large expansion of nerves in the extremities, face, or trunk. They can affect the brachial plexus or the lumbosacral plexus. When superficial they can cause cosmetic deformity to a distressing degree, and when a limb is affected, substantial expansion can compromise venous return and limb function.

Schwannomas are benign and slowly growing, well-encapsulated tumors composed of neoplastic Schwann cells in a collagenous matrix. They are the second most common tumor involving peripheral nerves and usually occur in patients

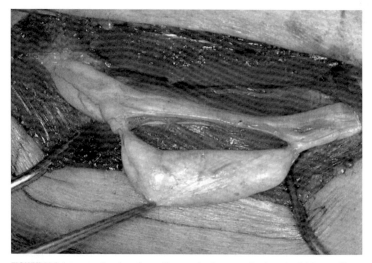

FIGURE 20.6 Intraoperative view of neurofibroma after its separation from the tibial nerve. The entering and exiting fascicles remain connected to the tumor but are divided at this point to free the tumor. This approach allows preservation of most of the nerve, which courses around the tumor outside its capsule and remains connected and functional. This patient has NF1 and suffered no deficit from the removal.

between 30 and 60 years of age. About 20% are found along the median, ulnar, or radial nerves. These tend to cause a mild (or no) neurological deficit, but pain can be a significant component of the clinical presentation. The classic distinction between neurofibromas and schwannomas holds that schwannomas are likely to arise from a small number of fascicles within the nerve, whereas neurofibromas arise more diffusely in the nerve and thus are more difficult to tease out surgically without nerve sacrifice.

In our experience schwannomas can usually be resected without sacrifice of nerve function by performing an intracapsular shelling out of the tumor (Fig. 20.6). Since these tumors are almost always histologically benign, any small remnants left behind in the approach rarely re-establish themselves to form recurrent tumor. Often the tumor arises from only one or two fascicles of the several hundred that make up the nerve, with most of the nerve bypassing the tumor albeit in a somewhat distorted course. Neurofibromas do appear to arise from a larger numbers of fascicles, although many of them have four feeding fascicles or fewer. Thus, they too can be resected in similar fashion with similar likelihood of preserving nerve function. Some neurofibromas run diffusely through the nerve as per the classical description, but the majority do not. Therefore, identity of a tumor as a neurofibroma should not preclude an attempt at resection as the nature of the tumor's origin and its resectability can only be determined at the time of surgical exposure.

Mutation of the *NF1* gene provokes the formation of neurofibromas. However, the alterations imposed by this syndrome are not limited to the induction of nerve sheath tumors. Patients are prone to have optic gliomas and frequently have short stature, neuropsychological abnormalities, a higher incidence of mental retardation, and dysplasia in the axial and appendicular skeleton as well as the skull. They have

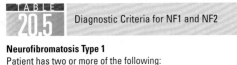

TABLE 20.5   Diagnostic Criteria for NF1 and NF2

Neurofibromatosis Type 1
Patient has two or more of the following:
 Six or more café-au-lait spots
   >1.5 cm in postpuberty
   >0.5 before puberty
 Two or more neurofibromas of any type or at least one plexiform neurofibroma
 Freckling in axilla or groin
 Optic glioma
 Two or more Lisch nodules (hamartomas of iris)
 One or more distinctive bone lesions, for example, sphenoid dysplasia or thinning of
   cortex of long bone
 One or more first-degree relatives with NF1
Neurofibromatosis Type 2
Confirmed NF2 has:
 Bilateral vestibular schwannomas
 or
 family history of NF2
 plus
 unilateral vestibular schwannoma at age <30 years or one or more of the following:
   Glioma
   Schwannoma
   Juvenile posterior subcapsular cortical opacities (in eye)

a higher incidence of intracranial glioma, usually astrocytoma, and of spinal cord ependymomas. The diagnostic criteria for NF1 (and for NF2) are given in Table 20.5.

NF2 is a separate, much less common, and somewhat misnamed condition caused by a completely different gene defect on chromosome 22. Patients with this disease do not get neurofibromas at all, but schwannomas that largely affect cranial nerves. They are also susceptible to the development of multiple cranial or spinal meningiomas and have some risk of developing intracranial glioma. The pathognomonic lesion of NF2 is a bilateral vestibular schwannoma leading to loss of hearing.

The malignant form of each of these tumors is termed a *neurofibrosarcoma* or malignant peripheral nerve sheath tumor (MPNST) as a more general descriptor. Although most schwannomas do not transform to a malignant tumor, melanotic schwannomas have a 10% chance of such transformation. For patients with NF1, the chance of developing an MPNST over the course of their lifetime is 10%. Such tumors are highly aggressive, invade locally, and can metastasize. Chemotherapy is ineffective, radiotherapy is palliative, and the main hope for treatment is early detection with a radical surgical removal. Two-thirds of MPNSTs arise from neurofibromas, usually in a patient with NF1. The 5-year survival rate is 15% to 20% in this category. Sporadic MPNSTs not associated with NF1 have a somewhat better survival rate with a 5-year survival rate of 50%. It is possible to acquire an MPNST after exposure of nerve to external beam irradiation. The treatment of these tumors, whatever their origin, is surgery which can be performed either as radical amputation of the involved limb, sparing of the limb with transection of the involved nerve, or selective resection with nerve sparing analogous to that performed for benign nerve sheath tumors. Although it is logical to suggest more radical strategies given the malignancy of this tumor type, we have had success in occasional patients treated with intracapsular resection because the MPNST may occupy only the core of the benign neurofibroma in which it arose and which has maintained benign histology around its periphery. Using this strategy, we have achieved recurrence-free survival exceeding 10 years in some patients. Thus, we do advocate using this approach to give the patient at least a chance of retention of function and save more aggressive resection for a second operation done for local recurrence.

In the past 5 years the classical categories of NF1 and NF2 have been joined by a third category, schwannomatosis. This occurs in patients with mutation of the *INI1* gene located on chromosome 22q at a separate locus from the *NF2* gene. Such patients have multiple schwannomas in peripheral, spinal, and cranial nerves. About one-third have segmental schwannomatosis limited to a single region of the body. Bilateral vestibular schwannomas have not yet been described in this disease, but unilateral involvement of the vestibular complex has been noted in a few patients. Schwannomatosis is not associated with learning disability and cannot be diagnosed without first ruling out the presence of a mutation in the *NF2* gene. Such patients present with pain syndromes that are quite amenable to relief by surgical resection (with nerve sparing, as above) of the offending tumor or tumors.

Recommended Readings

Armstrong TS, Vera-Bolanos E, Bekele BN, et al. Adult ependymal tumors: prognosis and the M. D. Anderson Cancer Center experience. *Neuro Oncol.* 2009;12:862–870.

Bhattacharyya AK, Perrin R, Guha A. Peripheral nerve tumors: management strategies and molecular insights. *J Neuro Oncol.* 2004; 69:335–349.

Bindal RK, Sawaya R, Leavens ME, et al. Surgical treatment of multiple brain metastases. *J Neurosurg.* 1993;79:210–216.

Bolton WD, Rice DC, Goodyear A, et al. Superior sulcus tumors with vertebral body involvement: a multimodality approach. *J Thoracic Cardiovasc Surg.* 2009;137: 1379–1387.

Cairncross JG, Macdonald D, Ludwin S, et al. Chemotherapy for anaplastic oligodendroglioma. National Cancer Institute of Canada clinical trials group. *J Clin Oncol.* 1998;12:2013–2021.

Cairncross JG, Ueki K, Zlatescu MC, et al. Specific genetic predictors of chemotherapeutic response and survival in patients with anaplastic oligodendrogliomas. *J Natl Cancer Inst.* 1998;90:1473–1479.

Chang EL, Selek U, Hassenbusch SJ III, et al. Outcome variation among "radioresistant" brain metastases treated with stereotactic radiosurgery. *Neurosurgery.* 2005;56:936–945.

Chi GH, Sciubba DM, Rhines LD, et al. Surgery for primary vertebral tumors: en bloc vs. intralesional resection. *Neurosurg Clin North Am.* 2008;19:111–117.

Chow TSF, McCutcheon IE. The surgical treatment of metastatic spine tumors within the intradural extramedullary compartment. *J Neurosurg.* 1996;85:225–230.

Colman H, Aldape K. Molecular predictors in glioblastoma: toward personalized therapy. *Arch Neurol.* 2008;65:877–883.

Dirks PB. Cancer: stem cells and brain tumors. *Nature.* 2006;444:687–688.

Fisher CG, DiPaola CP, Ryken TC, et al. A novel classification system for spinal instability in neoplastic disease: an evidence-based approach and expert consensus from the Spine Oncology Study Group. *Spine.* 2010;35:E1221–E1229.

Fourney DR, Abi-Said D, Rhines LD, et al. Simultaneous anterior-posterior approach to the thoracic and lumbar spine for the radical resection of tumors followed by reconstruction and stabilization. *J Neurosurg.* 2001;94:232–244.

Fourney DR, Rhines LD, Hentschel SJ, et al. En bloc resection of primary sacral tumors: classification of surgical approaches and outcome. *J Neurosurg Spine.* 2005;3:111–122.

Garces-Ambrossi GL, McGirt MJ, Mehta VA, et al. Factors associated with progression- free survival and long-term neurological outcome after resection of intramedullary spinal cord tumors: analysis of 101 consecutive cases. *J Neurosurg Spine.* 2009;11:591–599.

Gauthier H, Guilhaume MN, Bidard FC, et al. Survival of breast cancer patients with meningeal carcinomatosis. *Ann Oncol.* 2010;21:2183–2187.

Hanbali F, Fourney DR, Marmor E, et al. Spinal cord ependymoma: radical resection and outcome. *Neurosurgery.* 2002;51:1162–1174.

Harstad L, Hess KR, Groves MD. Prognostic factors and outcomes in patients with leptomeningeal melanomatosis. *Neuro Oncol.* 2008;10:1010–1018.

Hatiboglu MA, Weinberg JS, Suki D, et al. Impact of intraoperative high-field magnetic resonance imaging guidance on glioma surgery: a prospective volumetric analysis. *Neurosurgery.* 2009;64:1073–1081.

Hegi ME, Diserens AC, Gorlia T, et al. MGMT gene silencing and benefit from temozolomide in glioblastoma. *New Engl J Med.* 2005;352:997–1003.

Holman PJ, Suki D, McCutcheon IE, et al. Surgical management of metastatic disease of the lumbar spine: experience with 139 patients. *J Neurosurg Spine.* 2005;2: 550–563.

Jackson RJ, Fuller GN, Abi-Said D, et al. Limitations of stereotactic biopsy in the initial management of gliomas. *Neuro Oncol.* 2001;3:193–200.

Jackson RJ, Loh SC, Gokaslan Z. Metastatic renal cell carcinoma of the spine: surgical treatment and results. *J Neurosurg.* 2001;94:18–24.

Jiang H, Gomez-Manzano C, Lang FF, et al. Oncolytic adenovirus: preclinical and clinical studies in patients with human malignant gliomas. *Curr Gene Ther.* 2009; 9:422–427.

Karim AB, Afra D, Cornu P, et al. Randomized trial on the efficacy of radiotherapy for cerebral low grade glioma in the adult: European Organization for Research and Treatment of Cancer Study 22845 with the Medical Research Council study BRO4: an interim analysis. *Int J Radiat Oncol Biol Phys.* 2002;52:316–324.

Kim SS, McCutcheon IE, Suki D, et al. Awake craniotomy for brain tumors near eloquent cortex: correlation of intraoperative cortical mapping with neurological outcomes in 309 consecutive patients. *Neurosurgery.* 2009;64:836–846.

Kunwar S, Chang S, Westphal M, et al. Phase III randomized trial of CED of IL13-PE38QQR vs Gliadel wafers for recurrent glioblastoma. *Neuro Oncol.* 2010;12: 871–881.

Lacroix M, Abi-Said D, Fourney DF, et al. A multivariate analysis of 416 patients with glioblastoma multiforme: prognosis, extent of resection, and survival. *J Neurosurg.* 2001;95:190–198.

Louis DN, Ohgaki H, Wiestler OD, eds. *WHO Classification of Tumours of the Central Nervous System.* 4th ed. Lyon: International Agency for Research of Cancer; 2007.

Mahajan A, McCutcheon IE, Suki D, et al. Case-control study of stereotactic radiosurgery for recurrent glioblastoma multiforme. *J Neurosurg.* 2005;103:210–217.

Mehta M, Paleologos MA, Mikkelsen T, et al. The role of chemotherapy in the management of newly diagnosed brain metastases: a systematic review and evidence-based clinical practice guideline. *J Neuro Oncol.* 2010;96:71–83.

Mintz AH, Kestle J, Rathbone MP, et al. A randomized trial to assess the efficacy of surgery in addition to radiotherapy in patients with a single cerebral metastasis. *Cancer.* 1996;78:1470–1476.

Muldoon LL, Soussain C, Jahnke K, et al. Chemotherapy delivery issues in central nervous system malignancy: a reality check. *J Clin Oncol.* 2007;25:2295–2305.

Nieder C, Astner ST, Grosu AL, et al. The role of postoperative radiotherapy after resection of a single brain metastasis: combined analysis of 643 patients. *Strahlenther Onkol.* 2007;183:676–580.

Patchell RA, Tibbs PA, Regine WF, et al. Postoperative radiotherapy in the treatment of single metastases to the brain: a randomized trial. *JAMA.* 1998;280:1485–1489.

Patchell RA, Tibbs PA, Regine WF, et al. Direct decompressive surgical resection in the treatment of spinal cord compression caused by metastatic cancer: a randomised trial. *Lancet.* 2005;366:643–648.

Patchell RA, Tibbs PA, Walsh JW, et al. A randomized trial of surgery in the treatment of single metastases to the brain. *N Engl J Med.* 1990;322:494–500.

Patel AJ, Suki D, Hatiboglu MA, et al. Factors influencing the risk of local recurrence after resection of a single brain metastasis. *J Neurosurg.* 2010;113:181–189.

Plotkin SR, Stemmer-Rachamimov AO, Barker FG 2nd, et al. Hearing improvement after bevacizumab in patients with neurofibromatosis type 2. *New Engl J Med.* 2009;361:358–367.

Pollock BE, Brown PD, Foote RL, et al. Properly selected patients with multiple brain metastases may benefit from aggressive treatment of their intracranial disease. *J Neuro Oncol.* 2003;61:73–80.

Prabhu SS, Gasco J, Tummala S, et al. Intraoperative magnetic resonance imaging-guided tractography with integrated monopolar subcortical functional mapping for resection of brain tumors. *J Neurosurg.* 2011;114(3):719–726.

Ramirez C, Bowman C, Maurage CA, et al. Loss of 1p, 19q, and 10q heterozygosity prospectively predicts prognosis of oligodendroglial tumors–towards individualized tumor treatment? *Neuro Oncol.* 2010;12:490–499.

Rao G, Chang GJ, Suk I, et al. Midsacral amputation for en bloc resection of chordoma. *Neurosurgery.* 2010;66(3 Suppl Operative):41–44.

Rao G, Suki D, Charkrabarti I, et al. Surgical management of primary and metastatic sarcoma of the mobile spine. *J Neurosurg Spine.* 2008;9:120–128.

Rivera AL, Pelloski CE, Gilbert MR, et al. MGMT promoter methylation is predictive of response to radiotherapy and prognostic in the absence of adjuvant alkylating chemotherapy for glioblastoma. *Neuro Oncol.* 2010;12:116–121.

Saghal A, Bilsky M, Chang EL, et al. Stereotactic body radiotherapy for spinal metastases: current status, with a focus on its application in the postoperative patient. *J Neurosurg Spine.* 2011;14(2):151–166.

Sampson JH, Archer GE, Mitchell DA, et al. An epidermal growth factor receptor variant III-targeted vaccine is safe and immunogenic in patients with glioblastoma multiforme. *Mol Cancer Ther.* 2009; 8:2773–2779.

Shaw E, Arusell R, Scheithauer B, et al. Prospective randomized trial of low-versus high-dose radiation therapy in adults with supratentorial low-grade glioma: initial report of a North Central Cancer Treatment Group/Radiation Therapy Oncology Group/Eastern Cooperative Oncology Group study. *J Clin Oncol.* 2002; 20:2267–2276.

Shehadi JA, Sciubba DM, Suk I, et al. Surgical treatment strategies and outcome in patients with breast cancer metastatic to the spine: a review of 87 patients. *Eur Spine J.* 2007;16:1179–1192.

Smith JS, Chang EF, Lamborn KR, et al. Role of extent of resection in the long-term outcome of low grade hemispheric gliomas. *J Clin Oncol.* 2008;26:1338–1345.

Stupp R, Hegi ME, Mason WP, et al. Effects of radiotherapy with concomitant and adjuvant temozolomide versus radiotherapy alone on survival in glioblastoma in a randomised phase III study: 5-year analysis of the EORTC-NCIC trial. *Lancet.* 2009;10:459–466.

Suki D, Hatiboglu MA, Patel AJ, et al. Comparative risk of leptomeningeal dissemination of cancer after surgery or stereotactic radiosurgery for a single supratentorial solid tumor metastasis. *Neurosurgery.* 2010;64:664–676.

Sulman EP, Guerrero M, Aldape K. Beyond grade: molecular pathology of malignant gliomas. *Semin Radiat Oncol.* 2009; 19:142–149.

Vecht CJ, Haaxme-Reiche H, Noordijk EM, et al. Treatment of single brain metastasis: radiotherapy alone or combined with neurosurgery? *Ann Neurol.* 1993;33:583–590.

Walbert T, Groves MD. Known and emerging biomarkers of leptomeningeal metastasis and its response to treatment. *Future Oncol.* 2010;6:287–297.

Williams BJ, Fox BD, Sciubba DM, et al. Surgical management of prostate cancer metastatic to the spine. *J Neurosurg Spine.* 2009;10:414–422.

Yan H, Parsons DW, Jin G, et al. IDH1 and IDH2 mutations in gliomas. *New Engl J Med.* 2009;360:765–773.

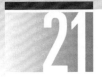

Cancer of Unknown Primary Site

Vanja Vaccaro and Gauri R. Varadhachary

Cancer of unknown primary site (CUP) is a heterogeneous group that comprises 3% to 4% of new cancer diagnoses and can pose a therapeutic challenge. Although chemotherapy is the primary treatment modality in patients with CUP, the surgeon may play an important role in both the diagnosis and the treatment of these patients. In particular, surgeons are often asked to evaluate patients with cancers that present as solitary metastases (lymph node(s) or liver as common presentations) or as carcinomatosis.

In this chapter, we define the presentation and clinical features of CUP; outline a practical approach to the diagnostic evaluation of patients with CUP, including the role of molecular profiling in the era of sophisticated immunohistochemistry; and discuss the role of surgery in various clinical scenarios.

DEFINITION AND GENERAL CONSIDERATIONS

CUP is defined by the presence of a biopsy-proven cancer for which the anatomical origin of the primary tumor is not revealed after a thorough medical history and physical examination (including breast and pelvic examination in women and testicular and prostate examination in men), routine laboratory tests, chest x-ray, computed tomography (CT) of the abdomen and pelvis, mammography in women, and prostate-specific antigen (PSA) test in men. The prevailing hypothesis in CUP is that the primary tumor either remains microscopic and escapes clinical detection or disappears after seeding the metastasis, which may be due to angiogenic incompetency of the primary tumor.

These tumors often are grouped according to histologic subtype. The major subtypes include squamous cell cancer, adenocarcinoma (including poorly differentiated adenocarcinoma), and poorly differentiated or undifferentiated neoplasm, the name given to a heterogeneous group of tumors of various cell origins. Table 21.1 lists the frequencies of each subtype (adenocarcinoma is the most common).

As found in large series, the most common locations of CUP metastases are the lymph nodes, bones, lungs, liver, and the peritoneum. Other metastatic sites include brain, meninges, pleura, subcutaneous tissues, adrenal glands, and kidney.

In most patients, the site of origin of the metastatic disease is never discerned. In others, the primary tumor site from which the metastases are derived is eventually identified during the lifetime of the patient through clinical examinations, surgery, or autopsy. Older studies report that in only 25% of CUP cases is the primary site identifiable during the patient's lifetime; this number is probably lower with sophisticated imaging techniques (where baseline studies have been negative). Metastases from squamous cell cancers typically originate in the head and neck region or the lungs, whereas metastatic adenocarcinomas originate in the lungs, breasts, thyroid gland, pancreas, liver, stomach, colon, or rectum.

The median survival of patients with CUP is 6 to 9 months. Specific subgroups of patients with metastatic CUP have considerably better prognoses than the group as a whole, when the patient is able to be treated with appropriate therapy.

Histopathology	Percentage of CUP Patients
Adenocarcinoma	60
Squamous cell carcinoma	5
Others:	35
Poorly differentiated adenocarcinoma	
Poorly differentiated carcinoma	
Poorly differentiated neoplasm	
Unclassified neoplasm	

CUP, cancer of unknown primary site.

This includes patients with squamous cell cancer metastatic to cervical lymph nodes, women with metastatic adenocarcinoma in axillary lymph nodes, men with undifferentiated cancer and elevated β-human chorionic gonadotropin (β-hCG) or alpha-fetoprotein (AFP) levels, women with peritoneal carcinomatosis, and patients with neuroendocrine CUP. These subgroups are discussed later in this chapter in more detail.

The therapeutic goal in evaluating patients with CUP is to identify those tumor types for which a cure or effective specific therapy is an option. In addition, local therapeutic options can potentially help with adequate disease control and palliation in selected patients.

HISTORY AND PHYSICAL EXAMINATION

In patients with CUP, a complete medical history and physical examination are essential. An individual history of malignancy or a family history of cancer may guide the surgeon in establishing the site of an occult primary tumor.

During physical examination of a patient with CUP, several anatomical sites warrant particular attention. The head and neck should be examined thoroughly, particularly when a diagnosis of squamous cell cancer has been made. This includes examination of the oropharynx, hypopharynx, nasopharynx, and larynx, typically assisted by indirect or fiberoptic laryngoscopy. The thyroid gland should be examined for enlargement or asymmetry. All nodal basins, including those of the head and neck and the supraclavicular, axillary, and inguinal regions, should be examined for palpable or enlarged lymph nodes.

In women, a careful breast examination and a thorough bimanual pelvic examination should be performed. For men, testicular and prostate examinations are particularly important. All patients should undergo a thorough skin examination and rectal examination.

LABORATORY STUDIES

Routine tests such as complete blood cell count, chemistry studies, liver function tests, and urinalysis should be performed in all patients, and stool should be checked for occult blood. Beyond these basic tests, the clinical laboratory has limited usefulness in the diagnostic evaluation of patients with CUP, but additional studies should be requested on the basis of histologic and radiologic findings. Serum tumor markers, although not specific enough to make a diagnosis, are helpful in following a patient's progress on treatment.

RADIOGRAPHIC EVALUATION

Radiographic evaluations of patients with CUP should be focused on identifying the primary tumor and delineating the extent of metastatic disease.

Chest X-ray and CT Scan of the Chest, Abdomen, and Pelvis

CT scan of the chest, abdomen, and pelvis is essential because it can help in locating the primary tumor, evaluating the extent of disease, and selecting the most favorable biopsy site.

Mammography

Women of childbearing age or older, particularly those with metastatic adenocarcinoma, should undergo mammography. Unfortunately, identifying subtle radiographic abnormalities is difficult in younger women, who often have extremely dense breast tissue. Magnetic resonance imaging (MRI) of the breast is indicated in women who present with isolated axillary adenopathy (if the mammogram and breast sonographic findings are negative).

Magnetic Resonance Imaging

In most cases, MRI is indicated if CT is contraindicated. Its most defined role in CUP is in women who present with isolated axillary lymph node metastases and suspected occult primary breast carcinoma. The results of several studies suggest that MRI of the breast can help with tumor detection in up to 75% of patients. This result can influence surgical management, with a negative breast MRI predicting a low yield at mastectomy.

Positron Emission Tomography

The role of positron emission tomography (PET) scan using 18F-fluoro-2-deoxy-D-glucose (18F-FDG PET) is controversial. PET imaging is recommended in patients with occult primary head and neck cancer (cervical CUP) and in those who present with a solitary potentially resectable CUP lesion. Several recent small studies have described the role of PET in patients who present with cervical CUP. The advantages of locating the primary tumor in patients who present with cervical lymphadenopathy (occult head and neck cancer) are (a) smaller postoperative radiation ports that can decrease early and late complications, (b) better surveillance for recurrence, and (c) improved prognostic determination. Rusthoven et al. reviewed 16 studies (1994 to 2003) of 302 patients with cervical lymph node metastases from unknown primary tumors. Conventional workup included panendoscopy, CT, or MRI, and, in 10 of these 16 studies, these tests were performed before diagnosis. They reported the overall sensitivity, specificity, and accuracy rates of FDG PET in detecting unknown primary tumors as 88.3%, 74.9%, and 78.8%, respectively. Approximately 25% of primary tumors that were not apparent after conventional workup were able to be identified on 18F-FDG PET, as were previously undetected regional or distant metastases in 27% of patients.

In general, an exhaustive search for the primary tumor site in these patients by radiographic evaluation can be expensive, inconvenient, and anxiety provoking for patients and often has no significant effect on patients' therapy or the ultimate course of their disease.

PATHOLOGIC EVALUATION

Fine-needle aspiration (FNA) biopsy has largely replaced core biopsy as the first pathologic test. This can be followed by core biopsy, incisional biopsy, or excisional biopsy as needed for more specific histologic identification. Good communication between the clinician and the pathologist is important because details of the medical history and physical examination can influence the pathologic review and facilitate submission of additional tissue, if necessary, for an accurate diagnosis.

Light Microscopy

Light microscopy (hematoxylin and eosin staining) is ordinarily sufficient to determine the cell of origin. About 60% of CUPs are found to be adenocarcinoma on light microscopy. An additional 5% are squamous cell carcinoma, and the remaining 35% are diagnosed as poorly differentiated adenocarcinoma, poorly differentiated carcinoma, or poorly differentiated neoplasm. Electron microscopy, which helps identify the ultrastructural features of the cell of origin, is rarely needed. For example, desmosomes and intracellular bridges are associated with squamous cell cancer, whereas tight junctions, microvilli, and acinar spaces are associated with adenocarcinoma. Premelanosomes are associated with melanoma, and neurosecretory granules are associated with small cell or neuroendocrine tumors. Lymphoma is typically characterized by an absence of junctions between the cells on electron microscopy. Electron microscopy can be time-consuming and expensive; therefore, with the availability of immunohistochemical stains, the need for it has diminished.

Immunohistochemical Analysis

Immunohistochemical analyses have become a routine addition to light microscopy, and a broad range of immunohistochemical markers are used to assist in the diagnosis after light microscopy. Common markers used for adenocarcinomas include cytokeratins (CKs) 7 and 20 and thyroid transcription factor (TTF-1). TTF-1, a nuclear protein, can be positive in lung and thyroid cancers. About 65% to 70% of lung adenocarcinomas and 25% of squamous cell lung cancers stain positive for TTF-1, and in patients with CUP, this test is helpful in differentiating between a primary lung tumor and metastatic adenocarcinoma (e.g., in patients presenting with metastatic pleural effusion). The CK marker combination pattern depicted in Figure 21.1 is also helpful.

Breast markers including estrogen receptor (ER), progesterone receptor (PR), Her-2/neu, and gross cystic disease fibrous protein should be checked in women who present with adenocarcinoma, especially isolated axillary adenopathy. Hep-par-1, a hepatocellular carcinoma marker, aids in the diagnosis of hepatocellular cancer, and CK-19 is sometimes used for cholangiocarcinoma. It can be difficult to distinguish metastatic cholangiocarcinoma, metastatic adenocarcinoma, and hepatocellular carcinoma in patients who present with liver-only metastatic disease. Other markers used in a directed fashion on the basis of past microscopy results include prostatic acid phosphatase and PSA for prostate cancer, and neuron-specific enolase and chromogranin for neuroendocrine cancers. Germ cell tumors often stain for β-hCG and AFP.

No immunohistochemical marker is 100% specific, and many of these tests (as well as serum markers) can be confusing and rarely help in the search for a primary tumor or in treatment planning.

Serum Tumor Markers and Cytogenetics

Unfortunately, patients with CUP typically have nonspecific overexpression of many serum tumor markers, including β-hCG, AFP, carcinoembryonic antigen, CA-125, CA 19–9, and CA 15–3. In patients who present with an undifferentiated carcinoma or a poorly differentiated carcinoma (especially with a midline tumor), β-hCG and AFP should be tested to rule out occult germ-line cancers. None of these markers has been found to have adequate specificity or sensitivity to consistently identify a primary tumor, nor the predictive value for either response to chemotherapy or survival.

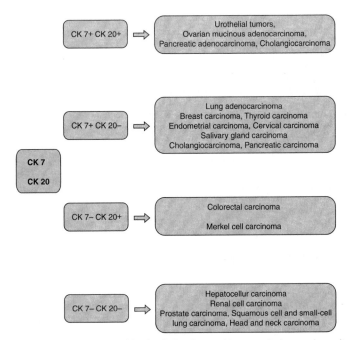

FIGURE 21.1 Approach to immunohistochemical markers used in cancer of unknown primary site.

Motzer et al. presented the molecular and cytogenetic results for 40 patients with CUP with poorly differentiated carcinoma. In 42% of patients (17), the diagnosis was made on the basis of genetic analysis. Thirty percent (12) of patients had cytogenetic changes characteristic of germ cell tumors (isochromosome 12p-I[12p]), increased 12p copy number, or deletion of the long arm of chromosome 12. These patients also responded better to cisplatin-based chemotherapy than did patients with other diagnoses (75% vs. 18%). Pantou et al. studied 20 biopsy specimens from patients with CUP and found that most samples had multiple complex cytogenetic patterns. Table 21.2 lists several common tumor markers and their roles in clinical evaluation of patients with CUP.

ROLE OF MOLECULAR PROFILING

The accurate diagnosis of the primary site in CUP would impact patients' prognosis and management, allowing site-specific therapy. Molecular profiling of tumors offers the chance of a systematic human cancer classification and is a promising technique to improve the site of origin diagnosis in CUP patients. Recently new molecular tests that identify molecular signatures of the tissue of origin are available.

Several studies have demonstrated the feasibility of using gene expression profiling with DNA microarray analysis to classify uncertain tumors according to their tissue of origin, by identifying gene subsets whose expression typifies each cancer class. These studies achieved accuracy in identifying the tissue of origin in

TABLE 21.2 Clinical Role of Selected Immunohistochemical Markers

Breast	ER, GCDFP-15, Mammaglobin, Her-2/neu
Lung	TTF-1, SP-A1
Muellerian, ovarian	ER, WT-1, PAX-8
Neuroendocrine	Chromogranin, synaptophysin, CD56
Germ cell	β-hCG, αFP, OCT¾, CKIT, CD30 (embryonal)
Urothelial	CK7, CK20, thrombomodulin
Kidney	RCC, CD10
Hepatocellular	Hep-par-1
Colorectal	CK7, CK20, CDX-2, CEA
Sarcoma	Desmin1, factor VIII2, CD31, smooth muscle actin for leiomyosarcoma, MyoD1 for rhabdomyosarcoma
Melanoma	S100, vimentin, HMB-45, tyrosinase and melan-A
Lymphoma	LCA, CD3, CD4, CD5, CD20, CD45

ER, estrogen receptor; GCDFP-15, gross cystic disease fibrous protein-15; TTF-1, thyroid transcription factor; SP-A1, surfactant protein A precursor; β-hCG, β-human chorionic gonadotropin; αFP, alpha-fetoprotein; CEA, carcinoembryonic antigen; LCA, leukocyte common antigen.

78% to 89% of tumors. Furthermore, it has been demonstrated that the patterns of gene expression remain consistent with the tissue of origin and are maintained in distant metastases, even if the metastases develop after a long interval; therefore, it is theoretically possible to build a comprehensive gene expression database spanning a majority of tumor types and use it as a clinical diagnostic tool.

Two main strategies have been used to identify the origin of tissue samples: the DNA microarray platforms and the quantitative reverse transcription real-time PCR-assays (qRT-PCR). In both strategies, messenger RNA (mRNA) is extracted from fresh frozen or formalin-fixed paraffin-embedded (FFPE) tumor tissue, purified, amplified, and tagged with fluorescent stains. Subsequently, it is hybridized to a DNA microarray consisting of hundreds or thousands of individual gene-specific probes complementary to multiple gene sequences. Relative levels of gene expression in the samples are estimated by measuring the fluorescence intensity for each probe. This kind of strategy can be used for the management of CUP by means of comparison of the multi-gene expression pattern of a CUP and assignment of the CUP specimen to the primary tumor type to which the CUP molecular signature most closely resembles. Microarray platforms have the advantage of being able to measure hundreds to thousands of transcripts in a single assay, but this technology requires fresh snap-frozen tissue and remains complex and time-consuming, and it is currently limited as a research tool. An accurate classification of multiple cancer types can be made using a reduced number of genes and a classification can be achieved using cheaper, faster, and more robust platforms for quantifying gene expression such as quantitative PCR. This requires shorter and simpler protocols, can be performed with equipments already present in most molecular diagnostics laboratories, and can be applied to FFPE tissue. In the clinic, real-time quantitative polymerase chain reaction (RT-PCR) is the "gold standard" for gene expression analysis. However, RT-PCR has a much lower capacity in measuring, at most, a few hundred genes from FFPE tissues and may be of lower quality than that obtained from frozen tissue; formalin fixation can cause formation of cross-links between proteins or between proteins and nucleic acids, which causes lower purity RNA when compared with frozen tissues. There are currently three assays commercially available in the United States to evaluate the tissue of origin in CUP patients (the Pathwork Tissue of Origin Test, which is a 1550-gene microarray-based test; Theros Cancer-TYPE ID, a 92-gene qRT-PCR assay; and the miRview mets test, a 48–microRNA qRT-PCR assay). Another microarray-based test, the 1900-gene CupPrint, is offered clinically in Europe but not in the United States. Finally, the CUP assay, a 10-gene qPCR assay, has been developed but is not yet clinically available.

Several independent studies have shown that it is feasible for a CUP to have its molecular signature studied by means of an array test, compared to the signatures of known solid tumors, and thus be genetically assigned to a primary tissue of origin with satisfactory accuracy. However, the routine use of a gene expression profile tool in the diagnosis and management of unknown primary cancer still has limitations. Since a primary cancer is not available, accuracy of the test cannot be determined easily. Also, there may be genomic differences that may exist between a CUP cancer and the solid known tumor counterpart with differences in therapeutic outcomes.

At this time, although a microarray-based gene expression profiling test will not obviate the need for thorough clinical investigation, it may facilitate more focused testing that would result in reduced cost, lower patient morbidity, and improved outcome. Therefore, the combination of gene expression profiling results in selected patients with a panel of immunohistochemistry markers may impact the diagnostic accuracy and the patient management in CUP cancers. This will be more important as specific targeted therapies emerge for known cancers which can then be applied to CUP subsets.

SPECIFIC DISEASE SITES

Metastatic Cancer to Cervical Lymph Nodes

Enlarged cervical lymph nodes are often found on biopsy to be positive for metastatic cancer. Patients with squamous cell cancer metastatic to cervical lymph nodes and an unknown primary tumor site have a better prognosis than do patients with CUP overall.

The neck comprises more than 25 nodal basins. These nodes have been grouped into six specific categories to standardize the pathologic evaluation of patients. The classification of cervical lymph nodes is shown in Table 21.3. The most common site of metastasis in patients with head and neck squamous cell cancer is the jugulodigastric or the level II upper internal jugular chain nodes, followed by the midjugular nodes. Metastasis to the other cervical nodal groups occurs with less frequency.

TABLE 21.3 Classification of Cervical Lymph Nodes

Level	Nodes
I	Submental nodes
II	Upper internal jugular chain nodes
III	Middle internal jugular chain nodes
IV	Lower internal jugular chain nodes
V	Spinal accessory nodes
	Transverse cervical nodes
VI	Tracheoesophageal groove nodes

In those patients with cervical lymph nodes from an occult squamous cell primary tumor, a careful head and neck examination is essential. Adequate lighting and mirrors must be used to visualize the entire oropharynx, hypopharynx, nasopharynx, and larynx. A CT scan of the head and neck (often including CT chest) is indicated to determine the primary tumor site and obtain complete staging information. As mentioned earlier in the text, some of these patients are also candidates for a PET/CT scan.

If no primary tumor is found on physical examination and imaging studies including a CT scan/PET, panendoscopy is a common next step. This is normally performed in the operating room with the patient under general anesthesia. Esophagoscopy, laryngoscopy, bronchoscopy, and nasopharyngoscopy are performed in an attempt to visualize the region and obtain biopsy specimens from the most common sites of occult squamous cell cancer in the head and neck region. Random biopsies of the most probable tumor site locations are performed on the basis of the location of the adenopathy.

Typical occult primary tumor sites in squamous cell cancer are the nasopharynx, the mid-base of the tongue, the pyriform sinus, and the tonsils. Table 21.4 shows the common pattern of cervical metastasis from different squamous cell tumors in the head and neck region. On the basis of the location of the nodal metastases, extrapolation of the likely source of the occult primary tumor is often possible, and the endoscopic examination should be focused on these locations. Bilateral tonsillectomy is an important part of the staging and evaluation process and it is not rare to see a small primary cancer hidden in the deep crypts of the tonsils.

If the primary tumor site cannot be identified on endoscopy, the standard approach is a combination of radical neck dissection and postoperative radiation therapy. The role of chemotherapy depends on the presence of bulky nodes (N3 disease), and neoadjuvant chemotherapy has not been well studied. On the basis of large series, the expected 5-year survival in these patients is 32% to 55%, and the overall rate of local control is 75% to 85%. Patients with extranodal extension or lymph nodes >6 cm (N3 disease) have higher rates of both local recurrence and distant metastases.

Patients with metastatic adenocarcinoma in cervical lymph nodes from an occult primary tumor have a less favorable outcome than do those with squamous cell cancer. Retrospective series have shown that lymphadenectomy and radiation therapy are much less effective in adenocarcinoma than in squamous cell carcinoma; the rate of local recurrence in these cases is nearly 100%, and the 5-year survival rate is 0% to 10%.

TABLE 21.4	Probable Sites of Primary Tumors According to the Location of the Cervical Metastases
Location of Nodes	**Primary Tumor Site**
Submental	Floor of the mouth, lips, or anterior tongue
Submaxillary	Retromolar trigone or glossopalatine pillar
Jugulodigastric	Hypopharynx, base of the tongue, tonsils, nasopharynx, or larynx
Low jugular	Thyroid, hypopharynx, or nasopharynx
Supraclavicular	Lung (40%), thyroid (20%), GI (12%), or GU (8%)
Posterior triangle	Nasopharynx

GI, gastrointestinal; GU, genitourinary.

Of particular interest is the presence of an enlarged Virchow's (supraclavicular) node, common in patients with metastatic adenocarcinoma. One study retrospectively reviewed 152 FNA biopsy samples of supraclavicular lymph nodes, comparing the sites of primary tumor when the metastasis was in the right versus the left supraclavicular node. Sixteen of 19 primary pelvic tumors metastasized to the left supraclavicular node, and all (6 of 6) primary abdominal malignancies metastasized to the left supraclavicular node. However, thoracic, breast, and head and neck malignancies did not differ in patterns of metastasis to the right and left supraclavicular nodes. On the basis of this information, the search for the primary tumor should be focused on the abdomen and pelvis in patients who present with adenocarcinoma in a left-sided Virchow's node.

Metastatic Cancer to Axillary Lymph Nodes

The histologic study of the tumor should be used to guide the evaluation of patients with cancer metastatic to axillary lymph nodes (lymphoma is not considered a CUP; metastatic melanoma with an unknown primary is discussed separately later in this chapter). Patients with squamous cell cancer metastatic to the axillary lymph nodes should undergo a careful skin examination; a chest x-ray; a thorough head and neck examination; and CT scans of the head, neck, and the chest to look for an occult squamous cell primary tumor.

Men with adenocarcinoma metastatic to an axillary lymph node and CUP should be evaluated for lung, gastrointestinal, and genitourinary primary tumors. Women with adenocarcinoma metastatic to the axillary lymph nodes should be evaluated similarly, although in women the likelihood of an occult breast primary tumor is high. Women with occult breast cancer who present with axillary metastases constitute approximately 0.5% of all women with breast cancer. When many such patients are treated for a presumptive diagnosis of breast cancer, the recurrence and survival results are similar to those of patients with a similar stage of breast cancer and a known primary tumor. A retrospective review of the mastectomy specimens from patients with occult primary tumors showed that in 50% to 65% of cases, the primary tumor was ultimately identified in the surgical specimen. Every woman should undergo a mammogram followed by breast sonography if the mammogram is negative (especially in younger patients with dense breasts). As discussed earlier, MRI of the breast is indicated in women who present with axillary adenopathy and CUP when mammogram and sonographic findings are negative.

The biopsy specimen from the lymph node should be subjected to routine histologic and immunohistochemical evaluation for ER, PR, and Her-2/neu. Although neither highly sensitive nor highly specific, the presence of ER or PR in this clinical scenario strongly suggests a breast primary tumor.

The treatment for women with adenocarcinoma metastatic to axillary lymph nodes has evolved dramatically over the last decade. The three general approaches are immediate mastectomy, observation, and radiation therapy. Immediate mastectomy is not performed in most patients if the imaging studies are negative because the chances of finding a primary are low. Observation with axillary dissection can result in recurrence in the breast (25% to 75%, depending on the study), requiring further therapy. The third approach is breast conservation therapy with locoregional radiation therapy, which has been shown to decrease the local recurrence rate and is the preferred approach for most patients at the M. D. Anderson Cancer Center. Our results show that in patients who have undergone axillary lymph node dissection alone, the incidence of local recurrence is 65% at 10 years, whereas a combination of axillary lymph node dissection and radiation therapy reduces the local recurrence rate to 25%. With this treatment, the overall survival rate was no different from that of patients with the same nodal stage of disease who had undergone mastectomy. The addition of adjuvant chemotherapy to surgery and radiation therapy increased the survival rate from 60% to 85% at 10 years. Tamoxifen should be part of the therapy for women of any age whose primary tumor (if identified) or axillary nodal metastases express ER or PR.

A retrospective study at the M. D. Anderson Cancer Center included 45 women with isolated axillary nodal metastases without a known primary tumor. The median follow-up duration was 7 years. Patients underwent either mastectomy or breast conservation therapy; external-beam radiation therapy was used in 71% of patients, and systemic chemotherapy was used in 73%. No significant difference was found between mastectomy and breast conservation in locoregional recurrence, distant metastases, or 5-year survival rate. Regardless of the surgical treatment used, the number of involved nodes was the only determinant of survival.

Cancer Metastatic to the Inguinal Nodes from an Unknown Primary Site

A relatively infrequent presentation of metastatic CUP is metastases to the inguinal lymph nodes. Excluding melanoma, the two most common histologic types are unclassified carcinoma and squamous cell carcinoma. Adenocarcinoma is rarely observed. In evaluating patients with inguinal metastases, a thorough investigation for the primary tumor should include examination of the skin of the lower extremities, perineum, buttocks, anal canal, and pelvic region. If the inguinal node is the solitary area of presentation, excision followed by local radiation therapy is the next preferred step. For bulky bilateral adenopathy, neoadjuvant chemotherapy followed by surgery, inguinal lymph node dissection, and radiation therapy can be considered if there are no other sites of metastatic disease. These patients are prone to lymphedema after multimodality therapy, so they should be educated regarding the risks and undergo treatment if lymphedema develops.

Peritoneal Carcinomatosis of Unknown Primary Site

Patients with peritoneal carcinomatosis of unknown primary site can present with ascites, bowel obstruction, or nonspecific gastrointestinal symptoms. The two subgroups in this category include (a) patients with mucin-producing adenocarcinoma with and without signet ring cells and (b) women with primary peritoneal carcinomatosis. Patients with mucin-producing adenocarcinoma often have multiple peritoneal implants, with the primary site most likely being the gastrointestinal tract (i.e., stomach, small bowel, appendix, or colon). Patients in this group have a poorer prognosis and respond poorly to currently available treatment regimens. These patients should undergo an upper endoscopy and colonoscopy to evaluate for a gastrointestinal primary tumor. If immunohistochemical analysis show a CK 20+, CK7−, CDX2+ pattern—a potential colon cancer profile—a colon cancer based treatment regimen should be considered.

The second subset is composed of women with primary peritoneal carcinomatosis. A histopathologic analysis of these patients reveals cells with serous papillary features and, on occasion, psammoma bodies. These patients may have elevated CA-125 levels but do not have obvious ovarian cancer (on CT pelvis and transvaginal sonography). Several studies have found that women who present with peritoneal carcinomatosis should be treated in a similar fashion to those with known advanced ovarian cancer. This includes maximal surgical cytoreduction at initial laparotomy, followed by platinum-based combination chemotherapy. One study found a prolonged median survival of 13 months in patients who had undergone paclitaxel and carboplatin-based chemotherapy, and 25% of the patients had progression-free survival of more than 2 years.

Unknown Primary Tumor with Metastatic Liver Disease

The surgeon is occasionally involved in the evaluation of patients who present with metastatic disease to the liver from an unknown primary tumor. The liver tumor may be discovered when the patient presents with symptoms on routine physical examination or incidentally on a radiologic study such as an abdominal sonogram or CT scan.

When patients present with metastatic disease to the liver and CUP, the most common cell type is adenocarcinoma (approximately 60% to 65%). However, anaplastic or poorly differentiated carcinoma, small-cell carcinoma, squamous cell carcinoma, neuroendocrine cancer, and unclassified tumors are also found. The likely primary tumors include gastrointestinal cancers (including pancreatic-biliary cancers), followed by a lung or breast tumor.

Most patients undergo a CT scan of the chest, abdomen, and pelvis; mammogram (in women); and an upper endoscopy and colonoscopy if suggested by marker data or symptoms. The overall survival of these patients is usually poor (median, 7 months), although a survival benefit (approximately 12 months) can be seen in patients who have a good performance status and respond to chemotherapy.

A subgroup of patients who present with CUP and liver metastases have low-grade neuroendocrine carcinoma. These may be diagnosed incidentally or when patients complain of hormonal symptoms (diarrhea, flushing, or nausea) or pain. Low-grade neuroendocrine cancers can remain indolent for several years with slow progression and may not need treatment for a long time (hormonal or other). Tumor markers, including serum chromogranin, neuron-specific enolase, and urine 5-HIAA, may be elevated. If a patient has carcinoid symptoms, endocrine therapy alone for hormone-related symptoms with somatostatin analogs should be used. Specific local therapies, such as right hepatectomy or chemoembolization, or systemic therapies, such as chemotherapy or more recently developed targeted therapy (anti-angiogenic agents, m-TOR inhibitors), are indicated if the patient is symptomatic with pain or uncontrolled endocrine symptoms.

CHEMOTHERAPY FOR METASTATIC CANCERS OF UNKNOWN PRIMARY SITE

Data from CUP trials are difficult to interpret because patients with CUP are a heterogeneous group. When chemotherapy is given to unselected groups of patients with metastatic CUP, an overall 5% to 10% 5-year survival rate can be anticipated, with median survival in most studies between 6 and 13 months. Patients with favorable subtypes (e.g., peritoneal carcinomatosis or lymph node-predominant disease) benefit from chemotherapy. Traditionally, cisplatin-based combination chemotherapy regimens have been used to treat patients with CUP. In a phase II study by Hainsworth et al., 55 patients with CUP were treated with paclitaxel, carboplatin, and oral etoposide every 21 days. Most were previously untreated, with only four having undergone previous chemotherapy. The overall response rate was 47%, the median overall survival was 13.4 months, and the regimen was well tolerated. Briasoulis et al. found comparable response rates and median overall survival in 77 patients with CUP with paclitaxel and carboplatin and without oral etoposide. In this study, patients with nodal or pleural disease and women with peritoneal carcinomatosis had a better response rate and an overall survival of 13 and 15 months, respectively. A phase II randomized trial by Culine et al. (the French Study Group on Carcinomas of Unknown Primary 01) studied 80 patients who were randomly assigned to receive either gemcitabine + cisplatin (GC) or irinotecan + cisplatin (IC). Seventy-eight patients were assessable for efficacy and toxicity. Objective responses were observed in 21 patients (55%) in the GC arm and in 15 patients (38%) in the IC arm. The median survival was 8 and 6 months in the GC and IC arms, respectively (median follow-up of 22 months).

Patients with poorly differentiated carcinoma, the possible germ cell equivalents, have traditionally undergone a trial of a cisplatin-based regimen. Patients with squamous cell cancer or neuroendocrine cancer have a significantly better response to chemotherapeutic agents than do patients with other tumor types. The role of second-line chemotherapy in CUP is poorly defined in the current era, therapies are chosen based on clues from presentation, immunohistochemistry, and response to first-line therapy.

Although cure is an unrealistic goal for many patients with metastatic CUP site, surgeons often are involved in the palliative care of such patients and in some selected cases are involved in planning definitive therapies for patients with locoregional disease. CUP is the epitome of personalized medicine and patients should be managed by a multidisciplinary team when necessary, to ensure improved survival and quality of life.

Recommended Readings

Briasoulis E, Kalofonos H, Bafaloukos D, et al. Carboplatin plus paclitaxel in unknown primary carcinoma: a phase II Hellenic Cooperative Oncology Group Study. *J Clin Oncol.* 2000;18:3101–3107.

Bugat R, Bataillard A, Lesimple T, et al. Summary of the Standards, Options and Recommendations for the management of patients with carcinoma of unknown primary site (2002). *Br J Cancer.* 2003;89(S1): S59–S66.

Culine S, Kramar A, Saghatchian M, et al. Development and validation of a prognostic model to predict the length of survival in patients with carcinomas of an unknown primary site. *J Clin Oncol.* 2002; 20:4679–4683.

Glover KY, Varadhachary GR, Lenzi R, et al. Unknown primary cancer. In: Abeloff MD, Armitage JO, Lichter AS, et al., eds. *Clinical Oncology.* 4th ed. Philadelphia, PA: Elsevier; 2008:2057–2074.

Greco FA, Hainsworth JD. One-hour paclitaxel, carboplatin, and extended-schedule etoposide in the treatment of carcinoma of unknown primary site. *Semin Oncol.* 1997;24:S19-101–S19-105.

Greco FA, Spigel DR, Yardley DA, et al. Molecular profiling in unknown primary cancer: accuracy of tissue of origin prediction. *Oncologist.* 2010;15(5):500–506.

Hainsworth JD, Burris HA III, Calvert SW, et al. Gemcitabine in the second-line therapy of patients with carcinoma of unknown primary site: a phase II trial of the Minnie Pearl Cancer Research Network. *Cancer Invest.* 2001;19:335–339.

Hainsworth J, Talantov D, Jatkoe T, et al. Gene profiling of tumour tissue in the diagnosis of patients with carcinoma of

unknown primary site: evaluation of the Veridex 10-gene molecular assay. *J Clin Oncol.* 2007;25(18S): abstract 21109.

Horlings HM, van Laar RK, Kerst JM, et al. Gene expression profiling to identify the histogenetic origin of metastatic adenocarcinomas of unknown primary. *J Clin Oncol.* 2008;26:4435–4441.

Joshi U, van der Hoeven JJ, Comans EF, et al. In search of an unknown primary tumour presenting with extracervical metastases: the diagnostic performance of FDG-PET. *Br J Radiol.* 2004;77:1000–1006.

Lassen U, Daugaard G, Eigtved A, et al. 18F-FDG whole body positron emission tomography (PET) in patients with unknown primary tumours (UPT). *Eur J Cancer.* 1999;35:1076–1082.

Ma XJ, Patel R, Wang X, et al. Molecular classification of human cancers using a 92-gene real-time quantitative polymerase chain reaction assay. *Arch Pathol Lab Med.* 2006;130:465–473.

Monzon FA, Koen TJ. Diagnosis of metastatic neoplasms: molecular approaches for identification of tissue of origin. *Arch Pathol Lab Med.* 2010;134(2):216–224.

Monzon FA, Medeiros F, Lyons-Weiler M, et al. Identification of tissue of origin in carcinoma of unknown primary with a microarray-based gene expression test. *Diagn Pathol.* 2010;5:3.

Morris EA, Schwartz LH, Dershaw DD, et al. MR imaging of the breast in patients with occult primary breast carcinoma. *Radiology.* 1997;205:437–440.

Motzer RJ, Rodriguez E, Reuter VE, et al. Molecular and cytogenetic studies in the diagnosis of patients with poorly differentiated carcinomas of unknown primary site. *J Clin Oncol.* 1995;13:274–282.

Olson JA Jr, Morris EA, Van Zee KJ, et al. Magnetic resonance imaging facilitates breast conservation for occult breast cancer. *Ann Surg Oncol.* 2000;7:411–415.

Pantou D, Tsarouha H, Papadopoulou A, et al. Cytogenetic profile of unknown primary tumors: clues for their pathogenesis and clinical management. *Neoplasia.* 2003;5:23–31.

Pavlidis N, Briasoulis E, Hainsworth J, et al. Diagnostic and therapeutic management of cancer of an unknown primary. *Eur J Cancer.* 2003;39:1990–2005.

Pentheroudakis G, Greco FA, Pavlidis N. Molecular assignment of tissue of origin in cancer of unknown primary may not predict response to therapy or outcome: a systematic literature review. *Cancer Treat Rev.* 2009;35(3):221–227.

Randall DA, Johnstone PA, Foss RD, et al. Tonsillectomy in diagnosis of the unknown primary tumor of the head and neck. *Otolaryngol Head Neck Surg.* 2000;122: 52–55.

Rubin BP, Skarin AT, Pisick E, et al. Use of cytokeratins 7 and 20 in determining the origin of metastatic carcinoma of unknown primary, with special emphasis on lung cancer. *Eur J Cancer Prev.* 2001; 10:77–82.

Rusthoven KE, Koshy M, Paulino AC. The role of fluorodeoxyglucose positron emission tomography in cervical lymph node metastases from an unknown primary tumor. *Cancer.* 2004;101:2641–2649.

Schelfout K, Kersschot E, Van Goethem M, et al. Breast MR imaging in a patient with unilateral axillary lymphadenopathy and unknown primary malignancy. *Eur Radiol.* 2003;13:2128–2132.

Tan D, Li Q, Deeb G, et al. Thyroid transcription factor-1 expression prevalence and its clinical implications in non-small cell lung cancer: a high-throughput tissue microarray and immunohistochemistry study. *Hum Pathol.* 2003;34:597–604.

Tothill RW, Kowalczyk A, Rischin D, et al. An expression-based site of origin diagnostic method designed for clinical application to cancer of unknown origin. *Cancer Res.* 2005;65:4031–4040.

Varadhachary GR, Talantov D, Raber MN, et al. Molecular profiling of carcinoma of unknown primary and correlation with clinical evaluation. *J Clin Oncol.* 2008;26: 4442–4448.

Surgical Emergencies in Cancer Patients

Brian Badgwell

An oncologic emergency is "an acute condition that is caused by cancer or the treatment of cancer and that requires intervention as soon as possible to avoid mortality or severe permanent morbidity." Cancer patients are at increased risk of emergent conditions due to the effects of their disease and treatments, including malnutrition, immunosuppression, and limited physiologic reserve.

The surgeon's role in oncologic emergencies is to make an assessment on whether a surgical solution is required, and if so, which one. The surgeon must also determine whether the benefits of the surgery outweigh the risks it imparts, including assessing the patient's suitability for surgery and whether the surgery is appropriate in the setting of the patient's overall prognosis. An oncologic emergency presents a complex clinical scenario in which multidisciplinary input and information about the patient's cancer and its treatment must be quickly obtained. Oncologic emergencies require physician-to-physician interaction; phone conversations between the consulting surgeon and low-level ancillary staff members are less than ideal substitutes. The consulting surgeon should not hesitate to contact the physician who is best informed of the patient's treatment history and prognosis, even if that physician is "off-service." At the onset of each consultation, the patient's hemodynamic stability must be assessed; a quick assessment, similar to the Advanced Trauma Life Support evaluation of trauma patients, can be used to evaluate the patient's airway, vital signs, and neurologic status.

For the purposes of this chapter, the spectrum of oncologic emergencies is categorized into surgical and medical emergencies, with an emphasis on surgical emergencies and intra-abdominal surgical emergencies in particular. As almost half of all cancers diagnosed are not amenable to cure, the distinction between oncologic emergencies and palliative care is sometimes difficult to distinguish. Therefore, this chapter also includes recent data about emergent surgical consultations for patients receiving palliative care.

ONCOLOGIC SURGICAL EMERGENCIES

Bowel Obstruction

Bowel obstruction is a frequent cause for general surgical evaluation and cancer patients are no exception. In cancer patients who have undergone intra-abdominal surgery, adhesions or hernias may cause bowel obstruction as may cancer itself. Determining whether the obstruction is due to adhesion formation or malignancy can be difficult. Such patients are treated according to commonly accepted surgical principles.

Generally, the approach to patients who present with bowel obstruction includes obtaining a history to help identify the etiology, location (gastric outlet, small bowel, large bowel, etc.), and degree of obstruction (partial, complete, or closed loop obstruction). The etiology of the obstruction may be mechanical (adhesions, hernias, malignancy, or intrinsic/extrinsic compression) or non-mechanical (pseudo-obstruction). Having information about the patient's treatment history (recent chemotherapy, prior surgeries, etc.) is critical to determining whether surgical intervention offers more benefit that risk. The goal of treatment is to perform surgical intervention before bowel ischemia occurs.

The first step in the physical examination is to assess the patient's hemodynamic status. The patient's abdomen should be examined to assess the severity of the obstruction, the possibility of underlying strangulation, and the presence of hernias. During the evaluation, the physician should determine whether a nasogastric tube, Foley catheter, or aggressive intravenous fluid resuscitation is necessary; laboratory findings may influence these decisions. Physical examination findings of fever, tachycardia, and/or leukocytosis can suggest ischemia or even perforation.

Initial imaging typically is an acute abdominal series (chest, supine abdomen, and upright abdomen plain-film x-rays) to evaluate the patient for intraperitoneal air and to help determine the cause and severity of the obstruction. Computed tomography (CT) can be a useful adjunct in determining the etiology, severity, and site of obstruction. A Gastrografin enema or sigmoidoscopy may be required to evaluate the patient for distal obstruction.

Malignant Bowel Obstruction

Malignant bowel obstruction is "the blockage of the small or large intestine in a patient with advanced cancer." In many patients, imaging studies do not clearly reveal whether the obstruction is due to direct tumor involvement or some other etiology. Up to one-third of bowel obstruction cases in cancer patients may be due to benign causes. Regardless of the cause, indicators of adverse outcome present at the time of initial evaluation upon which to base treatment decisions have not been firmly established. Given the paucity of prospective research and lack of evidence-based treatment algorithms, treatment decisions for patients with malignant bowel obstruction are largely based on retrospective reviews that highlight the considerable morbidity and mortality associated with surgery. According to Ripamonti et al., the rates of operative mortality and morbidity range from 9% to 40% and from 9% to 90%, respectively.

Because malignant bowel obstruction rarely requires immediate operative intervention, there is generally ample time to thoroughly evaluate the patient. CT can be used to help identify factors that are associated with diminished outcome in surgery, such as carcinomatosis and ascites. Although no absolute contraindications to surgery for malignant bowel obstruction have been identified, some factors that have been associated with poor surgical outcomes include previous abdominal surgery that revealed diffuse metastatic cancer; intra-abdominal carcinomatosis and imaging studies suggesting impaired gastrointestinal motility; ascites that rapidly recurs after drainage; extra-abdominal metastases that cause difficult-to-control symptoms; and previous irradiation of the abdomen/pelvis. Advanced age, hypoalbuminemia, and diminished performance status are also considered predictors of adverse surgical outcome. Patients who are not candidates for surgery may benefit from corticosteroids, antiemetics, octreotide, and analgesics.

Gastric Outlet Obstruction

Mortality rates of up to 30% have been reported in patients with malignant gastric outlet obstruction who undergo palliative gastrojejunostomy. Therefore, patients should be selected carefully for palliative gastrojejunostomy and considered for endoscopic stent placement when possible, although this option is heavily dependent on local availability and experience. Limited data from randomized trials, observational studies, and retrospective studies comparing stent placement to gastrojejunostomy revealed that patients in whom stents were placed had a shorter length of hospital stay and shorter time to liquid diet toleration; however, higher rate of recurrent obstructive symptoms were also seen. Some authors have recommended attempting stent placement in patients with a relatively short-life expectancy and pursuing gastrojejunostomy in patients with a relatively long-life expectancy.

Small Bowel Obstruction
The small bowel is the most frequent site of malignant bowel obstruction; small bowel obstruction occurs in two-thirds of patients with malignant bowel obstruction. Both the small and the large bowels are involved in approximately 20% of patients with malignant bowel obstruction. Surgery remains the mainstay of treatment as stents are difficult to place beyond the proximal small bowel. Surgery may involve a bypass procedure or resection. Determining the need for surgery can be difficult; not all partial bowel obstructions in cancer patients are due to direct tumor involvement, and partial obstructions may resolve with nonoperative therapy.

Large Bowel Obstruction
Endoscopic self-expandable metallic stents represent a significant advance in the treatment of malignant large bowel obstruction. A recent systematic review found that mortality rates among patients treated with expandable stents and patients treated with open surgery were similar; in addition, patients treated with expandable stents had a lower rate of serious adverse events and shorter length of hospital stay than patients treated with open surgery. Surgical options for malignant large bowel obstruction include bypass, resection of the obstructed area, or decompression of the obstruction with a diverting colostomy. Factors influencing choice of surgery include location of the obstruction; resectability of the obstructing lesion; the number and type of prior abdominal surgeries; and the baseline health status and overall oncologic prognosis of the patient.

Bowel Perforation
Cancer patients may be at increased risk of bowel perforation caused by direct tumor invasion or the side effects of chemotherapy, radiation, immunosuppression, or steroid administration. Because they are frequently subjected to endoscopic and interventional procedures, cancer patients are also at a risk for iatrogenic bowel perforation. Bowel perforation also may be caused by conditions unrelated to cancer or its treatments, such as diverticulitis, peptic ulcer disease, or appendicitis. Patients with bowel perforation are usually treated with prompt surgical intervention unless they have recently undergone certain treatments or have underlying oncologic issues which can increase the risk for morbidity and mortality with surgical intervention, such as pancytopenia associated with chemotherapy or end-stage disease. As with normal general surgical principles, patients who have diverticulitis with a contained abscess or perforation may be treated using a nonoperative approach.

Because the majority of cancer patients with bowel perforation have advanced or incurable cancer, factors such as the patient's prognosis, symptom burden, treatment history, and desires and the family's desires play equally important parts in managing the patient's bowel perforation. Most patients with bowel perforation are treated with surgery, but comfort, care and, non-operative management are also options in this complex clinical scenario.

Approximately 2% of colorectal cancer patients present with bowel perforation. Bowel perforation in colorectal cancer patients may be a direct result of transmural invasion of the bowel wall or less frequently a result of distal obstruction leading to proximal bowel dilation and perforation. Perforated colorectal cancers have been associated with both increased local and systemic recurrence. Operative mortality rates in cancer patients with bowel perforation approach 20%.

One chemotherapeutic agent that has been associated with bowel perforation is bevacizumab. Bevacizumab, a humanized monoclonal antibody to vascular endothelial cell growth factor, has demonstrated efficacy in combination with chemotherapy in patients with metastatic colorectal cancer and lung cancer. The incidence of bowel perforation in patients receiving bevacizumab is 1% to 2%, although it appears to vary across cancer types. Although infrequent, bevacizumab-associated bowel perforation is associated with 30-day mortality rates ranging from 13% to 50%. Emergency surgery in the setting of recent bevacizumab administration may be complicated by wound-healing difficulties and bleeding. To avoid the postoperative complications associated with bevacizumab use, most surgeons wait 6 weeks after bevacizumab therapy has stopped before proceeding with elective surgery. Stoma placement should be considered in patients with bevacizumab-associated bowel perforation who require surgery.

Cholecystitis

Risk factors for acalculous cholecystitis include immunosuppression, malnourishment, and systemic therapy; whether patients who receive systemic therapy are also at risk for calculous cholecystitis is unclear. Other risk factors for cholecystitis in cancer patients include hepatic embolization and biliary stent placement.

Cancer patients may have intra-abdominal fluid or malignant ascites that complicates the interpretation of pericholecystic fluid or gallbladder wall thickening on ultrasonography or CT. Hepatobiliary scintigraphy may be required to establish the correct diagnosis.

Not all cancer patients can undergo prompt laparoscopic cholecystectomy because of disease- and treatment-related issues such as recent chemotherapy, immunosuppression, neutropenia, malnutrition, comorbid conditions, and disease stage or prognosis. Given these concerns, some cancer patients with cholecystitis are best treated with cholecystostomy tube placement to avoid delaying treatment or performing a surgery that has a risk for conversion to an open procedure that may be inappropriate in the context of the patient's oncologic prognosis. Laparoscopic cholecystectomy and cholecystostomy tube removal have been described with low conversion rates.

Biliary Obstruction

Cancer patients presenting with emergent biliary obstruction and cholangitis are typically treated with endoscopic drainage and antibiotics. The treatment of stable patients with potentially resectable causes of biliary obstruction is described elsewhere in this book. Stable patients with unresectable causes of biliary obstruction may benefit from endoscopic, percutaneous, or surgical bypass procedures. In general, endoscopic or percutaneous methods of palliation are associated with less initial morbidity but shorter durability of palliation while surgical methods of palliation are associated with more initial morbidity but longer durability of palliation. The best approach to unresectable causes of biliary obstruction remains a matter of debate and depends on the capabilities of individual institutions.

Biliary obstruction from metastatic disease in the porta hepatis, which has been associated with a wide variety of cancers, often carries a very poor prognosis and prohibitively high rates of mortality and morbidity from surgery. Endoscopic or percutaneous biliary stent placement best accomplishes drainage and then consideration can be given to radiation therapy with or without chemotherapy.

Abdominal Pain in Neutropenic Patients

Neutropenia is a frequent sequela of chemotherapy. Abdominal pain in neutropenic patients can indicate any of a wide variety of conditions that are associated with significant mortality rates.

Surgeons who assist in diagnosing and managing abdominal pain in neutropenic patients must consider not only the broad spectrum of general surgical conditions that can cause abdominal pain but also conditions that are unique to neutropenic patients. One such condition is neutropenic enterocolitis, which is also referred to as neutropenic enteropathy, agranulocytic colitis, or if the disease is confined to the cecum, typhlitis. In a recent series of 60 patients from M. D. Anderson who presented with concomitant neutropenia and abdominal pain, neutropenic enterocolitis was found as the cause of abdominal pain in 28%, small bowel obstruction in 12%, and the cause remained uncertain in 35%. Less frequent conditions included *Clostridium difficile* colitis, diverticulitis, appendicitis, cholecystitis, colonic pseudo-obstruction, and splenic rupture. Thirty- and 90-day mortality rates for all patients in this series were 30% and 52%, respectively, and likely reflect the significant underlying disease and frequent comorbidities found in this patient population. Surgical intervention was performed in 15% and attempts were made to delay surgery until resolution of neutropenia. The clinical and pathologic criteria for diagnosing neutropenic enterocolitis have not been firmly established. A commonly accepted clinical diagnostic triad is the presence of neutropenia (<1,000 neutrophils/μL), abdominal pain, and bowel wall thickening on imaging. In patients with diarrhea, *C. difficile* colitis must be ruled out before a diagnosis of neutropenic enterocolitis can be made. Surgery is reserved for patients with perforation, sepsis, or a worsening of overall condition felt to be attributable to the enterocolitis.

In cancer patients with neutropenia, perioperative mortality rates have been documented to be as high as 41% to 57%. More recent reports of higher survival rates among neutropenic patients reflect efforts to delay surgery to allow the neutropenia to resolve and improvements in critical care, imaging, antibiotics, colony-stimulating factors, and white blood cell transfusions.

There are no formal recommendations for the medical treatment of neutropenia and abdominal pain, and many clinicians rely on recommendations from the Infectious Diseases Society of America for febrile neutropenia. These guidelines propose either monotherapy with cefepime, ceftazidime, a carbapenem, or piperacillin-tazobactam or duotherapy with an antipseudomonal β-lactam and an aminoglycoside. However, in the M. D. Anderson series noted above, the majority of patients with neutropenia and abdominal pain were treated with vancomycin for suspicion of gram-positive infection in the setting of severe sepsis, and metronidazole was often used because anaerobic species such as *Clostridium* are known to be involved in neutropenic enterocolitis. The use of antifungal agents in neutropenic patients has not been established, but the Infectious Diseases Society of America recommends that antifungal agents be considered in the setting of abdominal pain in patients that remain febrile or shows signs of infection concomitantly with neutropenia for ≥5 days, again based on recommendations for febrile neutropenia.

Gastrointestinal Bleeding

Gastrointestinal bleeding in cancer patients most commonly arises from benign causes such as peptic ulcer disease and gastritis. Primary tumors are rarely the source of brisk, uncontrollable hemorrhage. Gastric lymphoma patients who receive systemic chemotherapy have a high risk for gastrointestinal bleeding with reported rates of up to 11%. Metastatic tumors to the gastrointestinal tract, such as melanoma, can also cause gastrointestinal bleeding but more commonly cause chronic, relatively slow blood loss.

Standard surgical principles guide the management of gastrointestinal bleeding. After stabilization in the intensive care unit, initial diagnostic approaches are based on clinical signs indicating an upper or lower gastrointestinal source (such as coffee ground emesis, bright red blood per rectum, etc). In patients with upper gastrointestinal bleeding due to malignancy, use of endoscopy to control bleeding has good success rates and often allows for elective surgical intervention. Because postoperative mortality rates in patients who undergo surgery for bleeding gastric cancer approaches 10%, initial failed endoscopy should be followed by a second attempt if the patient is hemodynamically stable.

In patients in whom clinical signs indicate lower gastrointestinal bleeding, the initial diagnostic procedure is again endoscopy, which can also enable bleeding control and again convert an emergent surgical procedure into an elective one. In addition to endoscopy, nuclear red blood cell scans and angiography can be used adjunctively to help identify the source of lower gastrointestinal bleeding.

Anorectal Infections

Anorectal infections are rarely a source of major morbidity or mortality in patients who do not have cancer; but in patients who do have cancer, anorectal infections are a significant and potentially lethal condition. In the 1970s, mortality rates among immunosuppressed cancer patients with anorectal infections were reported to be as high as 50%; many of these infections were noted to be ulcerative but not associated with an abscess. The authors of these early reports recommended caution in proceeding with surgical intervention.

More recently, a National Cancer Institute study utilizing a selective surgical approach to anorectal infections in cancer patients revealed that 37% of patients required surgery and no patients died because of their anorectal infections. A recent M. D. Anderson study found that 58 of 100 patients with anorectal infections who underwent surgical oncology consultations were treated with operative intervention. Surgical intervention was most commonly associated with the identification of an abscess and erythema during physical examination. Necrotizing soft tissue infections were identified in only two patients but caused the only infection-related death.

Palliative Aspects of Surgical Oncologic Emergencies

Palliative surgery is defined as any procedure that is performed to reduce a patient's symptoms or improve their quality of life with no intent for cure, secondary to the patient's advanced or incurable malignancy. Surgical options offered in response to an oncologic emergency can differ depending on whether the patient's overall clinical goal is for palliation or cure. Inherently, surgical staff will want to address surgical emergencies with intent to cure; however, this can lead to inadvertent over-treatment in a patient where palliative care may be the more appropriate course. Also to be considered is the fact that if a patient's malignancy is determined to be incurable, they are not automatically disqualified from having surgical therapy, as a surgical procedure may significantly improve their quality of life. Thus it is important to identify the patient's prognosis and their overriding clinical goal at the onset of an emergent consult. A review by Krouse et al. showed that palliative surgical procedures accounted for 13% of all operations at one NCI-designated comprehensive cancer center and up to 21% of all operations performed by surgical oncologists. One recent study at M. D. Anderson attempted to determine the percentage of inpatients undergoing surgical evaluation who met the criteria for a surgical palliative evaluation. Surgical palliative evaluation was defined as a consultation with patients who had symptoms attributable to an advanced or incurable malignancy and/or the complications or toxicity of their treatments. In the study, 40% of all inpatient surgical oncology evaluations were requested for symptom palliation in patients with advanced or incurable malignancies. The most common reason for consultation was gastrointestinal obstruction (43% of patients). Ten percent of patients needed consultation for wound complications and/or infections and 8%

of patients needed consultation for gastrointestinal bleeding. Almost half of the patients had received systemic therapy within 6 weeks of needing a surgical palliative consultation. Palliative surgical procedures were performed in 27% of the patients. The 90-day morbidity and mortality rates were 40% and 7%, respectively; and the median overall survival of all patients who underwent palliative surgical evaluation was only 2.9 months.

MEDICAL EMERGENCIES

Superior Vena Cava Syndrome

- Superior vena cava obstruction can result from invasion, fibrosis, thrombosis, or external compression due to malignancy.
- Lung cancer, lymphoma, breast cancer, and thymic cancer are common malignant causes of superior vena cava syndrome. Lung cancer, the leading malignant cause of superior vena cava syndrome, accounts for 65% to 85% of cases. In the majority of patients, there is sufficient time to obtain a histologic diagnosis to guide therapy.
- Clinical symptoms of superior vena cava syndrome include dyspnea, cough, headache, and facial, neck, and/or chest wall venous engorgement. Cyanosis that worsens when the patient bends forward or is supine may also be present. Symptoms typically develop slowly and progress over a few weeks.
- CT angiography, the initial diagnostic test of choice in patients with suspected superior vena cava syndrome, can differentiate thrombosis from external compression, guide imaging-directed biopsy, and detect other emergent conditions such as spinal cord compression, pericardial metastases, and impending airway obstruction.
- Patients with superior vena cava syndrome may require diuretics, head elevation, steroids, intubation, and/or radiation therapy. In severe cases, vena cava stents can serve as temporizing measures during an ongoing workup.
- Further treatment involves tumor-specific therapy or thrombolysis. Any venous catheters must be removed.

Spinal Cord Compression

- The majority of patients with spinal cord compression present with back pain that may be exacerbated by movement, recumbency, coughing, sneezing, or straining.
- Progressive symptoms of spinal cord compression include weakness, numbness, urinary retention, and constipation.
- Magnetic resonance imaging is the diagnostic imaging study of choice.
- Treatment may involve steroids, radiation therapy, systemic therapy, and/or surgery.

Pericardial Tamponade

- Signs and symptoms of pericardial tamponade include chest pain, dyspnea, tachycardia, distant heart sounds, jugular venous distention, pulsus paradoxus, and ultimately hypotension.
- Electrocardiogram demonstrates low voltage. Echocardiography is the most useful test for diagnosing and evaluating the hemodynamic severity of a pericardial effusion.
- Pericardiocentesis can be performed under echocardiographic monitoring with drainage catheter placement and subsequent sclerosis therapy with tetracycline or thiotepa (an alkylating antiblastic agent).

- Surgical treatment of pericardial tamponade generally consists of subxiphoid pericardiotomy. However, in patients who have already undergone a subxiphoid approach, a transthoracic pleuropericardial window may be a better option.
- Radiation therapy can also be administered, particularly in patients with malignant effusions secondary to lymphoma.

Paraneoplastic Crises

Hypercalcemia

- Common etiologies of paraneoplastic crises include multiple myeloma and breast, lung, and kidney cancer, often in association with bone metastases.
- Elevated parathyroid hormone levels in association with hypophosphatemia indicate ectopic parathyroid hormone secretion.
- Hypercalcemia secondary to malignancy demonstrates elevated or normal serum phosphate levels.
- Electrocardiogram findings that indicate hypercalcemia include prolonged PR interval, shortened QT interval, and widened T waves. Arrhythmias that progress to bradycardia are also indicative of hypercalcemia.
- Symptomatic patients and patients with serum calcium levels >12 mg/dL require prompt treatment.
- The initial treatment for hypercalcemic patients is intravenous hydration followed by diuretics.
- Bisphosphonates can reduce bone resorption from metastatic disease but require 3 to 4 weeks to take effect.
- Plicamycin, an effective inhibitor of bone resorption, can take effect within 6 to 48 hours but has toxicities that can cause thrombocytopenia, hypotension, and hepatic and renal insufficiency.
- The main side effect of gallium nitrate, another effective bone resorption inhibitor, is nephrotoxicity.

Hyponatremia/Syndrome of Inappropriate Antidiuretic Hormone Secretion

- Hyponatremia/syndrome of inappropriate antidiuretic hormone secretion (SIADH) can result in mental status changes, nausea, headaches, seizures, comas, and ultimately death. Although SIADH is commonly associated with small-cell lung cancer, the syndrome may also be present in patients with prostate, adrenal, esophagus, pancreas, colon, and head and neck cancers.
- Pseudo-hyponatremia is due to hyperproteinemia, hyperglycemia, or hyperlipidemia.
- Chemotherapies such as vincristine and cyclophosphamide may be associated with hyponatremia.
- A low blood urea nitrogen level, hypouricemia, and hypophosphatemia are indicative of SIADH. SIADH treatment is tumor- and cause-specific. For example, SIADH symptoms associated with small-cell lung cancer may improve once the patient is treated with the appropriate chemotherapy while SIADH symptoms resulting from brain metastases may improve with the use of corticosteroids and radiation therapy. Treatment otherwise consists of restricting the patient's water intake to 500 to 1000 mL/day over several days to correct serum sodium levels. Further treatment may include demeclocycline, an antidiuretic hormone antagonist.
- Severe hyponatremia can be treated with a 3% hypertonic saline infusion and intravenous furosemide; the rate of correction should be limited to 0.5 to 1.0 mEq/hour to minimize the risk of central nervous system complications, such as osmotic demyelination.

Hypoglycemia
- Symptoms of hypoglycemia include mild manifestations including weakness, dizziness, and confusion and can progress to more severe symptoms such as seizures and coma.
- Hypoglycemia has many causes unrelated to cancer. However, hypoglycemia may be caused by insulinomas, adrenocortical tumors, hepatomas, sarcomas (fibrosarcoma, neurofibrosarcoma, and hemangiopericytoma), and mesotheliomas.
- When possible, hypoglycemia-causing tumors should be resected. Patients with unresectable insulin-secreting tumors may benefit from diazoxide, radiation therapy, diet modification, corticosteroids, glucagon, and/or growth hormone.

Tumor Lysis Syndrome
- Tumor lysis syndrome manifests as hyperuricemia, hyperkalemia, hyperphosphatemia, and hypocalcemia resulting from rapid cell lysis due to cytotoxic therapy. Acute renal failure is caused by the accumulation of uric acid or calcium phosphate in the renal tubules.
- Although tumor lysis syndrome most often occurs in lymphoma and leukemia patients after systemic chemotherapy, the syndrome may also occur in other cancer patients following radiation, hormonal, or ablative therapy.
- Preventive measures include intravenous hydration, urine alkalinization, and allopurinol administration.
- Treatment involves correcting electrolyte abnormalities, particularly hyperkalemia. Hemodialysis may be required.

Central Venous Catheter Sepsis
- Success rates of up to 80% have been reported for treating catheter-based infections with intravenous antibiotic therapy.
- However, catheter removal is the optimal treatment for patients with central venous catheter sepsis and is indicated for patients with persistently positive blood cultures, neutropenia, signs of systemic infection, a history of vascular grafts, or implanted prostheses.

Recommended Readings

Badgwell BD, Camp ER, Feig B, et al. Management of bevacizumab-associated bowel perforation: a case series and review of the literature. *Ann Oncol.* 2008; 19:577–582.

Badgwell BD, Chang GJ, Rodriguez-Bigas MA, et al. Management and outcomes of anorectal infection in the cancer patient. *Ann Surg Oncol.* 2009;16:2752–2758.

Badgwell BD, Cormier JN, Wray CJ, et al. Challenges in surgical management of abdominal pain in the neutropenic cancer patient. *Ann Surg.* 2008;248:104–109.

Badgwell BD, Smith K, Liu P, et al. Indicators of surgery and survival in oncology inpatients requiring surgical evaluation for palliation. *Support Care Cancer.* 2009;17:727–734.

Badgwell B, Feig BW, Ross MI, et al. Pneumoperitoneum in the cancer patient. *Ann Surg Oncol.* 2007;14:3141–3147.

Glenn J, Funkhouser WK, Schneider PS. Acute illnesses necessitating urgent abdominal surgery in neutropenic cancer patients: description of 14 cases and review of the literature. *Surgery.* 1989;105:778–789.

Helton W, Fisichella P. Intestinal Obstruction. In: *ACS Surgery: Principles and Practice.* New York: WebMD Professional Publishing; 2007:514–533.

Krouse RS. The international conference on malignant bowel obstruction: a meeting of the minds to advance palliative care research. *J Pain Symptom Manage.* 2007; 34:S1–S6.

Krouse RS, Nelson RA, Farrell BR, et al. Surgical palliation at a cancer center: incidence and outcomes. *Arch Surg.* 2001;136:773–778.

Lehrnbecher T, Marshall D, Gao C, et al. A second look at anorectal infections in cancer patients in a large cancer institute: the success of early intervention with antibiotics and surgery. *Infection.* 2002;30:272–276.

McCahill LE, Krouse R, Chu D, et al. Indications and use of palliative surgery-results of Society of Surgical Oncology survey. *Ann Surg Oncol.* 2002; 9:104–112.

Miner TJ. Palliative surgery for advanced cancer: lessons learned in patient selection and outcome assessment. *Am J Clin Oncol.* 2005; 28:411–414.

Miner TJ, Brennan MF, Jaques DP. A prospective, symptom related, outcomes analysis of 1022 palliative procedures for advanced cancer. *Ann Surg.* 2004; 240:719–726.

Musa MB, Katakkar SB, Khaliq A. Anorectal and perianal complications of hematologic malignant neoplasms. *Can J Surg.* 1975;18:579–583.

Osteen RT, Guyton S, Steele G, Jr, et al. Malignant intestinal obstruction. *Surgery.* 1980;87:611–615.

Ripamonti C, Twycross R, Baines M, et al. Clinical-practice recommendations for the management of bowel obstruction in patients with end-stage cancer. *Support Care Cancer.* 2001;9:223–233.

Rolston KV. The Infectious Diseases Society of America 2002 guidelines for the use of antimicrobial agents in patients with cancer and neutropenia: salient features and comments. *Clin Infect Dis.* 2004;39 Suppl 1:S44–S48.

Schimpff SC, Wiernik PH, Block JB. Rectal abscesses in cancer patients. *Lancet.* 1972; 2:844–847.

Starnes HF Jr, Moore FD Jr, Mentzer S, et al. Abdominal pain in neutropenic cancer patients. *Cancer.* 1986;57:616–621.

Wade DS, Douglass H Jr, Nava HR, et al. Abdominal pain in neutropenic patients. *Arch Surg.* 1990;125:1119–1127.

Watt AM, Faragher IG, Griffin TT, et al. Self-expanding metallic stents for relieving malignant colorectal obstruction: a systematic review. *Ann Surg.* 2007; 246: 24–30.

Wayne J, Bold R. Oncologic Emergencies. In: *The M. D. Anderson Surgical Oncology Handbook.* Philadelphia: Lippincott Williams & Wilkins; 2006:564–582.

Yeung SC, Escalante C. *Oncologic Emergencies.* In: *Cancer Medicine.* Hamilton: BC Decker Inc; 2006:2246–2265.

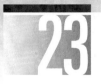

Principles of Radiation Oncology

Christopher Crane

Radiation oncology is the practice of using focused high-energy electromagnetic radiation to treat oncologic diseases. It can be delivered in a variety of different forms. Each type of radiation has different physical characteristics that offer unique advantages in individual patients, and the total radiation dose and its fractionation vary dependent on the clinical goals of each patient's overall treatment plan. Radiation therapy can be given concurrently with chemotherapy, as adjuvant or primary therapy, with resultant superior outcomes in the treatment of a wide range of malignancies. At M. D. Anderson Cancer Center, preoperative chemoradiation is preferred over postoperative, as it is offers less toxicity and improved tumor control.

BASIC RADIOBIOLOGY AND PRINCIPLES OF FRACTIONATION

Radiation kills tumor cells by irreversibly damaging their DNA; in general, the higher the total radiation dose is, the greater the likelihood the cells will be killed. Tissues and organs have known dose and volume tolerances to late radiation injury that must be respected to avoid permanent late toxicity. The total radiation dose and the technique used to deliver it are typically chosen in an effort to limit a patient's risk of developing late complications from radiation treatment. Some organs such as the liver, lungs, and kidneys can tolerate large tissue-ablative doses to small tissue volumes without disruption of function. This is because destruction of a small part of the organ does not affect its overall function. Known volumes of these organs can safely receive lower doses of radiation without impairing their function. Other organs, such as the spinal cord and gastrointestinal tract, cannot tolerate tissue-ablative doses delivered to one part of the organ without affecting its overall function. In these structures, the maximum radiation dose is the dose that will cause late injury to any part of the organ.

Four radiobiologic cellular processes—repair, repopulation, reoxygenation, and to a lesser extent, redistribution—dictate the optimization of fractionation.

Repair

All cells have the ability to repair some of the DNA damage caused by radiation. However, normal cells are able to repair sublethal DNA damage much more effectively than tumor cells; thus, delivering radiation in small daily fractions (1.8 to 2.0 Gy/day) can kill tumor cells without permanently harming normal cells. In general, smaller fractions of radiation enable a higher total radiation dose to be delivered. However, the normal cells' ability to repair DNA damage more effectively than tumor cells is generally lost with increasing doses per fraction, because the mounting double-strand DNA damage from higher doses overwhelms the cells' ability to repair it. Consequentially, lower total doses to the tumor can be safely delivered when large doses per fractions are used. Delivery of fraction doses as high as 25 Gy to small volumes may be clinically tolerable if no critical structures are near the target. For example, using stereotactic radiation therapy to deliver high doses per fraction to lung and liver tumors is tolerable because ablating the tissue surrounding such tumors does not affect organ function.

Repopulation

Repopulation refers to the ability of tumor cells to repopulate during a course of radiation treatment, if the time to deliver the full course of radiation is too long. The benefits of complete tumor eradication must be weighed against the acute toxicities of radiation if given too close together. Shortening the time period between radiation doses may increase the probability of killing all tumor clonogens. However, the amount to which these periods can be shortened in a course of standard fractionation radiotherapy is limited by acute toxicities to the tissues.

Redistribution

Redistribution refers to the distribution of tumor cells in different stages of the cell cycle. In each phase of the cell cycle, a cell has a different sensitivity to radiation. Redistribution is not routinely exploited in general radiation oncology practice.

Reoxygenation

Reoxygenation is the process in which hypoxic, radioresistant tumor cells become increasingly radiosensitive as they are exposed to oxygen with subsequent radiation fractions. Oxygen stabilizes radiation-produced free radicals, which lead to ionization, DNA strand breaks, and ultimately cell death in tumors. When a tumor reaches a diameter of 3 to 5 mm, it outgrows its blood supply and develops hypoxic areas that are radioresistant. When the tumor is irradiated, oxygenated (and thus radiosensitive) cells on the periphery of the tumor die, causing the tumor to shrink and allowing oxygen to diffuse to hypoxic areas, reducing treatment resistance.

Fractionation

Radiation oncologists fractionate total radiation doses to preserve normal cells and kill tumor cells. Fractionation is the process of dividing the total radiation dose into smaller, equal doses that are delivered over time. Fractionation exploits the inherent biological differences between normal cells and tumor cells. It allows normal cells time to recover between fractions, unlike tumor cells, which are less efficient in cellular damage repair. It also allows tumor cells in a relatively radioresistant phase of the cell cycle during one treatment to enter into a more sensitive phase of the cell cycle for the subsequent fraction.

Typically, radiation dose fractions are delivered daily over the course of 2 to 7 weeks. Standard radiation dose fractions range from 1.8 to 2 Gy. Hypofractionation refers to the delivery of larger doses per fraction of radiation (>2 Gy) over a shorter overall time. Hypofractionated regimens are typically given in the palliative care setting.

Accelerated fractionation refers to the delivery of standard fraction sizes given in a shorter overall time, often twice daily. Hyperfractionation refers to the delivery of a higher total radiation dose via smaller-than-standard doses per fraction. The goal of giving hyperfractionated treatment is to further exploit the difference in normal cells' and tumor cells' ability to repair sublethal DNA damage. For example, delivering 1.2 Gy twice daily may enable a 10% higher total dose to be delivered because the normal tissue can better tolerate the smaller dose fractions. Radiation fractions can be given twice daily without damaging normal tissues because the time required for these tissues to repair sublethal DNA damage is felt to be between 4 and 6 hours.

BASIC RADIATION PHYSICS

Radiation can be delivered externally via low- or high-energy beams or internally via implanted radiation sources. The method of radiation delivery depends on the type and location of the tumor, as well as the patient's overall health. Radiation is most commonly delivered with high-energy electromagnetic radiation (x-rays or photons) that penetrates tissues to varying degrees depending on the energy of the beams. Generally, beams with energies between 6 and 18 MV are used. The decision to use one type of beam versus another depends on the distance of the lesion from the skin's surface. In general, lesions closer to the surface of the skin are treated with lower-energy protons.

External Beam Radiation

External beam radiation can be delivered in the form of photons, electrons, or protons. Photon beams (x-rays or gamma rays) penetrate the body, irradiating both the tumor and the normal tissue. Electrons are subatomic negatively charged particles that only partially penetrate the body, depositing their energy at a depth that is dependent on the initial energy of the beam. Electron beams can be used to treat tumors within 6 cm of the surface of the skin. Protons are large subatomic particles that have a positive charge. The advantage of protons over electrons is that they deposit their energy at greater depths, enabling the treatment of tumors that are located farther away from the surface of the skin. The advantage of protons over photons is that there is no exit dose through the body, resulting in sparing of normal tissue.

Brachytherapy

Patients may also be treated with brachytherapy, the practice of directly delivering radiation by placing radioactive sources near the tumor or tumor bed. Brachytherapy offers advantages over external beam radiation because it can be used to deliver very high doses of radiation directly to the tumor while sparing surrounding normal tissues. In general, the level of radiation diminishes with the square of the distance from the radioactive source.

Factors that are considered when choosing a radioactive source for brachytherapy include the source's amount of radioactivity per gram ("specific activity"), its half-life of radioactive decay, and the energy of the photons or electrons it emits. Examples of tumors that are commonly treated with brachytherapy with curative intent include temporary cesium placement for cervical cancer, temporary iridium-192 placement for a variety of tumors, permanent iodine-125 seed implantation for prostate cancer, and permanent gold-198 seed implantation for a variety of malignancies.

RADIATION DOSIMETRY

In modern radiation oncology practice, radiographic imaging is used to plan treatment to target tumors while physically avoiding normal tissues to the greatest extent possible. Radiation treatment planning or "dosimetry" involves the creation of an optimized virtual treatment plan. Three-dimensional computed tomography (CT) images are used to design radiation fields and dose calculations, and blocking is used to block normal tissue structures (Fig. 23.1). A dose–volume histogram (Fig. 23.2) graphically represents the treated volumes of the tumor and regional target that receive various doses (Fig. 23.1).

Conventional radiotherapy delivers radiation in rectangular-shaped fields with additional blocks and wedges. Advanced radiation delivery techniques such as intensity-modulated radiation therapy (IMRT; Fig. 23.3) and stereotactic body radiation therapy deliver a radiation dose that conforms more precisely to the tumor than does a radiation dose delivered with conventional means. Both IMRT and stereotactic body radiation therapy involve inverse planning. The radiation oncologist contours the tumor target and any regional nodal targets as well as the

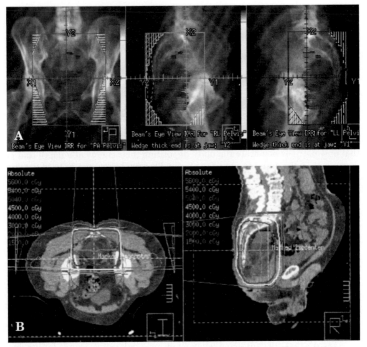

FIGURE 23.1 Three-dimensional plan for treatment fields (**A**) and dosimetry (**B**) for a patient receiving neoadjuvant chemoradiation. The lines surrounding the treatment volume in (**B**) represent the dose levels delivered to the planned volume and surrounding tissues.

organs at risk for radiation damage on a CT scan. Then, the computer optimizes the dose distribution in the context of the normal-tissue dose constraints that the radiation oncologist has specified. In IMRT, the radiation beam is divided into hundreds of tiny beams that turn on and off, resulting in highly customized dose distributions. This form of radiation planning and delivery is particularly useful for fractionated radiation therapy where high doses of radiation can be delivered while protecting critical structures.

IMAGE-GUIDED RADIATION THERAPY

In image-guided radiation therapy, imaging studies are used to verify that the radiation delivered during treatment is in accordance with the radiation delivery planned using the patient's initial CT scans. It ensures a more accurate setup in the delivery of the treatment to make sure that the tumor is not missed. Reasons for using image-guided radiation therapy include day-to-day set-up uncertainty, accurately positioning the patient over the course of treatment, adjusting treatment for organ motion during treatment, such as that due to gastric emptying or filling, and accounting for tumor shrinkage out of the planned field of radiation, which may occur with radiosensitive tumors such as lymphoma and anal cancer. Daily x-ray and/or cone beam CT studies, a limited CT scan obtained on

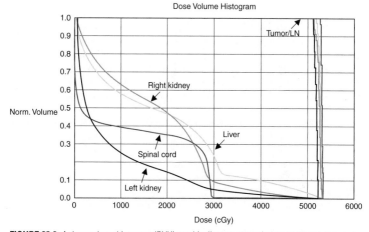

FIGURE 23.2 A dose volume histogram (DVH) graphically represents the treatment volumes and the various radiation doses received. Dose volume histograms enable radiation oncologists to objectively assess the safety of a radiation treatment plan and the adequacy of organ coverage.

the treatment machine immediately before treatment, are commonly used to guide radiation therapy.

CHEMORADIATION

Postoperative adjuvant chemoradiation was first used in the 1980s to treat rectal cancer patients. It has served as a model for other gastrointestinal sites. In virtually every tumor site where combined modality approaches are standard (e.g., head and neck cancer, breast cancer, sarcoma, rectal cancer), chemoradiation contributes to locoregional disease control of 90% or greater by eradicating microscopic residual disease in the tumor bed after complete tumor resection or reducing disease recurrence in regional lymph nodes. For most tumor sites, the patients who stand to benefit the most are those with T3 or T4 tumors, lymph node involvement, or microscopically close or positive surgical margins.

Preoperative chemoradiation has been shown to be more effective and less toxic than postoperative chemoradiation for many patients, likely because the chemotherapy is delivered with an intact blood supply and hypoxia-related chemoradiation resistance is avoided. The most oxygenated cells are at the periphery of the tumor. When treated in a preoperative setting, chemoradiation achieves tumor response rates of 80%. The resultant smaller tumors allow for increased resectability and a greater likelihood of attaining microscopically negative tumor margins (R0 resection). In contrast, with postoperative chemoradiation, these same peripheral tumor cells after surgery are in a hypoxic, radioresistant tumor bed and thus less responsive to the adjuvant treatment.

In the specific setting of gastrointestinal radiation, reduced acute toxicity with preoperative chemoradiation is related to a greater ability to avoid gastrointestinal mucosal irradiation. After gastrointestinal surgery, either small bowel is fixed in the tumor bed and/or the gastrointestinal tract anastomosis will have to be irradiated, which increases the risk of mucosal or anastomotic injury.

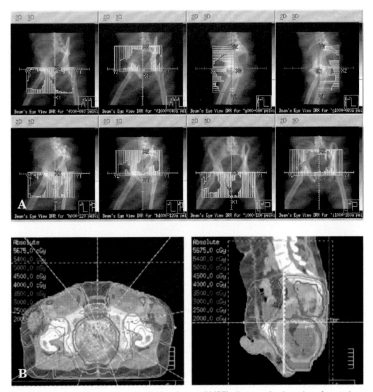

FIGURE 23.3 Intensity-modulated radiation therapy (IMRT) allows optimal sparing of normal tissues and the possibility of improved local tumor control with the use of higher radiation doses. IMRT for anal cancer is one of the best examples of the use of IMRT. IMRT spares the genitalia and thereby reduces toxicity and improves sexual function long term. Treatment fields (**A**) and dosimetry (**B**) for a typical IMRT plan are shown.

In contrast, with preoperative chemoradiation, the irradiated gastrointestinal tract with the targeted tumor is removed during surgery, and healthy bowel is used in the reconstruction, considerably lowering the possibility of late radiation injury to these structures. The assertion that preoperative chemoradiation offered advantages over postoperative chemoradiation was controversial until the question was successfully tested in a randomized phase III trial in rectal cancer patients. Patients who received preoperative chemoradiation had improved sphincter preservation, better local tumor control, and lower acute and late toxicity rates (such as anastomotic strictures and chronic diarrhea) than patients who received postoperative chemoradiation. In patients with pancreatic cancer, a single institution, prospective randomized trial showed that patients who received preoperative chemoradiation prior to undergoing pancreaticoduodenectomy for resection of malignancy had a decreased incidence of pancreatic anastomotic leaks presumably due to preoperative therapy-induced pancreatic fibrosis.

Preoperative chemoradiation also offers unique advantages in patients with poor performance status, high operative risk, or high distant metastasis risk. Most compelling is that preoperative chemoradiation offers the ability to treat virtually all patients who present with localized, resectable cancer with therapy that immediately addresses the limitations of curability—namely, micrometastatic disease. In contrast, delayed recovery from surgery can prevent the timely initiation of postoperative chemoradiation (optimally within 6 to 8 weeks after surgery), thus limiting its efficacy and enabling residual microscopic clonogens to repopulate to gross residual disease. An additional benefit of preoperative chemoradiation is that it facilitates patient selection for complex surgeries that have a significant risk of morbidity or mortality, identifying patients who would not do well with surgery.

RADIATION SIDE EFFECTS

In normal tissues, radiation reactions are classified as either acute reactions or late reactions. Acute radiation reactions are due to the temporary depletion of rapidly dividing cells. Common acute radiation reactions include skin desquamation, nausea, diarrhea, and reduced blood cell counts. After an acute radiation reaction, progenitor cells repopulate the tissue, and the effects of the acute reaction resolve. In contrast, late radiation reactions, which can include severe fibrosis, transverse myelitis of the spinal cord, blindness, and pulmonary fibrosis, are caused by microvasculature damage or the depletion of terminally differentiated cells.

RADIATION SAFETY

Time, distance, and shielding should be considered to protect healthcare personnel and patients from radioactive sources.

1. Healthcare personnel should minimize the amount of time they spend in close proximity to radiation sources. The highest levels of radiation exposure occur during procedures that require the use of fluoroscopy.
2. Since radioactivity falls off with the square of the distance, maximizing one's distance from the source diminishes his or her exposure to radiation. Radioactive sources should never be touched directly.
3. Shielding is an important aspect of radiation protection. All linear accelerators, CT scanners, and x-ray tubes are shielded in lead- and/or concrete-encased rooms; exposure to most hospital personnel is minimal. However, shielding is much more of a challenge for personnel who work more directly with radioactive sources. In general, lead aprons are effective protection against low-energy radiation sources such as diagnostic x-rays and fluoroscopy.

SUMMARY

Chemoradiation has been shown to improve locoregional control and survival in a variety of cancer patients. The use of preoperative chemoradiation is based on biologic factors such as tumor oxygenation and on clinical factors such as the avoidance of normal tissue irradiation and selection of the best candidates for curative surgery. The choice of radiation modality and treatment planning technique is based on the goal of achieving the optimal dose distribution. Typically, complex treatment plans are needed when the tumor is located near critical structures such as the spinal cord and bowel.

Recommended Readings

Crane CH, Varadhachary G, Wolff RA, et al. The argument for pre-operative chemoradiation for localized, radiographically resectable pancreatic cancer. *Best Pract Res Clin Gastroenterol.* 2006;20:365–382.

Krook JE, Moertel CG, Gunderson LL, et al. Effective surgical adjuvant therapy for high-risk rectal carcinoma. *New Engl J Med.* 1991;324:709–715.

Lowy AM, Lee JE, Pisters PW, et al. Prospective, randomized trial of octreotide to prevent pancreatic fistula after pancreaticoduodenectomy for malignant disease. *Ann Surg.* 1997;226:632–641.

NIH consensus conference. Adjuvant therapy for patients with colon and rectal cancer. *JAMA.* 1990;264:1444–1450.

Prolongation of the disease-free interval in surgically treated rectal carcinoma. Gastrointestinal Tumor Study Group. *N Engl J Med.* 1985;312:1465–1472.

Sauer R, Becker H, Hohenberger W, et al. Preoperative versus postoperative chemoradiotherapy for rectal cancer. *New Engl J Med.* 2004;351:1731–1740.

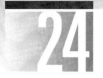

Reconstructive Surgery in Cancer Patients

**Justin M. Sacks, Matthew M. Hanasono,
Donald P. Baumann, Mark T. Villa,
Melissa A. Crosby, and Geoffrey L. Robb**

The goal of reconstructive surgery in cancer patients who have undergone extirpative surgery is to restore form and function. This goal is best accomplished by replacing the resected tissue—adipose, bone, nerve, skin, etc.—with similar tissue. Reconstructive options range from conservative measures such as primary closure and the use of local flaps and skin grafts to more complex methods of reconstruction, such as the use of pedicled flaps or microvascular free tissue transfer. This becomes necessary for the repair of complex defects (e.g., defects in regions that have been previously irradiated, regions in which surgery was previously performed, or regions that have a paucity of local structures).

GENERAL PRINCIPLES OF RECONSTRUCTIVE SURGERY

Reconstruction of oncologic defects is performed by primary closure, skin graft, local flaps, or microvascular free-tissue transfer. Selecting the appropriate reconstructive techniques is critical. The physiologic status of the patient must be considered and balanced with the overall reconstructive plan. For example, a patient with multiple comorbidities may not be able to tolerate a lengthy procedure involving protracted general anesthesia or multiple surgeries and should instead be treated with a more conservative type of reconstruction.

It is important that timing of reconstruction for surgical oncology defects is coordinated with tumor extirpation so as not to interfere with the ultimate goal of obtaining negative surgical margins. For example, reconstruction performed before final pathologic margin status is known to result in a negative oncologic outcome. Skin grafts, local flaps, or free flaps reconstruction can also interfere with lymphatic mapping and thus should be performed only after lymphatic mapping has been done. If the complete removal of a lesion results in a defect so large that it must be repaired immediately, the reconstructive surgeon should confer with the surgical oncologist preoperatively to coordinate the reconstructive process and determine which donor sites will be available to complete the reconstruction. The overall prognosis of the patient must also be taken into account when considering reconstruction for surgical defects. Reconstruction to improve a patient's quality of life is often considered even in a palliative scenario.

The timing of reconstruction is most often dictated by the status of the tumor and surgical margins. Immediate reconstruction refers to performing the final reconstruction at the time of the initial surgery, when the tumor is extirpated. Delayed reconstruction describes the practice of delaying final reconstruction until a later date, either for medical reasons or patient preference. For example, defects from surgery for most basal cell carcinomas can be repaired immediately if frozen tissue sections show negative margins, whereas reconstruction for defects from surgery for melanoma must be delayed until the tumor margin status is definitively determined, as margins cannot be established immediately because specific immunologic stains of the tissue samples must be performed. Certain mitigating factors such as advanced age, multiple comorbidities, or the need for locoregional control with adjuvant radiotherapy must also be considered in the timing and may warrant immediate reconstruction even without the knowledge of margin status.

Immediate and reliable vascularized tissue coverage is the primary goal of reconstruction following the excision of a neoplasm. When immediate reconstruction is performed, immediately after a tumor has been extirpated, tissue planes are readily accessible, and the wound bed has little or no fibrotic tissue. When the reconstruction is delayed, scar tissue, fibrosis, and wound contracture can inhibit optimal aesthetic and functional outcomes. If immediate reconstruction is not possible, the wound bed must be prepared for eventual reconstruction, with appropriate dressings, and debridement either before or at the time of the delayed reconstruction. Delayed wound reconstruction, while not optimal, is occasionally unavoidable, typically for defects with large soft-tissue deficits.

Surgical wounds are assessed based on their physical dimensions and components, their location, and patient's functional requirements. For example, the wound may be adjacent to critical structures. The reconstruction may need to account for loss of skin, subcutaneous tissue, fascia, muscle, nerves, bone, and/or mucosa. Aesthetic as well as functional parameters must also be considered. In addition, previous incisions must be taken into consideration because they may interfere with the planned reconstruction. The deleterious effects of radiation therapy, specifically as they relate to wound healing, must be considered. Specifically, radiation therapy can reduce vascularity in the wound bed, thus precluding the use of local tissue transfers. In such cases, the free tissue transfer of composite soft-tissue constructs can potentiate wound healing. Clinical and radiographic examinations of the structural components involved are required to plan a successful reconstruction.

RECONSTRUCTIVE TECHNIQUES

The core principle of the reconstructive algorithm is to progress from simple to more complex reconstructions on the basis of the specific wound requirements. The primary goal is to close a wound primarily with local tissue that will be tension-free and obliterate any dead-space. When primary closure is not feasible, skin grafts or local flaps of tissue can be used.

Skin grafts contain epidermis and variable amounts of dermis. A partial-thickness skin graft includes only one component of the dermis, whereas a full-thickness graft includes the entire dermis. Skin grafts require a vascularized bed for ingrowth, such as granulated tissue, fascia, muscle, or periosteum. Because full-thickness skin grafts contract less than split-thickness skin grafts, full-thickness grafts are preferable in regions where wound bed contraction is not desirable, such as the face, where wound bed contraction near ocular and nasal structures would compromise aesthetic and/or functional outcome. Aesthetic outcomes are inferior to those of local or free-tissue flap options in many instances.

Local flaps enable surgeons to reconstruct soft-tissue defects with similar tissue from an adjacent location. "Random" local flaps comprise adjacent skin and subcutaneous tissue and are based on a subdermal plexus vascular supply. By definition, random flaps do not have a distinct, named blood supply. In contrast, axial flaps (e.g., pectoralis major or rectus abdominis muscle flaps) are based on named blood vessels. An axial pattern flap and its named blood supply are elevated with an arterial and venous pedicle; these flaps are thus known as pedicled flaps. Axial flaps can be fasciocutaneous (deep muscle fascia with overlying skin), myocutaneous (deep muscle with skin), or osteocutaneous (bone with overlying skin), which enables reconstructive surgeons to repair defects with tissue that is similar to the resected tissue. These flaps have their own intrinsic blood supply and obliterate dead space, contour the wound, and cover neurovascular structures and bone.

Microvascular free tissue transfer involves harvesting a tissue construct and its named blood supply from a distant region of the body and placing it into a defect. Vascular anastomoses between the flap's major (donor) vessels and recipient vessels near the defect are performed under magnification provided by a surgical microscope or loupe. The decision to use a particular flap is based on the requirements for replacing missing skin, adipose tissue, fascia, muscle, and/or bone. The primary advantage of microvascular free tissue transfer is that tissue of a quality similar to that of the resected tissue can be moved from a remote part of the body, enabling optimal aesthetic and functional outcomes. Drawbacks of free tissue transfer are related to donor site morbidity and the potential for long operative times. However, when performed with appropriate technique and efficiency, free flaps are often the optimal choice for reconstruction for both form and function.

Tissue expansion is a process in which an inflatable prosthetic implant with a silicone shell is used to expand local and regional tissues so that they can eventually be advanced into the wound defect in a delayed fashion. The inflatable implant is inserted at the time of tumor extirpation or during a second procedure. At subsequent office visits, saline is injected through an integrated or remote port to gradually expand the implant. Once the tissue has been sufficiently expanded, it can be advanced into the defect. Because tissue expansion takes time, the method is not feasible for immediate reconstruction. Risks of tissue expansion include implant exposure, infection, and pain related to serial expansions.

HEAD AND NECK RECONSTRUCTION

The goals of reconstruction in the head and neck are to preserve function; resurface vital structures such as bone, mucosa, sinuses, nerves, and vessels; and maximize aesthetic outcomes. This can be accomplished with primary closure, skin grafts, local tissue, or free microvascular transfer. Each region of the head and neck has unique anatomical structures and functional dynamics that require special consideration for reconstruction.

SCALP

The scalp is a well-vascularized region composed of five layers: skin, subcutaneous tissue, the galea aponeurosis (a dense fibrous connective tissue layer interspersed between the frontalis, occipitalis, and temporalis muscles that fuses with the temporoparietal fascia at the temporal crest), loose areolar tissue, and the pericranium.

Defects of the scalp must be accurately assessed prior to reconstruction. This involves determining whether the defect is a full-thickness or partial-thickness defect and its size. Partial-thickness defects can be allowed to granulate and heal secondarily, or they can be covered with split-thickness skin grafts if an adequately vascularized wound bed, such as pericranium, can be accessed.

For full-thickness scalp defects <2 cm wide, primary closure can generally be accomplished with wide undermining below the galea. The resulting flaps can be lengthened further by scoring the galea, which enables several centimeters of scalp advancement. Scoring of the galea must be meticulously performed so as not to transect the subcutaneous blood vessels and compromise the flap. If primary closure cannot be accomplished, local rotation flaps are optimal for small defects ≤3 cm wide. Defects >3 cm but <5 cm can generally be reconstructed with rotation flaps and then skin grafting of the donor site on the pericranium. Larger defects may require multiple local flaps based on named blood vessels in the scalp, with further skin grafting of the donor sites.

Occasionally, skin cancers of the scalp can invade the underlying bone, necessitating removal of the outer-table or full-thickness calvarium, depending on the depth of tumor involvement. The repair of such defects requires autologous bone grafts such as split-calvarial grafts or prosthetic materials such as titanium mesh or methyl methacrylate in addition to free flaps. Surgical defects in irradiated regions of the scalp usually cannot be repaired with local flaps or tissue expansion. Instead, such defects are typically repaired with a free muscle flap (e.g., a latissimus dorsi or serratus anterior muscle-free flap) and skin grafts placed over the muscle.

FACE

Facial reconstruction can be divided into specific regions, each with its own anatomy and function: the forehead, periorbital region, cheek, nose, lips, and neck. Each region must be considered independently and collectively when defects cross facial zone boundaries.

Facial Skin

Facial skin defects secondary to skin cancer excisions tend to be several centimeters wide and can involve regions in which obtaining good aesthetic and functional results can be challenging. For instance, lesions in the lower eyelid need to be reconstructed appropriately so as not to cause ectropion of the lower eyelid.

Small superficial defects of the facial skin can often be closed primarily after an elliptical incision. Such an incision must be short and made in the direction of the facial skin-tension lines. If the wound cannot be closed primarily, the next option would be a local tissue flap based on a random blood supply, such as a transposition or rhomboid flap. Full-thickness skin grafts can be used instead if they match the thickness and color of the skin at the wound site. The best skin graft donor site for facial reconstruction is the region above the clavicle, as both the color and the texture of the skin there match that of the facial skin. Defects in the face >5 cm often require large fasciocutaneous rotation flaps from the cervical and deltopectoral region. In rare instances in which it is known that the patient will receive adjuvant radiation therapy or in which critical neurovascular structures are exposed and cannot be covered with local tissue, reconstruction with free tissue transfer may be necessary.

Forehead

The tissue layers of the forehead are similar to those of the scalp and include skin, subcutaneous tissue, frontalis muscle, loose areolar tissue, and pericranium. The superficial temporal, supraorbital, and supratrochlear vessels provide the blood supply to the forehead. Reconstruction options for forehead defects are limited owing to the inelasticity of the underlying soft tissues. Small defects in the forehead ≤2 cm wide can usually be corrected with primary closure. In patients with skin laxity in the forehead, wide surgical undermining of the skin surrounding the defect facilitates primary closure. Full-thickness skin grafts often can be placed onto vascularized muscle or pericranium to cover the exposed underlying structures.

Repairing forehead defects >2 cm generally requires the use of local flaps. Aesthetic considerations in the forehead region are the hairline and brow line, and these anatomical boundaries must be taken into account when performing local flap advancement. Local flaps must be designed within natural skin tension lines, with incisions being made in natural wrinkles or the hairline.

Defects larger than one-third the size of the forehead may require repair with thin, pliable fasciocutaneous free flaps such as a radial forearm or anterolateral thigh free flap. The relatively long vascular pedicle of the radial forearm flap allows versatility in insetting the flap, even in central forehead defects. Recipient blood vessels in this region in order of preference are the superficial temporal vessels, facial vessels, and great vessels in the neck. Vein grafting may be necessary if the facial vessels or great neck vessels are used.

Nose

The nose consists of nine aesthetic subunits: the dorsum, two sidewalls, the tip, the columella, two soft-triangles, and two alae. The adage to replace "like with like" is critical in this anatomical region. Nose defects involving <50% of an aesthetic subunit can be reconstructed with a local flap or full-thickness skin graft and the remaining subunit can be retained. However, the entire subunit should be reconstructed if the defect involves ≥50% of a subunit. Full-thickness defects of the nose comprise the external skin, cartilage, and nasal lining, and all three layers must be considered in repair. The nasal lining often can be reconstructed with local flaps obtained from the nasal mucosa. Cartilaginous structures can be reconstructed using cartilage grafts from the rib or ear. The nasolabial flap, which is based on the angular artery inferiorly or the dorsal branch of the ophthalmic artery superiorly, can be used to reconstruct defects in the lower nasal elements. Local flaps such as bilobed flaps can be used to reconstruct defects of the nasal sidewall and dorsum. The paramedian forehead flap, based on the supratrochlear artery, can be used to resurface the entire exterior nasal skin.

Lip

The skin of the lip is composed of dry and wet vermillion. The vermilion–cutaneous junction, the border between the red of the lip and surrounding skin, is a distinct anatomical line that must be meticulously reconstructed. Asymmetries at the vermillion–cutaneous junction of <1 mm will lead to visible irregularities in a reconstructed lip.

Defects less than one-third the width of the lower or upper lip are generally repaired with wedge resection and primary closure. For larger defects, a local flap, called a lip switch flap, must be considered. Lip switch flaps are pedicled flaps transferred from the lower or upper lip that are based on the labial branch of the facial artery. Lip switch flaps such as the Abbe or Estlander flap are used to repair defects that are between one and two thirds the width of the lip.

Defects larger than two thirds the width of the lip require bilateral rotation or advancement flaps, which recruit larger segments of tissue from adjacent cheek tissue. One such flap is the Karapandzic advancement flap, a neurovascular flap that preserves the elements of the facial nerve branches to the orbicularis oris. However, the use of advancement flaps can reduce the oral aperture, resulting in microstomia. Total lip defects can be reconstructed with a free radial forearm flap with a palmaris longus tendon graft to support the reconstructed lip and maintain lip height.

Ear

The outer ear is composed of skin closely adherent to an underlying cartilaginous framework. The surface anatomy of the ear consists of the helix, anti-helix, concha, tragus, and lobule. These structures must be preserved or reconstructed to maintain the inherent anatomy and contour of the ear.

Small defects in the skin of the helical rim can be repaired with excision of a triangular wedge and direct approximation. If the defect is small but direct approximation cannot be performed, the remaining helix can be reconstructed with local chondrocutaneous flaps; in this instance, the remaining helical rim is dissected off the scapha and advanced. Large defects of the helical rim can be covered with a postauricular or tubed flap. This is a staged procedure in which division and inset are performed 2 to 3 weeks after the initial transposition of the flap.

Small cartilage defects in the helical rim can be repaired using cartilage grafts taken from the contralateral ear. Large helical defects with missing cartilaginous components can be reconstructed using cartilage grafts from the ribs. These grafts can be sculpted to conform to the missing helical rim and covered with a pedicled temporoparietal fascia flap based on the superficial temporal artery. Alloplastic frameworks such as those composed of high-density polyethylene can also be used to repair cartilaginous defects in the ear, obviating the need for donor cartilage. Alloplastic implants should be covered with vascularized tissue such as a temporoparietal fascia flap.

The goal of reconstruction following total auriculectomy for an invasive cutaneous malignancy is to provide vascularized soft-tissue coverage of the exposed bone and tissue. Alternatively, a prosthetic ear can yield excellent aesthetic results. Osseointegrated appliances can also be constructed and are favored in bone that has not been previously irradiated.

Neck

The neck is a common site of primary cutaneous malignancies and of sentinel or completion lymph node dissections for cutaneous malignancies of the scalp and face. Defects in the neck from surgery for a primary cutaneous malignancy or lymph node dissection can usually be covered with an elevated deltopectoral or cervicofacial flap. Neck defects can also be covered with a pedicled pectoralis major muscle flap based on the thoracoacromial vessels; however, the bulk and limited reach of the pectoralis major muscle make it a second choice behind free flaps in the neck in some patients.

Defects whose size or location precludes repair with local flaps must be repaired with free flaps. A radial forearm, ulnar artery perforator, or anterolateral thigh free flap can be used to reconstruct neck defects in these instances. For all of these flaps, the recipient vessels can be the carotid and jugular systems; and if these cannot be used because of prior surgery or radiation, the transverse cervical vessels can be secondary donor and recipient vessels.

Oral Cavity

The oral cavity includes the tongue, floor of the mouth, alveolar ridges, retromolar trigone, palate, and buccal mucosa. Oral tumor resection results in a functional and aesthetic defect in the face and mouth. Defects involving any of these structures can compromise speech, chewing, swallowing, and breathing. The goal of reconstruction is to not only restore aesthetics, speech, and swallowing but also recreate an alveolar ridge suitable for dental rehabilitation so that chewing can be restored.

The radial forearm free flap is an excellent option for reconstructing thin mucosal defects, such as those in the floor of the mouth, buccal area, and palate, and for reconstructing the tongue after partial glossectomy. The lateral arm flap, which is supplied by the posterior radial collateral vessels, and the anterolateral thigh flap may also be appropriate choices provided they have a thin layer of sufficient subcutaneous fat.

For full-thickness cheek defects, the radial forearm flap or other fasciocutaneous flaps can be folded in on themselves to provide an internal and external lining. Total and near-total glossectomies require bulky flaps to potentially restore swallowing; for example, the rectus abdominis muscle flap or the anterolateral thigh flap plus a portion of the vastus lateralis muscle can provide adequate bulk for reconstructing large tongue defects. Speech and swallowing are key functional outcomes that must be considered when reconstructing glossectomy defects.

The resection of more locally advanced oral cancers that invade the maxilla or mandible can result in composite defects. The pedicled pectoralis major muscle flap can be used in these situations. In many patients, however, this flap's bulk, lack of pliability, and limited reach still make it a second choice behind free flaps in oral cavity reconstruction.

Mandible

The mandible plays a key role in mastication, deglutition, and phonation and structurally helps stabilize the airway. The most common indication for mandibular reconstruction is ablative surgery for neoplastic processes of the oral cavity and oropharynx. Ablative surgery includes enucleation, marginal resection, and segmental resection. Functional losses and aesthetic deformity depend on the size and location of the mandibular defect. Defects in the posterior body or ramus of the mandible are generally better tolerated than defects in the anterior mandible, which are associated with significant deformity and loss of function. Mastication and deglutition are often compromised following mandibulectomy because of the loss of structural support for the tongue and larynx. Airway compromise may result from a loss of airway stability and tongue support and necessitate tracheostomy. Malocclusion may develop as a result of a shift in the position of the mandible following mandibulectomy. Mandibular reconstruction following ablative surgery optimally preserves speech, swallowing, and airway integrity. It restores lower facial aesthetics and enables subsequent dental reconstruction.

In mandibulectomy defect repair, the functional and aesthetic results obtained with microvascular tissue transfer are superior to those obtained with nonvascularized bone grafts or pedicled tissue transfers. Smaller mandibulectomy defects may be reconstructed with nonvascularized grafts and metal plates, but such defects are rare. In most patients, mandibulectomy defects involve a large segment of the bony mandible, the internal oral lining, and/or the external skin. Free tissue transfer provides sufficient bony and soft tissue coverage with a reliable vascular supply. In general, vascularized bone flaps are used to reconstruct mandibulectomy defects >5 to 6 cm and composite defects. Vascularized bone flaps have high bone union rates because the flaps heal by primary bone healing, similar to how fractures heal. In contrast, nonvascularized bone grafts heal by osteoconduction.

The mainstay of mandibular reconstruction is the fibula flap. This flap provides up to 25 cm of bone, which is sufficient to reconstruct any mandibular defect. Furthermore, the shape of the fibula is relatively consistent, and osteotomies can be made at intervals to conform sections of the bone to a locking reconstruction plate modeled on the resected mandible. In addition, a skin paddle can be harvested to provide soft-tissue coverage. Harvest of the central fibula is well tolerated if 5 cm of proximal and distal fibula are preserved in situ for tibial stability. The length and caliber of the pedicle vessels are sufficiently large to be anastomosed to vessels in the neck.

The fibula flap is based on the peroneal artery and vein; therefore, its use requires that either the anterior or the posterior tibial vessels adequately perfuse the distal lower limb. An angiogram may be required to confirm this before harvest. Secondary flap sources for mandible reconstruction include the iliac crest, scapula, and radial forearm.

Maxilla

The maxilla is the predominant bony structure in the midface and contains or contributes to the palate, superior alveolar ridge, lateral nasal wall, orbital floor, and malar eminence. Historically, many maxillary defects secondary to tumor extirpation were not reconstructed because such repair would interfere with monitoring for tumor recurrence. Instead, maxillectomy defects were lined with skin grafts or allowed to re-epithelialize spontaneously, which facilitated monitoring for tumor recurrence. Prosthetic obturators were used in lieu of autologous tissue to isolate the oral cavity from the maxillary cavity and sometimes to restore the contour of the midface, because of concern that autologous tissue transfer could make the detection of early recurrences difficult.

More recently, with improved imaging modalities for detecting tumor recurrence, reconstructive surgeons can use autologous tissue to restore the midfacial contour, oronasal competence, and orbital support in patients with maxillectomy defects. However, the optimal tissue to use for reconstruction in this area depends on the specific defect, again with the idea of replacing resected tissue with similar tissue. Muscle or myocutaneous free flaps (e.g., the rectus abdominis free flap), fasciocutaneous free flaps (e.g., the anterolateral thigh and radial forearm fasciocutaneous free flaps), and osseous or osseocutaneous free flaps (e.g., the fibula and iliac free flaps) have all been used for maxilla reconstruction.

Pharynx and Esophagus

The goal of pharyngeal and esophageal reconstruction is to restore swallowing and speech. Reconstruction of the pharynx and proximal esophagus is challenging. Most patients who require reconstruction also receive radiation therapy, which complicates reconstructive efforts.

Traditional methods of pharyngeal and esophageal reconstruction, including the use of tubed deltopectoral flaps or procedures such as a gastric pull-up or colonic interposition, have given way to immediate reconstruction with jejunal segment, radial forearm, and anterolateral thigh free flaps. Pharyngeal and esophageal reconstruction with the anterolateral thigh free flap has been shown to result in a slightly better functional outcome than reconstruction with the jejunal free flap. The jejunal free flap offers the benefit of a secretory surface, which can help reduce symptoms of xerostomia, but swallowing is often interrupted by disordered peristalsis within the flap, and speech tends to be less robust and understandable. Furthermore, harvest of a jejunal flap requires laparotomy and bowel anastomosis. Anterolateral thigh free flaps and jejunal free flaps have similar rates of stricture formation and fistula formation. Both options are superior to non-microvascular alternatives. After immediate pharynx and esophagus reconstruction, a tracheoesophageal puncture is generally performed for speech restoration.

BREAST RECONSTRUCTION

The treatment for breast cancer involves multiple modalities, including surgery (resective and reconstructive), systemic therapy (chemotherapy and/or hormonal therapy), and potentially radiation therapy. The order and amount to which these therapies are used varies on a case by case basis. From a reconstructive standpoint, one must consider the amount of breast parenchyma removed (mastectomy versus partial mastectomy), the amount of skin remaining after surgical resection (skin-sparing versus simple mastectomy), whether radiation may be required or has already been given, and the use and timing of systemic therapy, specifically chemotherapy.

The overall goals of breast reconstruction are to restore the form and contour of the resected breast and to achieve symmetry with the contralateral breast. Each type of breast reconstruction has its advantages and disadvantages. There is no one approach to breast reconstruction that is appropriate in all patients. Some aspects to consider in helping a patient choose the right reconstructive option are as follows: (a) the patient's desires and expectations, (b) the treatment that they have undergone and still have to undergo, (c) their willingness to undergo surgery again, and (d) their overall prognosis with the disease. In general, breast reconstruction is a process that entails—two to four surgical procedures over the course of 4 to 12 months. (There are certain instances in which a single-stage reconstruction may be possible.) These procedures include the initial breast reconstruction, any subsequent operations for achieving breast symmetry, and nipple reconstruction.

When counseling patients on reconstructive options it is important to remember that the primary focus of treatment is treating the cancer. Reconstruction is important, but it is a secondary goal. Women can often feel overwhelmed by all of the treatment options, not only in treating their cancer but also in the reconstruction. It is important to remember that every patient has different expectations for her body following treatment for breast cancer. Counseling patients on all options for reconstruction (including not undergoing reconstruction), and then allowing patients to make their own decisions, leads to highest long-term satisfactions rates post-treatment for breast cancer. It is additionally important to give patients a realistic idea of what to expect after reconstruction.

Timing Considerations for Breast Reconstruction

An important aspect to discuss with patients is the timing of breast reconstruction. This is based not only on the patient's wishes but also on the characteristics of the disease. Immediate reconstruction takes place at the time of the breast cancer surgery. Delayed reconstruction takes place later, after the treatment for the cancer is complete (Fig. 24.1). Immediate reconstruction results in the best aesthetic outcomes if postmastectomy radiation therapy is not needed. But if postmastectomy radiation therapy is required, delayed reconstruction is preferred as it avoids potential aesthetic and radiation delivery problems. Unfortunately this is often not known until the surgical pathology returns well after the surgery is over.

At M. D. Anderson, the employment of two variations of delayed reconstruction, "delayed-immediate" and "delayed-delayed", are now commonly used to answer this conundrum. These two variations are performed with the goal of preserving the breast skin envelope for an optimal aesthetic outcome while taking into account the possibility that a patient may need to receive adjuvant radiation therapy. Delayed-immediate breast reconstruction is a two-staged approach that optimizes treatment when the need for adjuvant radiation therapy has yet to be determined. In the first stage, after a skin sparing mastectomy is performed, a tissue expander is placed until it is known whether or not adjuvant radiation therapy is necessary. Once pathologic review comes back, if radiation is not required, then patients undergo immediate reconstruction. If radiation is required, then the patients undergo radiation and have their final reconstruction after their oncologic treatment is finished. In delayed-delayed breast reconstruction, the need for adjuvant radiation therapy is known before mastectomy, and a tissue expander is placed at the time of mastectomy to preserve the skin envelope. Typically in both delayed-immediate and delayed-delayed breast reconstruction, the tissue expander is removed after radiation therapy has been completed, and breast reconstruction is performed with autologous tissue from the abdomen, back, buttock or thigh or a permanent implant.

Reconstruction After Partial Mastectomy

In a partial mastectomy, only the portion of the breast that contains the cancer is removed, and the remainder of the breast tissue is left in place. This is performed with the expectation that adjuvant radiation will be required to complete treatment. For the most part, reconstruction is not required because little or no skin and only a portion of breast tissue are removed during a partial mastectomy. When larger portions of tissue are removed or when women have very large breasts, so that the volume of tissue removed is only a small percentage of the overall total volume, the remaining breast tissue can sometimes be rearranged to fill the defect. If the remaining breast tissue volume is insufficient, additional tissue may be brought to the breast, usually from the back or the abdomen. Immediate reconstruction is preferred in patients who undergo partial mastectomy.

A

B

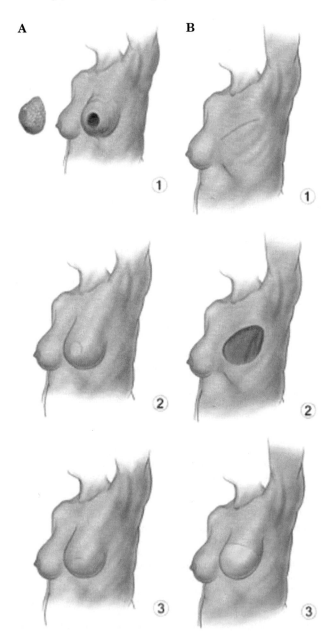

FIGURE 24.1 Immediate reconstruction (**A**) is performed at the time of the breast cancer surgery. Delayed reconstruction (**B**) is performed after the patient has completed breast cancer treatment.

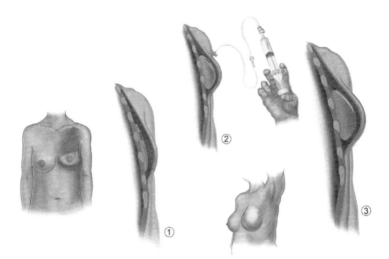

FIGURE 24.2 Staged breast reconstruction consisting of a tissue expander place submuscularly followed by permanent implant placement. (1) The tissue expander is placed under the muscle followed by serial expansion, (2) the tissue expander is replaced with a permanent implant, and (3) the unlabeled images reflect pre- and post-reconstruction states.

Reconstruction After Mastectomy

The vast majority of breast reconstructions are performed using tissue expanders and implants; latissimus dorsi myocutaneous flaps and implants; or abdominal tissue-based flaps. A staged reconstruction consisting of tissue expansion followed by permanent implant placement is the most common method of breast reconstruction (Fig. 24.2). For tissue expansion, an expander is placed under the pectoral muscle either immediately after mastectomy or as a delayed procedure. The overlying incisions are allowed to heal, and then saline solution is injected into the expander weekly or every other week until the desired final volume is achieved.

Implant-Based Reconstruction

After the patient has completed and recovered from all oncologic treatment, a second-stage operation is performed to remove the tissue expander and place the permanent breast implant.

The advantages of implant-based reconstruction are that it is simple, requires less operating room time than reconstruction with flaps, and is suitable for women who are not able to undergo reconstruction utilizing autologous tissue flaps. The disadvantages of implant-based reconstruction include the potential for infection, capsular contracture, and implant rupture; in addition, young patients may need to undergo implant replacement several times over the course of their lives. Implant-based reconstruction is a poor choice for patients who have received radiation therapy, as it leads to significantly higher risks of fluid collection, infection, capsular contracture, and implant extrusion.

Another type of implant-based reconstruction employs a latissimus dorsi flap with or without a skin component over an implant (Fig. 24.3). The latissimus dorsi is a broad, fan-shaped muscle that originates on the back and inserts at the shoulder. Because most women do not have enough tissue volume on their backs for

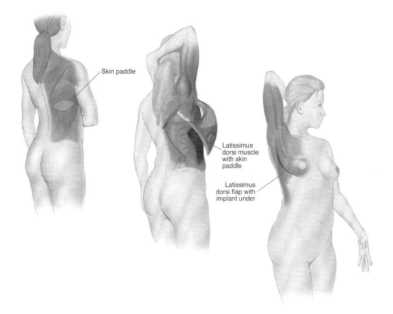

Skin paddle

Latissimus
dorsi muscle
with skin
paddle

Latissimus
dorsi flap with
implant under

FIGURE 24.3 The latissimus dorsi muscle flap with skin component (myocutaneous flap). The flap comprising the latissimus dorsi muscle and some of the overlying skin is rotated anteriorly to the chest. An implant can be placed under this flap for appropriate volume reconstruction.

complete breast reconstruction, the latissimus dorsi flap is rarely used alone to reconstruct the breast. Instead, the latissimus dorsi muscle with some of the overlying skin is rotated anteriorly to the chest to cover an implant, facilitate closure of the mastectomy defect, and give the reconstructed breast a more natural contour. The implants used in reconstruction with a latissimus dorsi muscle flap are generally the same as those used after tissue expansion.

The primary advantage of using the latissimus dorsi flap in implant-based breast reconstruction is that the flap can provide sufficient tissue to cover the implant without the need for tissue expansion, and thus a staged approach may not be required. The drawbacks of using the latissimus dorsi flap include longer surgery and recovery times than with implant-only reconstructive surgery, a scar on the back, and potential arm weakness following surgery. Regardless, the approach is a viable option for women who are thin and thus are not candidates for an abdominal flap. It is particularly useful in those who have received radiation therapy or in whom other types of reconstruction have failed.

Autologous Tissue Reconstruction

In autologous tissue reconstruction, the patient's own skin, fat, and muscle are transferred from one area of the body to the chest to reconstruct one or both breast mounds, usually without the need for a supplemental prosthesis or implant. Autologous reconstruction can be performed with a pedicled flap or a free flap. The most common donor site for the tissues used for breast reconstruction is the abdomen. The tissue either remains attached to the body on a vascular pedicle and is transposed into position (a "pedicled" flap) or is completely detached from the abdomen and then reattached in the chest using microvascular surgery for anastomoses between donor and recipient vessels (a "free flap" or "free tissue transfer").

Transverse Rectus Abdominis Myocutaneous Flap

The harvest of the classic transverse rectus abdominis myocutaneous (TRAM) flap for breast reconstruction involves isolating the skin and subcutaneous tissue located between the pubic bone and the umbilicus, and then an entire rectus abdominis muscle. The superior epigastric vessels, which supply blood to the muscle and overlying tissue, remain attached. A tunnel is created in the subcutaneous tissue between the abdomen and breast cavities (through the inframammary crease), and the flap is passed through this tunnel and rotated into the breast cavity.

A variation of the classic TRAM flap is the free TRAM flap (Fig. 24.4). In breast reconstruction with a free TRAM flap, the deep inferior epigastric vessels are divided when the flap is harvested and then reattached in the chest under an operating microscope. The advantages of the free TRAM flap include its relatively large skin area and tissue volume available for reconstruction. While these techniques are originally described as taking the entire width of the rectus abdominis muscle, as time has progressed, efforts to take less and less muscle have resulted in several refinements to the technique including the muscle-sparing TRAM flap, in which only a small amount of muscle is taken with the blood supply; the deep inferior epigastric artery perforator flap, in which the blood supply is dissected out completely and no muscle is taken with the flap; and the superficial inferior epigastric artery flap (Fig. 24.5).

Other Flaps

Autologous tissue flaps for breast reconstruction can also be harvested from other sites, including the buttocks or thighs (Fig. 24.6). These flaps are reserved for patients in whom the abdomen is not available as a donor site. Overall, breast reconstruction with autologous tissue produces the best long-term results. However, these procedures are of greater magnitude, are associated with longer operative and recovery times, and have a small but present risk of failure.

Nipple and Areola Reconstruction

Nipple-areolar reconstruction, if desired, is performed as a separate procedure after the reconstructed breast has attained its final shape and position. A nipple position on the breast mound is determined based on symmetry with the contralateral breast, and a three-dimensional nipple is constructed with a local skin flap, usually from the breast itself (Fig. 24.7). After the reconstructed nipple has had the opportunity to heal, a "new" areola is tattooed around the reconstructed nipple. Other options include tattooing a nipple areolar complex directly on top of the reconstructed breast without the three-dimensional reconstruction.

RECONSTRUCTION OF THE TRUNK

The chest and abdominal wall account for roughly one-third of the entire surface area of the human adult body. As with surgical defects in the head and neck, surgical defects in the trunk can expose or compromise critical anatomical structures. When possible, cutaneous defects in the trunk resulting from cancer resection are usually repaired with wide undermining of the adjacent subcutaneous tissue down to the deep investing fascia and local flap advancement. Resection of neoplasms that involve the full thickness of the abdominal wall or chest wall requires the use of pedicled or free flaps for defect repair.

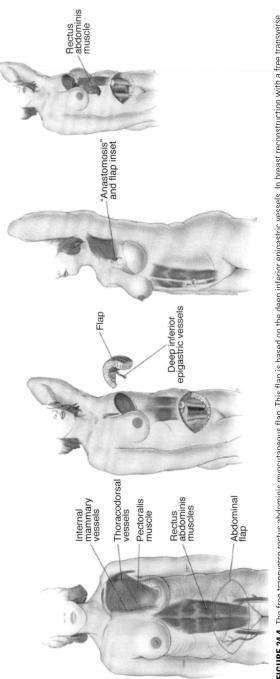

FIGURE 24.4 The free transverse rectus abdominis myocutaneous flap. This flap is based on the deep inferior epigastric vessels. In breast reconstruction with a free transverse rectus abdominis myocutaneous flap, the deep inferior epigastric vessels are divided at the time of flap harvest and then reattached to recipient vessels (e.g., internal mammary vessels) in the chest under an operating microscope.

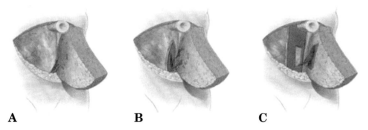

FIGURE 24.5 (**A**) The superficial inferior epigastric artery (SIEA) flap is based on blood vessels that run under the skin and whose harvest does not require dissection into the rectus abdominis fascia or muscle. (**B**) The deep inferior epigastric artery perforator (DIEP) flap is based on a dissection of the blood vessels that pass through the rectus abdominis muscle; no muscle or fascia is taken when the flap is harvested. (**C**) In breast reconstruction with a muscle-sparing transverse rectus abdominis myocutaneous flap, only a small amount of rectus muscle is taken with the deep inferior epigastric vessels.

Thorax

The incidence of skin cancer on the chest wall is comparatively low. Depending on the extent of the defect, thoracic reconstruction must account for the pleural cavity, skeletal support (ribs and sternum), and soft-tissue coverage of the chest and axilla. Forming an airtight seal at the time of wound closure is crucial to preserving the intrathoracic negative pressure gradient. Skeletal stabilization with prosthetic materials to reduce the risk of paradoxical chest wall motion (flail chest) is warranted for resections involving either ≥4 rib segments or chest wall cavities >6 cm in diameter.

The majority of chest wall defects can be repaired with local or regional myocutaneous flaps. Flap options for sternal wound coverage include the rectus abdominis flap based on the superior epigastric vessels and the pectoralis major flap either as a pedicled flap based on the thoracoacromial vessels or as a turnover flap based on the internal mammary perforator vessels. Options for axillary coverage include the pectoralis major and latissimus dorsi flaps. The latissimus dorsi and trapezius muscle flaps can be used to cover defects in the posterior thorax.

Chest wall defects can be classified as either full-thickness or partial-thickness defects. Partial-thickness defects possess an intact bony wall and thus do not require extensive reconstruction or the use of muscle flaps, while full-thickness defects require complex reconstruction to maintain the intrathoracic negative pressure gradient, mostly with flap closure. Many full-thickness chest wall defects can be repaired with a pedicled flap from the abdomen such as a pedicled TRAM flap or vertical rectus abdominis myocutaneous flap, which can be extended up as far as the axilla or clavicle and whose donor sites can be closed primarily. A pedicled flap from either the abdomen or the back, such as a latissimus dorsi myocutaneous flap, can also be used to repair large full-thickness defects. If the skin defect is too large for the latissimus dorsi myocutaneous flap, then muscle alone is typically transposed and covered with a skin graft.

Abdomen

Most cutaneous defects that result from ablative oncologic surgery in the abdomen can be closed primarily because of the laxity of the skin and subcutaneous tissue in the region. Large fasciocutaneous flaps based on myocutaneous perforator vessels can be raised off the abdominal wall and closed in layers to obliterate dead space. If the defect involves the fascia of the abdominal wall, the goal of

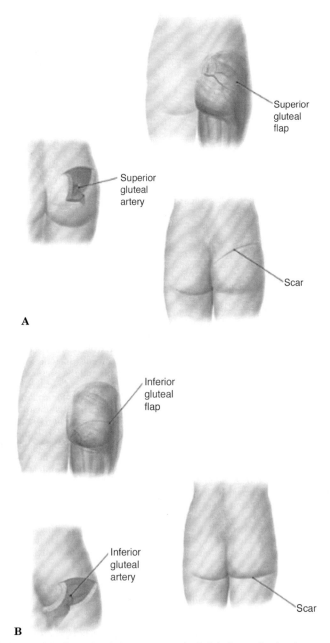

FIGURE 24.6 Other flap options for breast reconstruction include the superior gluteal artery perforator flap (**A**) and the inferior gluteal artery perforator (**B**) flap.

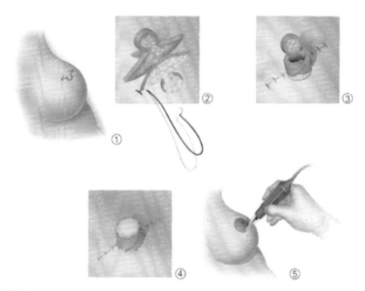

FIGURE 24.7 Local tissue flaps on the reconstructed breast mound are used to reconstruct the nipple. A local skin flap is reflected up and folded to reconstruct a three-dimensional nipple (2–4). Areola pigmentation is performed once the reconstructed nipple has healed (5).

reconstruction is to restore the integrity and continuity of the abdominal wall. To enable primary closure when there is a paucity of fascia, component separation, in which the layers of the abdominal wall fascia and muscle are separated to increase medialization of the rectus components, is often employed. If the fascial defect is larger than what a lateral component separation can account for, then autologous fascial grafts can be taken from the tensor fascia lata in the thigh if required. Acellular dermal matrix, a bioprosthetic mesh, has also been proven to effectively restore abdominal wall integrity. Pedicled flaps such as the anterolateral thigh myocutaneous flap can be used to obliterate dead space and reconstruct skin, subcutaneous tissue, and fascial elements. Free tissue transfer is rarely necessary to repair abdominal wall defects but remains an option if the available local or regional tissue is insufficient for defect repair.

Perineum

Perineal reconstruction presents a unique challenge because the form and function of the perineal surface is distinct from those of other surfaces of the body. The perineum is important for pregnancy, intercourse, hip mobility, and bowel and bladder motility. Perineal skin and fatty tissue are very sensitive to pressure and touch and are durable, elastic, and weight-bearing. In addition, the perineal skin is softly padded, pigmented, and hair-bearing, which makes it impossible to match with distant tissue. Treatment for skin cancers such as Bowen disease and invasive squamous cell carcinoma, which involve the skin and subcutaneous tissues only, results in defects of the vulvoperineal surface.

Superficial surgical defects of the perineum can be repaired with split-thickness skin grafts. Split-thickness skin grafts are especially useful if the status of excision margins is uncertain and the risk of local recurrence is high as it can be excised and repeated if further resection is required. Skin grafts generally provide better aesthetic outcomes than other tissue options but carry a higher risk of reconstruction failure because of fluid collection below the graft or shear. Partial- and full-thickness skin grafts can both be obtained from the suprapubic area and should incorporate as much of the pubic hairline as possible to conceal the donor site. Full-thickness skin grafts can be harvested from the abdominal wall, provided that site has sufficient redundant tissue, and used to cover large surface-area defects in the perineum.

Irradiated Perineum

A local or regional flap should be used to repair defects in regions of irradiated perineum. Small skin defects in the perineum can be repaired with a local rotation flap such as a rhomboid skin flap. Rotation flaps are most effective when used in the lateral and posterior aspects of the perineal area, which have the most skin laxity. Larger defects may require regional sensate fasciocutaneous flaps such as a posterior thigh fasciocutaneous flap or muscle flaps such as a pedicled gracilis muscle flap. In these cases, patients must avoid putting pressure on the area of the pedicle for several weeks. Larger defects of the perineum can also be reconstructed with a pedicled anterolateral thigh myocutaneous flap, in which variable amounts of skin, adipose tissue, and fascia and vastus lateralis muscle are elevated and transferred to fill and re-contour soft-tissue defects.

RECONSTRUCTION IN THE EXTREMITIES

The role of the reconstructive surgery in the extremities is to preserve both form and function. Multimodality therapy, incorporating chemotherapy and radiation therapy with surgery, has expanded the indications for limb salvage in patients with cancers of the extremities. Amputation is now reserved for treating advanced or metastatic disease where limb salvage is not possible. In line with advances in oncologic imaging and treatment, there have been tremendous advances in reconstructive techniques for repairing both soft-tissue and bony defects in the extremities. Pedicled flaps and free tissue transfers have revolutionized reconstruction for defects in the extremities.

Reconstructive surgery following extirpative surgery to treat cutaneous malignancies in the extremities generally involves primary closure, skin grafts, or local or regional cutaneous and myocutaneous flaps. Defects from surgery for soft-tissue and bony neoplasms, such as sarcomas, which are less common than cutaneous malignancies in the extremities, generally require reconstruction with pedicled or free flaps. Adjuvant therapy often decreases tumor size and facilitates limb sparing, but the radiation therapy used may also hinder wound healing and necessitate a non-irradiated tissue flap closure to provide coverage of the nerves, vessels, and bone.

Requirements for replacing various tissues in the extremities, including bone, nerves, muscle, soft tissues, and skin, must be anticipated before reconstruction. Bony defects can be repaired with limb shortening with or without later bone transport for lengthening, allografts, bone grafts, or vascularized bone flaps. Free and pedicled muscle flaps not only provide well-vascularized wound coverage but can also be neurotized and provide functional muscle. Fasciocutaneous flaps, myocutaneous flaps, and muscle flaps covered with split-thickness skin grafts can be used to replace resected soft tissue and skin.

Microsurgical techniques can be used to repair damaged nerves, thereby restoring motor and sensory functions. Primary nerve repair performed at the time of tumor resection results in the best functional outcome. If the nerve deficit is too large to perform a tension-free repair, nerve grafting may be necessary. The donor nerve is typically the sural nerve, which provides sensation to the lateral foot and can provide as much as 40 cm of nerve from one leg with minimal morbidity.

Limb sparing, however, must be weighed against performing an oncologically adequate resection. In addition, preserving a limb that is nonfunctional, insensate, or painful provides little if any benefit over amputation. Indications for amputation include major neurovascular or extensive muscle involvement of the limb by the tumor resulting in a nonfunctional limb following tumor resection; infection and fractures that could compromise reconstruction and delay adjuvant therapy; poor nutrition and other serious medical conditions; a lack of patient motivation for rehabilitation; and the need for multiple surgeries. Patients must understand before they undergo limb reconstructive surgery that poor functional outcomes, tumor recurrence, or infections and other wound complications may ultimately lead to amputation.

Upper Extremity`

At a minimum, functional upper limb reconstruction should provide a stable shoulder joint, restore elbow flexion, and ensure median nerve sensibility. Flap coverage is indicated for upper-extremity defects with extensive tissue loss and for the coverage of vital structures such as bones, tendons, nerves, and major vessels when skin grafts would be unlikely to adhere or provide durable coverage or would lead to significant scarring and impaired function. For example, contracture of the scar tissue from incisions placed parallel to the axis of the limb across joints can result in a decreased range of motion and may require z-plasty procedures or interposition of a pliable flap for contracture release. Similarly, tendons that have been stripped bare of paratenon are poor recipients for skin grafts and their function can be compromised if adherence occurs, thus preventing their free gliding movement. Following the amputation of a digit or limb, fillet flaps, in which the bone has been partially or totally removed, can be used to cover the distal stump with well-vascularized tissue.

Proximal Arm

Upper limb wounds can be covered with distant pedicled flaps from the trunk and pelvis, including the groin flap, which is supplied by the superficial circumflex iliac vessels; the anterior chest wall flap, which is supplied by the intercostal or thoracoepigastric vessels; and epigastric or abdominal flaps, which are supplied by the superficial inferior epigastric vessels or random-pattern blood flow. These flaps generally require 2 to 3 weeks (or more) of immobilization for neovascularization. After neovascularization has occurred, the donor pedicle is divided.

The pedicled pectoralis major flap, which is based on the thoracoacromial vessels, can be used to repair defects in the anterior shoulder or provide tissue coverage of an amputation site. The pedicled latissimus dorsi flap, which is based on the thoracodorsal vessels, can be used to repair defects in the shoulder, axilla, and upper arm. The pedicled latissimus dorsi muscle flap can be extended to the olecranon, antecubital fossa, and posterior axilla and can be used as a functional muscle transfer to restore elbow flexion or extension in many patients.

Forearm and Elbow

Soft-tissue defects in the forearm and elbow can be reconstructed with a pedicled radial forearm fasciocutaneous flap based on the radial artery and its venae comitantes. An Allen test should be performed prior to surgery to determine whether the ulnar and radial vessels in the hand are patent. If a single vessel is inadequate to perfuse the hand, vein grafting can be performed to re-establish blood flow as needed. If pedicled flaps are not available or large enough to cover the defect, then free-tissue transfer should be considered.

Many muscle, myocutaneous, and fasciocutaneous free flaps can be used to repair defects in the upper extremity. The rectus abdominis, latissimus dorsi, serratus anterior, and gracilis (often the flap of choice for innervated functional reconstruction) muscle or myocutaneous free flaps and the radial forearm, ulnar forearm, lateral arm, anterolateral thigh, dorsalis pedis, and scapular/parascapular fasciocutaneous free flaps have all been successfully used in upper-extremity reconstruction. In addition, the first and second toes have both been successfully transferred to replace the thumb, and fibula and iliac crest osseous flaps have been used to reconstruct the long bones of the upper limb. Angiography may be indicated before harvesting a fibula flap if distal perfusion to the foot is in question.

Hand

The first and second most common malignant tumors in the hand are squamous cell carcinoma and melanoma, respectively. Skin cancer can affect any surface of the hand. Intrinsic characteristics of the nail beds and the palmar and dorsal skin surfaces warrant different reconstructive approaches. Because the hand is crucial to the functions of everyday life, a baseline functional assessment should be performed before tumor excision. As a general principle, digit length should be preserved to the greatest extent possible during oncologic resection. Additionally, the skin of the dorsum of the hand has moderate laxity; is thin, mobile, and pliable; and protects the superficial extensor tendons. Reconstruction of this area should take these characteristics into account with the goal of preserving these functions.

Small defects in the hand can be closed primarily. Every attempt should be made to preserve the paratenon to minimize scarring around the tendon and to optimize functional outcomes. Defects >2 cm can be resurfaced with skin grafts provided the paratenon has been preserved. Full-thickness skin grafts provide a better contour match and result in less contracture than split-thickness skin grafts. When the paratenon cannot be preserved, local flaps such as rotation, advancement, transposition (rhomboid), and cross-finger flaps can be used.

The temporoparietal fascia flap, which is based on the superficial temporal artery, and a skin graft can be used to reconstruct the dorsal hand and provide a suitable surface against which the underlying tendons can glide. Large defects in the dorsum, in which tendons are exposed and the paratenon is absent, can be reconstructed with the reverse-flow pedicled radial forearm flap. However, harvesting the flap destroys a major vessel that supplies blood to the hand, and the donor site typically must be covered with a skin graft. Alternatives to the reverse-flow pedicled radial forearm flap include the anterolateral thigh and lateral arm free flaps.

Defects in the distal cutaneous or subungual regions of the fingertips that result from wide surgical excision must be repaired in a way that maintains function. Typically, this means preserving as much length of the involved digit as possible. The cross-finger flap can be used to cover defects ≤3 cm long and ≤2 cm wide on any of the phalanges. Defects that result from the removal of the nail plate and excision of the nail bed can be resurfaced with full-thickness skin grafts. In contrast to the skin on the dorsum of the hand, palmar skin is glabrous and thick and receives significant sensory innervation. Most palmar defects are resurfaced with full-thickness skin grafts; larger palmar defects can be reconstructed using the pedicled reverse radial forearm fasciocutaneous flap. When amputation is necessary, it is generally performed at the distal interphalangeal or middle phalangeal level. In middle phalangeal-level amputations, finger flexion is maintained by preserving the insertion of the flexor digitorum superficial tendon into the base of the second phalynx. Repair of the amputation defect involves the use of full-thickness skin grafts or local flaps.

The reconstructed limb, hand, or digit must have adequate sensory and motor function; otherwise, reconstruction may be more of a detriment than a benefit to the patient's quality of life. Primary nerve repair or a nerve graft is often needed to preserve adequate function. Epineural or interfascicular repairs are also typically performed depending on the nerve and location. Tendon transfers, in which functionally expendable muscle and/or tendon units are rerouted to replace functionally critical units, are also possible.

Lower Extremity

Defects in the groin and proximal medial or anterior thigh can often be closed with a pedicled rectus abdominis muscle or myocutaneous flap supplied by the deep inferior epigastric vessels. Large defects in other areas of the thigh are typically reconstructed with adjacent muscle flaps, including the rectus abdominis and latissimus dorsi muscle flaps, or myocutaneous free flaps. The femoral and deep femoral vessels are usually good recipient vessels for free flaps. End-to-side anastomoses are commonly performed in the lower extremity to preserve blood flow to the distal limb.

Osteotomy defects in the knee, distal femur, and proximal tibia are usually reconstructed with an allograft or endoprosthesis. Soft-tissue coverage of defects in the knee, upper third of the lower leg, or first 15 cm of the thigh above the knee can be achieved with pedicled gastrocnemius muscle flaps. The medial or lateral heads of the gastrocnemius can be separated and used as pedicled muscle flaps, or both heads can be used to provide muscle flap coverage. A pedicled gastrocnemius muscle flap receives its blood supply from the sural artery and vein, which are branches of the popliteal vessels. Larger defects in the anterior knee can be repaired using a reverse anterolateral thigh flap. If both heads of the gastrocnemius muscle are to be used for reconstruction, the soleus muscle must be preserved to provide plantar flexion of the foot. Defects in the middle third of the leg can be reliably repaired with soleus muscle flaps. As with the gastrocnemius muscle, the soleus muscle can be split down its median raphe, and the medial and lateral heads of the muscle can be used separately. If the soleus muscle is to be used for reconstruction, then the gastrocnemius muscle must be preserved to maintain plantar flexion. Alternatively, one head of the soleus muscle and one head of the gastrocnemius muscle can be used for reconstruction, which spares plantar flexion. Reconstructing the distal third of the leg with local or regional muscle flaps is not usually possible because local tissues lack laxity. Generally, all but the smallest wounds in this region must be repaired with fasciocutaneous, muscle, or myocutaneous free flaps.

Foot

Small defects in the foot can be repaired with skin grafts and local flaps. These defects can be covered with fasciocutaneous perforator flaps based on single perforating vessels that can be harvested with varying amounts of skin, subcutaneous tissue, and fascia. However, larger defects in the foot must be repaired using microvascular free tissue transfer. Many large defects can be repaired with a free muscle flap, such as a gracilis muscle or serratus anterior muscle free flap, and covered with a skin graft. The largest defects may require repair with a rectus abdominis or latissimus dorsi muscle free flap and skin graft coverage.

The design of muscle flaps used for foot reconstruction must take into account the expected atrophy of the muscle with time; too much flap bulk is usually unfavorable for ambulation and may necessitate revision surgery and/or special orthotic footwear. Fasciocutaneous flaps such as the radial forearm flap are also used for foot reconstruction and can be designed to include sensory innervation. Muscle and fasciocutaneous flaps are susceptible to pressure ulceration and so must be vigilantly monitored for the breakdown of skin and soft tissue.

Plantar sensation must be reestablished after nerve resection in lower limb reconstruction. Without protective plantar sensation, the lower limb is prone to ulceration and injury that can lead to infection and ultimately amputation. However, if plantar sensation cannot be reestablished, good extremity management may allow a patient to maintain the foot as a "bioprosthesis." Proximal nerve resection and repair yield poorer functional restoration than does distal reconstruction. In addition, postoperative immobilization of the affected extremity is necessary for approximately 7 to 10 days after nerve repair. Reinnervation, which usually occurs at a rate no faster than 1 mm/day, can be detected by testing for an advancing Tinel sign and performing nerve conduction studies. If reinnervation is expected to take >12 to 18 months, muscle stimulation to maintain motor end-plate function can be attempted.

Patients who undergo free tissue transfer and bony reconstruction of the lower extremity usually require a period of bedrest during which the affected extremity remains elevated. Deep venous thrombosis must be prevented during this time. After 5 to 7 days of bedrest, patients can sit and dangle the affected extremity for 15 to 30 minutes at a time. Standing and crutch-assisted ambulation with gradual weight bearing is then allowed with the flap gently wrapped with an elastic bandage to help contour the flap and prevent venous pooling.

SUMMARY

Reconstruction for oncologic defects requires attention to both aesthetic and functional requirements. These defects can be routinely and safely reconstructed using multidisciplinary and systematic approaches and following oncological principles. The ultimate goal of reconstructive surgery is a healed wound with minimal patient morbidity. Coordinated and specialized reconstructive techniques optimize aesthetic and functional outcomes.

Recommended Readings

Head and Neck Reconstruction

Ariyan S. The pectoralis major myocutaneous flap for reconstruction in the head and neck. *Plast Reconstr Surg.* 1979;63:73–81.

Burget GC, Menick FJ. Nasal reconstruction: seeking a fourth dimension. *Plast Reconstr Surg.* 1986;78:145–157.

Hanasono MM, Sacks JM, Goel N, et al. The anterolateral thigh free flap for skull base reconstruction. *Otolaryngol Head Neck Surg.* 2009;140(6):855–860.

Hidalgo DA. Fibula free flap: a new method of mandible reconstruction. *Plast Reconstr Surg.* 1989;87:71–78.

Newman MI, Hanasono MM, Disa JJ, et al. Scalp reconstruction: a fifteen-year experience. *Ann Plast Surg.* 2004;52:501–506.

Robb GL, Lewin JS, Deschler DG, et al. Speech and swallowing outcomes in reconstructions of the pharynx and cervical esophagus. *Head Neck.* 2003;25:232–244.

Yu P, Chang DW, Miller MJ, et al. Analysis of 49 cases of flap compromise in 1310 free flaps for head and neck reconstruction. *Head Neck.* 2009;31(1):45–51.

Yu P, Hanasono MM, Skoracki RJ, et al. Pharyngoesophageal reconstruction with the anterolateral thigh flap after total laryngopharyngectomy. *Cancer.* 2010;116(7):1718–1724.

Yu P, Lewin JS, Reece GP, et al. Comparison of clinical and functional outcomes and hospital costs following pharyngoesophageal reconstruction with the anterolateral thigh free flap versus the jejunal flap. *Plast Reconstr Surg.* 2006;117(3):968–974.

Zafereo ME, Weber RS, Lewin JS, et al. Complications and functional outcomes following complex oropharyngeal reconstruction. *Head Neck.* 2010;32(8):1003–1011.

Breast Reconstruction

Bostwick J. *Plastic and Reconstructive Breast Surgery.* 2nd ed. St. Louis, MO: Quality Medical Publishing; 2000.

Kroll SS, Reece GP. *The Well-informed Patient's Guide to Breast Reconstruction.* Houston, TX: The University of Texas M. D. Anderson Cancer Center; 2002.

Kroll SS, Schusterman MA, Reece GP, et al. Choice of flap and incidence of free flap success. *Plast Reconstr Surg.* 1996;98:459–463.

Kronowitz SJ. Immediate versus delayed reconstruction. *Clin Plast Surg.* 2007;34(1): 39–50.

Kronowitz SJ. Delayed-immediate breast reconstruction: technical and timing considerations. *Plast Reconstr Surg.* 2010; 125(2):463–474.

Kronowitz SJ, Kuerer HM, Buchholz TA, et al. A management algorithm and practical oncoplastic surgical techniques for repairing partial mastectomy defects. *Plast Reconstr Surg.* 2008;122(6):1631–1647.

Kronowitz SJ, Robb GL, Youssef A, et al. Optimizing autologous breast reconstruction in thin patients. *Plast Reconstr Surg.* 2003;112:1768–1778.

Miller MJ, Rock CS, Robb GL. Aesthetic breast reconstruction using a combination of free transverse rectus abdominis musculocutaneous flaps and breast implants. *Ann Plast Surg.* 1996;37:258–264.

Tran NV, Evans GR, Kroll SS, et al. Postoperative adjuvant irradiation: effects on transverse rectus abdominis muscle flap breast reconstruction. *Plast Reconstr Surg.* 2000;106:313–317.

Trunk and Perineum Reconstruction

Arnold PG, Pairolero PC. Chest wall reconstruction: an account of 500 consecutive patients. *Plastic Reconstr Surg.* 1996;98: 804–810.

Buchel EW, Finical S, Johnson C. Pelvic reconstruction using vertical rectus abdominis musculocutaneous flaps. *Ann Plast Surg.* 2004;52:22–26.

Butler CE, Gündeslioglu AO, Rodriguez-Bigas MA. Outcomes of immediate vertical rectus abdominis myocutaneous flap reconstruction for irradiated abdominoperineal resection defects. *J Am Coll Surg.* 2008;206(4):694–703.

Chang RR, Mehrara BJ, Hu QY, et al. Reconstruction of complex oncologic chest wall defects: a 10-year experience. *Plastic Reconstr Surg.* 2004;52:471–479.

Garvey PB, Rhines LD, Dong W, et al. Immediate soft-tissue reconstruction for complex defects of the spine following surgery for spinal neoplasms. *Plast Reconstr Surg.* 2010;125(5):1460–1466.

McCraw JB, Papp C, Ye Z, et al. Reconstruction of the perineum after tumor surgery. *Surg Oncol Clin N Am.* 1997;6:177–189.

Extremity Reconstruction

Barwick WJ, Goldberg JA, Scully SP, et al. Vascularized tissue transfer for closure of irradiated wounds after soft tissue sarcoma resection. *Ann Surg.* 1992;216:591–595.

Brennan MF. Management of extremity soft-tissue sarcoma. *Am J Surg.* 1989;158: 71–78.

Cordeiro PG, Neves RI, Hidalgo DA. The role of free tissue transfer following oncologic resection in the lower extremity. *Ann Plast Surg.* 1994;33:9–16.

Evans GRD, Goldberg DP. Principles of extremity microvascular reconstruction. In: Schusterman MA, ed. *Microsurgical Reconstruction of the Cancer Patient.* Philadelphia, PA: Lippincott-Raven; 1997: 233–247.

Gidumal R, Wood MB, Sim FH, et al. Vascularized bone transfer of limb salvage and reconstruction after resection of aggressive bone lesions. *J Reconstr Microsurg.* 1987;3:183–188.

Hidalgo DA, Carrasquillo IM. The treatment of lower extremity sarcomas with wide excision, radiotherapy, and free-flap reconstruction. *Plast Reconstr Surg.* 1992; 89:96–101.

Reece GP, Schusterman MA, Pollock RE, et al. Immediate versus delayed free-tissue transfer salvage of the lower extremity in soft tissue sarcoma patients. *Ann Surg Oncol.* 1994;1:11–17.

Robb GL, Reece GP. Lower extremity reconstruction. In: Schusterman MA, ed. *Microsurgical Reconstruction of the Cancer Patient.* Philadelphia, PA: Lippincott-Raven; 1997:289–322.

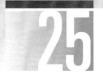

Targeted Cancer Therapy

Mark J. Truty

INTRODUCTION

The term "personalized medicine" first gained wide popularity in 1999 after staff writers of the *Wall Street Journal* published an article, "New Era of Personalized Medicine—Targeting Drugs for Each Unique Genetic Profile," which was later reprinted in the *Oncologist*. In this publication, the authors described the use of new bioinformatics from single-nucleotide polymorphism (SNP) analysis on cancer drug development. Since that initial publication there has been widespread hope and enthusiasm for the future of oncologic patient care (Fig. 25.1). Traditional cancer therapy has centered on clinical rather than biologic variables, and on evidence of efficacy obtained from large epidemiologic trials. Unfortunately, such variables and large cohort studies take into account neither the vast molecular variability of individuals within a population nor the significant biological heterogeneity of the cancers themselves. Oncologists have long recognized that each individual's cancer is different from every other in etiology, clinical presentation, response and tolerance to therapy, recurrence, and ultimately prognosis. Personalized oncology attempts to provide an objective basis for the utilization of these differences in order to provide interventions that are clinically effective and less toxic. The knowledge of the molecular profile of both the patient and their cancer is necessary to guide the selectivity of therapy for any individual. In this new "omics" era, it is now possible to gather the specificities of the genome, transcriptome, and proteome of individuals and their respective malignancies with clinically available, high-throughput methods. Personalized cancer therapy is the systematic use of this molecular information to optimize a specific patient's care. Personalized cancer therapy reaches beyond traditional clinical oncology by taking advantage of recent advances in our molecular understanding of cancer and applying it selectively for the largest clinical impact. The ambitious goal of personalized cancer therapy is to tailor care for individual patients using a biologically based and hypothesis-driven approach. Such an approach relies on targeted therapies.

Traditional cytotoxic chemotherapy is based on the principle that cancer is the uncontrolled growth of cells coupled with the hallmarks of malignancy: invasion and metastasis. Traditional cytotoxic chemotherapeutic drugs have direct effects on cell division and/or DNA synthesis preferentially affecting rapidly dividing malignant cells; however, these drugs also have detrimental effects on normal cells that lead to significant toxicity and a narrow therapeutic index. Although cytotoxic chemotherapy is potentially curative for hematologic malignancies, it is palliative for the majority of solid tumors. Therefore, cytotoxic chemotherapy is often combined in multimodal therapy (with radiation therapy and/or surgery) in most circumstances today. The ideal therapeutic agent would be selective for the cancer cells themselves while sparing normal tissues. The concept of using agents to selectively target tumors is not based in modern discovery. Nearly a century earlier a "magic bullet" hypothesis was proposed by Paul Erlich in which he reasoned that if a compound could be made that selectively targeted a disease then a drug could be made to be delivered along with that selective agent that would specifically kill the targeted disease. It was his work in pathology where he visualized the differential affinities of chemical dyes for specific biological structures that he conjectured that

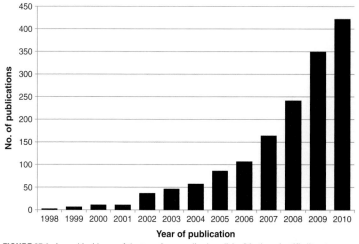

FIGURE 25.1 Annual incidence of the term "personalized medicine" in the scientific literature (PubMed search, May 2010).

the biological effect of a chemical compound depends on its chemical composition and the cell on which it acts. By connecting chemistry with biology and medicine, a century of research and development into targeted chemotherapeutics was inspired.

The three major classes of targeted cancer agents currently in clinical use are small molecule therapies, monoclonal antibodies, and cancer vaccines. Other modalities such as immunomodulatory agents are also being investigated and are considered forms of targeted agents (Table 25.1). Although all targeted cancer therapies behave as "biological agents," this specific term should be reserved for substances made from living organisms (monoclonal antibodies, vaccines, interleukins, etc.). Many of these targeted agents are used in combination with more traditional cytotoxic regimens as well as with radiation therapy and/or surgical extirpation to treat solid tumors. Targets refer to any number of biological molecular compounds including DNA, RNA, proteins, sugar moieties, lipids, receptors, enzymes, and hormones (Fig. 25.2). Nothing provides more compelling validation for the identification of targets in oncology than the emerging knowledge about the genetics of human disease over the last several decades. Therefore, target identification is the most important aspect of targeted oncologic drug development.

TARGETED CANCER DRUG DEVELOPMENT

New oncologic drug development is moving away from the traditional approach of assessing a potential candidate molecule's effect on tumor growth, as most drugs identified in this fashion have demonstrated clear limitations in clinical efficacy. Drug identification now focuses on screening a candidate compound's effects on novel molecular targets or specific pathways and determining whether such effects cause a gain or loss in function that reverses or delays cancer progression. Thus, initial efficacy screening is based on the cancer cell selectivity of a novel target or critical pathway. Ideally, such manipulation of target function would cause a clinically measurable phenotypic change that could be demonstrated throughout

(*text continue on page 621*)

TABLE 25.1 Major Classes of Targeted Cancer Therapies Approved by the U.S. Food and Drug Administration

Generic Drug Name	Trade Name	Type of Therapy	Approved Tumor Types	Mechanism of Action
Signal Transduction Inhibitors				
Cetuximab	Erbitux®	Monoclonal antibody	SCCHN, Metastatic colorectal cancer	EGFR inhibitor
Crizotinib	Xalkori®	Small molecule	EML4-ALK fusion + advanced NSCLC	ALK inhibitor
Dasatinib	Sprycel®	Small molecule	CML, ALL	Multi-TK inhibitor
Erlotinib	Tarceva®	Small molecule	Metastatic NSCLC, Metastatic pancreatic cancer	EGFR/TK inhibitor
Everolimus	Afinitor®	Small molecule	Advanced giant cell astrocytoma, Advanced renal cell cancer Advanced pancreatic neuroendocrine cancer	mTOR inhibitor
Gefitinib	Iressa®	Small molecule	Metastatic NSCLC	EGFR/TK inhibitor
Imatinib mesylate	Gleevec®	Small molecule	GIST, CML, ALL, Dermatofibrosarcoma protuberans, Myeloproliferative disorders	Multi-TK inhibitor
Ipilimumab	Yervoy®	Monoclonal antibody	Metastatic Melanoma	CTLA-4 Inhibitor
Lapatinib	Tykerb®	Small molecule	Metastatic breast cancer	Multi-TK inhibitor
Nilotinib	Tasigna®	Small molecule	CML	Multi-TK inhibitor
Panitumumab	Vectibix®	Monoclonal antibody	Metastatic colorectal cancer	EGFR inhibitor
Temsirolimus	Torisel®	Small molecule	Advanced renal cell cancer	mTOR inhibitor
Trastuzumab	Herceptin®	Monoclonal antibody	HER2+ breast cancer, Metastatic HER2+ gastric/GEJ cancers	HER2 inhibitor
Vemurafenib	Zelboraf	Small molecule	V600E mutation + advanced melanoma	B-raf inhibitor

Epigenetic/Transcriptional Control Agents

Alitretinoin	Panretin®	Small molecule	AIDS-related Kaposi's sarcoma	Retinoic A & X receptor activator
Azacitidine	Vidaza®	Small molecule	Myelodysplastic syndrome	Demethylating agent
Bexarotene	Targretin®	Small molecule	Refractory cutaneous T-cell lymphoma	Retinoic X receptor activator
Romidepsin	Istodax®	Small molecule	Refractory cutaneous T-cell lymphoma	HDAC inhibitor
Tretinoin	Vesanoid®	Small molecule	Acute promyelocytic leukemia	Retinoic receptor activator
Vorinostat	Zolinza®	Small molecule	Refractory cutaneous T-cell lymphoma	HDAC inhibitor

Apoptosis Inducers

Bortezomib	Valcade®	Small molecule	Multiple myeloma, Mantle cell lymphoma	Proteosome inhibitor
Pralatrexate	Folotyn®	Small molecule	Refractory peripheral T-cell lymphoma	DNA synthesis inhibitor

Angiogenesis Inhibitors

Bevacizumab	Avastin®	Monoclonal antibody	Glioblastoma, Metastatic colorectal cancer, Metastatic NSCLC, Advanced renal cell cancer	VEGF inhibitor
Pazotinib	Votrient®	Small molecule	Advanced renal cell cancer	Multi-TK inhibitor
Sorafenib	Nexavar®	Small molecule	Advanced renal cell cancer, Advanced hepatocellular cancer	VEGF/TK inhibitor
Sunitinib	Sutent®	Small molecule	GIST, Metastatic renal cell cancer, Advanced pancreatic neuroendocrine cancer	VEGF/TK inhibitor
Vandetanib	Zactima®	Small molecule	Medullary Thyroid Cancer	VEGF/EGF/Multi-TK Inhibitor

Immunocytotoxic Agents

Alemtuzumab	Campath®	Monoclonal antibody	B-cell chronic lymphocytic leukemia	CD52 inhibitor
Ofatumumab	Arzerra®	Monoclonal antibody	Refractory chronic lymphocytic leukemia	CD20 inhibitor
Rituximab	Rituxan®	Monoclonal antibody	B-cell non-Hodgkin's lymphoma, CLL	CD20 inhibitor

(continued)

TABLE 25.1 Major Classes of Targeted Cancer Therapies Approved by the U.S. Food and Drug Administration[a] (*continued*)

Generic Drug Name	Trade Name	Type of Therapy	Approved Tumor Types	Mechanism of Action
Ligand-Directed Agents				
131I-Tositumomab	Bexxar®	Radiolabeled mono-clonal antibody	Refractory non-Hodgkin's lymphoma	CD20 inhibitor and Iodine-131
Brentuximab vedotin	Adcetris	Monoclonal antibody-drug conjugate	Anaplastic large cell lymphoma and Hodgkin lymphoma	CD30 bound Monomethyl auristatin E
Denileukin Diftitox	Ontak®	Conjugated small molecule	Refractory cutaneous T-cell lymphoma	Interleukin-2 and Diphtheria toxin
Ibritumomab Tiuxetan	Zevalin®	Radiolabeled mono-clonal antibody	Refractory B-cell non-Hodgkin's lymphoma	CD20 inhibitor and Yttrium-90 or Indium-111
Prophylactic Vaccines				
Bivalent human papillomavirus	Cervarix®	Vaccine	Cervical cancer	Immune response to viral antigens
Quadrivalent recombinant human papillomavirus	Gardasil®	Vaccine	Cervical cancer, Vulvar cancer, Vaginal cancer	Immune response to viral antigens
Recombinant hepatitis B surface antigen	—	Vaccine	Hepatocellular cancer	Immune response to viral antigen
Therapeutic Vaccines				
Bacillus Calmette–Guérin	—	Vaccine	Superficial bladder cancer	Local immune response
Sipuleucel-T	Provenge®	Vaccine	Prostate cancer	Immune response to PAP

GIST, gastrointestinal stromal tumor; CML, chronic myelogenous leukemia; ALL, acute lymphoblastic leukemia; TK, tyrosine kinase; HER2, human epidermal growth factor receptor 2; GEJ, gastroesophageal junction; NSCLC, non–small cell lung cancer; EGFR, epidermal growth factor receptor; SCCHN, squamous cell carcinoma of the head and neck; mTOR, mammalian target of rapamycin; HDAC, histone deacetylase; VEGF, vascular endothelial growth factor; PAP, prostatic acid phosphatase.
[a]Data obtained from www.fda.gov/Drugs.

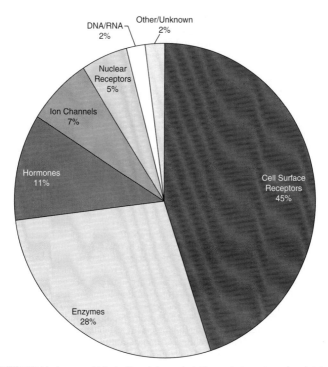

FIGURE 25.2 Most common biological targets in oncologic therapy by percentage of market share.

treatment with validated biomarkers or other functional assays. One of the major factors responsible for failure in modern oncologic therapy is inappropriate target selection; therefore, target identification and validation are critical steps in new targeted oncologic drug discovery. Targets can be either previously established (i.e., targets for which there is lengthy and sound scientific understanding of how the target functions in both normal and malignant physiology) or newly discovered as a result of drug discovery campaigns or basic scientific research and clinical validation. To be pharmaceutically useful, targets need to be "druggable"; that is, targets need to be accessible to potential agents and bind to them in a way that elicits a beneficial biological effect.

There are two major approaches to target identification: a systems approach and a molecular approach. A systems approach to target identification includes obtaining information about potential new targets from clinical trials and in vivo animal model studies. Although systems approaches lead to most clinically pertinent discoveries, the methodology is too protracted to facilitate the rapid identification of targets needed in oncological drug discovery. Therefore, the majority of current target discovery strategies utilize a molecular approach to identify potential new targets by mining the scientific literature of genomic, microarray, and proteomic databases. Such methods enable a large number of potentially significant compounds to be rapidly screened and identified. Targeted drug discovery and development are resource-intensive, and only a small fraction of compounds investigated for use in humans are eventually approved. Due to the significant cost and time needed to discover, develop, and obtain approval for pharmaceuticals, most new, approved targeted oncologic drugs are based on reformulations of existing active compounds.

All targeted therapies undergoing development go through similar stages: target identification; lead drug identification and formulation; candidate drug preclinical toxicity testing; pharmacokinetic/pharmacodynamic studies and preclinical efficacy testing in animal models; phase I dosing studies and target efficacy testing; and subsequent initial phase II and larger phase III trials. All of these stages depend on several prerequisites: that a target exists and can be identified, that a drug can be synthesized to affect that target, that the synthesized drug can be optimized for potency and limited toxicity, and that the drug effects on the target can be monitored with simple minimally invasive testing. The goal in the first stage of drug development, target identification, is to identify a target for a potential therapy. As all malignancies have developed multiple mutations, a multitude of potential targets exist for an individual patient and his or her malignancy. The focus in the second stage, lead identification, is to identify a chemical class of compounds (a "lead") that will interact with a target in a way that potentially impacts the disease studied. Using high-throughput analytical chemistry screening of large proprietary chemical libraries obtained from third-party suppliers or synthesized directly, hundreds to thousands of candidate compounds are tested, usually by means of binding assays that examine chemical similarity and potency, for their ability to modify the target. In the third stage of drug development, lead optimization, researchers chemically modify the structure of the lead for more precise and specific binding affinity. The fourth stage of drug development, candidate nomination, is used to identify a candidate drug that meets pre-established criteria for preclinical toxicity testing and pharmaceutical formulation studies. Once a candidate drug has passed the rigors of the initial preclinical analysis and gathered enough scientific merit for further development as an investigational new drug, clinical testing of this novel agent ensues. Targeted cancer therapies are the largest and fastest growing class of cancer drugs in terms of sales due to the decreased growth of revenues from traditional cytotoxic therapies, as a result of patent expiration, and a shift of focus toward the molecular targeted cancer market. Thus, a reasonable understanding of the mechanisms and uses of these agents is a requisite for all surgical oncologists.

SMALL MOLECULE TARGETED THERAPY

Among the most actively developed and utilized drugs are the small molecule therapies. Small molecule targeted therapies typically block the growth, invasion, and metastasis of specific malignancies by directly interfering with enzymes, specific receptors, or other molecules involved in tumor growth and progression; however, they can also act as mimetics and activate certain anticancer pathways such as apoptosis. By directly targeting the molecular mechanisms and cellular components that are specifically responsible for tumor growth, these agents promise improved efficacy over other traditional types of treatment and are potentially less toxic to normal tissues. Small molecule agents can translocate through plasma membranes and interact with the cytoplasmic domain of cell surface receptors and intracellular signaling molecules. For example, various small molecule inhibitors have been generated to target cancer-cell proliferation and survival pathways such as Ras, MEK, PI3K, mTOR, Src, and VEGF. Small molecule therapies are developed to be as monospecific as possible to avoid the detrimental side effects that typically manifest with traditional nonspecific therapies. However, small molecule therapies are generally thought to be less specific for certain molecular targets. Although this lower specificity may lead to exacerbated and often unexpected toxicities, it is also potentially advantageous because it may enable these agents to inhibit several signaling pathways involved in the cancer process at once. The adverse effects generally associated with small molecule agents are typically mild and usually consist of cutaneous (rash, acne, dry skin, and pruritus) or gastrointestinal (diarrhea, nausea, vomiting, and anorexia) manifestations. Compared to traditional cytotoxic chemotherapy, small molecule agents are typically less expensive and more convenient to administer because many are available as oral agents. Small molecule agents are typically taken daily because of their short half-life. Most of the small molecule agents approved by the U.S. Food and Drug Administration (FDA) are used for the treatment of solid tumors; although some of the small molecule agents are indicated for the treatment of hematological malignancies.

Small molecule targeted therapies represent a highly profitable class of anticancer therapies for major pharmaceutical companies as they have been approved for various tumor types. The promise of extraordinary financial rewards has driven the considerable pipeline activity for small molecule targeted therapies within oncologic drug development in recent years. The examination of the small molecule targeted cancer therapies within phase III trials offers significant insight into how rapid this new wave of personalized oncology is developing. Several hundred small molecule targeted therapies are currently in development for cancer, with more than 50 currently being investigated in formal clinical trials. The majority of these agents target G-protein-coupled receptors and protein kinases with single-target signal transduction inhibitors and/or multitargeted inhibitors accounting for more than 25% of the pipeline, respectively. These two classes each contain a number of agents with novel mechanisms of action. The protein kinases that have been targeted most intensively for drug development are plasma membrane-associated protein tyrosine kinases, along with peptide mimetics and antisense oligonucleotides.

As critical signaling molecules, protein tyrosine kinases have proven to be excellent targets for small molecule inhibitors that compete with ATP (adenosine triphosphate) and inhibit kinase activity and have emerged as indispensable for studying targeted therapy. Researchers continue to develop other small molecule kinase inhibitors against other kinases that are more selective and capable of overcoming the drug resistance of initial candidate compounds. Over 50 distinct targets are currently being tested in phase I clinical trials. Most small molecule inhibitors of tyrosine kinases are ATP mimetics. For example, imatinib mesylate (Gleevec, Novartis AG, Basel, CH), which in 2002 became one of the first successful small molecule inhibitors to be approved for cancer treatment, inactivates the kinase activity of the BCR–ABL oncogene fusion protein and has shown remarkable efficacy in the treatment of patients with Philadelphia chromosome-positive chronic myelogenous leukemia. Imatinib mesylate is also a multitarget inhibitor of other tyrosine kinases such as c-KIT and PDGFR (platelet-derived growth factor receptor), which are found in most gastrointestinal stromal tumors, glioblastomas, and dermatofibrosarcoma protuberans tumors. Due to the pluripotent nature of inhibition of these agents, the small molecule inhibitors of tyrosine kinase have been found to be useful in a variety of malignancies. As a result, other tyrosine kinase inhibitors targeting the VEGF and PDGFR receptors have been developed. Sorafenib (Nexavar, Bayer AG, Leverkusen, DE) and sunitinib (Sutent, Pfizer, New York, NY) were approved in 2005 and 2006, respectively, for the treatment of gastrointestinal stromal tumors and renal cell carcinoma with sorafenib also being approved for advanced hepatocellular carcinoma in 2007. The FDA recently approved epidermal growth factor receptor (EGFR) inhibitors such as gefitinib (Iressa, AstraZeneca,

Paddington, UK) for non–small cell lung cancer and erlotinib (Tarceva, Genentech, San Francisco, CA) for non–small cell lung cancer and pancreatic cancer. These particular drugs highlight the modern personalized approach to oncology. With the clinical availability of EGFR testing, these agents can be used selectively in patients whose tumors will most likely have a response, thus fulfilling the goal of personalized targeted therapy.

Several small molecule inhibitors have essentially completely changed the paradigm of treatment for several solid tumors, specifically GIST and pancreatic neuroendocrine cancers. Imatinib has served as the hallmark example of the exciting possibilities that targeted cancer therapies can offer. The introduction of this agent has prompted revision of the management algorithms that have traditionally guided the treatment of these tumors. Historically, even after a complete oncologic surgical resection, the vast majority of patients would relapse leading to markedly limited long-term survival. With current therapy using this potent small molecule inhibitor against the KIT protein–tyrosine kinase which is constitutively activated in more than 90% of these tumors (and to a lesser extent the inhibition of platelet-derived growth factor receptor alpha-tyrosine kinase—another target of imatinib identified in a small subset of GIST tumors), imatinib has been shown to induce significant responses and/or stabilization of disease in a large proportion of patients studied in clinical trials. Furthermore, the dramatic responses seen have led to new evidence-based guidelines recommending this agent as first-line therapy in borderline resectable disease to improve resectability as well as its use in the adjuvant postoperative setting to minimize recurrence. As a result, a multidisciplinary treatment of this disease has emerged which has led to changes in sequencing strategy for each therapeutic intervention (i.e., surgery first vs. targeted therapy first). Similar changes in treatment paradigms are also now being investigated for other tumor types. For example, everolimus (Afinitor, Novartis) has recently (2011) received FDA approval for advanced pancreatic neuroendocrine cancers, based on treatment with this targeted agent showing significant improvements in progression-free survival compared to placebo. Traditional therapies have had essentially no efficacy for this malignancy and the introduction of this agent will certainly alter the management and course of this disease.

Several malignancies are thought to be due in part to epigenetic mechanisms such as transcriptional gene silencing. Epigenetic changes, which are changes in gene expression without associated changes in DNA structure, are potentially reversible. As a result, there is significant interest in identifying compounds that have selective effects on transcriptional control in cancer. DNA demethylating agents that can re-express genes that have been silenced by hypermethylation have been recently identified as intriguing candidate compounds. When given to patients at low doses, DNA demethylating agents exhibit significant antitumor activity. The FDA has approved the use of two such agents, azacytidine (Vidaza, Celgene, Summit, NJ) and decitabine (Dacogen, Eisai, Tokyo, Japan), as elective treatments for myelodysplastic syndrome. Histone deacetylase (HDAC) inhibitors constitute another promising group of epigenetic agents. Cells must control the coiling and uncoiling of DNA around histones in order to effect gene expression which is accomplished with the assistance of histone acetylases (leading to transcriptionally active chromatin) and histone deacetylases (leading to transcriptionally silenced chromatin). As one of the major epigenetic mechanisms for controlling gene expression, HDAC inhibitors result in hyperacetylation of histones, thereby affecting gene expression that has been shown to induce differentiation, cell cycle arrest, and apoptosis. However, the pleiotropic nature of HDAC inhibitors raises the possibility that their antitumor abilities are accompanied by other, less desirable effects as nonhistone proteins such as transcription factors which are also targets for acetylation with varying functional effects. However, many phase I clinical trials have indicated that HDAC inhibitors are well tolerated. The first drugs of this type, vorinostat (Zolinza, Patheon, Research Triangle Park, NC) and romidepsin (Istodax, Celgene), have been approved in 2006 and 2009, respectively, for the treatment of cutaneous T-cell lymphoma. Several other compounds of this type are currently in early phase clinical development as potential treatments for solid and hematological cancers both as monotherapy and in combination with traditional cytotoxic agents.

MONOCLONAL ANTIBODY THERAPY

Molecularly targeted therapies account for the three leading anticancer brands; as a result, drug developers have tried to capitalize on the success of this class of therapy by incorporating these targeted biological agents into their pipelines. Currently, there are over 100 biological targeted therapies in development for cancer, and immunologic agents (monoclonal antibodies specifically) represent the majority of these therapies. Monoclonal antibodies have benefited from higher initial approval success rates than other new chemical entities including small molecule agents in the field of oncology. More than 50% of the therapeutic monoclonal antibodies that have entered commercially sponsored clinical development are indicated for cancer treatment.

Many tumor cells express unusual antigens that are inappropriate for the cell type or its environment or that are normally present only during fetal development. Cancer cells display cell surface receptors that are rare or absent on the surfaces of healthy cells, and many of these cell surface receptors are responsible for activating cellular signal transduction pathways that cause unregulated growth and division. For example, ErbB2 is a constitutively active cell surface receptor that is produced at abnormally high levels in approximately 30% of breast cancers (known as human epidermal growth factor receptor 2 (HER2)-positive breast cancer).

Monoclonal antibodies, which target tumor-associated antigens, are a form of passive immunotherapy. Tumor antigens are derived from self-proteins that are either mutated or otherwise differentially expressed in normal and tumor cells. The advent of hybridoma technology enabled the production of monoclonal antibodies. Initial therapeutic antibodies were simple murine analogues resulting in these initial monoclonal antibodies being highly immunogenic in humans. Additionally, they had a short half-life due to immune complex formation, limited penetration to tumor sites, and displayed inadequate induction of immune effector responses in humans. This limited their clinical applicability. Significant advances in antibody engineering led to the development of chimeric, humanized and fully human monoclonal antibodies that remedied many of these initial problems. Recombinant DNA technology, transgenic mice and phage display have replaced hybridoma technology. There are four major types of monoclonal antibodies: murine (-omab), chimeric (-ximab), humanized (-zumab), and human (-mumab). Antibodies are categorized into five classes based on the sequence of constant regions of their heavy chain: IgM, IgD, IgG, IgE, and IgA. These classes are based on the sequence of the constant regions of their heavy chain. Within these chains are constant and variable regions. The constant region, which constitutes the Fc (fragment, crystallizable) domain, ensures that each antibody generates an appropriate immune response for a given antigen by binding to a specific class of Fc receptors and other immune molecules such as complement proteins. Antibodies are linked to immune effector functions by the Fc fragment. The variable regions, which constitute the Fab (fragment, antigen binding) domain, allow antigen specificity. IgG, composed of two heavy and two light chains, is the antibody most frequently used for biological cancer therapy. The putative mechanisms of monoclonal antibody-based cancer therapy can be classified as direct or indirect. Monoclonal antibody therapy has direct effects on tumor cells by blocking the function (e.g., ligand binding, cell cycle progression, DNA repair, angiogenesis, receptor internalization, and proteolytic cleavage of receptors) or stimulating the function (e.g., apoptosis) of their targeted signaling molecules or receptors. The indirect action of monoclonal antibodies is mediated by the immune system and is dependent on Ig-mediated mechanisms to activate immune-effector function, including complement-dependent cytotoxicity and antibody-dependent cellular cytotoxicity.

Monoclonal antibodies are usually well tolerated by cancer patients. Most of the observed adverse effects are mild and similar to those associated with small molecule therapies, including dermatological manifestations (acne, rash, dry skin, and pruritus). Infusion-related manifestations (fever, chill, and asthenia) are also seen. Monoclonal antibodies have none of the bone marrow-suppressive properties of cytotoxic chemotherapy. Monoclonal antibodies are larger than small molecule agents and are administered intravenously. Because of their size, mono-clonal antibodies do not cross the blood–brain barrier; however, they can be administered intratumorally to treat lesions in the central nervous system. Mono-clonal antibodies cannot pass through the cellular membrane and thus can act only on molecules that are expressed on the cell surface. The major advantage of thera-peutic monoclonal antibodies in cancer treatment is dependent on their ability to bind antigens expressed on the tumor cell surface with a highly specific selectivity, and this antigen-binding affinity is associated with the biological potency of these agents.

Some of the most effective monoclonal antibodies are used to treat hemato-logical cancers. In 1997, the first therapeutic antibody, rituximab (Rituxan, Genentech), was approved by the FDA for the treatment of B-cell non-Hodgkin's lymphoma. Rituximab targets the CD20 surface antigen, which is found on most B-cell lymphomas. CD20 is securely anchored in the cell membrane, where it is protected from antigen loss. Anti-CD20 antibodies such as rituximab affect the regulation of the cell cycle and induce a number of signaling events that lead to the induction of apoptosis. Anti-CD20 antibodies may also indirectly inhibit tumor growth and progression by inducing complement-dependent cytotoxicity and antibody-dependent cellular cytotoxicity. Since the introduction of ritux-imab, other monoclonal antibodies have become standard first- and second-line therapies for a number of hematological malignancies, and some monoclonal antibodies are now used to treat solid tumors. In 1998, the FDA approved trastu-zumab (Herceptin, Genentech), a genetically engineered monoclonal antibody that inhibits the proliferation of HER2+ tumor cells, for use in patients with met-astatic breast cancer. This agent has enjoyed marked clinical success for several HER2+ malignancies including breast as well as in HER2+ subsets of gastric cancer.

Another promising approach to treating solid tumors is to target the tumor microenvironment, in particular the endothelium of tumor blood vessels. Treat-ment with a monoclonal antibody targeting VEGF, a key mediator of tumor angio-genesis, can dramatically suppresses tumor growth. Bevacizumab (Avastin, Genentech), a humanized variant of an anti-VEGF antibody, was approved as a first-line treatment for patients with metastatic colorectal cancer in 2004. Block-ing angiogenesis is an effective strategy for treating cancers, can be used in vari-ous tumor types and settings, and has minimal toxic effects on normal tissue. However, these antiangiogenic agents should be used with some caution as they have been associated with specific adverse events that include gastrointestinal perforation, fistula formation, delayed wound healing, hemorrhage, and arterial thromboembolic events. Antiangiogenic therapies have become a fixture in oncology. As an example, Bevacizumab (Avastin, Genentech), is the top-selling molecularly targeted cancer therapy brand, and will most likely remain a leading drug over the next decade due to indication expansion across a number of tumor types.

As most cancer cells share the majority of common features with the normal host cells from which they are derived, the high levels of selective toxicity needed cannot be achieved with traditional anticancer chemotherapeutics without increased toxicities against normal tissue. As a result, often suboptimal doses of cytotoxic cancer chemotherapeutics are administered resulting in failure of therapy, development of drug resistance, and ultimately metastatic disease and death. The selective toxicity of an anticancer drug can be increased either by increasing the amount of the drug that reaches the cancer tissue or by decreasing the concentration of drug that normal tissues are exposed to. Ligand-directed therapy, which enables tumor specificity and limits toxicity to normal tissue, shows promise against cancers. Ligand-directed therapy can deliver higher doses of a drug to the tumor tissue and may overcome obstacles presented by cytotoxic chemotherapy. Monoclonal antibodies can be conjugated with toxins, radioisotopes, cytokines, DNA molecules, or even small molecule agents to selectively target tumor cells while limiting normal tissue toxicity. Several ligand-directed monoclonal antibodies bound to either radiation sources or toxins such as tositumomab/I 131 (Bexxar, GlaxoSmithKline, London, UK), ibritumomab tiuxetan (Zevalin, Spectrum Pharmaceuticals, Irvine, CA), and denileukin diftitox (Ontak, Ligand Pharmaceuticals, Lenexa, KS) have been approved by the FDA for follicular lymphoma, B-cell lymphoma, and cutaneous T-cell lymphoma, respectively.

CANCER VACCINE THERAPY

The successful treatment of cancer patients with monoclonal antibodies has spawned various other forms of promising biologic therapies. Immunotherapeutics are biologically targeted agents that take advantage of a patient's innate tumor response through the use of cancer vaccines and other immunomodulatory agents. The identification of tumor-specific antigens, tumor-specific lymphocytes, and tumor-specific T-cell responses in cancer patients led to the development of immunotherapies aimed at augmenting antitumor immune responses. Innumerable innate and adaptive immune effector cells and molecules participate in the recognition and destruction of cells that have undergone malignant transformation, a process that is known as cancer immunosurveillance. However, cancer cells avoid such immunosurveillance mechanisms through the outgrowth of poorly immunogenic tumor cell variants and through immunosubversion. At the time most human cancers are diagnosed, tolerogenic signals outweigh immunogenic signals mainly because of tumor-induced suppression. Tumor cells can evade the immune system through the downregulation of major histocompatibility complex class molecules and cellular components involved in the antigen processing and presentation machinery, as well as through the secretion of inhibitor cytokines and the expression of coinhibitory molecules.

Cancer vaccines are a form of active immunotherapy; they are meant to trigger the patients' innate immune response to fight cancer. Cancer vaccines target one or more specific tumor antigens. Various forms of vaccines have been utilized, including irradiated tumor cells, tumor cell extracts, and tumor proteins or antigens expressed in naked plasmids or viral vectors. Much of the initial work in cancer vaccine therapy was performed in melanoma, which is the most immunogenic solid malignancy. As subset of melanomas are diagnosed as metastatic lesions with no evidence of a primary tumor, suggesting that local immune effector functions lead to the regression of primary melanomas. There are two broad types of cancer vaccines: preventive (or prophylactic) vaccines, which are intended to prevent cancer from developing in otherwise healthy people; and treatment (or therapeutic) vaccines, which are intended to treat existing cancers. In 1981, the FDA approved the hepatitis B vaccine that protects against chronic HBV infection. Chronic HBV infection can lead to hepatocellular cancer, making this the first cancer preventive vaccine to be successfully developed and marketed. The next prophylactic cancer vaccine was not approved until 2006, when the FDA approved the Human Papillomavirus (HPV) quadrivalent vaccine (Gardasil, Merck, Whitehouse Station, NJ), which protects against infection by two subtypes of HPV (16 and 18), that cause approximately 70% of all cases of cervical cancers worldwide. In 2008, the FDA expanded this approval to include its use in the prevention of HPV-associated vulvar and vaginal cancers. Unlike traditional vaccines, which are often typically composed of weakened, whole microbes, the viral tumor antigens used for the HPV vaccine are not infectious, but still are sufficiently immunogenic enough to be able to stimulate the production of antibodies.

The initial proof-of-concept of using cancer vaccines for therapeutic indications involved the use of the Bacillus Calmette–Guérin (BCG) tuberculosis vaccine for the topical treatment of bladder carcinoma. Currently, BCG vaccine therapy is the only FDA-approved agent for the primary therapy treatment of in situ bladder cancer and has replaced cystectomy as the initial treatment of choice in most patients. More recently another therapeutic cancer vaccine is sipuleucel-T (Provenge, Dendreon, Seattle, WA), which was approved for the treatment of asymptomatic or minimally symptomatic metastatic, castrate-resistant (hormone refractory) prostate cancer in 2010. The vaccine is generated by culturing patients' autologous peripheral blood mononuclear cells with a recombinant fusion protein containing granulocyte macrophage colony stimulating factor and the prostate tumor-antigen, prostatic acid phosphatase. Sipuleucel-T is not curative but has been found in trials to lead to prolonged survival compared to placebo.

Although vaccines have been successful in the induction of protective immunity to pathogenic microorganisms due to the immune recognition of foreign antigens expressed by these pathogens, the fact that cancer cells arise from one's own tissue poses a significant challenge for cancer immunotherapy. Two significant biological obstacles that limit the efficacy of cancer vaccines are the strength of immunological tolerance and the intrinsic limitations on the ability of the immune effector cells to expand in number in response to antigenic stimulation. There are strict biological limits imposed on the immune system to prevent excessive immune effector cell activation and expansion, and these same biological restrictions limit cancer vaccines. Immunotherapeutic agents that can circumvent many of the biological restrictions have been invented and formulated and proven to be biologically active, including dendritic cell activators and growth factors, vaccine adjuvants, T-cell stimulators and growth factors, genetically modified T-cells, immune checkpoint inhibitors, and agents to neutralize or inhibit suppressive cells, cytokines, and enzymes. Tumor antigens, most of which are shared by normal cells and perceived by the immune system, typically evoke weak immune responses because tolerance prevents generation of immune responses to normal cells. Mutated tumor antigens are the only truly unique antigens, and these are strongly immunogenic, and elicit robust immune responses, and have been the focus of most cancer vaccine development. However, only a handful of such mutated tumor antigens are currently known. In this context, cancer can be viewed as an autoimmune phenomenon in which tolerance to self prevents effective immune responses to tumor antigen. The development of a prioritized list of cancer vaccine target antigens, using well-vetted criteria generated by expert panels, is currently in progress. The elucidation and weighting of criteria to assess cancer antigens will assist investigators in the immunotherapy field in determining the characteristics and the experimental data required to select the most promising antigens for further development and testing as vaccines in clinical trials.

Despite the large number of preclinical studies and ongoing clinical trials investigating tumor antigens as anticancer vaccines, few clinical data exist regarding the actual capacity of anticancer vaccines to induce effective antitumor activity are available. In clinical trials, serologically effective vaccines have stimulated high-frequency, high-avidity T-cell responses but ultimately failed to control tumor growth. The use of vaccine adjuncts such as granulocyte macrophage colony stimulating factor to recruit dendritic cells and high-dose interleukin-2 or the incorporation of dendritic cells themselves into vaccine constructs may provide the immunological impetus necessary to overcome the baseline tumor immunosuppressive activity and initiate a successful antitumor response. As cancer vaccines typically fail in patients with heavy tumor burdens, they should be reserved for patients with early or minimal residual disease or used as an adjuvant therapy following surgical resection or debulking and only in the setting of a clinical trial.

FUTURE DIRECTIONS IN TARGETED CANCER THERAPY

Targeted approaches to cancer therapy are continuing to evolve. Whether these approaches utilize small molecule agents, monoclonal antibodies, or cancer vaccines will be determined by the specificity of the targets identified. However, the major challenge with targeted approaches is biological. Tumor instability, which can lead to therapy resistance, is the Achilles' heel of targeted therapy. Thus, today's therapeutic oncologic target is tomorrow's resistant mutant. Because it is unclear whether tumors will develop resistance to small molecule agents, monoclonal antibodies, or cancer vaccines, it is also unknown whether these targeted therapies will have lasting effects. However, the recent clinical successes of these targeted therapies have established them as the cornerstone of modern cancer treatment. The simultaneous use of multiple distinct classes of agents that target one specific pathway could be thought of as one of the promising strategies for maximally inhibiting target molecules and overcoming the limitations of and resistance inherent to any single blockade. As the oncogenic progression in most cancers is a multistep process, and molecular pathogenesis is not linked to the defect of a single target, the initial promise of single targeted therapy seems at least theoretically to be an ineffective and adverse strategy and cannot be expected to yield optimal outcomes. Therefore, the use of multitargeted therapies, which overcome issues of tumor heterogeneity while maintaining the selectivity of treatment and minimizing resistance, is most likely the strategy for cancer treatment in the immediate future. Targeted cancer therapy has significantly changed the way many cancer patients are currently treated. In addition to serological biomarker evaluation, molecular profiling is now incorporated into the baseline histological assessment of many patients' cancers. The short-term, intermittent intravenous administration of traditional high-dose cytotoxic chemotherapy is being replaced with the long-term, continuous oral administration of low-dose targeted therapies. While the traditional oncological endpoints (response and survival rates) remain, biomarkers are being developed to assess treatment, and treatment is increasingly aimed at achieving metabolic and functional stability rather than anatomic stability. The ultimate goal of cancer therapy is also changing, moving from disease eradication to disease control. More patients are living longer in a pharmacological homeostasis with their cancers.

The implementation of personalized cancer therapy will require dramatic reform, including, but not limited to, changes in: health care infrastructure;

diagnostic and therapeutic business models; reimbursement policies from government and private payers; and regulatory oversight. It will also rely on electronic medical records, tissue banks, biodatabases, and additional affiliations between major academic cancer centers, pharmaceutical industries, and local health care providers. The future of health care administration must embrace personalized cancer therapy as an integrated, coordinated, evidence-based approach to individualizing cancer patient care. As a result of this potential health care model shift, we are seeing significant changes in occurring in health care policies.

Simply defined, personalized medicine is the use of information from genomes and their derivatives to guide medical decision-making. Because autopsy studies show the actual incidence of cancer to be far greater than that reported in life, we must consider and question the utility of using genetic data to predict the likelihood of a future malignancy. Furthermore, other than the few previously mentioned prophylactic vaccines, therapeutic interventions have not been shown to be effective for the majority of malignancies. As more genetic data are generated and with this information, now freely available electronically, significant medical, legal, and ethical implications have arisen. As a direct result of these rapid developments, the Genetic Information Non-Discrimination Act (GINA) passed into law in 2008, prohibits discrimination on the basis of genetic information with respect to health insurance and employment. Additional important legislation in the Genomic and Personalized Medicine Act of 2007, which did not make it through initial congressional approval aimed to create the necessary resources and integrate government stakeholders to advance and regulate this new field of medicine. The last decade has experienced a steady embrace of personalized medicine by senior government officials, industry leadership, health care providers, and the public. It is now appropriate to reflect on and summarize the achievements and advances that have been made to reach the lofty goals inherent in the term "personalized medicine." The stated aim of the Genomics and Personalized Medicine Act is "To secure the promise of personalized medicine for all Americans by expanding and accelerating genomics research and initiatives to improve the accuracy of disease diagnosis, increase the safety of drugs, and identify novel treatments, and for other purposes." Interestingly, the new bill that has been put forth for pending congressional debate and discussion is the first iteration to formally define the term "personalized medicine." However, the bill limits its definition of "personalized medicine" to "any clinical practice model that emphasizes the systematic use of preventive, diagnostic, and therapeutic interventions that use genome and family history information to improve health outcomes." It also calls for the creation of an Office of Personalized Healthcare and several committees to address translational challenges of personalized medicine, the standardization of the collection of human biological samples, the funding of further research and education on personalized medicine, and the creation of a national biobank. As a result of these extraordinary changes in medicine, oncology, and health care policy, treating physicians need to be at the center of this discussion involved in both the scientific as well as the political aspects in order to assist and guide us into this new realm of personalized targeted oncology.

Recommended Readings

Arora A, Scholar EM. Role of tyrosine kinase inhibitors in cancer therapy. *J Pharmacol Exp Ther.* 2005;315:971–979.

Barr E, Sings HL. Prophylactic HPV vaccines: new interventions for cancer control. *Vaccine.* 2008;26:6244–6257.

Bishton M, Kenealy M, Johnstone R, et al. Epigenetic targets in hematological malignancies: combination therapies with HDACs and demethylating agents. *Expert Rev Anticancer Ther.* 2007;7:1439–1449.

Buchdunger E, O'Reilly T, Wood J. Pharmacology of imatinib (STI571). *Eur J Cancer.* 2002;38(suppl 5):S28–S36.

Cheever MA, Allison JP, Ferris AS, et al. The prioritization of cancer antigens: a national cancer institute pilot project for the acceleration of translational research. *Clin Cancer Res.* 2009;15:5323–5337.

Demidem A, Lam T, Alas S, et al. Chimeric anti-CD20 (IDEC-C2B8) monoclonal antibody sensitizes a B cell lymphoma cell line to cell killing by cytotoxic drugs. *Cancer Biother Radiopharm.* 1997;12:177–186.

Druker BJ. STI571 (Gleevec) as a paradigm for cancer therapy. *Trends Mol Med.* 2002; 8:S14–S18.

Dunkelberger JR, Song WC. Complement and its role in innate and adaptive immune responses. *Cell Res.* 2010;20:34–50.

Dunn GP, Bruce AT, Ikeda H, et al. Cancer immunoediting: from immunosurveillance to tumor escape. *Nat Immunol.* 2002;3:991–998.

Dunn GP, Old LJ, Schreiber RD. The immunobiology of cancer immunosurveillance and immunoediting. *Immunity.* 2004;21:137–148.

Esteller M. Cancer epigenomics: DNA methylomes and histone-modification maps. *Nat Rev Genet.* 2007;8:286–298.

Garland SM, Hernandez-Avila M, Wheeler CM, et al. Quadrivalent vaccine against human papillomavirus to prevent anogenital diseases. *N Engl J Med.* 2007;356: 1928–1943.

Goodman VL, Rock EP, Dagher R, et al. Approval summary: sunitinib for the treatment of imatinib refractory or intolerant gastrointestinal stromal tumors and advanced renal cell carcinoma. *Clin Cancer Res.* 2007;13:1367–1373.

Grillo-Lopez AJ, Hedrick E, Rashford M, et al. Rituximab: ongoing and future clinical development. *Semin Oncol.* 2002;29:105–112.

H.R.5440—Genomics and Personalized Medicine Act. 2011. Available at: http://www.opencongress.org/bill/111-h5440. Accessed May 11, 2011.

Harari D, Yarden Y. Molecular mechanisms underlying ErbB2/HER2 action in breast cancer. *Oncogene.* 2000;19:6102–6114.

Hersey P. Immunotherapy of melanoma. *Asia Pac J Clin Oncol.* 2010;6(suppl 1):S2–S8.

Higano CS, Schellhammer PF, Small EJ, et al. Integrated data from 2 randomized, double-blind, placebo-controlled, phase 3 trials of active cellular immunotherapy with sipuleucel-T in advanced prostate cancer. *Cancer.* 2009;115:3670–3679.

Hogquist KA, Baldwin TA, Jameson SC. Central tolerance: learning self-control in the thymus. *Nat Rev Immunol.* 2005;5:772–782.

Hurwitz H, Fehrenbacher L, Novotny W, et al. Bevacizumab plus irinotecan, fluorouracil, and leucovorin for metastatic colorectal cancer. *N Engl J Med.* 2004;350:2335–2342.

Jiang S, ed. *Regulatory T Cells and Clinical Application.* London: Springer; 2008.

Kaminskas E, Farrell A, Abraham S, et al. Approval summary: azacitidine for treatment of myelodysplastic syndrome subtypes. *Clin Cancer Res.* 2005;11: 3604–3608.

Kohler G, Milstein C. Continuous cultures of fused cells secreting antibody of predefined specificity. *Nature.* 1975;256:495–497.

Lamm DL. Optimal BCG treatment of superficial bladder cancer as defined by American trials. *Eur Urol.* 1992;21(suppl 2):12–16.

Langreth R, Waldholz M. New era of personalized medicine: targeting drugs for each unique genetic profile. *Oncologist.* 1999; 4:426–427.

Morton DL, Malmgren RA, Holmes EC, et al. Demonstration of antibodies against human malignant melanoma by immunofluorescence. *Surgery.* 1968;64:233–240.

Mukherji B, Chakraborty NG, Sivanandham M. T-cell clones that react against autologous human tumors. *Immunol Rev.* 1990; 116:33–62.

Ollila DW, Kelley MC, Gammon G, et al. Overview of melanoma vaccines: active specific immunotherapy for melanoma patients. *Semin Surg Oncol.* 1998;14:328–336.

Pietras RJ, Fendly BM, Chazin VR, et al. Antibody to HER-2/neu receptor blocks DNA repair after cisplatin in human breast and ovarian cancer cells. *Oncogene.* 1994;9:1829–1838.

Reichert JM, Rosensweig CJ, Faden LB, et al. Monoclonal antibody successes in the clinic. *Nat Biotechnol.* 2005;23:1073–1078.

Senger DR, Van de Water L, Brown LF, et al. Vascular permeability factor (VPF, VEGF) in tumor biology. *Cancer Metastasis Rev.* 1993;12:303–324.

Weiner LM, Dhodapkar MV, Ferrone S. Monoclonal antibodies for cancer immunotherapy. *Lancet.* 2009;373:1033–1040.

Whiteside TL. Immune responses to malignancies. *J Allergy Clin Immunol.* 2010; 125:S272–S283.

Yang Y, Adelstein SJ, Kassis AI. Target discovery from data mining approaches. *Drug Discov Today.* 2009;14:147–154.

Yao JC, Shah MH, Tetsuhide I, et al. Everolimus for advanced pancreatic neuroendocrine tumors. *N Engl J Med.* 2011; 364:514.

Zhao L, Liu Z, Fan D. Overview of mimotopes and related strategies in tumor vaccine development. *Expert Rev Vaccines.* 2008; 7:1547–1555.

Zitvogel L, Tesniere A, Kroemer G. Cancer despite immunosurveillance: immunoselection and immunosubversion. *Nat Rev Immunol.* 2006;6:715–727.

26 Pharmacotherapy of Cancer

Andrea Landgraf Oholendt

A basic understanding of cancer pharmacotherapy and related toxicities is mandatory for the full integration of the surgical oncologist into a multidisciplinary cancer care program. To intelligently discuss surgical options with patients, knowledge of the available treatment regimens and their potential for toxicity is essential.

This chapter includes a discussion of basic principles of chemotherapy, an overview of the mechanisms of drug action and drug resistance, a tabular listing of the drugs available and their common toxicities, and a tabular listing of approved biological agents used in oncology. Finally, a summary of cancer pain management and the treatment of chemotherapy-induced emesis (CIE) is included.

The reader should be aware that a complete discussion of cancer chemotherapy is beyond the scope of this brief overview. The drug and dosage regimens listed are representative examples only and do not constitute a listing of all available protocols. For specific prescribing information, the practitioner is advised to consult individual manufacturer package inserts or one of the referenced texts.

BASIC PRINCIPLES OF CHEMOTHERAPY

Cancer chemotherapeutic agents are the result of drug design and, largely, empiricism. Their use has been developed based on an understanding of tumor growth characteristics, the cell cycle, drug mechanisms of action, and drug resistance. It is hoped that new techniques and advances in molecular biology will allow improvements in drug design to extend the possibility of complete chemotherapeutic response and possibly the cure of patients currently deemed beyond salvage.

Tumor Growth and Kinetics

Kinetic aspects of tumor growth have been well described. Two concepts that underscore our knowledge of the kinetics of tumor growth are Skipper laws and Gompertzian growth. Skipper laws apply to cells in the proliferating compartment of a tumor. First, the doubling time of proliferating cells is constant, creating a straight line on a semilog plot. Second, cell kill by a particular drug at a given dose is constant, irrespective of body burden. In most solid tumors, however, only a portion of cells within the tumor—the growth fraction—is proliferating at any given time. This partially accounts for the refractory nature of many solid tumors to chemotherapy.

Human tumors follow a pattern of Gompertzian, rather than straight line, growth. Gompertzian growth describes a cell population decreasing as a result of cell death and increasing because of proliferation. Also, cell subpopulations may have ceased to proliferate but have not died, further swaying the growth curve from a straight semilog plot. The normal Gompertzian growth curve is sigmoid in shape. Maximum tumor growth rate occurs at approximately 30% of maximum tumor volume, where nutrient and oxygen supply to the greatest number of tumor cells is optimized. This portion of the curve is also where drug efficacy against a particular tumor may best be estimated.

The cell cycle is an important fundamental concept to understand when designing chemotherapeutic agents and treatment regimens. The cell cycle is divided into five components. The resting or nonproliferating cell is in the G0 phase. Upon entering the active portion of the cycle following stimulation, DNA synthesis occurs during the S phase and is followed by the postsynthetic G2 phase. Mitosis occurs during the M phase, which precedes the postmitotic G1 phase.

The cell cycle becomes important in drug selection because cells in the growth fraction are more susceptible to certain agents. In a broad sense, antineoplastic agents may be classified on the basis of their activity in relation to the cell cycle. Most antimetabolites, etoposide, hydroxyurea, vinca alkaloids, and bleomycin are cell cycle-specific agents that are most effective against tumors with a high growth fraction. In contrast, alkylating agents, antineoplastic antibiotics, fluorouracil, floxuridine, and procarbazine exert their effect independent of the cell cycle and generally show more activity against slow-growing tumors.

Drug Mechanisms and Therapeutics

Knowledge of the basic mechanisms of action of chemotherapeutic agents is critical in selecting drugs for an effective chemotherapy combination regimen, minimizing toxicity and drug interactions, and preventing emergence of drug-resistant clones. Agents may damage the DNA template by alkylation, cross-linking, double-strand cleavage by topoisomerase II, intercalation, and blockage of RNA synthesis. Spindle poisons may arrest mitosis. Antimetabolites block enzymes necessary for DNA synthesis. Hormonal agents and their antagonists may influence cellular signal transduction, and biological response modifiers may influence the host's immune response to the tumor alone or in the context of concomitantly administered drugs. Antibody-based therapeutics have revolutionized the care of some cancer patients, including those with colon cancer, breast cancer, and certain leukemias and lymphomas. These therapies explicitly target cancer cells based on structural and biological properties that differ from normal cells. They include unconjugated antibodies or antibodies that have toxic materials attached that can deliver radiation or immunotoxins directly to cancer cells. Unconjugated antibodies, such as rituximab and trastuzumab, exert their cytotoxicity by invoking immune responses against the targeted cells. Conjugated antibodies, such as Zevalin and Bexxar, deliver toxic compounds directly to tumor sites, thus resulting in cell death. In addition to antibody-based therapies, orally available small molecule targeted therapies have been created, such as imatinib mesylate, erlotinib, and sorafenib. Imatinib mesylate is a protein tyrosine kinase inhibitor of bcr/abl, an abnormality found in some patients with chronic myelogenous leukemia. Erlotinib inhibits the intracellular phosphorylation of the tyrosine kinase associated with the epidermal growth factor receptor while sorafenib prevents tumor cell angiogenesis and proliferation by inhibiting multiple other intracellular tyrosine kinases.

Combination chemotherapy is frequently used in an effort to forestall the development of drug resistance to antineoplastic agents and to achieve synergism with reduced toxicity. The Goldie–Coldman hypothesis assumes that at the time of diagnosis, most tumors possess resistant clones. Multiple mechanisms of drug resistance develop during cancer progression. The most well studied of these involves the *mdr* gene, which codes for membrane-bound *P*-glycoprotein. *P*-glycoprotein serves as a channel through which cellular toxins (i.e., chemotherapeutic agents) may be excreted from the cell. Additional mechanisms of drug resistance are decreased drug transport into cells, reduction of drug activation, drug metabolism enhancement, development of alternative metabolic pathways, drug inhibition of enzyme targets overcome by gene amplification, and impairment of drug binding to a target. A single drug may be subject to one or more mechanisms.

Interestingly, normal human cells never develop drug resistance. As a result, several caveats of combination chemotherapy have emerged. Drugs shown to be active as single agents should be chosen, and drugs selected for combined use should have different mechanisms of action. Ideally, drugs with different dose-limiting toxicities should be administered together, although toxicity overlap may necessitate dose reduction, as with myelosuppression. Finally, drug combinations with similar patterns of resistance should be avoided.

Different patterns of chemotherapy administration are used in particular settings with specific goals. Induction chemotherapy is usually high dose and given in combination to induce complete remission. Consolidation is a repetition of an induction regimen in a complete responder to prolong remission or increase the cure rate. Chemotherapy given with an intent similar to that of consolidation but with higher doses than induction or with different agents at high doses is known as intensification. Maintenance regimens are low-dose, long-term protocols intended to delay tumor cell regrowth after complete remission. Induction, consolidation, intensification, and maintenance usually apply to hematologic malignancies but may also describe solid tumor regimens.

Neoadjuvant treatment in the preoperative or perioperative period is used more commonly with solid tumors, such as locally advanced breast carcinoma, soft-tissue sarcomas of the extremities, and, more recently, rectal carcinoma and squamous cell carcinoma of the head and neck. It is often given in combination with radiation therapy to improve survival, resectability, and organ preservation.

Palliative chemotherapy may be given to control symptoms or, if the toxicity profile is favorable, prolong life for incurable patients. Salvage chemotherapy involves the use of a potentially curative, high-dose protocol in patients failing or recurring after different standard treatment plans have been attempted.

Adjuvant chemotherapy is administered following curative surgery or radiation therapy as a short-course, high-dose regimen to destroy a low number of residual tumor cells. Several factors determine the effectiveness of adjuvant regimens, including tumor burden, drug dose and schedule, combination chemotherapy, and drug resistance. The drug(s) must be active locally against residual cells and distantly against clinically occult metastatic deposits. Extensive literature supports the use of adjuvant chemotherapy for breast, colon, rectal, and anal carcinomas and for ovarian germ cell tumors, osteosarcoma, and pediatric solid tumors. No definitive benefit has been reported yet for pancreatic, gastric, and testicular carcinomas or for cervical cancer and melanoma, although investigative adjuvant therapy protocols are ongoing and open for patient enrollment in these disease sites.

Most chemotherapeutic agents exhibit very steep dose–response profiles and have low therapeutic indices, making a high-dose, short-term administration desirable. This can be accomplished through regional dose intensification. One example is intraperitoneal chemotherapy for ovarian cancer with high risk of peritoneal recurrence or for primary tumors that manifest as intraperitoneal disease, such as pseudomyxoma peritonei and peritoneal mesothelioma. Another type of regional dose intensification is intra-arterial therapy, which requires regional tumor confinement and a unique tumor blood supply and is most commonly used in hepatic artery infusion for primary or metastatic liver tumors that are surgically unresectable. Intra-arterial chemotherapy has also been used for gliomas of the brain and some head and neck tumors. Isolated perfusion of a specific anatomical site, usually the extremities, is one more type of regional dose intensification that allows for the delivery of very high doses of chemotherapy to the involved site with little systemic toxicity; it is often combined with hyperthermia. The largest body of literature discusses its use in all stages of melanoma, although limb perfusion for extremity sarcoma has been reported.

CHEMOTHERAPEUTIC AGENTS

Fundamental knowledge of the drugs available for cancer treatment, their mechanisms of action, general dose ranges, dominant toxicities, and indications for use are important to the general surgeon caring for cancer patients. Table 26.1 lists the available agents and their mechanisms of action, doses, and toxicities. Table 26.2 lists the available biological agents, as well as their U.S. Food and Drug Administration (FDA) indications and dosages. Table 26.3 lists commonly used combination chemotherapeutic regimens.

(*text continue on page 654*)

TABLE 26.1

Cancer Chemotherapeutic Agents: Mechanisms, Doses, and Toxicities

Drug	Dose and Schedule	Toxicity
Alkylating Agents		
Altretamine (hexamethylmelamine, Hexalen®)	260 mg/m² PO in divided doses × 14–21 d	Nausea and vomiting, myelosuppression, paresthesias, CNS toxicity
Bendamustine (Treanda®)	100–120 mg/m², days 1–2 every 21–28 d	Myelosuppression, nausea and vomiting, infusion reactions, dermatologic toxicity
Busulfan (Myleran®)	4–8 mg PO daily	Myelosuppression, pulmonary fibrosis, aplastic anemia, skin hyperpigmentation
Carmustine (BCNU, BiCNU®)	150–200 mg/m² IV every 6–8 wk	Delayed myelosuppression, nausea and vomiting, hepatotoxicity
Chlorambucil (Leukeran®)	0.1–0.2 mg/kg/d PO × 3–6 wk (average 4–10 mg/d)	Myelosuppression, pulmonary fibrosis, hepatotoxicity
Carboplatin (Paraplatin®)	300–360 mg/m² IV every 4 wk or target area under the curve (AUC) of 4–6 mg/dL every 3–4 wk, AUC 2 mg/dL weekly during radiation[a]	Myelosuppression, nausea and vomiting, peripheral neuropathy, ototoxicity, hypersensitivity
Cisplatin (Platinol®, Platinol®-AQ)	40–120 mg/m² IV every 3–4 wk 20 mg/m²/d IV × 5 d every 3–4 wk; 20–40 mg/m² IV weekly during radiation[a]	Nephrotoxicity, nausea and vomiting, peripheral neuropathy, myelosuppression, ototoxicity
Cyclophosphamide (Cytoxan®, Neosar®)	40–50 mg/kg IV in divided doses over 2–5 d, 1–5 mg/kg/d PO	Myelosuppression, hemorrhagic cystitis, immunosuppression, alopecia, stomatitis, SIADH
Dacarbazine (DTIC-Dome®)	2.0–4.5 mg/kg/d IV × 10 250 mg/m²/d IV × 5 d (melanoma), 150 mg/m²/d IV × 5 d 375 mg/m² IV every 15 d (Hodgkin disease)	Myelosuppression, nausea and vomiting, flu-like syndrome, hepatoxicity, alopecia, seizures

Drug	Dose	Toxicity
Ifosfamide (Ifex®)	1.2 g/m² IV daily × 5 d every 3 wk	Myelosuppression, hemorrhagic cystitis, somnolence, confusion
Lomustine (CCNU, CeeNU®)	130 mg/m² PO every 6 wk	Delayed myelosuppression, nausea and vomiting, hepatotoxicity, neurotoxicity, nephrotoxicity
Mechlorethamine (Nitrogen mustard, Mustargen®)	0.4 mg/kg IV single dose or in divided doses of 0.1–0.2 mg/kg/d	Myelosuppression, nausea and vomiting, phlebitis, gonadal dysfunction
Melphalan (Alkeran®)	2–6 mg PO daily × 14–21 d, 10 mg PO daily × 7–10 d, 16 mg/m² IV every 2–4 wk	Myelosuppression, stomatitis, nausea and vomiting, gonadal dysfunction
Oxaliplatin (Eloxatin®)	85–130 mg/m² IV every 2–3 wk	Myelosuppression, nausea and vomiting, hypersensitivity, peripheral neuropathy, cold sensitivity
Procarbazine (Matulane®)	50 mg/m² IV weekly during radiation[a] 1–6 mg/kg/d PO daily 100 mg/m²/d PO × 14 d	Myelosuppression, nausea and vomiting, lethargy, depression, pares-thesias, headache, flu-like syndrome
Streptozocin (Zanosar®)	500 mg/m²/d IV × 5 d, 1,000–1,500 mg/m² IV weekly	Renal toxicity, nausea and vomiting, diarrhea, altered glucose metabolism, liver dysfunction
Temozolomide (Temodar®)	75–150 mg/m²/d PO/IV × 5 d every 28 d	Myelosuppression, nausea and vomiting, alopecia, asthenia, rash
Thiotepa (Thioplex®)	0.3–0.4 mg/kg IV every 1–4 wk	Myelosuppression, nausea and vomiting, mucositis, skin rashes
Antimetabolites		
Capecitabine (Xeloda®)	2,000–2,500 mg/m²/d PO × 14 d every 21 d 1,650 mg/m²/d PO during radiation[a]	Diarrhea, stomatitis, nausea and vomiting, hand-foot syndrome, myelosuppression
Cladribine (Leustatin®)	0.09–0.1 mg/kg/d IV continuous infusion × 7 d every 4 wk	Myelosuppression, fever, rash
Clofarabine (Clolar®)	52 mg/m² IV × 5 d every 2–6 wk	Nausea and vomiting, diarrhea, myelosuppression, pruritus, rigors, der-matitis, abdominal pain, infection
Cytarabine (Ara-C, Cytosar®, DepoCyt™)	100–200 mg/m²/d IV infusion × 5–7 d 1–3 g/m² IV every 12 h × 4–12 doses	Myelosuppression, nausea and vomiting, diarrhea, hepatotoxicity, fever, conjunctivitis, CNS toxicity
Fludarabine (Fludara®)	25 mg/m²/d IV × 5 d every 4 wk	Myelosuppression, nausea and vomiting, fever, malaise, pulmonary infiltrates

(*continued*)

TABLE 26.1 Cancer Chemotherapeutic Agents: Mechanisms, Doses, and Toxicities (*continued*)

Drug	Dose and Schedule	Toxicity
Floxuridine (FUDR®)	0.1–0.6 mg/kg/d × 5–14 d continuous arterial infusion	Hepatotoxicity, gastritis, nausea and vomiting, diarrhea
5-Fluorouracil (5-FU, Adrucil®)	300–500 mg/m²/d IV × 3–5 d 10–15 mg/kg IV weekly 200–300 mg/m²/d IV continuous infusion	Stomatitis, myelosuppression, diarrhea, nausea and vomiting, cerebellar ataxia
Gemcitabine (Gemzar®)	1,000–1,250 mg/m² IV weekly × 3 wk every 28 d; 300–350 mg/m² IV weekly during radiation[a]	Myelosuppression, fever, flu-like syndrome, rash, pulmonary toxicity, mild nausea and vomiting
Hydroxyurea (Hydrea®)	80 mg/kg PO every 3 d, 20–30 mg/kg PO daily	Myelosuppression, nausea and vomiting, rash
6-Mercaptopurine (6-MP, Purinethol®)	1.5–2.5 mg/kg/d PO (average 100–200 mg/d)	Myelosuppression, nausea and vomiting, anorexia, diarrhea, hepatotoxicity
Methotrexate (MTX, Mexate®, Rheumatrex®)	2.5–5.0 mg PO daily (low dose), 50 mg/m² IV every 2–3 wk (low dose), 1–12 g/m² IV every 1–3 wk (high dose), 5–10 mg/m² (max 15 mg) intrathecal every 3–7 d	Mucositis, myelosuppression, pulmonary fibrosis, hepatotoxicity, nephrotoxicity, diarrhea, skin erythema
Pemetrexed (Alimta®)	500–600 mg/m² IV every 21 d	Myelosuppression, fatigue, nausea and vomiting, diarrhea, rash, infection
Pentostatin (Nipent®)	4 mg/m² IV every other wk	Nephrotoxicity, CNS depression, myelosuppression, nausea and vomiting, conjunctivitis
Pralatrexate (Folotyn®)	30 mg/m² IV weekly × 6 wk every 7 wk	Myelosuppression, nausea and vomiting, stomatitis, dyspnea, edema
6-Thioguanine (6-TG, Tabloid®)	2 mg/kg PO daily	Myelosuppression, hepatotoxicity, stomatitis

Histone Deacetylase Inhibitors and Demethylating Agents

Azacitidine (Vidaza®)	75–100 mg/m² SC × 7 d every 4 wk	Nausea and vomiting, myelosuppression, pyrexia, diarrhea, constipation, fatigue, ecchymosis
Decitabine (Dacogen®)	15 mg/m² IV Q 8 h × 3 d every 6 wk 20 mg/m² IV daily × 5 d every 4 wk	Myelosuppression, nausea and vomiting, pyrexia, edema
Nelarabine (Arranon®)	1,500 mg/m² IV days 1, 3, 5 every 21 d 650 mg/m² IV daily × 5 day every 21 d (pediatric)	CNS toxicity, myelosuppression, nausea and vomiting, edema, peripheral neuropathy
Romidepsin (Istodax®)	14 mg/m² IV days 1, 8, 15 every 28 d	Nausea and vomiting, myelosuppression, anorexia, asthenia
Vorinostat (Zolinza®)	400 mg PO daily	Myelosuppression, nausea and vomiting, diarrhea, dysgeusia, QTc prolongation

Natural Products *Antitumor Antibiotics*

Bleomycin (Blenoxane®)	10–20 U/m² IV, IM, or SC once to twice weekly	Pneumonitis, pulmonary fibrosis, fever, hypersensitivity, hyperpigmentation, alopecia
Dactinomycin (Actinomycin D, Cosmegen®)	0.5 mg/d IV × 5 d max 0.012–0.015 mg/kg/d IV × 5 d max (children)	Stomatitis, myelosuppression, anorexia, nausea and vomiting, diarrhea, alopecia
Doxorubicin (Adriamycin PFS®, Adriamycin RDF™)	40–75 mg/m² IV every 21 d 20–30 mg/m²/d IV × 3 d, every 3–4 wk	Myelosuppression, cardiotoxicity, stomatitis, alopecia, nausea and vomiting
Doxorubicin Liposomal (Doxil®)	20–50 mg/m² IV every 3–4 wk	Same as above
Epirubicin (Ellence®)	100–120 mg/m² IV every 3–4 wk	Myelosuppression, nausea and vomiting, cardiotoxicity, alopecia
Idarubicin (Idamycin®)	12 mg/m²/d IV × 3 d every 3 wk	Myelosuppression, nausea and vomiting, stomatitis, alopecia, cardiotoxicity
Mitomycin C (Mutamycin®)	20 mg/m² IV every 6–8 wk	Myelosuppression, nausea and vomiting, anorexia, alopecia, stomatitis
Mitoxantrone (Novantrone®)	12 mg/m²/d IV × 3 d 12–14 mg/m² IV every 3 wk	Myelosuppression, cardiotoxicity, alopecia, stomatitis, nausea and vomiting

(continued)

TABLE 26.1	Cancer Chemotherapeutic Agents: Mechanisms, Doses, and Toxicities (*continued*)

Drug	Dose and Schedule	Toxicity
Mitotic Inhibitors		
Estramustine (Emcyt®)	10–16 mg/kg PO daily	Myelosuppression, ischemic heart disease, thrombophlebitis, hepatotoxicity, nausea and vomiting
Docetaxel (Taxotere®)	60–100 mg/m² IV every 21 d	Myelosuppression, fluid retention, hypersensitivity, peripheral neuropathy, onycholysis, alopecia
Ixabepilone (Ixempra®)	40 mg/m² IV every 21 d	Myelosuppression, nausea and vomiting, alopecia, hypersensitivity, peripheral neuropathy, mucositis
Paclitaxel (Taxol®)	135–175 mg/m²/d IV infusion every 3 wk 80 mg/m² IV infusion weekly	Myelosuppression, peripheral neuropathy, alopecia, mucositis, anaphylaxis, onycholysis
Paclitaxel Protein Bound (Abraxane®)	260 mg/m² IV every 3 wk	Same as above
Vinblastine (Velban®)	3–18.5 mg/m² IV every 1–2 wk	Myelosuppression, paralytic ileus, alopecia, nausea, stomatitis
Vincristine (Vincasar®)	0.03–1.4 mg/m² IV weekly (2.0 mg/wk max)	Peripheral neuropathy, paralytic ileus, SIADH, myelosuppression
Vinorelbine (Navelbine®)	25–30 mg/m² IV weekly	Peripheral neuropathy, myelosuppression, nausea and vomiting, hepatic dysfunction
Topoisomerase Inhibitors		
Etoposide (VP–16, VePesid®, etopoPHOS®)	35–100 mg/m²/d IV × 3–5 d 100 mg/m²/d PO × 5 d	Myelosuppression, nausea and vomiting, diarrhea, fever, hypotension with infusion, alopecia
Irinotecan (CPT-11, Camptosar®)	125 mg/m² IV weekly 350 mg/m² IV every 3 wk	Myelosuppression, diarrhea, nausea and vomiting, anorexia
Teniposide (Vumon®)	60 mg/m²/d IV × 5 d every 3 wk 50–100 mg/m² IV once weekly	Myelosuppression, nausea and vomiting, alopecia, hepatotoxicity, hypotension with infusion
Topotecan (Hycamtin®)	1.25–1.5 mg/m²/d IV × 5 d	Myelosuppression, fever, flu-like syndrome, nausea and vomiting

Enzymes

Asparaginase (Elspar®, Kidrolase®)	6,000 IU/m² IM 3 × wk 1,000 IU/kg/d IV × 10 d	Allergic reactions, nausea and vomiting, liver dysfunction, CNS depression, hyperglycemia
Pegaspargase (Oncaspar®)	2,500 IU/m² IM every 14 d	Hypersensitivity reactions, hepatotoxicity, fever, nausea and vomiting

Miscellaneous Agents

Arsenic trioxide (Trisenox™)	0.15 mg/kg daily up to 60 doses (induction) 0.15 mg/kg daily × 25 doses (consolidation)	APL differentiation syndrome, nausea and vomiting, pyrexia, edema, diarrhea, ECG abnormalities, electrolyte abnormalities
Bortezomib (Velcade®)	1.3 mg/m² IV twice weekly for 2 wk followed by a 10-d rest period (21-d cycle)	Fatigue, pyrexia, nausea and vomiting, thrombocytopenia, anemia, hypotension, diarrhea, constipation, peripheral neuropathy
Temsirolimus (Torisel®)	25 mg IV weekly	Rash, mucositis, hypersensitivity, asthenia, edema, nausea and vomiting, myelosuppression, hyperlipidemia, hyperglycemia

Hormonal Agents *Adrenocorticoids*

Dexamethasone (Decadron®)	0.5–4.0 mg PO, IV, IM daily	Fluid retention, hyperglycemia, hypertension, infection
Methylprednisolone (Depo-Medrol®, Medrol®, Solu-Medrol®)	4–200 mg/d PO, IV daily	Fluid retention, hyperglycemia, hypertension, infection
Prednisone (Deltasone®)	5–100 mg/d PO	Same as above

Estrogens

Diethylstilbestrol (DES)	1–15 mg/d PO	Fluid retention, feminization, uterine bleeding, nausea and vomiting, thromboembolism
Estradiol (Climara®, Estrace®)	0.6–30 mg PO daily	Same as above

Progestins

Medroxyprogesterone (Provera®, Depo-Provera®)	400–1,000 mg IM weekly	Weight gain, fluid retention, feminization, cardiovascular effects
Megestrol (Megace®)	40–320 mg/d PO	Same as above

(*continued*)

TABLE 26.1 Cancer Chemotherapeutic Agents: Mechanisms, Doses, and Toxicities (*continued*)

Drug	Dose and Schedule	Toxicity
Antiestrogens		
Tamoxifen (Nolvadex®)	20–40 mg/d PO	Hot flashes, nausea and vomiting, altered menses
Toremifene (Fareston®)	60 mg PO daily	Same as above
Fulvestrant (Faslodex®)	250 mg IM monthly	Nausea and vomiting, constipation, diarrhea, headache, back pain, hot flushes, pharyngitis
Aromatase Inhibitors		
Aminoglutethimide (Cytadren®)	250 mg PO BID–QID	Rash, hot flushes, fever, drowsiness, nausea, anorexia
Anastrozole (Arimidex®)	1 mg PO daily	Same as above
Exemestane (Aromasin®)	25 mg PO daily	Same as above
Letrozole (Femara®)	2.5 mg PO daily	Same as above
Androgens		
Testosterone (Androderm®, Depo®-Testosterone)	200–400 mg IM every 2–4 wk (long acting)	Masculinization, amenorrhea, gynecomastia, nausea, water retention, changes in libido, skin hypersensitivity, hepatotoxicity
Methyltestosterone (Android®, Testred®)	50–200 mg PO daily	Same as above
Fluoxymesterone (Android-F®, Halotestin®)	10–40 mg PO daily	Same as above

Antiandrogens

Bicalutamide (Casodex®)	50 mg PO daily	Hot flashes, decreased libido, impotence, diarrhea, nausea and vomiting, gynecomastia, hepatotoxicity
Flutamide (Eulexin®)	250 mg PO tid	Same as above
Nilutamide (Nilandron®)	150–300 mg PO daily	Same as above

LHRH Analogs

Leuprolide (Lupron® Depot)	1 mg SC daily, 7.5 mg IM monthly, 22.5 mg IM every 3 mo, or 30 mg IM every 4 mo, 22.5 mg IM every 3 mo	Hot flashes, menstrual irregularity, sexual dysfunction, edema
Goserelin (Zoladex®)	3.6–10.8 mg implant SC every 1–3 mo	Same as above
Triptorelin (Trelstar® Depot, Trelstar® LA)	3.75 mg IM monthly (Depot) or 11.75 mg IM every 84 d (LA)	Same as above
Abarelix (Plenaxis®)	100 mg IM on days 1, 15, 29, and every 4 wk thereafter	Same as above

[a]Non-FDA–approved dose; PO, orally; CNS, central nervous system; IV, intravenously; SIADH, syndrome of inappropriate antidiuretic secretion; SC, subcutaneously; IM, intramuscularly; BID, twice daily; QID, four times daily; tid, three times daily; APL, acute promyelocytic leukemia; ECG, echocardiogram; LHRH, luteinizing hormone-releasing hormone.

TABLE 26.2 Biological Agents Used in Oncology

Cytokine	Indications	Dose and Schedule	Toxicity
Interferon-alfa-2b (Roferon®-A, Intron A®)	Melanoma, hairy-cell l eukemia, Kaposi sarcoma, chronic hepatitis B and C	2–50 million IU/m^2/d or 3 × per wk	Flu-like syndrome, anorexia, depression, fatigue
Interleukin-2 (Aldesleukin, Proleukin®)	Renal cell carcinoma, metastatic melanoma	600,000–720,000 IU/kg every 8 h × 14 doses	Chills, fever, edema, hepatotoxicity, nephrotoxicity, hypotension, mental status changes, anemia, thrombocytopenia, diarrhea, nausea and vomiting
Interleukin-11 (Oprelvekin, Neumega®)	Thrombocytopenia	50 μg/kg SC once daily	Fluid retention, peripheral edema, dyspnea, tachycardia, atrial arrhythmias, dizziness
Filgrastim (G-CSF, Neupogen®)	Nonmyeloid malignancy, neutropenia	5–10 μg/kg IV or SC daily	Hypersensitivity, bone pain, fever, malaise
Pegfilgrastim (pegylated G-CSF, Neulasta®)	Nonmyeloid malignancy, neutropenia	6 mg SC once per chemotherapy cycle 24 h after chemotherapy	Bone pain, nausea and vomiting, fever, fatigue
Sargramostim (GM-CSF) (Leukine®)	Acceleration of myeloid recovery BMT failure or engraftment delay Induction for acute myelogenous leukemia Mobilization after autologous peripheral blood progenitor cells	250 μg/m^2/d IV or SC	Rash, fluid retention, bone pain, cardiac arrhythmia, dyspnea, hypersensitivity

Drug	Indication	Dose	Side Effects
Epoetin alfa (Erythropoietin; Epogen®, Procrit®)	Anemia associated with chronic renal failure, cancer chemotherapy, or AIDS treatments. Reduction of blood transfusions in surgery patients.	Initial dose: 50–300 U/kg IV or SC 3 × per wk or 40,000–60,000 U SC weekly	Hypertension, hypersensitivity, fever, tachycardia, nausea, thrombotic events
Darbepoetin (Aranesp®)	Anemia associated with chronic renal failure and cancer chemotherapy	Initial dose: 2.25–4.5 μg/kg SC weekly or 200–300 μg SC every 2 wk	Same as above
Monoclonal Antibody			
Bevacizumab (Avastin®)	Colorectal cancer Breast cancer Non–small cell lung cancer Renal cell carcinoma Glioblastoma	5–15 mg/kg IV infusion every 2–3 wk	Infusion-related reactions, nausea and vomiting, hypertension, proteinuria, gastrointestinal perforation, wound healing complications, thrombotic events
Cetuximab (Erbitux®)	Colorectal cancer Head and neck cancer	400 mg/m² IV infusion (loading dose), then 250 mg/m² IV infusion weekly **OR** 500 mg/m² IV every 2 wk[a]	Infusion-related reactions, skin rash, paronychia, nausea and vomiting, constipation, diarrhea, hypomagnesemia
Panitumumab (Vectibix®)	Colorectal Cancer	6 mg/kg IV every 14 d	Same as above
Rituximab (Rituxan®)	Non-Hodgkin lymphoma Chronic lymphocytic leukemia	375 mg/m² IV infusion weekly × 4–8 doses (NHL) 375 mg/m² IV cycle 1, then 500 mg/m² IV cycles 2–6 (CLL)	Hypersensitivity, infusion-related fever and chills/rigors, hypotension, myelosuppression, tumor lysis syndrome, Hepatitis B reactivation
Trastuzumab (Herceptin®)	Breast cancer	Initial dose: 4 mg/kg IV infusion Maintenance dose: 2 mg/kg IV infusion weekly **OR** 8 mg/kg IV infusion Maintenance dose: 6 mg/kg IV infusion every 3 wk[a]	Infusion-related fever and chills, cardiac dysfunction, including dyspnea, cough, peripheral edema; hypersensitivity; diarrhea

(continued)

TABLE
26.2   Biological Agents Used in Oncology (continued)

Cytokine	Indications	Dose and Schedule	Toxicity
Alemtuzumab (Campath®)	B-cell chronic lymphocytic leukemia	Initial dose: 3 mg/d IV infusion, if tolerated increase to 10 mg/d IV, if tolerated increase to 30 mg/d IV 3 × per wk	Infusion-related fever, chills, rash, nausea, hypotension, shortness of breath, opportunistic infections, neutropenia, thrombocytopenia
Ofatumumab (Arzerra™)	Chronic lymphocytic leukemia	300 mg IV week 1, then 2,000 mg IV weekly × 7 wk, then 2,000 mg IV every 4 wk × 4 doses	Infusion-related fever and chills, rash, myelosuppression, infection, Hepatitis B reactivation
Immunotoxin			
Denileukin diftitox (Ontak®)	Cutaneous T-cell lymphoma	9 or 18 μg/kg/d IV × 5 d, repeat every 21 d	Acute hypersensitivity, including hypotension, dyspnea, rash, chest pain, tachycardia; vascular leak syndrome; confusion; nausea and vomiting; diarrhea
Radiopharmaceutical			
Tositumomab and Iodine 131/ Tositumomab (Bexxar®)	Non-Hodgkin lymphoma	Dosimetric step: Tositumomab 450 mg IV followed by iodine I-131 tositumomab (5 mCi iodine I-131, 35 mg tositumomab) IV Therapeutic step: Tositumomab 450 mg IV followed by iodine I-131 tositumomab (iodine I-131 to deliver 75 cGy and 35 mg tositumomab) IV	Myelosuppression, asthenia, fever, chills, cough, pain, infection, nausea and vomiting, human-antimurine antibodies, secondary malignancies

Drug	Indication	Dosing	Adverse Effects
Ibritumomab tiuxetan (Zevalin®)	Non-Hodgkin lymphoma	Dosimetric step: Rituximab 250 mg/m² IV followed by Indium-111 ibritumomab tiuxetan (5 mCi) IV Therapeutic step: Rituximab 250 mg/m² IV followed by yttrium-90 ibritumomab tiuxetan 0.4 mCi/kg (maximum 32 mCi) IV	Myelosuppression, asthenia, infusion-related reactions, nausea and vomiting, cough, secondary malignancies
Tyrosine Kinase Inhibitors			
Dasatinib (Sprycel®)	Chronic myeloid leukemia Ph+ acute lymphoblastic leukemia	100–140 mg PO daily 140 mg PO daily	Myelosuppression, edema, diarrhea, rash, fatigue, nausea and vomiting, hemorrhage, headache, dyspnea
Erlotinib (Tarceva®)	Non–small cell lung cancer Pancreatic cancer	150 mg PO daily 100 mg PO daily	Rash, diarrhea, fatigue, cough, nausea and vomiting, conjunctivitis, increased hepatic transaminases
Imatinib (Gleevec®)	Chronic myeloid leukemia, Ph+ acute lymphoblastic leukemia, myelodysplastic syndrome, gastrointestinal stromal tumors	400–800 mg PO daily	Fluid retention, muscle cramps, nausea and vomiting, diarrhea, fatigue, hepatotoxicity, myelosuppression
Lapatinib (Tykerb®)	Breast cancer	1,250 mg PO daily	Hepatotoxicity, cardiotoxicity, hand-foot syndrome, rash, diarrhea, nausea and vomiting, myelosuppression
Nilotinib (Tasigna®)	Chronic myeloid leukemia	400 mg PO BID	Rash, nausea and vomiting, myelosuppression, pruritus, fatigue, QTc prolongation
Pazopanib (Votrient™)	Renal cell carcinoma	800 mg PO daily	Diarrhea, hypertension, nausea and vomiting, anorexia, depigmentation, hepatotoxicity, cardiotoxicity
Sorafenib (Nexavar®)	Renal cell carcinoma Hepatocellular carcinoma	400 mg PO BID	Rash, hand-foot syndrome, alopecia, diarrhea, nausea and vomiting, myelosuppression, cardiotoxicity
Sunitinib (Sutent®)	Renal cell carcinoma, gastrointestinal stromal tumor	50 mg PO daily × 4 wk every 6 wk	Cardiotoxicity, diarrhea, nausea and vomiting, mucositis, hair/skin depigmentation, hypothyroidism

(continued)

	Biological Agents Used in Oncology (continued)		

TABLE 26.2

Cytokine	Indications	Dose and Schedule	Toxicity
Miscellaneous Agents			
Everolimus (Afinitor®)	Renal cell carcinoma	10 mg PO daily	Mucositis, asthenia, diarrhea, hair depigmentation, nausea and vomiting, cardiotoxicity, hepatotoxicity
Lenalidomide (Revlimid®)	Myelodysplastic syndrome Multiple myeloma	10 mg PO daily 25 mg PO daily for 21 d every 28 d	Myelosuppression, venous thromboembolism, diarrhea, pruritus, rash, fatigue, teratogenic
Thalidomide (Thalomid®)	Multiple myeloma	200–400 mg PO daily	Myelosuppression, venous thromboembolism, peripheral neuropathy, pruritus, constipation, rash, fatigue, teratogenic

aNon-FDA–approved dose; SC, subcutaneously; IV, intravenously; BMT, bone marrow transplant; Ph+, Philadelphia chromosome positive.

Acronym	Cancer Use	Agents
ABH	Melanoma	Dactinomycin, carmustine, hydroxyurea
ABV	Hodgkin lymphoma	Doxorubicin, bleomycin, vinblastine
ABVD	Hodgkin lymphoma	Doxorubicin, bleomycin, vinblastine, dacarbazine
AC	Breast, sarcoma, neuroblastoma	Doxorubicin, cyclophosphamide
ACE, CAE	Small-cell lung	Cyclophosphamide, doxorubicin, etoposide
AP	Ovarian, endometrial	Doxorubicin, cisplatin
ASHAP	Hodgkin lymphoma	Doxorubicin, methylprednisolone, cisplatin, cytarabine
AVADOX	Esophageal, gastric	Bevacizumab, docetaxel, capecitabine
BEACOPP	Hodgkin lymphoma	Bleomycin, etoposide, doxorubicin, cyclophosphamide, vincristine, procarbazine, prednisone, filgrastim
BEAM	Bone marrow transplant	Carmustine, etoposide, cytarabine, melphalan
BEP	Testicular	Bleomycin, etoposide, cisplatin
BHD	Melanoma	Carmustine, hydroxyurea, dacarbazine
Bold-IFN	Melanoma	Bleomycin, vincristine, lomustine, dacarbazine, interferon alfa 2b
BOP	Testicular	Bleomycin, vincristine, cisplatin
BuCy	Bone marrow transplant	Busulfan, cyclophosphamide
CAF	Breast	Cyclophosphamide, doxorubicin, fluorouracil
CAV	Small-cell lung	Cyclophosphamide, doxorubicin, vincristine
CAVE	Small-cell lung	Cyclophosphamide, doxorubicin, vincristine, etoposide
CE	Head and neck	Carboplatin, etoposide
CF	Small-cell lung	Cisplatin, fluorouracil
CGI	Bladder	Cisplatin, gemcitabine, ifosfamide

(continued)

TABLE 26.3 Commonly Used Combination Chemotherapeutic Regimens (*continued*)

Acronym	Cancer Use	Agents
CHOP	Non-Hodgkin lymphoma	Cyclophosphamide, doxorubicin, vincristine, prednisone
CHOP-Bleo	Non-Hodgkin lymphoma	Cyclophosphamide, doxorubicin, vincristine, prednisone, bleomycin
CMF	Breast	Methotrexate, fluorouracil, cyclophosphamide
CODOX-M	Non-Hodgkin lymphoma	Cyclophosphamide, vincristine, methotrexate, leucovorin, cytarabine
COPP	Hodgkin lymphoma	Cyclophosphamide, vincristine, prednisone, procarbazine
CVD	Prostate	Cyclophosphamide, vincristine, dexamethasone
CVD	Melanoma	Cyclophosphamide, vincristine, dacarbazine
CVD + IL-21	Melanoma, sarcoma (bone or soft tissue)	Cisplatin, vinblastine, dacarbazine, aldesleukin, interferon-α cyclophosphamide, vincristine, doxorubicin, dacarbazine
Cy-TBI	Bone marrow transplant	Cyclophosphamide, total body irradiation
DCF	Esophageal, gastric	Docetaxel, cisplatin, fluorouracil
DCTER	Acute myelogenous leukemia, myelodysplastic syndrome	Daunorubicin, cytarabine, thioguanine, etoposide
DI	Soft-tissue sarcoma	Doxorubicin, ifosfamide
DOX	Esophageal, gastric	Docetaxel, oxaliplatin, capecitabine
DT-PACE	Multiple myeloma	Dexamethasone, thalidomide, cisplatin, doxorubicin, cyclophosphamide, etoposide
EAP	Gastric, small bowel	Etoposide, doxorubicin, cisplatin
ECF	Esophageal, gastric	Epirubicin, cisplatin, fluorouracil
EFP	Gastric, small bowel	Etoposide, fluorouracil, cisplatin
ELF	Gastric	Etoposide, leucovorin, fluorouracil
EOX	Esophageal, gastric	Epirubicin, oxiliplatin, capecitabine
EP	Testicular	Etoposide, cisplatin

EPOCH	Non-Hodgkin lymphoma	Doxorubicin, etoposide, vincristine, cyclophosphamide, prednisone
ESHAP	Non-Hodgkin lymphoma	Methylprednisolone, etoposide, cytarabine, cisplatin
FA	Acute myelogenous leukemia	Fludarabine, cytarabine
FAC	Breast	Fluorouracil, doxorubicin, cyclophosphamide
FCR	Non-Hodgkin lymphoma, chronic lymphocytic leukemia	Rituximab, fludarabine, cyclophosphamide
FEC	Breast	Fluorouracil, epirubicin, cyclophosphamide
FLAG	Acute myelogenous leukemia	Fludarabine, cytarabine
bFLOX	Colorectal	Oxaliplatin, fluorouracil, leucovorin
FND	Non-Hodgkin lymphoma	Fludarabine, mitoxantrone, dexamethasone
FOLFOX	Colorectal	Oxaliplatin, fluorouracil, leucovorin
FOLFIRI	Colorectal	Irinotecan, fluorouracil, leucovorin
FU/LV	Colorectal	Fluorouracil, leucovorin
GemCis	Pancreatic	Gemcitabine, cisplatin
GemOx	Pancreatic	Gemcitabine, oxaliplatin
GTP	Bladder	Gemcitabine, paclitaxel, cisplatin
GTX	Pancreatic	Gemcitabine, docetaxel, capecitabine
HyperCVAD	Acute lymphocytic leukemia, non-Hodgkin lymphoma, multiple myeloma	Cyclophosphamide, doxorubicin, vincristine, dexamethasone
IA	Acute myelogenous leukemia	Idarubicin, cytarabine
IGEV	Hodgkin lymphoma	Ifosfamide, gemcitabine, vinorelbine, prednisolone
ITP	Bladder	Ifosfamide, paclitaxel, cisplatin
IVAC	Non-Hodgkin lymphoma	Etoposide, ifosfamide, mesna, cytarabine, methotrexate
KAVE	Prostate	Ketoconazole, doxorubicin, vincristine, estramustine
MACOP-B	Non-Hodgkin lymphoma	Methotrexate, leucovorin, doxorubicin, prednisone, cyclophosphamide, vincristine, bleomycin
MAID	Soft-tissue sarcoma	Mesna, doxorubicin, ifosfamide, dacarbazine

(continued)

TABLE 26.3

Commonly Used Combination Chemotherapeutic Regimens (*continued*)

Acronym	Cancer Use	Agents
m-BACOD	Non-Hodgkin lymphoma	Methotrexate, leucovorin, doxorubicin, cyclophosphamide, vincristine, bleomycin, dexamethasone
MICE (ICE)	Sarcoma, non-Hodgkin lymphoma	Ifosfamide, carboplatin, etoposide, mesna
MBC	Head and neck	Methotrexate, bleomycin, cisplatin
MINE	Non-Hodgkin lymphoma	Mesna, ifosfamide, mitoxantrone, etoposide
MOPP	Hodgkin lymphoma	Mechlorethamine, vincristine, procarbazine, prednisone
MP	Multiple myeloma	Melphalan, prednisone
MP	Prostate	Mitoxantrone, prednisone
M-VAC	Bladder	Methotrexate, vinblastine, doxorubicin, cisplatin
PAC	Ovarian, endometrial	Cisplatin, doxorubicin, cyclophosphamide
PAD	Multiple myeloma	Bortezomib, doxorubicin, dexamethasone
PE	Small-cell lung	Cisplatin, etoposide
PI	Small-cell lung	Cisplatin, irinotecan
POMB	Testicular	Cisplatin, vincristine, methotrexate, bleomycin
R-CHOP	Non-Hodgkin lymphoma	Rituximab, cyclophosphamide, doxorubicin, vincristine, prednisone
Stanford V	Hodgkin lymphoma	Doxorubicin, vinblastine, mechlorethamine, vincristine, bleomycin, etoposide, prednisone
TAC	Breast	Docetaxel, doxorubicin, cyclophosphamide
TCF	Esophageal	Paclitaxel, cisplatin, fluorouracil
TE	Prostate	Docetaxel, estramustine
TIP	Head and neck, testicular	Paclitaxel, ifosfamide, mesna, cisplatin
TEC	Prostate	Paclitaxel, estramustine, carboplatin

TEE	Prostate	Paclitaxel, estramustine, etoposide
T-FOX	Esophageal, gastric	Docetaxel, fluorouracil, oxaliplatin
TMP	Bladder	Paclitaxel, methotrexate, cisplatin
TPF	Head and neck	Cisplatin, docetaxel, fluorouracil
TPFC	Head and neck	Cisplatin, docetaxel, fluorouracil, cetuximab
TT-R	Non-Hodgkin lymphoma	Rituximab, paclitaxel, topotecan
VAC	Sarcoma	Vincristine, dactinomycin, cyclophosphamide
VAD	Multiple myeloma	Vincristine, doxorubicin, dexamethasone
VB	Testicular	Vinblastine, bleomycin
VC	Non–small cell lung	Vinorelbine, cisplatin
VeIP	Testicular	Vinblastine, cisplatin, ifosfamide
VIP	Testicular, genitourinary	Etoposide, cisplatin, ifosfamide, mesna
VTD	Multiple myeloma	Bortezomib, thalidomide, dexamethasone
XELIRI	Colorectal	Irinotecan, capecitabine
XELOX	Colorectal	Oxaliplatin, capecitabine
5 + 2	Acute myelogenous leukemia	Cytarabine, daunorubicin or mitoxantrone
7 + 3	Acute myelogenous leukemia	Cytarabine, daunorubicin or idarubicin or mitoxantrone

MANAGEMENT OF CANCER PAIN

The vast majority of patients with advanced cancer, and as many as 60% of patients with any stage of disease, experience significant pain. However, cancer pain is frequently undertreated for a multitude of reasons and fears that are largely unfounded. Effective management of cancer pain is achieved best with a multidisciplinary approach, including pain specialists, oncologists, nurses, pharmacists, physiatrists, physical and occupational therapists, psychologists, psychiatrists, primary care physicians, social workers, clergy, and hospice caregivers. Open lines of communication are of paramount importance to the successful management of cancer pain.

Cancer pain may be due to direct tumor involvement of bone, nerves, viscera, blood vessels, or mucous membranes and can occur postoperatively, after radiation therapy or after chemotherapy. Narcotic use should follow the basic principles of cancer pain management, beginning with an agent that has the potential to provide relief; individualization of the agent, route, dose, and schedule; titration to efficacy; and provision of relief for breakthrough pain. Side effects should be anticipated and treated. Change from one route of administration to another should be done with equianalgesic doses, and the oral route should be used whenever possible. In cancer patients receiving chemotherapy, combination analgesics employing an acetaminophen component may not be the best choice for treatment of chronic pain secondary to the risk of masking a neutropenic fever and the risk of acetaminophen toxicity if large doses are required. In addition, combination products using an aspirin or ibuprofen component are discouraged secondary to the antiplatelet and antipyretic effects. The nonsteroidal anti-inflammatory agents are a useful adjunct to the treatment of cancer pain but must be used with caution secondary to the antiplatelet effects. The practitioner should be aware of various adjuncts to pain management, including steroids, antidepressants, anxiolytics, and neuroleptics, as well as neuroablative, neurostimulatory, and anesthetic procedures.

Table 26.4 is a compilation of various nonnarcotic and narcotic analgesic agents for treating cancer pain and includes dose ranges and expected toxicities.

MANAGEMENT OF CIE

Because many surgical patients receive neoadjuvant and adjuvant chemotherapy, the surgeon may be required to treat CIE, which often results in a dose-limiting toxicity that may lead patients to refuse further therapy. Three physiological areas are included in the pathogenesis of CIE: (a) the emetic center in the lateral reticular formation of the medulla, (b) vagal and splanchnic afferents from the gastrointestinal tract to the central nervous system, and (c) the chemoreceptor trigger zone in the area postrema of the medulla. Chemotherapeutic agents and their metabolites may trigger the latter two directly.

Three patterns of emesis tend to occur in association with chemotherapy. Acute emesis occurs within 24 hours of chemotherapy. Delayed emesis occurs more than 24 hours after the cessation of chemotherapy administration and is predisposed by female gender, high-dose cisplatin, and prior episodes of acute emesis. Anticipatory emesis may occur before retreatment in patients whose prior episodes of emesis were poorly controlled, occurring in up to 25% of patients who received prior chemotherapy. Younger age and history of motion sickness also predispose patients to CIE.

An emetogenic potential is assigned to individual chemotherapy agents and is categorized as high, moderate, low, and minimal emetogenic risk. Table 26.5 lists the emetogenic potential of many of the chemotherapeutic agents. When chemotherapy agents are combined, the agent with the highest level of emetogenicity will determine the overall emetogenic potential of the chemotherapy regimen. Once the

(*text continue on page 658*)

TABLE
26.4

Nonnarcotic and Narcotic Analgesic Agents Used for Treating Cancer Pain

Drug	How Supplied	Dose and Schedule	Toxicity
Nonnarcotics			
Acetaminophen (Tylenol®)	Various tablets, liquid, and suppository strengths	650–1,000 mg PO every 6 h	Hepatic and renal impairment
Celecoxib (Celebrex®)	Capsules: 100 and 200 mg	100–400 mg PO daily	Dyspepsia, heartburn, nausea, gastrointestinal bleeding, renal dysfunction
Ibuprofen (Advil®, Motrin®)	Tablets: 50, 100, 200, 400, 600, and 800 mg Suspension: 100 mg/5 mL	200–400 mg PO every 4–6 h	Same as above
Ketorolac (Toradol®)	Injection: 15 and 30 mg/mL Tablets: 10 mg	15–30 mg IV/IM every 6 h, 10 mg PO every 6 h (limit therapy to 5 d)	Same as above
Nabumetone (Relafen®)	Tablets: 500 and 750 mg	100–2,000 mg PO daily	Same as above
Naproxen (Naprosyn®, Aleve®)	Tablets: 125, 220, 250, 275, 375, 500, and 750 mg Suspension: 125 mg/5 mL	250–500 mg PO twice daily	Same as above
Tramadol (Ultram®, Ultram® ER, Ryzolt™, Ultracet®)	Tablets: 50 mg Extended-release tablets: 100, 200, 300 mg Tablets: 37.5 mg with acetaminophen	50–100 mg PO every 4–6 h 100–300 mg PO Daily 37.5–75 mg PO every 4–6 h	Dizziness, nausea, constipation, headache
Narcotics			
Codeine	Tablets: 15, 30, and 60 mg Oral solution: 12 mg/5 mL with acetaminophen Tablets: 15, 30, and 60 mg with acetaminophen Injection: 30 and 60 mg	15–60 mg PO, IM, IV, or SC every 4–6 h, 50–100 mcg IM/IV every 1–2 h	Sedation, constipation, nausea, respiratory depression; occurs with all narcotic analgesics
Fentanyl (Duragesic®, Fentora®, Aciq®, Sublimaze®)	Lozenges: 100, 200, 300, 400, 600, 800, 1,200, and 1,600 mcg Transdermal patch: 12, 25, 50, 75, and 100 μg/h Injection: 50 mcg/5 mL	200–400 mcg PO every 2–3 h Apply one patch (25–300 mcg/h) every 72 h	Same as above
Levorphanol (Levo-Dromoran®)	Tablets: 2 mg Injection: 2 mg/mL	1–4 mg PO/IV/IM/SC every 4–8 h	Same as above

(continued)

TABLE 26.4 Nonnarcotic and Narcotic Analgesic Agents Used for Treating Cancer Pain (*continued*)

Drug	How Supplied	Dose and Schedule	Toxicity
Hydrocodone (Lortab®, Vicodin®)	Tablets: 2.5, 5, 7.5, and 10 mg with acetaminophen Oral elixir: 2.5 mg with acetaminophen/5 mL, 7.5, 10, mg with acetaminophen/15 mL	5–10 mg PO every 4–6 h	Same as above
Hydromorphone (Dilaudid®)	Tablets: 2, 4, and 8 mg Injection: 1, 2, 4, and 10 mg/ mL Oral liquid: 5 mg/5 mL Suppository: 3 mg	2–4 mg PO every 3–4 h, 0.5–2 mg IV/IM every 3–4 h	Same as above
Methadone (Dolophine®)	Tablets: 5, 10, and 40 mg Oral solution: 1, 2, and 10 mg/mL Injection: 10 mg/mL	2.5–20 mg PO every 3–4 h, 5–15 mg IV/IM every 3–4 h	As above: delayed toxicity, QT prolongation
Meperidine (Demerol®)	Tablets: 50 and 100 mg Oral syrup: 50 mg/5 mL Injection: 25, 50, 75, and 100 mg/mL	50–150 mg PO every 3–4 h, 25–100 mg IV/IM every 3–4 h	As above: seizures from normeperidine metabolite accumulation
Morphine (MSIR® MS Contin®, Kadian®, Avinza™, Oramorph® SR)	Tablets: 15, and 30 mg Oral solution: 10 and 20 mg/5 mL Extended-release tablets/capsules: 15, 20, 30, 45, 50, 60, 75, 80, 90, 100, 120, and 200 mg Injection: 0.5, 1, 2, 4, 8, 10, 15, 25, and 50 mg/mL Suppositories: 5, 10, 20, and 30 mg	10–30 mg PO every 3–4 h, 30–200 mg PO every 8–24 h, 2–10 mg IV/IM every 3–4 h	Same as above
Oxycodone (Percocet®, Tylox®, Roxicet™, OxyContin®)	Tablet/capsule: 5, 15, 30 mg Oral solution: 1 and 20 mg/mL Tablets: 2.5, 5, 7.5, and 10 mg with acetaminophen Controlled-release tablets: 10, 20, 40, 60, 80, and 160 mg	5–10 mg PO every 4–6 h, 20–160 mg PO every 8–12 h	Same as above
Oxymorphone (Opana®, Opana® ER)	Tablets: 5, 10 mg Extended-release tablets/capsules: 5, 7.5, 10, 15, 20, 30, 40 mg Injection: 1 mg/mL Suppositories: 5 mg	5–20 mg PO every 4–6 h, 5–20 mg PO every 12 h, 0.5–1.5 mg IV/IM/SC every 4–6 h	Same as above

PO, orally; IM, intramuscularly; IV, intravenously; SC, subcutaneously.

TABLE 26.5 Emetogenic Potential of Individual Chemotherapeutic Agents

Frequency of Emesis[a]	Agents	
High emetic risk (>90% frequency of emesis)	AC combination (Doxorubicin or Epirubicin with cyclophosphamide) Carmustine >250 mg/m^2 Cisplatin ≥50 mg/m^2	Cyclophosphamide >1,500 mg/m^2 Dacarbazine Mechlorethamine Streptozocin
Moderate emetogenic risk (30%–90% frequency of emesis)	Aldesleukin >12–15 million IU/m^2 Altretamine Amifostine >300 mg/m^2 Arsenic trioxide Azacitidine Bendamustine Busulfan Carboplatin Carmustine ≤250 mg/m^2 Cisplatin <50 mg/m^2 Clofarabine Cyclophosphamide ≤1,500 mg/m^2 Cytarabine >200 mg/m^2 Dactinomycin	Daunorubicin Doxorubicin Epirubicin Idarubicin Ifosfamide Interferon alfa ≥10 million IU/m^2 Irinotecan Melphalan Methotrexate 250–>1,000 mg/m^2 Oxaliplatin Temozolomide
Low emetogenic risk (10%–30% frequency of emesis)	Amifostine <300 mg/m^2 Aldesleukin ≤12 million IU/m^2 Cytarabine 100–200 mg/m^2 Docetaxel Doxorubicin (liposomal) Etoposide 5-Fluorouracil Floxuridine Gemcitabine Interferon alfa >5 <10 million IU/m^2 Ixabepilone	Methotrexate >50 <250 mg/m^2 Mitomycin Mitoxantrone Paclitaxel Paclitaxel (albumin) Pemetrexed Pentostatin Romidepsin Topotecan
Minimal emetogenic risk (<10% frequency of emesis)	Alemtuzumab Asparaginase Bevacizumab Bleomycin Bortezomib Cetuximab Cladribine Cytarabine <100 mg/m^2 Decitabine Denileukin diftitox Fludarabine Interferon alfa ≤5 million IU/m^2	Methotrexate ≤50 mg/m^2 Nelarabine Panitumumab Pegaspargase Rituximab Temsirolimus Trastuzumab Valrubicin Vinblastine Vincristine Vinorelbine

[a]Proportion of patients who experience emesis in the absence of effective antiemetic prophylaxis.
Adapted from: Ettinger DS, Kloth DD, Kris MG, et al. NCCN Antiemesis Clinical Practice Guidelines in Oncology. Version 2.2010, National Comprehensive Cancer Network, 2010. The University of Texas M.D. Anderson Cancer Center. Antiemetic Guidelines for Chemotherapy-Induced Nausea and Vomiting (CINV). 2008.

TABLE 26.6	General Recommendations for Treatment of Acute and Delayed Chemotherapy-induced Emesis	

Emetogenicity Level	Acute Emesis	Delayed Emesis
High	5-HT3 antagonist + corticosteroid + aprepitant ± lorazepam	Aprepitant + corticosteroid ± lorazepam
Moderate	5-HT3 antagonist + corticosteroid ± aprepitant ± lorazepam	5-HT3 antagonist **OR** corticosteroid **OR** aprepitant ± corticosteroid ± lorazepam
Low	Corticosteroid **OR** metoclopramide **OR** phenothiazine ± lorazepam	No routine prophylaxis recommended
Minimal	No routine prophylaxis recommended	No routine prophylaxis recommended

Adapted from: Ettinger DS, Kloth DD, Kris MG, et al. NCCN Antiemesis Clinical Practice Guidelines in Oncology. Version 2.2010, National Comprehensive Cancer Network, 2010. The University of Texas M.D. Anderson Cancer Center. Antiemetic Guidelines for Chemotherapy-Induced Nausea and Vomiting (CINV). 2008.

level of emetogenicity is determined, the recommended agents for prevention of acute and delayed emesis for the chemotherapy combination can be ascertained from available antiemetic guidelines (Table 26.6). The emetogenic potential of many agents is dose-dependent; therefore, additional antiemetic prophylaxis/treatment may be required with higher chemotherapy dosages.

The treatment of CIE experienced a revolution with the introduction of the first selective serotonin antagonist, ondansetron. Currently, there are four FDA-approved selective serotonin antagonists available for the treatment and prevention of CIE (ondansetron, dolasetron, granisetron, and palonosetron). Palonosetron is the only selective serotonin antagonist FDA approved for the prevention of acute and delayed nausea and vomiting. These agents have also found great utility in the prevention of postoperative nausea and vomiting and radiation therapy-induced nausea and vomiting. Intravenous (IV) administration is not necessary in most cases of noncisplatin-induced emesis, as the oral administration is comparable (palonosetron is only available for IV administration). They also have the advantage of not causing sedation and therefore can be safely administered in combination with other agents. High-dose IV metoclopramide is effective in treating CIE, although less so than ondansetron, but its extrapyramidal side effects can be a significant problem. These extrapyramidal side effects may occur with any of the antidopaminergic agents, including metoclopramide, haloperidol, droperidol, and the phenothiazines. The extrapyramidal side effects can be treated/prevented by coadministration or pretreatment with an anticholinergic such as benztropine or diphenhydramine. Standard phenothiazines are less effective but serve as useful adjuncts in the treatment of CIE. Corticosteroids, especially dexamethasone and methylprednisolone, act via a mechanism that is still unclear. In combination with other agents, corticosteroids dramatically improve antiemetic efficacy and may reduce the incidence of unwanted side effects by permitting dosage reduction. Corticosteroids are especially useful in treating/preventing delayed emesis. Aprepitant is a substance P/neurokinin (NK) 1 receptor antagonist. It is FDA-approved for prevention of acute and delayed CIE with initial and repeated courses of highly emetogenic chemotherapy, as well as for postoperative nausea and vomiting. For CIE, aprepitant must be used in combination with a serotonin receptor antagonist

TABLE 26.7 Antiemetic Agents for Chemotherapy-induced Emesis

Drug	Class/Mechanism	Dose and Schedule	Toxicity
Ondansetron (Zofran®, Zofran® ODT™)	Selective serotonin receptor antagonist	8–24 mg IV daily, 4–8 mg PO every 8 h	Headache, constipation, dizziness, fatigue, ECG changes
Granisetron (Kytril®)	Selective serotonin receptor antagonist	1–2 mg IV daily, 2 mg PO daily	Same as above
Granisetron (Sancuso®)	Selective serotonin receptor antagonist	3.1 mg/24 h patch apply 24–48 prior to chemo and wear up to 7 d	Same as above
Dolasetron (Anzemet®)	Selective serotonin receptor antagonist	100 mg IV or PO daily	Same as above
Palonosetron (Aloxi®)	Selective serotonin receptor antagonist	0.25 mg IV day 1 of chemotherapy	Same as above
Aprepitant (Emend®)	Substance P/Neurokinin 1 receptor antagonist	125 mg PO day 1, 80 mg PO daily days 2 and 3	Fatigue, hiccups, diarrhea, increased hepatic enzymes, drug interactions
Fosaprepitant (Emend® for Injection)	Substance P/Neurokinin 1 receptor antagonist	40 mg PO 3 h prior to anesthesia 115 mg IV day 1, 80 mg PO daily days 2 and 3, 150 mg IV day 1	Fatigue, hiccups, diarrhea, increased hepatic enzymes, drug interactions
Metoclopramide (Reglan®)	Other—dopamine antagonist	0.5–2 mg/kg IV every 3–4 h for highly emetogenic agents 10–40 mg PO/IV every 4–6 h for less emetogenic agents	Diarrhea, dystonia, akathisia, extrapyramidal effects, sedation, ECG changes
Haloperidol (Haldol®)	Other—dopamine antagonist	1–3 mg IV or PO every 3–6 h	Dystonia, akathisia, hypotension, sedation, extrapyramidal effects, ECG changes
Droperidol (Inapsine®)	Other—dopamine antagonist	0.5–2.0 mg IV every 4 h	Same as above

(continued)

TABLE
26.7

Antiemetic Agents for Chemotherapy-induced Emesis (continued)

Drug	Class/Mechanism	Dose and Schedule	Toxicity
Prochlorperazine (Compazine®)	Phenothiazine—dopamine antagonist	10 mg PO or IV every 4–6 h, 25 mg PR every 6 h	Dystonia, extrapyramidal effects, sedation, anticholinergic effects (dry mouth, dizziness, blurred vision, etc.)
Promethazine (Phenergan®)	Phenothiazine—dopamine antagonist	12.5–25 mg PO/IV/PR every 4–6 h	Same as above
Chlorpromazine (Thorazine®)	Phenothiazine—dopamine antagonist	25–50 mg PO every 4–6 h	Same as above
Dexamethasone (Decadron®)	Other—corticosteroid	10–20 mg IV daily 4 mg PO every 6–12 h	Hyperglycemia, euphoria, insomnia, psychosis, gastrointestinal upset
Methylprednisolone (Depo-Medrol®, Medrol®, Solu-Medrol®)	Other—corticosteroid	250–500 mg IV daily	Same as above
Lorazepam (Ativan®)	Other—benzodiazepine	0.5–2 mg IV/PO/SL every 4–8 h	Sedation, amnesia, confusion
Diphenhydramine (Benadryl®)	Antihistamine/anticholinergic	25–50 mg IV or PO every 4–6 h	Sedation, anticholinergic effects (dry mouth, dizziness, blurred vision, etc.)
Dronabinol (Marinol®)	Other—cannabinoid	5–10 mg/m² PO every 4–6 h	Drowsiness, dizziness, euphoria, dysphoria, hypotension, hallucinations
Nabilone (Cesamet®)	Other—cannabinoid	1–2 mg PO twice daily	Drowsiness, dizziness, euphoria, dysphoria, hypotension, hallucinations
Olanzapine (Zyprexa®)	Other—serotonin receptor and dopamine antagonists	2.5–5 mg PO twice daily	Fatigue, restlessness, memory changes, weight gain, constipation, extrapyramidal effects, hyperglycemia

IV, intravenously; PO, orally; ECG, electrocardiogram; PR, as needed; SL, sublingually.

and a corticosteroid. It is not indicated as treatment for breakthrough nausea or emesis. Due to interactions with the CYP450 system, aprepitant has a potential to interact with many medications. Lorazepam, a benzodiazepine, is useful in the prevention of anticipatory emesis and may reduce the incidence of dystonic reactions to metoclopramide. Most importantly, combinations of these agents, specifically ondansetron, dexamethasone, lorazepam, and metoclopramide, increase antiemetic efficacy and reduce troublesome side effects through presumed synergistic activity. Table 26.7 lists available and commonly used antiemetic agents with their dose ranges and the known major side effects.

Recommended Readings

Ciavarella S, Milano A, Dammacco F, et al. Targeted therapies in cancer. *BioDrugs.* 2010;24(2):77–88.

DeVita V, Hellman S, Rosenberg S, eds. *Cancer: Principles and Practice of Oncology.* 8th ed. Philadelphia, PA: Lippincott; 2008.

Dy SM, Asch SM, Naeim A, et al. Evidence-based standards for cancer pain management. *J Clin Oncol.* 2008;26:3879–3885.

Ettinger DS, Kloth DD, Kris MG, et al. NCCN Clinical Practice Guidelines in Oncology, Antiemesis. Version 2.2010. National Comprehensive Cancer Network, 2010. Available at: http://www.nccn.org.

Navari RM. Pharmacological management of chemotherapy-induced nausea and vomiting: focus on recent developments. *Drugs.* 2009;69(5):515–533.

Pazdur R, ed. *Cancer Management: A Multidisciplinary Approach.* 12th ed. Melville, NY: PRR, Inc.; 2009.

Perry M, ed. *The Chemotherapy Source Book.* 4th ed. Philadelphia, PA: Lippincott Williams & Wilkins; 2008.

Swarm R, Pickar A, Benedetti C, et al. NCCN Clinical Practice Guidelines in Oncology, Adult Cancer Pain. V.1.2010. National Comprehensive Cancer Network, 2010. Available at: http://www.nccn.org.

Note: Page number followed by f and t indicates figure and table respectively.